TREMORS

TREMORS

EDITED BY

CLAUDIA M. TESTA
Department of Neurology, University of North Carolina at Chapel Hill, Chapel Hill, NC, USA

DIETRICH HAUBENBERGER
Department of Neurosciences, University of California San Diego, La Jolla, CA, USA

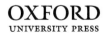

OXFORD
UNIVERSITY PRESS

OXFORD
UNIVERSITY PRESS

Oxford University Press is a department of the University of Oxford. It furthers
the University's objective of excellence in research, scholarship, and education
by publishing worldwide. Oxford is a registered trade mark of Oxford University
Press in the UK and certain other countries.

Published in the United States of America by Oxford University Press
198 Madison Avenue, New York, NY 10016, United States of America.

Library of Congress Cataloging-in-Publication Data
Names: Testa, Claudia M., editor. | Haubenberger, Dietrich, editor.
Title: Tremors / [edited by] Claudia M. Testa, Dietrich Haubenberger.
Description: New York, NY : Oxford University Press, [2022] |
Includes bibliographical references and index.
Identifiers: LCCN 2021051185 (print) | LCCN 2021051186 (ebook) |
ISBN 9780197529652 (hardback) | ISBN 9780197641149 (epub) |
ISBN 9780197602591
Subjects: MESH: Tremor
Classification: LCC RC346 (print) | LCC RC346 (ebook) | NLM WL 340 |
DDC 616.8—dc23/eng/20211209
LC record available at https://lccn.loc.gov/2021051185
LC ebook record available at https://lccn.loc.gov/2021051186

DOI: 10.1093/med/9780197529652.001.0001

1 3 5 7 9 8 6 4 2

Printed by Marquis, Canada

CONTENTS

ACKNOWLEDGMENTS

The editors thank our colleagues, especially those in the Tremor Research Group and the MDS Tremor Task Force for their mentorship, collegiality, and inspiration. We also thank the many patients and families who are the driving force behind all work in this field.

The editors thank Dr. Matthew Frosch for a thoughtful and thorough guest edit of the neuropathology chapter.

Dr. Testa wishes to thank her family for their enduring support, and Craig Panner of OUP for his dogged belief in this book from the beginning.

Dr. Haubenberger thanks Simona, Theodor, and Avi, for their endless patience during evening- and weekend-hours dedicated to this book.

CONTRIBUTORS

Peter G. Bain, MA, MD, FRCP
Reader & Honorary Consultant Neurologist
Department of Brain Sciences
Imperial College London
London, UK

Jos Becktepe, MD
Managing Senior Physician
Department of Neurology
University Hospital Schleswig-Holstein,
Campus Kiel
Kiel, DE

Yarema B. Bezchlibnyk, MD, PhD, FRCSC
Assistant Professor
Department of Neurosurgery and Brain
Repair
University of South Florida
Tampa, FL, USA

Christopher Y. Caughman, MD
Assistant Professor
Department of Neurology
Emory University
Atlanta, GA, USA

Deepa Dash, MD, DM
Clinical Fellow, Movement Disorders
Parkinson's Disease and Movement Disorders
Centre, Division of Neurology, Department
of Medicine
The Ottawa Hospital and the University of
Ottawa
Ottawa, CA

Günther Deuschl, PhD
Department of Neurology
Christian-Albrecht University
Kiel, Germany

Michiel F. Dirkx, MD, PhD
Post-doctoral Researcher
Donders Institute for Brain, Cognition and
Behaviour, Centre for Cognitive Neuroimaging
Radboud University
Nijmegen, NL

Nicolas Dohse, BS
Sidney Kimmel Medical College at Thomas
Jefferson University
Philadelphia, PA, USA

Rodger J. Elble, MD, PhD
Professor
Department of Neurology
Southern Illinois University School of
Medicine
Springfield, IL, USA

Alberto J. Espay, MD, MSc
Professor
Department of Neurology and Rehabilitation
Medicine
University of Cincinnati
Cincinnati, OH, USA

Stewart A. Factor, DO
Professor of Neurology, Director of the
Movement Disorders Program, Vance Lanier
Chair for Neurology
Emory University
Atlanta, GA, USA

Alfonso Fasano, MD, PhD
Professor, Clinician Investigator
Department of Medicine, Division of
Neurology
University of Toronto, Krembil Brain Institute
Toronto, ON, CA

Shaila Ghanekar, BS
Department of Neurology
University of South Florida Morsani College of
Medicine
Tampa, FL, USA

Clifton L. Gooch, MD
Chair, USF Neurology and Vice-President of
Clinical and Translational Research, Tampa
General Hospital
Neurology
University of South Florida
Tampa, FL, USA

Mark Hallett, MD, DM (hon)
Chief, Human Motor Control Section
National Institute of Neurological Disorders
and Stroke
National Institutes of Health
Bethesda, MD, USA

Dietrich Haubenberger, MHSc, MD
Voluntary Associate Clinical Professor
Department of Neurosciences
University of California San Diego
San Diego, CA, USA

Kristoffer Haugarvoll, MD, PhD
Consultant Neurologist
Neuro-SysMed, Neurology
Haukeland University Hospital
Bergen, NO

Rick C. Helmich, MD, PhD
Principle Investigator, Neurologist
Donders Institute for Brain, Cognition and
Behaviour, Department of Neurology, Centre
of Expertise for Parkinson and Movement
Disorders
Radboud University Medical Centre
Nijmegen, NL

H. A. Jinnah, MD, PhD
Professor
Departments of Neurology, Human Genetics,
and Pediatrics
Emory University School of Medicine
Atlanta, GA, USA

Sheng-Han Kuo, MD
Assistant Professor
Department of Neurology
Columbia University
New York, NY, USA

Peter A. LeWitt, MD, MMedSc
Professor and Sastry Foundation Endowed Chair
in Neurology
Departments of Neurology,
Wayne State University School of Medicine and
Henry Ford Hospital
Detroit, Michigan, USA

Laura de Lima Xavier, MD
Neurologist
Department of Neurology
UNC Chapel Hill
Carrboro, NC, US

Elan D. Louis, MD, MS
Professor and Chair
Department of Neurology
University of Texas Southwestern Medical Center
Dallas, TX, USA

Shabbir Merchant, MD
Assistant Professor
Department of Neurology
Harvard Medical School. Beth Israel Deaconess
Medical Center
Boston, MA, USA

Tiago A. Mestre, MD, MSc, PhD
Associate Professor
Division of Neurology, Department of Neurology
University of Ottawa, the Ottawa Hospital
Research Institute
Ottawa, ON, CA

William Ondo, MD
Professor
Department of Neurology
Methodist Neurological Institute and Weill
Cornell Medical School
Houston, TX, USA

Ming-Kai Pan, MD, PhD
Assistant Professor and Clinical Research
Director
Department and Graduate Institute of
Pharmacology
National Taiwan University College of Medicine
Taipei, TW

Margi Patel, MD
Neurologist
Baylor Scott & White Medical Center
Lakeway, TX, USA

Owen A. Ross, PhD
Associate Professor
Department of Neuroscience
Mayo Clinic
Jacksonville, FL, USA

Petra Schwingenschuh, MD
Associate Professor
Department of Neurology
Medical University of Graz
Graz, AT

Aasef G. Shaikh, MD, PhD
Neurology
University Hospitals
Cleveland
Moreland Hills, OH, USA

Holly Shill, MD, FAAN
Professor
Department of Neurology
Barrow Neurological Institute
Phoenix, AZ, USA

Aparna Wagle Shukla, MD
Professor
Department of Neurology
University of Florida
Gainesville, FL, USA

Kristina Simonyan, MD, PhD, Dr Med
Associate Professor
Otolaryngology—Head and Neck Surgery
Harvard Medical School, Massachusetts Eye and Ear
Boston, MA, USA

Claudia M. Testa, MD, PhD
Professor
Department of Neurology
University of North Carolina at Chapel Hill
Chapel Hill, NC, USA

Felipe Vial, MD
Staff Neurologist
Department of Neurology
Clinica Alemana—Universidad del Desarrollo
Santiago, CL

Chen-Ya Yang, MD, MPH
Attending Physician and Lecturer
Department of Physical Medicine and
Rehabilitation
Taichung Veterans General Hospital, Chiayi and
Wanqiao Branch / National Yang Ming Chiao
Tung University
Chiayi, TW

Theresa A. Zesiewicz, MD
Professor
Department of Neurology
University of South Florida Morsani College of
Medicine
Tampa, FL, USA

INTRODUCTION

Descriptions of tremor encompass ancient civilizations to the present day. Significant work has been done in all fundamental areas: nosology and classification; pathophysiology; and etiology. This work drives improved recognition and treatment of tremors, and accelerating growth in new therapeutics development.

This book is grouped into three sections. The initial section, "Tremor Foundations," presents work across research modalities, providing an overview on the underpinnings of tremor as symptom and disease. The breadth of work remaining in tremor pathophysiology and etiology does not render the area intractable; on the contrary, recent developments in the understanding of tremor pathology, pathophysiology, genetics, aided by groundbreaking discoveries using neuroimaging techniques, allow glimpses into future breakthroughs to come. The following section, "The Family of Tremors" presents the full extended range of tremor presentation, spanning isolated tremors, tremor as one of several features of a neurological disorder, as well as other hyperkinetic movement phenotypes commonly referred to, mimicking, or framed as tremors. The final section, "Tremor in the Clinic," reviews the growing knowledge range of clinical topics in tremors. Advances in assessing tremor bring pathophysiology concepts into clinical use, and have opened up an active era in new therapeutic development. Clinical research in tremors also now encompasses more holistic treatment approaches, novel treatment modalities, and diversity and inclusivity, all areas likely to feed back into basic etiology and pathophysiology research of this common movement disorder.

The sections all connect across key concepts in defining and working with tremors: nosology is critical to create a shared language; definitions are not hard lines, but ways to frame research hypotheses and to best direct prognosis and treatment especially in the absence of clear etiologies; ideally, classification systems exist in dynamic conversation with research and clinical experience.[1] Creating tremor syndromes and discussing them together with syndromes characterized by other hyperkinetic rhythmical or pseudo-rhythmical movements is ultimately about pragmatic utility in the clinic and in research: how does this help direct and advance research progress? How do syndrome classifications help get patients connected to the best treatment pathways? State-of-the-art clinical care, together with work to further elucidate the causes and pathways of tremors will ultimately shift tremor syndrome definitions as well as inform new therapeutics development.

Tremor is one of the most common movement disorders. This dynamic, rich topic is sure to see continued rapid growth in research and clinical care options.

REFERENCE

1. MacMahon B, Pugh TF. Causes and entities of disease. In: Clark DW, MacMahon B, eds. *Preventive Medicine*. Vol 1. Little, Brown; 1987: 11–18.

SECTION 1

Tremor Foundations

The system detailed in Chapter 2 serves a shared framework for later sections, but is inherently imperfect, and subject to healthy challenges and likely future evolution. The two-axes system is heavily weighted to Axis 1, external features that define clinical tremor syndromes, but Chapters 6 and 7 illustrate the growth in data on Axis 2 etiologically defined genetic and acquired tremors. Idiopathic tremors are detailed in the next section.

This section opens with the historical context for recognizing and defining tremor, and a review of a contemporary tremor classification system. The basic underpinnings of tremor are detailed in Chapters 3–5, each using a different experimental lens to illuminate current understanding and knowledge gaps in tremor neuropathology.

1

Tremor

History, Background, Basic Definitions

ELAN D. LOUIS

FIRST DESCRIPTIONS

Human beings, under certain circumstances, may develop repetitive and oscillatory movements (i.e., tremors).[1] Indeed, one may find evidence of this phenomenon across the ancient world. For example, in Ayurvedic medicine, a system that developed in India approximately 3,000 years ago, the word "kampa" denoted tremor, and "kampavata" was an imbalance due to tremor.[1,2] In the Edwin Smith Surgical papyrus, a medical-surgical case-based text that dates back at least to the Middle Kingdom in Egypt, hieroglyphs denoting tremor or shuddering were used numerous times[1] (Figure 1.1). In Greece, the Aphorisms of Hippocrates contain the following reference to tremor—"when tremors occur in ardent fevers, they are terminated by delirium".[1]

Over time, observations of and knowledge about tremors grew, and, eventually, it became apparent that tremors occurred in different circumstances and under different conditions. Thus, the notion that some tremors occurred at rest, while others occurred with action began to take form. As such, the distinction between these two forms of tremor has been credited to Galen of Pergamon (AD 129–216), who, in his treatise on tremor, used different terms to distinguish between action tremor and rest tremor.[1] This observation would be repeated and expanded upon by later authors: Sylvius de la Boe (AD 1680), Van Swieten (AD 1745), and Sauvages (AD 1768).[1]

In the 1600s, medicine as a field began to move away from the mere identification of symptoms and signs to a greater appreciation of the constellation of such symptoms and signs within certain individuals, how these inter-related and connected symptoms and signs developed over time, and how these symptoms and signs could be linked to changes in underlying organs.[1] As such, physicians noted that certain maladies could appropriately be viewed as "diseases"—individuals who suffered from a particular malady therefore shared a common set of symptoms, signs, natural history, and underlying organ pathology. With regards to tremor, physicians took note of the fact that shaking was not a mere symptom or sign, and that certain diseases were characterized by specific types of tremor, a reproducible natural history, and, in some instances, what seemed to be identifiable causes. One of these diseases was essential tremor (ET), which is the most common of the tremor disorders.[3] Given this high prevalence, its nosological history deserves special attention.

Physicians in the nineteenth century began to note that within certain families, individuals were stricken with what seemed to be the same type of tremor malady: action tremor.[1] It furthermore seemed that the individuals with this tremor shared a general clinical resemblance (e.g., location of tremor, severity of tremor, age of onset, and natural history of tremor), and that it seemed reasonable to designate a distinct disease entity for individuals with this type of action tremor. The tremor had no obvious cause, and when it was mild it seemed to be no more than a constitutional anomaly or an inherent, indispensable feature of the individual and their family.[1] The word "essential" was applied to a number of different diseases in the nineteenth century (e.g., essential convulsions, essential paralysis) when the problem had no readily identifiable cause and, in the framework of the time, seemed to be an inherent characteristic of an individual, such as having a short stature, having green eyes, or shaking. Thus, at that time, the term "essential" began to be applied to this type of tremor.[1]

The term "essential tremor" was initially used in 1874 by Pietro Burresi, a physician in Italy. Burresi, a professor of medicine at the University of Siena, described an 18-year-old man with severe, isolated action tremor.[4] Tremor, which was present in the arms, occurred during voluntary movements. It was also present in the head.

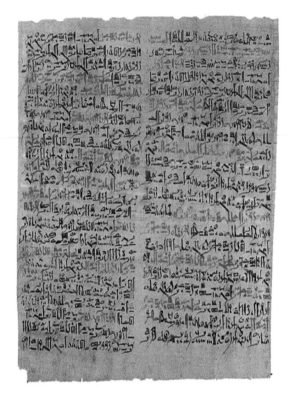

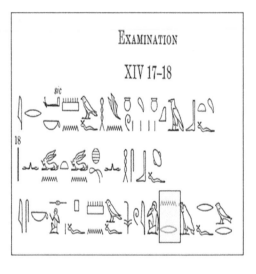

FIGURE 1.1: On the Left is a Portion of Edwin Smith's Surgical Papyrus. On the right is text describing the examination of a patient who is shaking. The text highlighted in yellow is the root of the word "to tremble," which is the rippled water glyph over the open mouth glyph.

No other family members had tremor; hence, the tremor did not seem to be familial. Burresi proposed the term *tremore semplice essenziale* (i.e., simple essential tremor).[4] Important in his discussion was the notable absence of paralysis or other central nervous system signs.[4] The term "essential tremor" was increasingly adopted, and by the last decade of the nineteenth century and the early years of the twentieth, the term began to appear more regularly in the medical literature. Authors wrote about this entity, characterizing it as a chronic or lifelong condition, whose main clinical feature, action tremor, occurred in relative isolation of other neurological signs.[4-6] This tremor disorder was often observed in families, but not in all instances, such as the case Burresi reported; therefore, "familial" is variably used as a qualifier.

TREMOR AS A SYMPTOM, TREMOR AS A SIGN, TREMOR DIAGNOSES

As previously discussed, under certain circumstances, humans may complain of shaking, and as such, tremor is a *symptom*. The symptom term "tremor" may be used by patients to denote the physical examination finding of tremor, or shivering, myoclonus, ataxia, or internal shaky sensations. Tremor may also be observable on visual inspection or recorded on electromyography or accelerometry and, as such, tremor is also a *sign*. Third, there are *diseases* and *families of diseases* in which tremor on examination is a prominent and/or central finding. Hence, to avoid confusion, it is important to distinguish symptoms (patient experiences), signs (examination or objective testing features), and diseases (constellations of symptoms and signs that are characterized by patterns in natural history and are linked to underlying causes and pathophysiologies).[7] Thus, to note that "essential tremor was seen on examination" is a confusing statement as it applies a disease label to a physical examination finding. It is more accurate to note that "action tremor was seen on examination." This potentially confusing word usage occurs in other areas of movement disorders, where, for example, "dystonia" is used to denote both a physical examination finding as well as a diagnosis.[8] Those who study and treat tremor, however, do not need to fall prey to this vagueness: distinguishing between usages of the term "tremor" is enabled by common features of tremor symptoms and signs.

Patients use a variety of terms to denote a *symptom* of tremor—"shaking," "shakiness," "nervous," "weak," "nodding," or "bobble" (to refer to head tremor), "quaver" (to refer to voice tremor), "quiver" or "tremble" (to refer to body tremor).[9] As a *physical examination finding* or *sign*, tremor may take a number of forms, with a main separation being between action tremor (i.e., tremor that occurs during a voluntary contraction of skeletal muscle) and rest tremor (i.e., tremor that occurs in a body part that is supported against gravity and is inactive).[10] Action tremor may be further subdivided into postural tremor (tremor that occurs when the body part is held motionless against the force of gravity), kinetic tremor (tremor that occurs during a voluntary movement), intention tremor (tremor that occurs when approaching a target), and isometric tremor (tremor that occurs when a muscle contracts against a rigid, stationary object).[10] As a *diagnosis*, there are a number of diseases that are characterized by tremor. For example, in Parkinson disease, a cardinal feature is rest tremor although patients often also exhibit postural and kinetic tremors.[10–12] In ET, the cardinal feature is kinetic tremor,[13] although patients often exhibit postural tremor,[13] intention tremor,[14,15] and in some instances, rest tremor as well.[16]

WHAT EXACTLY IS A "TREMOR"?

The first step in terms of identifying and classifying tremor is to recognize that tremors have two key features. This is, aside from being involuntary, they are rhythmic (i.e., regularly recurring) and oscillatory (i.e., rotating around a central plane). As such, the recent expert classification of tremor, published in 2018, defined tremor as follows: "tremor is an involuntary, rhythmic, oscillatory movement of a body part".[17] This being stated, there are a number of tremor disorders that were noted in the same publication to be "partly rhythmic" (e.g., palatal tremor),[17] leading some experts to question whether tremors should be defined sensu stricto as "rhythmic" movements. If one views a definition as something that marks a boundary or limit, then movements that are not rhythmic should either not be classified as "tremor" or tremor itself should not be classified

as "rhythmic." If one views a definition as something that establishes the character of something, then one may be more incorporative. While on the one hand, these are issues of nosology, in the absence of known etiologies or pathophysiologies classification is the beginning of treatment and hence, these issues merit serious consideration. This author refers to movements that are not strictly rhythmic and oscillatory as "tremulous," although there are other approaches to this thorny area. To summarize, we have phrased the question, "what is tremor"? This topic is still debated, although there is general agreement that the core features that are under consideration are "oscillatory" and "rhythmic."

SYNDROME OR DISEASE?

Previously, we have been discussing tremor as a physical examination finding as well as tremor disorders as diagnostic entities. Two forces have resulted in recent years in a reconsideration of tremor disorders with respect to their position as diagnostic entities.

The first is dealing with clinical heterogeneity, and we will use ET as an example. While in the past ET was often viewed as a mono-symptomatic condition, this is increasing being viewed as outdated.[18–21] Clinical and pharmacological-response differences across patients are becoming increasingly apparent and a large literature documenting such differences has evolved in the past decade.[18–21] Clinical differences revolve around the variable presence of a range of motor features (various tremors, gait abnormalities, eye motion abnormalities, co-occurrence of cerebellar features, and dystonia) and non-motor features (cognitive, psychiatric, sensory) across patients. Recognition of this heterogeneity has raised several questions. First, is there one "ET" or more than one "ET"? A recent coinage of a new term, ET-plus,[17] was an attempt, albeit problematic,[22–26] to deal with this heterogeneity by creating two subtypes with the label "ET." The attempt was based on the notion that ET might be a syndrome rather than a disease. Such attempts should be lauded although they should be more data-derived and scientifically formulated.[22] Second, what are the boundaries of ET? Third, is there even something we can encapsulate and refer to as ET?

The second issue relates to the transition from a two-layered approach to defining disease to a three-layered approach, which is occurring across all fields of medicine at present. As previously discussed, in the 1600s, medicine as a field began to move from the mere identification of symptoms and signs to a greater appreciation of the constellation of such symptoms and signs within certain individuals and how these developed over time, a paradigm shift that has been attributed to Dr. Thomas Sydenham and others. In the ensuing century, Dr. Giovanni Morgagni and others demonstrated how these symptoms and signs could be linked to changes in underlying organs—a second paradigm shift.[1,7] As such, "disease" was defined in two layers—organ-based changes (i.e., pathology and pathophysiology) and resulting clinical features. At present, a third layer is generally considered—that of underlying cause or "etiology." Research and knowledge about the genetic causes of diseases over the past half-century have spurred this on. Thus, all diseases are now viewed as having an underlying genetic cause, an environmental one, or a combination of the two. Those diseases for which we cannot at present apply such a designation are viewed as having a cryptogenic cause. Thus, an evolving view of disease is now three-layered: etiology, pathogenesis, and clinical. As such, diseases may be seen as a series of longitudinal events that start with a cause, then develop into a series of tissue-based changes (including molecular pathological changes), which then result in a set of clinical features.

These two forces have resulted in recent years in a reconsideration of tremor disorders with respect to their position as diagnostic entities. With respect to ET, for example, there is a discussion as to whether it is a syndrome or disease/family of diseases. Those who argue that it is a syndrome indicate that it is impossible to encapsulate all of the heterogeneity of ET into a single entity and that the clinical entity we refer to as "ET" is no more than a constellation of clinical features that are loosely held together.[27] This author and others refer to ET as a family of diseases rather than a syndrome with the understanding that certain causes will eventually be linkable to certain pathologies and certain clinical features, albeit at the moment, the nature of these links is not clear.[28]

COMMONALITIES OF THOUGHT

While it is important to recognize and understand sources of controversy, it is equally important to recognize areas in which there is a commonality of thought. With respect to tremor, there are certainly areas of commonality

and general consensus. Thus, tremor disorders are, first of all, generally viewed as disorders that are broadly characterized by their involuntary, rhythmic, and oscillatory nature. Second, tremor disorders are generally distinguishable as such from other broad categories of involuntary movement. Third, there is heterogeneity and complexity in these disorders which makes it difficult at times to classify and conveniently encapsulate them. A final issue for consideration is the general agreement that tremor disorders are incredibly common. Enhanced physiological tremor, for example, is found in the vast majority of individuals in the general population,[29-31] and prevalence studies, though presenting variable numbers due to methodological differences across studies, indicate that 4–6% of all adults have ET,[3,32] with as many as 20% in older age groups,[3,33,34] and Parkinson disease in 0.05–0.25% of adults.[35] In addition to their high prevalence, common tremor disorders impact function and quality of life, another indicator of their public health importance. Of additional public health importance is that tremor is a feature of several devastating neurological conditions such as Parkinson disease, and tremor in and of itself may be associated with considerable functional difficulty.[36-38] Thus, on multiple levels, tremors are conditions that require serious consideration.

TREMOR IN THE MAINSTREAM

Another way to judge the importance of a disease is to see how much it is part of mainstream life and/or how much it has figured into human history. Previously, we discussed commentary on tremor that dates back to ancient times as well as medical writings on tremor that similarly date back. In more recent history, including that of the United States, one may also find evidence of tremor. For instance, three (5.4%) of the 56 signers of the Declaration of Independence had ET: John Adams (1735–1826), Samuel Adams (1722–1803), and Stephen Hopkins (1707–1785).[39,40] Stephen Hopkins was said to have commented while he signed the document that although his hand shook, his heart remained resolute and steady. John Quincy Adams (1767–1848), the sixth president of the United States and son of John Adams, also had tremor.

In more recent times, Adolf Hitler developed a condition toward the end of his life that was characterized by a parkinsonian-type tremor in his left hand, and this condition likely affected his behavior, actions, and decision-making during the Second World War.[41] The opening up of a second front with Russia in June of 1941 may have been linked with a desire to finalize victory in a limited time window, driven by his advancing disease.

Franklin Delano Roosevelt (1882–1945), on the other side of the conflict during the Second World War, was noted in 1943 to have an action tremor that affected his handwriting. There were others in the family with tremor as well. In late 1944, Senator Harry Truman (1884–1972), upon meeting his new boss, had noted that Roosevelt, while pouring cream into his tea, got more in the saucer than in his cup.[42]

The American actress Katherine Hepburn (1907–2003) is also said to have had ET, with the tremor affecting cranial structures (head and voice) prominently. Other prominent individuals too numerous to list here have had parkinsonism with its accompanying tremor.

In our own field of neurology there is a relevant history as well. Silas Weir Mitchell (1829–1914) is recognized as one of the most important figures in American neurology, remembered for his seminal descriptions of causalgia and phantom limb syndrome as well as his research on peripheral nerve injuries and gunshot wounds.[43] Mitchell had action tremor, and later in life his handwriting became so tremulous so that it was virtually illegible.[43]

SUMMARY

Human beings have been shaking for thousands of years and have been documenting their experiences with tremor during this time. Tremors are extraordinarily common. Tremor disorders are also heterogeneous. Greater appreciation of this heterogeneity has fueled recent controversies on how to best classify, subdivide, and name tremors. Research on these disorders is active, and it is hoped that this research will result in a greater understanding of their underlying etiologies and pathophysiological mechanisms, generating the next evolution in tremor experience, nosology, and classification.

REFERENCES

1. Louis ED. Essential tremor. *Arch Neurol.* 2000;57(10):1522–1524.
2. Gourie-Devi M, Ramu MG, Venkataram BS. Treatment of Parkinson's disease in "Ayurveda" (ancient Indian system of medicine): discussion paper. *J R Soc Med.* 1991;84(8):491–492.
3. Louis ED, Ferreira JJ. How common is the most common adult movement disorder? Update on the worldwide prevalence of essential tremor. *Mov Disord.* 2010;25(5):534–541.
4. Louis ED, et al. Historical underpinnings of the term essential tremor in the late 19th century. *Neurology.* 2008;71(11):856–859.
5. Critchley M. Observations of essential (heredofamilial) tremor. *Brain.* 1949;72:113–139.
6. Critchley E. Clinical manifestations of essential tremor. *J Neurol Neurosurg Psychiatry.* 1972;35(3):365–372.
7. Battista Morgagni G. *De sedibus et causis morborum per anatomen indagatis libri quinque.* ex Thypographia Remondiniana; 1761.
8. Balint B, et al. Dystonia. *Nat Rev Dis Primers.* 2018;4(1):25.
9. Louis ED, et al. Differences in the prevalence of essential tremor among elderly African Americans, whites, and Hispanics in northern Manhattan, NY. *Arch Neurol.* 1995;52(12):1201–1205.
10. Louis ED. Tremor. *Continuum (Minneap Minn).* 2019;25(4):959–975.
11. Lance JW, Schwab RS, Peterson EA. Action tremor and the cogwheel phenomenon in Parkinson's disease. *Brain.* 1963;86:95–110.
12. Reich SG. Does this patient have Parkinson disease or essential tremor? *Clin Geriatr Med.* 2020;36(1):25–34.
13. Louis ED. The primary type of tremor in essential tremor is kinetic rather than postural: cross-sectional observation of tremor phenomenology in 369 cases. *Eur J Neurol.* 2013;20(4):725–727.
14. Louis ED, Frucht SJ, Rios E. Intention tremor in essential tremor: prevalence and association with disease duration. *Mov Disord.* 2009;24(4):626–627.
15. Deuschl G, et al. Essential tremor and cerebellar dysfunction clinical and kinematic analysis of intention tremor. *Brain.* 2000;123(Pt 8):1568–1580.
16. Louis ED, Hernandez N, Michalec M. Prevalence and correlates of rest tremor in essential tremor: cross-sectional survey of 831 patients across four distinct cohorts. *Eur J Neurol.* 2015;22(6):927–932.
17. Bhatia KP, et al. Consensus statement on the classification of tremors: from the task force on tremor of the International Parkinson and Movement Disorder Society. *Mov Disord.* 2018;33(1):75–87.
18. Louis ED. The evolving definition of essential tremor: what are we dealing with? *Parkinsonism Relat Disord.* 2018;46(Suppl 1):S87–S91.
19. Benito-Leon J. Essential tremor: from a monosymptomatic disorder to a more complex entity. *Neuroepidemiology.* 2008;31(3):191–192.
20. Galvin JE. When a tremor is not just a tremor: cognitive and functional decline in essential tremor, a more complex disorder than we thought. *J Am Med Dir Assoc.* 2009;10(4):218–220.
21. Jankovic J. Essential tremor: a heterogenous disorder. *Mov Disord.* 2002;17(4):638–644.

22. Louis ED, et al. Essential tremor-plus: a contro-versial new concept. *Lancet Neurol.* 2020;19(3): 266–270.

23. Louis ED. "Essential Tremor Plus": A problematic concept: implications for clinical and epidemiological studies of essential tremor. *Neuroepidemiology.* 2020;54(2):180–184.

24. Louis ED. Essential tremor: "Plus" or "Minus." Perhaps now is the time to adopt the term "the essential tremors." *Parkinsonism Relat Disord.* 2018;56:111–112.

25. Prasad S, Pal PK. Reclassifying essential tremor: implications for the future of past research. *Mov Disord.* 2019;34(3):437.

26. Vidailhet M. Essential tremor-plus: a temporary label. *Lancet Neurol.* 2020;19(3):202–203.

27. Elble RJ. The essential tremor syndromes. *Curr Opin Neurol.* 2016;29(4):507–512.

28. Lenka A, Louis ED. Do we belittle essential tremor by calling it a syndrome rather than a disease: yes. *Front Neurol.* 2020;11:522687.

29. Louis ED, et al. How normal is "normal"? Mild tremor in a multiethnic cohort of normal subjects. *Arch Neurol.* 1998;55(2):222–227.

30. Louis ED, et al. Tremor in normal adults: a population-based study of 1158 adults in the Faroe Islands. *J Neurol Sci.* 2019;400:169–174.

31. Elble RJ. Tremor in ostensibly normal elderly people. *Mov Disord.* 1998;13(3):457–464.

32. Dogu O, et al. Prevalence of essential tremor: door-to-door neurologic exams in Mersin Province, Turkey. *Neurology.* 2003;61(12):1804–1806.

33. Louis ED, Thawani SP, Andrews HF. Prevalence of essential tremor in a multiethnic, community-based study in northern Manhattan, New York, N.Y. *Neuroepidemiology.* 2009;32(3):208–214.

34. Khatter AS, Kurth MC, Brewer MA, et al. Prevalence of tremor and Parkinson's disease. *Parkinsonism Relat Disord.* 1996;2(4):205–208.

35. Abbas MM, Xu Z, Tan LCS. Epidemiology of Parkinson's disease—east versus west. *Mov Disord Clin Pract.* 2018;5(1):14–28.

36. Bain PG, et al. Assessing the impact of essential tremor on upper limb function. *J Neurol.* 1993;241(1):54–61.

37. Busenbark KL, et al. Is essential tremor benign? *Neurology.* 1991;41(12):1982–1983.

38. Heroux ME, et al. Upper-extremity disability in essential tremor. *Arch Phys Med Rehabil.* 2006;87(5):661–670.

39. Louis ED. Samuel Adams' tremor. *Neurology.* 2001;56(9):1201–1205.

40. Louis ED, Kavanagh P. John Adams' essential tremor. *Mov Disord.* 2005;20(12):1537–1542.

41. Gupta R, et al. Understanding the influence of Parkinson Disease on Adolf Hitler's decision-making during World War II. *World Neurosurg.* 2015;84(5):1447–1452.

42. Lomazow S. The untold neurological disease of Franklin Delano Roosevelt (1882–1945). *J Med Biogr.* 2009;17(4):235–240.

43. Louis ED. Silas Weir Mitchell's essential tremor. *Mov Disord.* 2007;22(9):1217–1222.

Clinical Classification of Tremor Syndromes

JOS BECKTEPE AND GÜNTHER DEUSCHL

CLINICAL CLASSIFICATION OF TREMOR SYNDROMES

Tremor is the most common movement disorder, but classifying tremor syndromes correctly can be challenging even for experienced movement disorder experts. For most tremor disorders, no objective measure exists, so the diagnosis relies solely on the clinical skills and experience of the examiner. Various classification schemes for tremors have been applied in the past, and most were based either on phenomenology, presumed etiology, or anatomy/physiology.

In 1853, Romberg listed the tremor etiologies as follows: mercury, alcohol, senile tremor, febrile tremor, and paralysis agitans.[1] Oppenheim in 1911 added the description of tremor phenomenology (rest, during movement/intention, and with mental excitement) and suggested certain maneuvers for the examination of tremor (e.g., raising arms, touching the nose, bringing water to the mouth) that are still applied nowadays.[2] In 1972, Fahn classified tremors depending on their relationship to voluntary motor activity and differentiated between normal physiological tremor and pathological tremors.[3] The 1998 consensus statement on the classification of tremors by the Movement Disorder Society developed the first complete classification scheme, including activation condition and syndromic classifications.[4] The main critique of the 1998 MDS criteria was the lack of an internal consistency. Some tremors were classified based on their clinical phenomenology, like orthostatic tremor or primary writing tremor, while other tremors were defined according to their presumed etiology (like parkinsonian tremor) or their anatomical origin (like cerebellar tremor). These classification inconsistencies prove inadequate, especially for multietiological tremor syndromes like essential tremor.

The 2018 updated consensus criteria overcame this inconsistency by consequently applying a two-axis approach.[5] Axis 1 comprises the clinical phenomenology and Axis 2 the etiology.

These two axes are not dependent on each other so Axis 1 syndromes can be combined with various Axis 2 etiologies. Also, when developing additional signs, an Axis 1 syndrome may evolve into another over time.

Axis 1

The definition of tremor is an involuntary, rhythmic, oscillating movement of a body part. On Axis 1 the clinical features of the tremor patient are described. Since the medical treatment of most tremor syndromes is only symptomatic and based on the clinical syndrome, an exact phenotyping of the tremor syndrome is crucial to clinical diagnosis. This assessment includes the patient's history, the tremor characteristics in terms of localization, activation conditions and tremor frequency, the examination of additional neurological or systemic signs, and, possibly, additional laboratory tests (electrophysiology, imaging, serum or tissue biomarkers; see Figure 2.1). These tremor syndromes are based only on Axis I features (Table 2.1).

Historical features

The patient's history guides the diagnostic procedure. The age at onset should be documented as precisely as possible and can be categorized into the following age groups: infancy (birth to 2 years); childhood (3–12 years); adolescence (13–20 years); early adulthood (21–45 years); middle adulthood (46–60 years); and late adulthood (>60 years). The sequence of body part involvement (e.g., whether hands were affected prior to the neck or the other way around) and the dynamic of progress should be asked for. Information about exacerbating conditions (like cognitive/emotional stress, physical activity of other body parts, specific tasks or limb positions) and relieving factors (medication, alcohol sensitivity) are of diagnostic value as well. The family history should include tremor and

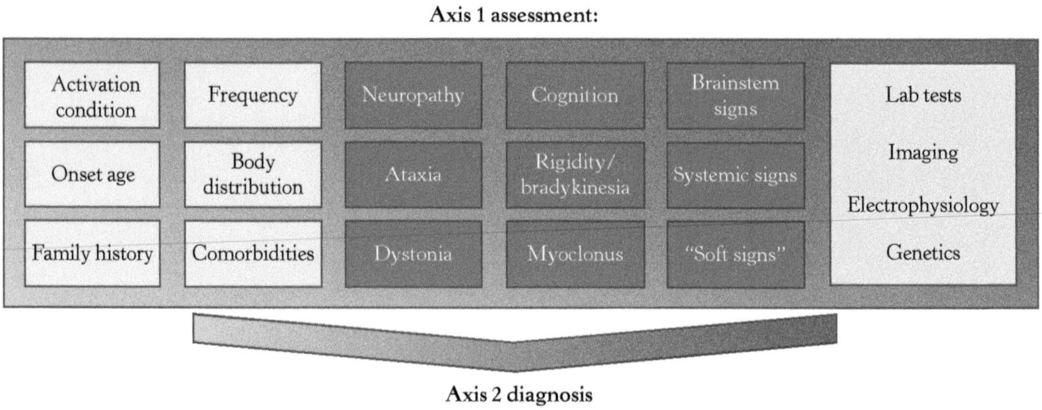

Axis 1 assessment:

FIGURE 2.1: Axis 1 Tremor Assessment. Axis 1 classification of tremor is based on clinical features from the patient's medical history, physical examination, and possibly additional laboratory tests.

any other movement disorders as well as other hereditary conditions.

Clinical features

The clinical features of tremor are described regarding the anatomical distribution of tremor, the activation conditions, and the tremor frequency.

Anatomical distribution of tremor

The anatomical distribution of tremor can be focal (involves one single body region like head, voice, chin, one extremity etc.), segmental (two or more neighboring body regions affected, like head and arm, bi-brachial, etc.) hemitremor or generalized (upper and lower body parts affected).

Activation conditions

The activation conditions are of utmost importance for the classification of tremors, and standardized maneuvers should be applied for the clinical examination. The two main activation classifications are rest tremor and action tremor.

Rest tremor: In general, rest tremor should be examined in complete relaxation of the affected body part. However, the examination of rest tremor of the hands is not standardized and certain possible methods of examination are commonly used: with arms resting on the knees or on the armrest in prone-/semi-prone position or dangling loosely from the armrest. The forearms should not actively be supinated because isometric muscle contraction provokes postural tremor, which may be misinterpreted as rest tremor. Since sensitivity and specificity for

detecting rest tremor may vary for these different rest positions, the preferred hand position should depend on the purpose of examination.[6] By definition, the semi-prone position is not at rest and, despite possibly higher sensitivity, must be reproduced during complete rest with the hand dangling from the armrest.[6] Rest tremor of the head and legs should be examined in a supine position.

Rest tremor in Parkinson disease (PD) is typically provoked by mental (e.g., serial seven-task stroop test) or physical (e.g., walking, movements of other body parts) activation[7] and the therapeutic effect of levodopa on PD rest tremor is reduced by cognitive stress.[8] Accordingly, rest tremor assessment should include a cognitive stress paradigm to avoid overestimation of treatment effects in real life.[8] In contrast to this, rest tremor in PD is suppressed, at least transiently, by voluntary activation of the trembling body part in >90% of the patients[9] and will possibly re-emerge in postural position after a mean latency of 9 seconds.[10,11] Testing this rest tremor suppression helps to distinguish between PD tremor and essential tremor (ET), since ET is not suppressed by voluntary movement.[9]

Action tremor is any tremor that is triggered by voluntary contraction of muscle and is further divided into postural, kinetic and isometric tremor.

Postural tremor occurs while maintaining any position against gravity (this includes orthostatic tremor), although the amplitude may vary in different limb positions.[12] Upper limb postural tremor is the most common action tremor and is typically examined with the arms outstretched or

TABLE 2.1 AXIS 1 ISOLATED AND COMBINED TREMOR SYNDROMES

Isolated tremor syndromes	ET	1) isolated tremor syndrome of bilateral upper limb action tremor 2) at least 3 years' duration 3) with or without tremor in other locations (e.g., head, voice, or lower limbs) 4) absence of other neurological signs, such as dystonia, ataxia, or parkinsonism.
	Isolated segmental postural or kinetic tremor	Typically involves the upper limbs, but may also involve the head, voice, tongue, and face
	Isolated rest tremor	Most commonly occurs in an upper or lower limb or as a hemitremor, but may occur elsewhere (e.g., lips, jaw, or tongue); absence of other neurological signs (rigor, akinesia, dystonia)
	Isolated focal tremors	Isolated voice tremor is a visible and/or audible tremor of the vocal apparatus Isolated head tremor is a shaking of the head in yes-yes, no-no, or variable directions
		Palatal tremor is characterized by rhythmic movement of the soft palate at 0.5 to 5 Hz
	Task- and position-specific tremor	Tremor occurring during a specific task or posture, e.g., writing, sports (tennis, golf), musical instrument
	Primary orthostatic tremor	Generalized high-frequency (13–18 Hz) isolated tremor syndrome that occurs when standing; electrophysiological confirmation of the tremor frequency is needed
Borderline	ET-plus	ET and additional neurological signs of uncertain significance (e.g., impaired tandem gait, questionable dystonic posturing, memory impairment, rest tremor) that do not suffice to make an additional syndrome classification or diagnosis
Combined tremor syndromes	Pseudo-orthostatic tremor	Orthostatic tremors with a frequency <13Hz; usually associated with other signs, e.g., parkinsonism, ataxia and dystonia
	Dystonic tremor	Tremor in a body part affected by dystonia is labeled as dystonic tremor; when tremor and dystonia are found in different body parts, this is called tremor associated with dystonia
	Tremor combined with parkinsonism	Typically, a unilateral or asymmetrical 4- to 7-Hz rest tremor of the hand ("pill-rolling" tremor), lower limb, jaw, tongue, or foot (classic parkinsonian tremor); postural or kinetic tremors with the same or different frequency as the rest tremor may coexist in patients with parkinsonism as well
	Intention tremor	Tremor during goal-directed movements at <5 Hz, with or without other localizing signs
	Holmes tremor	Rest, postural, and intention tremor that usually emerges from proximal and distal rhythmic muscle contractions at low frequency (<5 Hz)
	Myorhythmia	Rhythmic movement disorder of cranial or limb muscles at rest or during action with a frequency of 1 to 4 Hz. Usually associated with localizing brainstem signs and with a diagnosable etiology
Others	Functional tremor	Characterized by distractibility, frequency entrainment, or antagonistic muscle coactivation
	Indeterminate tremor	Tremors that do not fit into an established syndrome or that need further observation to clarify

with flexed elbows and hands kept in front of the chest ("batwing position"). Postural tremor of the legs can be examined in the sitting or supine position with one leg extended, and postural tremor of the head can be examined in supine position and when lifting the head.

Position-specific postural tremor occurs only when the affected body part is brought into a specific posture or position. In contrast to task-specific kinetic tremor, no associated task is needed to induce the tremor: the position itself triggers the occurrence of the shaking.[13]

Kinetic tremor embodies simple kinetic tremor, intention tremor, and task-specific kinetic tremor. Simple kinetic tremor occurs during purposeless active movements (e.g., waving the hands) and shows no relevant amplitude alteration within the movement. Intention tremor occurs during visually guided goal-directed movements and is characterized by an amplitude increase during the deceleration and target phase.[14] Intention tremor of the upper limbs is most common, but intention tremor of the head and the legs may occur as well.[15,16]

Task-specific kinetic tremors occur only when the patient performs a specific and usually skilled task. The most frequent task-specific kinetic tremors are primary writing tremor[17] and primary voice tremor, but musician's and sportsperson's task-specific tremor were described as well.

Tremor frequency

The tremor frequency is often used to characterize tremor, and it can be categorized as <4, 4 to 8, 8 to 12, and >12 Hz. Accelerometric or electromyographic measures provide the most accurate information about the tremor frequency. The frequency of the most common tremor syndromes (like ET and PD tremor) lies between 4 and 8 Hz, so in general the frequency alone is not helpful to differentiate tremor entities (Figure 2.2). Exceptions are as follows:

Holmes tremor has a frequency below 5 Hz.
Myorhythmia has a 1 to 4 Hz frequency.
Primary orthostatic tremor has a 13 to 18 Hz frequency.

Additional signs

During the clinical examination, special emphasis should be placed on the presence of additional symptoms beyond the tremor. Neurological signs to look for include, but are not limited to, cerebellar signs, dystonic posturings, akinesia, signs of peripheral neuropathy, and brainstem signs. In addition to neurological symptoms, systemic signs of illness (e.g., diabetes mellitus as a clue for concomitant neuropathy and neuropathic tremor) should be considered for finding an etiology. Accordingly, Axis 1 entities may be separated into isolated and combined tremor syndromes depending on the presence of additional neurologic signs (Table 2.1).

Apart from the occurrence of undoubted "hard" additional neurological signs, the presence of signs of uncertain significance ("soft signs") was integrated into the tremor classification as

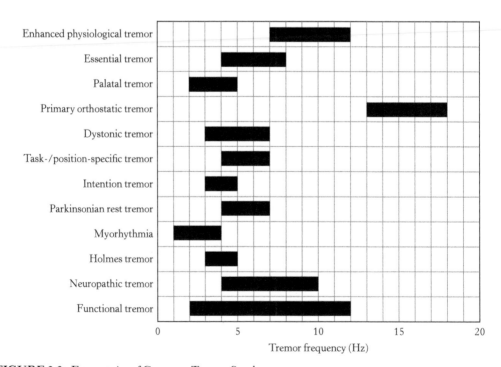

FIGURE 2.2: Frequencies of Common Tremor Syndromes.

well. These soft signs are defined as "additional signs that do not suffice to make an additional syndrome classification or diagnosis."[5] The applicability and clinical meaning of these signs is currently controversial, and the interrater agreement on the presence of such signs is at best moderate.[18,19] But the threshold for considering a sign as soft versus significant for ataxia, parkinsonism, dystonia, etc. is critically important in the classification and treatment of tremors. Therefore, "hard criteria" for the interpretation of such soft signs need urgently to be established.

Other data that may contribute
Imaging

Magnetic resonance imaging is always indicated when a structural brain anomaly, like a focal lesion, or neurodegenerative or metabolic brain abnormalities are supposed to be causal for the tremor. This accounts especially for unilateral or focal tremor syndromes combined with other signs (like ataxia, dystonia, parkinsonism, or dementia) or when a positive family history for neuropsychiatric symptoms combined with movement disorders is prevalent. Structural abnormalities will most likely be localized in the cerebellum, brain stem, or basal ganglia. In patients with an isolated tremor syndrome, structural neuroimaging is usually not recommended, but there may be exceptions; for example, a sudden onset of symptoms.

In general, *lesions of various origin (mostly brainstem and basal ganglia lesions)* may be found causative in unilateral tremor syndromes (e.g., Holmes tremor).

Depending on the combined tremor syndrome, typical MRI abnormalities point toward a specific etiology, although reliable data from larger samples regarding sensitivity and specificity of these signs are lacking:

- *Splenium and middle cerebral peduncle (MCP) sign* in fragile X–associated tremor ataxia syndrome (FXTAS, combined with ataxia and neuropsychiatric symptoms)[20]
- *Hot cross bun sign* in multiple system atrophy (combined with parkinsonism, ataxia, or neurovegetative symptoms)[21] or spinocerebellar ataxias (especially SCA 2, 7, 8, combined with ataxia and other signs)[22]
- *Hummingbird/penguin silhouette/ morning glory flower sign* in progressive supranuclear palsy (combined with parkinsonism, supranuclear gaze palsy)[23]

- *Giant panda sign* in Wilson's disease (combined with dystonia, parkinsonism)[24]

Presynaptic dopamine transporter imaging (^{123}I-FP-CIT SPECT (DAT-SPECT)) is indicated to help differentiate between parkinsonism-associated tremor and ET,[25] dystonic tremor, or isolated rest tremor (scans without evidence of dopaminergic deficit, or SWEDD) when the clinical examination is not clear.

Serum tests: Tremor can be provoked by several states of systemic homeostatic imbalance, like hyperthyroidism, hypoglycemia, or renal or liver failure. The resulting tremor is usually an isolated (or combined with systemic signs) bilateral action tremor. The new tremor classification does not encompass "enhanced physiological tremor" as a specific Axis 1 syndrome because its concept is always associated with an etiology. The diagnosis of enhanced physiological tremor is confirmed when a specific Axis 2 etiology is found (e.g., hyperthyroidism, sympathomimetic drugs) and when the tremor is normalized with successful management. Therefore, basic lab tests including electrolytes, glucose, thyroid, and liver and renal function should be performed in every patient with a newly diagnosed tremor syndrome. In special cases, further laboratory tests are required (Table 2.2; basic lab tests in bold).

Use of polygraphic tremor analysis

The polygraphic (combined electromyographic and accelerometric) tremor analysis provides an objective and reproducible measure of tremor. While isolated electromyographic or accelerometric measures provide information about the tremor amplitude and frequency, deeper information about peripheral and central components of the tremor can be achieved by the combined polygraphic analysis.[26,27] However, the diagnostic value depends on the experience of the examiner. For the differential diagnosis of the most frequent upper limb tremor syndromes (like ET and parkinsonian tremor) the tremor frequency alone is not helpful because the frequencies of different syndromes overlap (Figure 2.2). More advanced mathematical analyses for an accelerometric-based differentiation of tremor syndromes were developed,[28] but to date no application available for clinical routine has been provided.

In a clinical context, there are four situations where polymyography is helpful in the classification of the tremor syndrome.

TABLE 2.2: ACQUIRED TREMOR ETIOLOGIES AND INDICATIVE TESTS*

Tremor etiology	Test
Hyperthyroidism	**Thyroid levels (T3, T4, TSH)**
Metabolic imbalance, hypocalcemia, hypokalemia	**Electrolytes (Na, K, Ca, Cl)**
Hypo-/hyperparathyroidism	Parathormone
Pheochromocytoma	Serum catecholamines
Paraproteinemia	Immune electrophoresis
Autoimmune neuropathies	Cerebrospinal fluid (CSF) examination, NCS, nerve biopsy
Alcoholism, hepatocellular degeneration	**Liver enzymes**
Hypoglycemia	**Glucose**
Paraneoplasia (e.g., paraneoplastic cerebellar degeneration)	Serum and CSF examination for onconeuronal antibodies and cell surface antibodies (e.g., anti-Yo (PCA-1), anti-Ri (ANNA-2), anti-Tr/DNER, anti-amphiphysin, anti-GAD, anti-GluR1)
Arsenic, bismuth, bromine, mercury, lead, alcohol, certain drugs	Toxicological assessment

* Basic Lab Tests Marked in Bold should be Performed in Every Newly Diagnosed Tremor Patient

1. When a functional genesis is suspected, the polygraphic tremor analysis provides an objective measure of features that are suggestive of functional tremor. These include distractibility, accuracy of tapping performance for a given frequency, a positive entrainment or increase of frequency/amplitude variability on the contralateral side, increase of total power after weight loading, response to contralateral ballistic movements, tonic muscle coactivation at the onset of tremor, and a high interlimb coherence in bilateral tremors. By applying these laboratory-supported criteria in a standardized test battery, a sensitivity of 89.5% and a specificity of 95.9% for the distinction of functional from organic tremor were shown.[29]

2. For the diagnosis of primary orthostatic tremor, confirmation of the 13- to 18-Hz frequency, which is highly coherent among affected extremities, is needed. Orthostatic tremor with a slower frequency should be termed "pseudo-orthostatic tremor."

3. For differentiating cortical myoclonus or asterixis from tremor, note that myoclonus is characterized by short-lasting (<50–100ms), irregular EMG bursts of agonists and antagonists, often followed by a silent period. Additionally, rhythmic cortical myoclonus typically has a frequency greater than 8 Hz.

4. For distinguishing enhanced physiological tremor from ET, note that while ET always has a central origin, enhanced physiological tremor has mainly mechanical and mechanical-reflex components. These peripheral components depend on the mass of the oscillating extremity, and by applying additional weight the accelerometric frequency will decrease. In tremors with a central origin, both EMG and accelerometric signal will remain unchanged after weight loading. Hence, a decrease of tremor frequency after weight loading is a specific finding for a tremor with peripheral origin. About 10% of enhanced physiological tremors have a central origin as well. In these cases, EMG frequency will remain unchanged after inertial loading because the central generator cannot be modulated from the periphery, but the frequency of the mechanical component will decrease.

Axis 2

On Axis 2 the specific etiology of the tremor syndromes is described. Etiologies can be acquired, genetic, or idiopathic.

Table 2.2 provides an overview of important acquired tremor etiologies and indicative lab tests. Most acquired causes for tremor are potentially reversible, and finding the underlying disease may be crucial for starting an adequate treatment.

A genetic cause underlies many tremor disorders; inheritance includes autosomal dominant and recessive, X-linked, and mitochondrial patterns, as well as chromosomal abnormalities. Usually, these patients exhibit tremor syndromes combined with other neurologic or systemic symptoms. Table 2.3 summarizes some important monogenetic entities that might present with combined tremor syndromes (for detailed reviews, see[30,31]). However, tremor may precede the appearance of other neurologic signs for a long time, or these additional signs may be so discreet that they are overseen by the examiner. These patients may then be labeled as having isolated tremor syndrome (often ET) on Axis 1 at the beginning.

Additionally, in many tremor syndromes, including the large group of ETs, a positive family history for tremor is frequently reported but no causal mutations are known, suggesting more complex heritability patterns.

In the clinical routine, genetic tests should be considered only in patients with combined tremor syndromes and a positive family history for movement disorders, neuropathy, or neuropsychiatric symptoms. In patients with isolated tremor syndromes, genetic tests are not recommended, since no disease-causing genes for isolated tremor syndromes are known.[32]

In most patients with isolated tremor syndromes, the etiology remains idiopathic. This includes ET; isolated segmental, postural, or kinetic tremor; isolated rest tremor; isolated focal tremors; task- and position-specific tremors; and primary orthostatic tremor.

APPLYING THE CLASSIFICATION SYSTEM: HOW CLASSIFICATIONS MAY EVOLVE

When applying the classification system, Axis 1 and Axis 2 diagnosis may change over time due to further assessments and/or exhibition of further signs. The two axes are not dependent of each other, however, and Axis 1 syndromes can be combined with various Axis 2 etiologies. The first step is to label the patient with an accurate Axis 1 syndrome diagnosis. As an example, we consider that tremor in a patient who presents with a rest tremor of one upper limb for 2 years without further hard signs of parkinsonism or dystonia will be labeled as isolated rest tremor on Axis 1. When further diagnostics, including presynaptic dopaminergic tracer imaging in

this case, remain normal, the etiology on Axis 2 remains idiopathic; this patient might formerly have been labeled as SWEDD. Within a year, the patient develops a rest tremor on the other hand and postural tremor on both hands as well. The Axis 1 diagnosis is now ET-plus rest tremor. The Axis 2 diagnosis is still idiopathic. After another year, a mild dystonic posturing of the right arm is recognized, and tremor and dystonic posturing improve when the patient touches her right shoulder. Now that Axis 1 diagnosis is dystonic tremor. The patient reports that her grandson and granddaughter were seen for a generalized DYT-TOR1A dystonia. Now genetic testing for DYT-TOR1A is performed in the patient as well and confirms a GAG deletion. So now the patient has a dystonic tremor syndrome (Axis 1) caused by DYT-TOR1A mutation (Axis 2).[33]

Similarly, a patient who presents with action tremor of both upper limbs for 4 years without further signs might be labeled as having ET (Axis 1) with idiopathic etiology (Axis 2). When the patient develops questionable signs of ataxia, Axis 1 diagnosis is changed toward ET-plus. Next, a brain MRI is performed and shows a characteristic splenium and MCP sign. Genetic testing confirms expansion of the CGG triplet repeat within the *FMR1* gene, so the etiology is now FXTAS.[34]

WEAKNESSES AND KNOWLEDGE GAPS AFFECTING THE CURRENT CLASSIFICATION SYSTEM

This current tremor classification reflects the status of our current knowledge about tremors. Given the increasing scientific interest regarding this symptom, further development is likely. One of the main weaknesses is that the separation of tremor syndromes is based on clinical symptoms rather than a deep understanding of pathophysiology, pathoanatomy, genetics, or any other strong data showing the neuropathologic basis of the symptoms.

Already, much discussion has emerged around the subclassification of ET and ET-plus, which reflects at best moderate consensus about a gray area of "soft signs" in tremor phenotyping. Two groups found independently that, among all ET patients, those with ET-plus are more frequent than those with the closer definition of ET alone.[35,36] One of the authors of the consensus statement has criticized the definition of ET-plus[19,37] as lacking a scientific basis. However, the

TABLE 2.3: COMBINED TREMOR SYNDROMES WITH MONOGENETIC INHERITANCE

Tremor combined with	Gene or karyotype	Inheritance pattern	Onset age (range), yrs	Main tremor phenomenology	Clinical features	Indicative diagnostics
Parkinsonism						
PARK-LRRK2	*LRRK2*	AD	>50 (28–82)	Parkinsonian rest tremor, in >60% initial symptom	Slow progress, phenotype similar to sporadic PD; almost all LRRK2-patients exhibit tremor during disease progress	DAT-SPECT: decreased uptake
PARK-Parkin	*PRKN*	AR	31 (3–81)	Parkinsonian rest tremor, dystonic action tremor	Slow progress, dystonic features, dopa-induced motor fluctuations	DAT-SPECT: decreased uptake
Dystonia						
DYT-TOR1A	*TOR1A*	AD	12 (4–64)	Dystonic rest and action tremor of upper limbs/ head, also writing tremor and Holmes-like tremor phenomenology reported	Isolated generalized dystonia, mostly starting focally in lower extremities; cases with focal/ segmental dystonia reported	
DYT-GCH1	*GCH1*	AD	6 (0–50)	Dystonic action tremor, parkinsonian rest tremor	Dopa-responsive combined dystonia, often with parkinsonism, diurnal fluctuation, starts in lower extremities, pyramidal signs, psychiatric symptoms	Dopa-test: marked improvement CSF pterin analysis: low tetrahydro-biopterin, low neopterin phenylalanine loading test: high post-dose phenylalanine levels
DYT-THAP1	*THAP1*	AD	16 (5–38)	Dystonic action tremor of head/upper limbs	Mostly starting at cervical region/upper limbs, laryngeal dystonia and sometimes generalization	
DYT-ANO3	*ANO3*	AD	19–69	Action tremor of upper limbs/ head	Cranio-cervical or segmental dystonia; tremor might precede dystonic symptoms	

Tremor combined with	Gene or karyotype	Inheritance pattern	Onset age (range), yrs	Main tremor phenomenology	Clinical features	Indicative diagnostics
DYT-GNAL	*GNAL*	AD	30 (7–53)	Action tremor of upper limbs/ head	Cervical or cranial dystonia; tremor might precede dystonic symptoms	
Wilson disease	*ATP7B*	AR	15–21 (till 70)	Dystonic action tremor, parkinsonian rest tremor, tongue tremor	Dysarthria (~60%) dystonia (~40%) tremor (~35%) rigidity/akinesia (~15 %) choreoathetosis (~15%) epileptic seizures (5%)	Serum: low copper and ceruloplasmin, elevated liver function Urine: high copper. MRI: "face of the giant panda"
Ataxia/Neuropathy						
SCA-ATXN2	*ATXN2*	AD	32 (1–66)	Postural limb tremor, rest tremor	Ataxia, neuropathy, cognitive deficits, parkinsonism, myoclonus	Brain MRI: atrophy of cerebellum, pons, cervical spine; (DAT-SPECT might show decreased uptake)
SCA-ATXN3	*ATXN3*	AD	36 (4–70)	Parkinsonian rest tremor, slow orthostatic tremor	Ataxia, parkinsonism, dystonia, chorea	Brain MRI: pontocerebellar atrophy
SCA-CACNA1A	*CACNA1A*	AD	>50	Postural tremor	Ataxia, rarely parkinsonism	Brain MRI: cerebellar atrophy
SCA-PPP2R2B	*PPP2R2B*	AD	38 (8–55)	Action tremor of upper limbs/ head, rarely parkinsonian rest tremor	Ataxia, parkinsonism, cognitive deficits	Brain MRI: cerebellar atrophy; DAT-SPECT might show decreased uptake
SCA-FGF14	*FGF14*	AD	12–20	Action tremor of upper limbs	Ataxia, orofacial dyskinesia, cognitive deficits	Brain MRI: cerebellar atrophy
Friedreich ataxia	*FXN*	AR	5–25 (late onsets till 70yrs reported)	Action tremor of upper limbs, head	Ataxia, pyramidal signs, sensorimotor neuropathy, chorea	Brain/spine MRI: initially normal, in advanced stages atrophy of cervical spine and cerebellum; nerve-conduction test: reduced or absent SNAP and normal motor conduction velocity (>40m/s)
Fragile X tremor/ ataxia syndrome (FXTAS)	*FMR1*	XL	>50 (50–90)	Intention tremor of upper limbs, postural and rest tremor also reported	Ataxia, cognitive decline, neuropathy, vestibular and autonomic dysfunction, premature ovarian failure in female relatives	Brain MRI: splenium and MCP sign; white matter hyperintensities, brain atrophy

Continued

TABLE 2.3: CONTINUED

Tremor combined with	Gene or karyotype	Inheritance pattern	Onset age (range), yrs	Main tremor phenomenology	Clinical features	Indicative diagnostics
Spinal and bulbar muscle atrophy (Kennedy disease)	*AR*	XL	40 (18–64)	High-frequency postural tremor of hands and legs	Degeneration of lower motor neurons with fasciculations, dysarthria, dysphagia, muscle weakness, gynecomastia, testicular atrophy, diabetes mellitus	EMG: signs of acute and chronic denervation
Klinefelter syndrome	47, XXY	QCA	0–30	Postural and intention tremor of upper limbs, sometimes also voice, head, leg tremor	Tall stature, hypergonadotropic hypogonadism, infertility	Serum: hypergonadotropic hypogonadism

AD = autosomal dominant; AR = autosomal recessive; CSF = cerebrospinal fluid; DAT-SPECT = ^{123}I-FP-CIT SPECT; EMG = electromyography; MRI = magnetic resonance imaging; SNAP = sensory nerve action potential; QCA = Quantitative chromosomal abnormality; XL = X-chromosomal linked

lack of a unifying scientific basis for determining the phenotype range of ET or ET-plus is the justification for outlining this clinical subgrouping: despite considerable efforts (reviewed in[38,39]), we have currently only negative findings regarding the genetics, pathoanatomy, biochemistry, and other attempts to objectively provide etiologic or pathologic underpinnings of the condition known as ET. The most likely reason is that ET is a syndrome with heterogeneous etiologies. The consensus group recommends subclassifying ET patients with soft signs or additional unusual features, with the expectation that deeper phenotyping of the clinical features will allow researchers to associate specific subgroups with objective etiology findings like genetic mutations. Therefore, the term ET-plus is a placeholder until we find better underpinnings of the causes.[40]

Many studies mention the occurrence of soft signs (dystonic posturing, cerebellar signs, cognitive changes) in ET and other tremor syndromes, but these do not suffice to make a clear diagnosis of dystonia, cerebellar disease, or dementia. To date, recognition of such soft signs is at the clinician's discretion and therefore very subjective; hence, a unifying definition of such signs is needed.

The overarching MDS classification of all existing tremor syndromes within one schematic[4,5]

has opened communication at least on well-defined tremor syndromes among and between clinicians and scientists, but it remains a mainly clinical definition. It represents the current clinical knowledge and will be modified as soon as we have more objective data on the etiology and pathophysiology of this unique symptomatology.

REFERENCES

1. Romberg MH. *A Manual of the Nervous Diseases of Man.* Vol. 2. Sydenham Society. 1853.
2. Oppenheim H. *Textbook of Nervous Diseases for Physicians and Students.* 5th ed. Bruce A. GE Stechert & Company; 1911;2:1237.
3. Fahn S. Differential diagnosis of tremors. *Med Clin N Am.* 1972;56(6):1363–1375.
4. Deuschl G, Bain P, Brin M. Consensus statement of the Movement Disorder Society on Tremor. Ad Hoc Scientific Committee. *Mov Disord.* 1998;13(Suppl. 3):2–23.
5. Bhatia KP, Bain P, Bajaj N, et al. Consensus statement on the classification of tremors, from the task force on tremor of the international Parkinson and Movement Disorder Society. *Mov Disord.* 2018.
6. Wilken M, Bruno V, Rossi M, Ameghino L, Deuschl G, Merello M. Sensitivity and specificity of different hand positions to assess upper limb rest tremor. *Mov Disord.* 2019.

7. Raethjen J, Austermann K, Witt K, Zeuner KE, Papengut F, Deuschl G. Provocation of Parkinsonian tremor. *Mov Disord.* 2008;23(7):1019–1023.

8. Zach H, Dirkx MF, Pasman JW, Bloem BR, Helmich RC. Cognitive stress reduces the effect of levodopa on Parkinson's Resting Tremor. *CNS Neurosci Ther.* 2017;23(3):209–215.

9. Papengut F, Raethjen J, Binder A, Deuschl G. Rest tremor suppression may separate essential from parkinsonian rest tremor. *Parkinsonism Relat Disord.* 2013;19(7):693–697.

10. Belvisi D, Conte A, Bologna M, et al. Re-emergent tremor in Parkinson's disease. *Parkinsonism Relat Disord.* 2017;36:41–46.

11. Jankovic J, Schwartz KS, Ondo W. Re-emergent tremor of Parkinson's disease. *J Neurol Neurosurg Psychiatry.* 1999;67(5):646–650.

12. Sanes JN, Hallett M. Limb positioning and magnitude of essential tremor and other pathological tremors. *Mov Disord.* 1990;5(4):304–309.

13. Schaefer SM, Hallett M, Karp BP, DiCapua DB, Tinaz S. Positional tremor and its treatment. *Mov Disord Clin Pract.* 2017;4(5):768–771.

14. Deuschl G, Wenzelburger R, Löffler K, Raethjen J, Stolze H. Essential tremor and cerebellar dysfunction clinical and kinematic analysis of intention tremor. *Brain.* 2000;123(8):1568–1580.

15. Kestenbaum M, Michalec M, Yu Q, Pullman SL, Louis ED. Intention tremor of the legs in essential tremor: prevalence and clinical correlates. *Mov Disord Clin Pract.* 2015;2(1):24–28.

16. Leegwater-Kim J, Louis ED, Pullman SL, et al. Intention tremor of the head in patients with essential tremor. *Mov Disord.* 2006;21(11):2001–2005.

17. Bain PG, Findley LJ, Britton TC, et al. Primary writing tremor. *Brain.* 1995;118(Pt 6):1461–1472.

18. Fearon C, Espay AJ, Lang AE, et al. Soft signs in movement disorders: friends or foes? *J Neurol Neurosurg Psychiatry.* 2019;90(8):961–962.

19. Louis ED, Bares M, Benito-Leon J, et al. Essential tremor-plus: a controversial new concept. *Lancet Neurol.* 2020;19(3):266–270.

20. Hall DA, Robertson E, Shelton AL, et al. Update on the clinical, radiographic, and neurobehavioral manifestations in FXTAS and FMR1 premutation carriers. *Cerebellum.* 2016;15(5):578–586.

21. Shrivastava A. The hot cross bun sign. *Radiology.* 2007;245(2):606–607.

22. Lee YC, Liu CS, Wu HM, Wang PS, Chang MH, Soong BW. The "hot cross bun" sign in patients with spinocerebellar ataxia. *Eur J Neurol.* 2009;16(4):513–516.

23. Berg D, Steinberger JD, Warren Olanow C, Naidich TP, Yousry TA. Milestones in magnetic resonance imaging and transcranial sonography of movement disorders. *Mov Disord.* 2011;26(6):979–992.

24. Prashanth L, Sinha S, Taly A, Vasudev M. Do MRI features distinguish Wilson's disease from other early onset extrapyramidal

disorders? An analysis of 100 cases. *Mov Disord.* 2010;25(6):672–678.

25. Benamer TS, Patterson J, Grosset DG, et al. Accurate differentiation of parkinsonism and essential tremor using visual assessment of [123I]-FP-CIT SPECT imaging: the [123I]-FP-CIT study group. *Mov Disord.* 2000;15(3):503–510.

26. Elble RJ, McNames J. Using portable transducers to measure tremor severity. *Tremor Other Hyperkinet Mov.* 2016;6.

27. Lauk M, Timmer J, Lücking C, Honerkamp J, Deuschl G. A software for recording and analysis of human tremor. *Comput Methods Programs Biomed.* 1999;60(1):65–77.

28. di Biase L, Brittain J-S, Shah SA, et al. Tremor stability index: a new tool for differential diagnosis in tremor syndromes. *Brain.* 2017;140(7):1977–1986.

29. Schwingenschuh P, Saifee TA, Katschnig-Winter P, et al. Validation of "laboratory-supported" criteria for functional (psychogenic) tremor. *Mov Disord.* 2016;31(4):555–562.

30. Magrinelli F, Latorre A, Balint B, et al. Isolated and combined genetic tremor syndromes: a critical appraisal based on the 2018 MDS criteria. *Parkinsonism Relat Disord.* 2020;77:121–140.

31. Ure RJ, Dhanju S, Lang AE, Fasano A. Unusual tremor syndromes: know in order to recognise. *J Neurol Neurosurg Psychiatry.* 2016;87(11):1191–1203.

32. Wardt Jvd, van der Stouwe AMM, Dirkx M, et al. Systematic clinical approach for diagnosing upper limb tremor. *J Neurol Neurosurg Psychiatry.* 2020;91(8):822–830.

33. Cáceres-Redondo MT, Carrillo F, Palomar FJ, Mir P. DYT-1 gene dystonic tremor presenting as a "scan without evidence of dopaminergic deficit." *Mov Disord.* 2012;27(11):1469.

34. Apartis E, Blancher A, Meissner WG, et al. FXTAS: new insights and the need for revised diagnostic criteria. *Neurology.* 2012;79(18):1898–1907.

35. Prasad S, Rastogi B, Shah A, et al. DTI in essential tremor with and without rest tremor: two sides of the same coin? *Mov Disord.* 2018;33(11):1820–1821.

36. Rajalingam R, Breen DP, Lang AE, Fasano A. Essential tremor plus is more common than essential tremor: insights from the reclassification of a cohort of patients with lower limb tremor. *Parkinsonism Relat Disord.* 2018;56:109–110.

37. Louis ED. Rising problems with the term "ET-plus": time for the term makers to go back to the drawing board. *Tremor Other Hyperkinet Mov.* 2020;10:28.

38. Deuschl G, Elble R. Essential tremor—neurodegenerative or nondegenerative disease towards a working definition of ET. *Mov Disord.* 2009;24(14):2033–2041.

39. Elble R, Deuschl G. Milestones in tremor research. *Mov Disord.* 2011;26(6):1096–1105.

40. Vidailhet M. Essential tremor-plus: a temporary label. *Lancet Neurol.* 2020;19(3):202.

Neuroanatomy and Physiological Mechanism of Tremor

MING-KAI PAN

INTRODUCTION

Tremor, by definition, is an involuntary rhythmic movement of one or more body parts. Therefore, there are two key factors involved in the tremor generation mechanism: a *rhythm-generating network* driven by a single or interconnected areas with pacemaking neurons; and a *motor-specific network* that permits only the oscillations manifested as tremor without interacting with other rhythm-related brain functions, such as memory formation, learning, and sleeping. In rhythm generation, *olivocerebellum* (inferior olive, Purkinje cells, and deep cerebellar nuclei) and the *Guillain-Mollaret triangle* (deep cerebellar nuclei, red nucleus, and inferior olive) are the two major circuits. The oscillations arise, maintain, and propagate in the motor network that normally regulates motor coordination (cerebellum), sensory feedback (sensory cortex), motor planning (premotor cortex), pattern generation (basal ganglia), and motor output (primary motor cortex). There are also important relay structures in the motor networks, including thalamus and pons. By integrating the two key factors of tremor, the *cerebro-ponto-cerebello-thalamo-cortical circuit* and the *cortico-basal ganglia circuit* are the two major contributors of tremor pathophysiology in the central nervous system. In addition to centrally driven tremor mechanisms, there are also peripheral mechanisms generating physiological or enhanced physiological tremor. The peripheral mechanisms include skeletomuscular mechanical components and the spinal reflex circuit. The central and peripheral mechanisms are interconnected by the corticospinal projections and spinocerebellar feedback. **Figure 3.1** summarizes the contributing networks involved in tremor, with additional notations of pacemaking ion channels.

CENTRAL NETWORKS OF RHYTHMIC MOVEMENTS

There are several basic components necessary to generate a stable oscillatory network. First, there should be pacemaking neurons with intrinsic firing properties. Second, these neurons should generate stable firing frequencies for tremor, either through self-control or through reciprocal interactions among other pacemaking neurons in the network. Third, there should be a mechanism to generate significant synchrony among pacing neurons for observable effects, i.e., tremor. Finally, feedback and inhibitory innervations should be included in biological oscillatory networks to avoid uncontrolled positive feedback or easy perturbation without inhibitory filtering. Based on these principles, neuroscientists have made great progress elucidating neuronal oscillatory networks in various brain functions, such as alpha rhythm of cerebral oscillations, hippocampal ripples for memory consolidation, and spindle waves for sleep.

Unlike sleep and memory consolidation, tremor can be characterized by body area involved, and by activation condition.[1] The two main activation conditions are (1) action, with voluntary muscle contraction; and (2) rest, when muscles are relaxed. Overlapping neural mechanisms are involved in tremors that occur under different activation conditions.

Oscillatory networks: Where does tremor originate?

Similar to other oscillatory networks, self-pacing neurons for motor rhythm generation can either work as a dominant source, or work with other types of autonomous neurons in an interconnected network to determine a final output frequency. The rhythm-generating mechanism of tremor predominantly implicates the olivocerebellar circuitry, which has important roles in both normal volitional movement and action tremor. Other areas such as the thalamus may also be involved in generating oscillations, particularly in pathologic conditions. The basal ganglia have a clear but poorly understood role in generating rest tremor.

The olivocerebellar circuit

The olivocerebellum is composed of the *inferior olive (IO)*, cerebellar cortex *Purkinje cells (PCs)*, and *deep cerebellar nuclei (DCN)* of the cerebellar subcortical area. Neurons in the IO send glutamatergic axons, called climbing fibers, to PCs. PCs then send GABAergic outputs to DCN neurons,

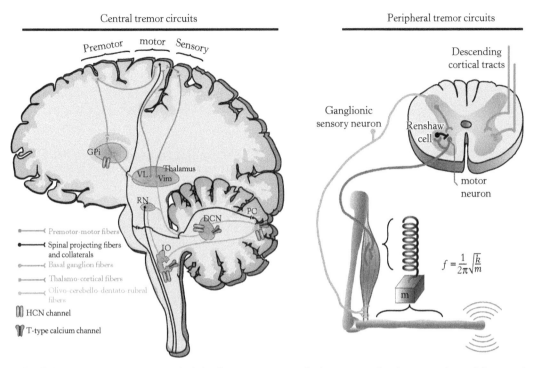

FIGURE 3.1: Tremor Circuitry. The left column summarizes the locations and major connections of the central tremor circuitry. Neurons capable of generating pace-making properties, especially those equipped with HCN or T-type calcium channels, are marked. The right column illustrates the peripheral tremor circuits, emphasizing the interaction between neural feedback loops and intrinsic oscillatory properties related to the mechanics of limb structures. Abbreviations: GPi = Globus pallidus internus; VL = ventral lateral nucleus; Vim = ventral intermediate nucleus; RN = red nucleus; DCN = deep cerebellar nucleus; PC = Purkinje cell; IO = inferior olive; k = overall elastic index of the system; m = mass of the musculoskeletal system; HCN = Hyperpolarization-activated cyclic nucleotide–gated.

the major outputs of the cerebellum, use thalamic relays to connect with cerebral cortex. PCs and these principal neurons in the IO and the DCN all have pacemaking properties required for rhythm generation. Patients with action tremor, especially essential tremor (ET), may experience tremor disappearance after strokes in olivocerebellar areas.[2–4]

Inferior olive

The IO is considered a major oscillatory generator in the tremor circuitry. Rhythmicity and synchrony, two essential factors to generate oscillations, are found in the IO. IO neurons have intrinsic rhythmic firing properties. IO neurons are also equipped with "electrical synapses" via gap junctions that promote synchrony among IO neurons. Harmaline, a chemical that enhances IO rhythmicity and synchronicity, has a profound acute tremor effect in rodents, cat and primates.[5–9]

The IO receives major cortical inputs from the cerebral cortices, including the premotor and primary sensory cortices. The IO also receives direct sensory inputs from spino-olivary tracts and from trigeminal nuclei. Other afferent fibers

come from deep nuclei, including the DCN and red nucleus. The IO sends climbing-fiber efferents to cerebellar cortex PCs.

Neuronal Firing Properties. IO neurons typically generate action potentials at 1~12 Hz in rodent and cat, with an average at ~ 4 Hz. The firing frequency is based on the interplay between hyperpolarization-activated cyclic nucleotide-gated (HCN) channels and T-type calcium channels. IO innervation of PCs helps generate complex spikes in PCs.

Ion channel properties. Rhythmic firings of IO neurons are built by two major components: HCN and T-type calcium channels. HCN channels regulate subthreshold oscillations of neuronal membrane potentials. During membrane potential hyperpolarization, HCN channels provide ramping depolarizing currents, which lead to rhythmic oscillations of membrane potentials in many pacemaking neurons and cardiomyocytes.[10] The kinetics of HCN channels are also regulated by cAMP and beta-adrenergic stimulation, which explains increased heart rate during stress. IO HCN channels are not only rhythm-generating, but also act as band-pass filters to select input signals biased to 2-10 Hz.[11] In awake mice, HCN channels synchronize oscillatory rhythm and stabilize the frequencies of complex spikes in PCs.[12]

T-type calcium channels in IO can generate depolarization passing through the action-potential generation threshold and calcium influx to maintain a cluster of action potentials.[11] This property is also a key component of oscillation generation in many pacemaking neurons, including thalamic,[13,14] subthalamic neurons[15] and PCs.[14] In the IO, T-type calcium channels serve as amplifiers of oscillations initially triggered by HCN channels[11] via a positive feedback cycle: calcium influx depolarizes neurons, and depolarization promotes more T-type calcium channels to open until spontaneous channel inactivation occurs. Activation of T-type calcium channels drives subthreshold oscillations above threshold and generates trains (bursts) of action potentials. Bursts not only promote synchronization in neighboring neurons but also send strong outputs toward PCs and reliably generate complex spikes.[16]

Electrical synapses. One of the most unique properties of IO neurons is gap-junction electrical synapses. Using electrical synapses, an IO neuron can transduce its subthreshold oscillations to its neighbors with minimal delay, whereas regular synapses only allow neurotransmitter releases from all-or-none action potentials, with the time delay of vesicle release and frequency distortion by neurotransmitter receptor kinetics. Electrical synapses enable maximal IO neuron synchronization.

Evidence of human IO involvement in tremor. IO hypertrophy has been associated with palatal or oculopalatal tremor.[17-20] Excessive climbing-fiber synapses from the IO to the PCs are also observed in human cerebellar pathology of ET cases.[21,22] It should be noted that tremor can have different causes and not all tremor patients have IO pathology.[23,24]

Purkinje cells

PCs are the sole cell type of cerebellar cortical output. All inputs from the premotor cortex or the IO require direct or indirect communication with PCs in order to be transmitted out of the cerebellar cortex to the DCN, and from there out of the cerebellum. Moreover, PCs are one of the few projecting neuron types that use GABA as their main neurotransmitter. PCs receive two types of glutamatergic inputs. One is from IO climbing fibers. The other is from the parallel fibers of granule cells, located in the cerebellar cortex right below the PC layer. PCs are also pacemaking cells with much higher intrinsic firing rates than IO neurons. Recent evidence suggests that

synchronization of PCs plays a key role in the pathophysiology of action tremor.[5,25]

Neuronal Firing Properties. PCs are among the fastest-firing neurons in the brain. A PC typically fires at 60–80 Hz in a simple-spike (regular firing) mode, and easily goes up to 140 Hz in awake behaving mice. When receiving inputs from the IO, PCs can generate transient complex spikes (bursts) whose intra-burst firing frequency is ~ 400 Hz.[5]

Ion channel properties. Similar to IO cells, PCs also express HCN channels and exhibit pacemaking properties. In PCs, glutamatergic inputs from climbing fibers activate T-type calcium channels and generate complex spikes that play a major role in the generation of tremor in mice.[5,26] Parallel fibers from granule cells to PCs activate mGluR1 channels. These two glutamatergic inputs, when occurring together, activate additional P/Q type calcium channels that trigger long-term depression of PCs, cause plasticity changes, and modulate the simple-spike firing frequencies. To achieve ultrafast burst firings of action potentials, PCs equip resurgent sodium channels and allow sodium channels to bypass inactive states and open repetitively in a single depolarizing episode.[27,28] Notably, PCs and the principal neurons of the subthalamic nucleus are two neuron types expressing resurgent sodium channels, and both structures have roles in tremor pathophysiology and therapeutics.[27,29]

Deep cerebellar nuclei

DCNs include the fastigial (medial cerebellar) nucleus, interpose nuclei (globose and emboliform nuclei), and dentate (lateral cerebellar) nucleus. They all receive cerebellar cortical inputs from PCs and regulate various type of motor control including oculo-vestibular coupling (fastigial), axial movement (interpose), and limb coordination (dentate). DCN neurons widely innervate brainstem reticular nuclei and red nucleus, and send fibers to major relay neurons including in the thalamus. In terms of tremor, IO-generated oscillations are relayed through PCs to the DCN and then to further structures such as the thalamus. Notably, DCN neurons also innervate the IO with GABAergic axons, which control the conductance of gap junctions and thus the synchronization between IO neurons.[30] Models suggest that loss of DCN-to-IO GABAergic innervation may be the pathophysiology of IO hypertrophy linked to palatal tremor.[17] The IO-PC-DCN-IO circuit forms a closed oscillatory loop. Topographical differences in tremor may involve different oscillatory circuits of cerebellar cortices and DCN subregions.

Neuronal Firing Properties. Averaged DCN firing rates in rodents and cats are 20–40 Hz, but can be as high as 170 Hz during evoked conditions.[31,32]

Ion channel properties. As with the IO and PCs, DCN neurons are equipped with HCN and T-type calcium channels for self-pacing. Moreover, DCN neurons have unique rebound firing properties. DCN neurons receive GABAergic innervations from PCs, whose firings lead to transient pauses of neuronal activity by GABAergic hyperpolarization, followed by activation of T-type calcium channels and therefore rebound burst firings.

Tremor generating properties of the olivocerebellar IO-PC-DCN circuit

In summary, the IO sends climbing fibers to innervate PCs, which generate complex spikes in response to climbing-fiber inputs. PC complex spikes provide strong inputs to the DCN, causing a transient pause of DCN firings and then rebounded burst firings. The precise firing times in the IO, PC, and DCN neurons are further tuned by the subthreshold oscillations of membrane potentials related to the intrinsic firing properties of each area. The final oscillatory frequencies are also regulated by neurotransmitters. GABAergic inputs from PCs forbid DCN intrinsic firings not aligned with the circuitry frequency, and DCN-to-IO GABAergic inputs generate similar effects on the IO with additional regulation of IO-to-IO synchrony via gap-junction modulations. Glutamatergic inputs from the IO to the DCN promote the frequency alignment toward the desired final output frequency.[33]

Guillain-Mollaret triangle

Besides the IO-PC-DCN circuit, another circuit involves the dentate nuclei of the DCN, red nucleus, and IO. Each dentate nucleus heavily innervates the contralateral red nucleus, which sends fibers to the spinal cord and collaterals to bilateral IOs. The IO regulates dentate nuclei neurons indirectly through PCs, and sends sparse collaterals directly to the dentate.[26,34] This dentato-rubro (red nucleus)-IO brainstem loop is referred to as the Guillain-Mollaret triangle. The Guillain-Mollaret triangle also forms a closed loop with pacemaking IO and DCN neurons; therefore, it is capable of generating frequency-dependent oscillations. Based on the computational modeling, the triangle can further augment IO-PC-DCN-generated DCN firings that are coherent with the oscillations in the triangle using the excitatory IO-to-DCN inputs.[33] The overlapping IO-PC-DCN and Guillain-Mollaret triangle circuits may work together to generate final tremor frequency, but the detailed coordinating mechanism remains to be elucidated.

Thalamus

The thalamus is not considered part of the oscillatory generator in volitional movement. However, it is an established target in treating various types of tremor. The thalamus likely serves as a central node in the information relay that allows pathological frequencies to propagate from the cerebellum/basal ganglia toward the motor cortex. Another important question is whether the thalamus itself is an oscillatory source of tremor. The reticular nucleus of the thalamus has long been identified as a pacemaker for sleep spindles and delta oscillations during sleep. However, evidence is limited on whether thalamic relay neurons in the VIM (cerebellar thalamus) or VA/VL (basal ganglia thalamus) also have pacing properties. Slice recordings in mice do not reveal spontaneous firings in the VIM, VL, and VM neurons, but more evidence is required to draw a conclusion.

Basal ganglia

Basal ganglia play a crucial role in parkinsonian rest tremor. Deep brain stimulation (DBS) in the *subthalamic nucleus (STN)* or the *globus pallidus internus (GPi)* consistently suppresses rest tremor.[35] Moreover, lesioning therapies using MRI-guided focus ultrasound (MRIgFUS) at the STN or GPi have DBS-comparable efficacy.[35] Therefore, the STN and GPi are active and essential components in rest tremor pathophysiology. In terms of rhythm generation, STN neurons have self-pacing properties and ion channel compositions similar to cerebellar PCs, including HCN and T-type calcium channels and the unique resurgent sodium channels for ultrafast burst-firing.[15,36] In fact, the STN is the key generator of abnormal beta oscillations at 13–40 Hz, a key electrophysiological signature detected in the cortical-basal ganglia circuitry of patients with Parkinson disease.[37–45] Specifically, the glutamatergic cortico-subthalamic "hyperdirect" pathway triggers rhythmic firings of STN neurons via GluN2A-containing NMDA receptors and generates beta oscillations.[46,47] GPi neurons also have HCN channels for self-pacing.[48–50] and participate in the propagation of beta oscillations in the basal ganglia circuitry.

Subthalamic nucleus

While STN neurons are capable of generating oscillations, current evidence suggests that the STN is not the rhythm generator for rest tremor. Many studies suggest that STN oscillations at the tremor frequency are less correlated with rest tremor,[51–55] although STN-tremor coherence has been observed.[56] Instead, oscillatory patterns showing stronger STN theta (4–7 Hz) power and weaker beta (13–30 Hz) power are positively correlated with rest tremor[51]. Consistently, using combined non-linear spectral information (e.g., considering the whole frequency dynamics of STN instead of the tremor frequency alone), STN local field potentials, especially high-frequency components (>200 Hz), can be used to identify tremor in STN-DBS patients.[53,55] These data suggest that the STN actively participates in rest tremor, but is not the direct tremor generator that oscillates at the tremor frequency.

Globus pallidus internus

GPi neurons, on the other hand, can fire at tremor frequency. 10–40% of recorded GPi neurons in parkinsonian tremor patients fire at the tremor frequency and coherent with tremor.[57-60] Notably, GPi-electromyography (EMG) coherence in these studies is all intermittent, and tremor may appear prior to the rhythmic GPi firings. In this context, the GPi is less likely to participate in tremor initiation than in tremor maintenance or feedback[57]. Further information is required to clarify the exact role of the GPi in parkinsonian rest tremor.

As compared to the cerebello-thalamo-cortical circuit and its role in action tremor, basal ganglia and parkinsonian rest tremor are much less understood. One of the key obstacles is that there are very few animal studies, including one study in monkeys[61] and one study in mice,[62] reported generating rest tremor.

Cerebello-thalamo-cortical circuits in rest tremor

Although the IO-PC-DCN olivocerebellar circuit and its thalamo-cortical transmissions are mainly associated with action or postural tremor, the cerebello-thalamo-cortical circuit also participates in rest tremor. Magnetoencephalography (MEG) study shows clear cerebellar oscillations at the frequency of parkinsonian rest tremor and significant MEG-EMG coherence.[63] VIM activities are highly coherent with rest tremor.[64,65] These data suggest that cerebellar circuits may be the generator of tremor-related oscillations and the basal ganglia may be the switch to turn tremor on/off.[64,66,67] This dimmer (cerebellum)-switch (basal ganglia) model may explain the confusing findings of basal ganglia oscillations in parkinsonian rest tremor.

Summary

IO neurons, PCs, and DCN neurons of the olivocerebellum all have intrinsic firing properties and form the IO-PC-DCN circuit involved in rhythm generation of action tremor. This olivocerebellar circuit may require support of Guillain-Mollaret triangle, a dentato-rubro-olivary brainstem loop. Thalamus is also required to propagate DCN output to the cerebral cortex, which loops back via the cortico-ponto-cerebello pathway to from a close oscillatory circuitry. In the basal ganglia, the GPi and STN are active contributors to parkinsonian rest tremor, but their roles in tremor oscillatory generation remain largely unclear. Current theory suggests that the basal ganglia serve as the switch to turn tremor on or off, while the cerebellar circuit remains the generating source of tremor oscillations.

PATHOPHYSIOLOGY OF AUGMENTED OSCILLATIONS IN THE CEREBELLAR-BASED CIRCUITS FOR TREMOR

The pacemaking properties of cerebellar circuits play important roles in generating volitional rhythmic movements. There are several mechanisms that drive the normal oscillatory circuits to pathological states that then lead to involuntary tremor. These mechanisms include *enhanced automaticity and synchrony in the inferior olive, increased Purkinje cell synchrony by increasing IO-to-PC innervations,* and *disruption of GABAergic transmission in the olivocerebellar circuits.* In addition, channelopathies could also increase neuronal automaticity to the pathological states.

Enhanced automaticity and synchrony in the inferior olive

Harmaline is a beta-carboline alkaloid that can induce acute transient action tremor in rodents, cats, pigs, and monkeys.[68] Harmaline-induced tremor is widely used as an animal model for ET. There are limited data on harmaline and tremor in humans. One group observed increased blood levels of harmane and other beta-carboline alkaloids associated with increased risk of ET.[69,70]

Mechanistically, harmaline enhances IO automaticity and synchrony by promoting burst firings, rebound firings, and inter-burst silencing around 3–12 Hz.[5,7,8] In brain slices, harmaline hyperpolarizes IO neurons, which increases the availability of HCN and T-type calcium channels and therefore creates excessive rhythmic IO bursting.[8] Harmaline also creates super-synchrony of IO neurons via electrical coupling by gap junctions.[8] Notably, knocking out a central gap-junction protein, connexin-36, did not abolish harmaline-induced mouse tremor,[6] while T-type calcium channel knockout did.[9] Therefore, T-type calcium channels may be a key mechanism in generating harmaline-induced action tremor. T-type calcium channel blockers have therapeutic effects on nicotine-induced tremor[71] and have been under development for other tremor syndromes.

Another proposed mechanism of increased IO synchrony is the loss of GABAergic innervations from the DCN to the IO.[17] Loss of such GABAergic innervations can lead to loss of the inhibitory control of IO electrical coupling,[30] which may then lead to IO over-synchrony, IO hypertrophy, and palatal or oculopalatal tremor.[17]

Increased PC synchrony by increasing IO-to-PC innervations

One reported neuropathology finding in ET is an excessive innervation of climbing fibers to PCs.[21,22,26] This climbing-fiber overgrowth, also known as pruning deficits, is correlated to the reduced expression of GluRδ2 protein in PCs.[26] A mouse model with GluRδ2 deficiency recapitulates climbing-fiber pruning deficits and develops action tremor.[26] Climbing-fiber overgrowth causes excessive synchronization and oscillations of PCs, as measured using cerebellar local field potentials. Blocking PC oscillatory activities can suppress the tremor, whereas induced cerebellar oscillations by rhythmic PC activation induces tremor in normal mice.[26] The observations in mice are supported by human findings using cerebellar electroencephalography (EEG) to detect cerebellar oscillations in ET patients.[26] These observations support an IO-to-PC tremor generation mechanism. More studies are required to confirm the proposed pathophysiology validity. The findings are summarized in Figure 3.2 and Video 3.1.

Disruption of GABAergic transmission in olivocerebellar circuits

GABA-related mechanisms are a hypothesized key tremor generation mechanism. In a mouse model with homozygous $GABA_A$ receptor knockout, action tremor responsive to alcohol, primidone, and propranolol was observed.[72] A follow-up study found that a PC-specific $GABA_A$ receptor knockout is sufficient to induce an action tremor phenotype,[73] implicating the inhibitory control of PC from nearby interneurons in the molecular layers. Such a GABAergic mechanism has been proposed in action tremor related to alcohol withdrawal.[74] In ET patients, one study showed reduction of GABA receptor expression and mRNA in the dentate nuclei of the DCN[75]. Disruption of GABAergic input from the DCN to the IO, as mentioned previously, may lead to IO hypertrophy and palatal tremor.[17] Changes in the GABA-related system in ET were observed via flumazenil PET,[76] showing abnormalities in the cerebellum, ventrolateral thalamus, and premotor cortex. Computational modeling also emphasizes the importance of the GABA system in the cerebellar circuits.[33]

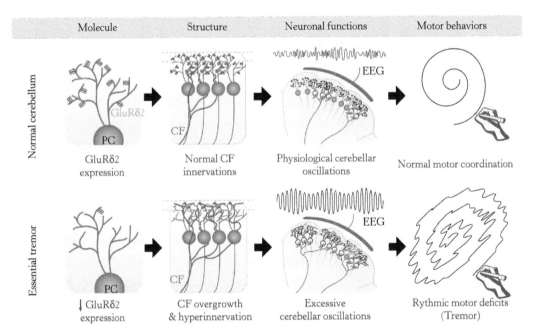

Molecule	Structure	Neuronal functions	Motor behaviors

Normal cerebellum:
GluRδ2 expression — Normal CF innervations — Physiological cerebellar oscillations (EEG) — Normal motor coordination

Essential tremor:
↓ GluRδ2 expression — CF overgrowth & hyperinnervation — Excessive cerebellar oscillations (EEG) — Rythmic motor deficits (Tremor)

FIGURE 3.2: An IO-to-PC Mechanism of Essential Tremor. Reduced expression of GluRδ2 proteins in cerebellar PCs leads to CF overgrowth, which causes excessive cerebellar oscillations and drives tremor. Abbreviations: PC = Purkinje cell; CF = climbing fiber; EEG = electroencephalography.

The graph is modified from Pan et al. *Science Translational Medicine* 2020, 15;12(526):eaay1769. DOI: 10.1126/scitranslmed.aay1769, Supplementary Figure 18.

Mutations of ion channels supporting pacemaking properties

HCN channels play a key role in frequency generation in the IO-PC-DCN circuit. Notably, beta-adrenergic receptors can positively modulate HCN channels via cGMP pathways. The HCN channel increases channel conductance when exposed to beta-sympathomimetics or stress. This mechanism contributes to enhanced physiological tremor and augmented action tremor in ET. Caffeine, which directly stimulates cAMP pathways, also acts on HCN channels and contributes to increased heart rate and enhanced physiological tremor.[77,78] In a rat model, mutations of the *HCN1* gene, which encodes one of the four HCN channels subunits, can lead to ET-like tremor when co-expressed with *tm* mutation.[79] Notably, *HCN* gene mutations have not yet been reported in human tremor syndromes.

T-type calcium channels are responsible for rebound firings and amplification of rhythmicity, and play a crucial role in IO oscillatory mechanisms, IO-to-PC communication, and PC-to-DCN firings. Mutations of *CACNA1G* ($CaV_{3.1}$), encoding one subtype of T-type calcium channel, were found by whole genome sequencing in families with three or more cases of ET, not ET-plus,[1] with at least one case showing early onset of definite or probable ET (age <= 50 years).[80]

Genetic variants in sodium channel subunit encoding genes *SCN4A* and *SCA11A*, as well as the potassium channel subunit encoding gene *KCNS2* (Kv9.2), have been described in single ET families.[80–82] The *SCN4A* disease-associated variant was reported in a family with ET and episodic pain, and the *SCN11A* variant in a family with ET and epilepsy. Notably, these channelopathies are gain-of-function mutations to enhance oscillatory networks. For example, increased Kv9.2 conductance caused by the point mutation Kv9.2-D379E, in collaboration with T-type calcium channels, triggers stronger and self-sustained rebound firings and increases oscillatory activities.[68]

MAINTENANCE AND PROPAGATION OF OSCILLATIONS IN THE TREMOR CIRCUITS

While the generators of rhythmic oscillations are the key components that lead to tremor, other non-pacemaking structures are also important to relay neuronal oscillations within central tremor circuits, gate oscillations among different motor scenarios, or send oscillatory outputs to muscles. In action tremor pathophysiology, neuronal oscillations flow in the cerebro-ponto-cerebello-thalamo-cortical circuit that contains other non-pacemaking structures including the pons, cerebral cortex, and thalamus. In rest tremor, the STN-pallido-thalamic circuit is involved but with a less understood role. Notably, the cerebro-ponto-cerebello-thalamo-cortical circuit also participates in rest tremor.[66,83]

Cerebro-ponto-cerebello-thalamo-cortical circuits

Premotor cortex

The premotor cortex, including the medial premotor cortex (supplementary motor area, SMA), lateral premotor cortex, and cingulate motor area, participates in motor preparation and is strongly involved in generating volitional rhythmic movement.[84] These subregions connect strongly to the primary motor cortex, receive inputs from the cerebellum,[85,86] and send fibers directly to the spinal cord (from the SMA)[87] and basal ganglia (from the cingulate motor area).[85] The premotor cortex also sends outputs to the pons, which in turn innervates the cerebellum via pontine mossy fibers.

In ET, fMRI studies showed abnormalities in the SMA, including increased SMA gray mater volume, decreased SMA functional connectivity to the primary motor cortex, and increased SMA–spinal cord functional connectivity.[88] EEG- or MEG-based studies showed involvement of the premotor cortex in volitional mimicked tremor, ET, and parkinsonian rest tremor[63,84,89,90].

Pons

The pons is the major relay of the cortico-ponto-cerebellar pathway, connecting the premotor cortex to the cerebellum. In fact, more than half of the ventral pons (basis pontis) participates in this relay function. Pons abnormalities are reported to cause action tremor.[91,92]

Cerebellum

The cerebellar circuitry is known for its roles in motor coordination. Finely-tuned motor coordination requires precise control of each participating muscle, which needs to work properly in space and time. Specifically, tremor involves repetitive and alternating muscle contraction of agonists and antagonists. Cerebellar dysfunction has been associated with dystonia, which generates agonist and antagonist co-contractions, supporting active roles for the cerebellum in coordinating muscles for tremor,[93,94] particularly action tremor. Action tremor encompasses kinetic tremor, i.e, tremor with actions, and postural tremor, when the body part is held in an active posture against gravity.[1]

In rodents, the olivocerebellum contributes to the regulation of multi-joint movement.[95] Climbing fibers from the IO synchronize nearby PCs in a timely manner in micro-domains, to provide proper coordination in various limb positions.[95] In the pathological olivocerebellum with increased oscillatory properties, activation of the IO-PC-DCN network during action can lead to manifested network oscillations and thus kinetic tremor. Moreover, the computational load of cerebellar motor coordination is significantly increased for precise movement. Cerebellar lesions frequently cause dysmetria with a key feature of terminal crescendo (increase in amplitude) at the moment that requires precise targeting, such as touching the examiner's finger. This phenomenon can be rhythmic and is known as intention tremor, a type of action tremor.[96] Besides its role in movement, the cerebellum also receives sensory feedback from the spinal cord and cortical sensory area via their mossy fiber projections. These sensory feedbacks are known to play crucial roles in maintaining gait, balance, and posture. Indeed, the cerebellum also actively participates in postural tremor.[97,98] Taken together, the cerebellum is responsible for motor coordination and is a key player in action tremor.

Interestingly, there is also strong fMRI and EEG evidence of cerebellar involvement in rest tremor.[63,66,99] Parkinsonian patients with rest tremor also show synaptic pathology from climbing-fiber-to-PC.[21] Unfortunately, currently no animal models reliably recapitulate rest tremor for further investigation.

The cerebellum sends glutamatergic outputs toward the thalamus, the next key player in the central network of tremor.

Thalamus

The thalamus, as a critical relay between the cerebellum to the premotor and primary motor cortices (Figure 3.1, left column, blue and purple lines) as well as between the basal ganglia and motor cortex (Figure 3.1, left column, green and purple lines), is regarded as a crucial component of tremor circuits. The ventral intermediate nucleus (VIM) of the thalamus is the major relay of cerebellar inputs to the motor cortex, while the ventral anterior nucleus (VA) and ventral lateral nucleus (VL) of the thalamus receive inputs from the GPi that are relayed to the premotor and primary motor cortices. Thalamotomy or thalamic DBS produces consistent therapeutic benefits in ET, vocal tremor, parkinsonian tremor, and Holmes tremor.[65,100,101] Intra-operative recordings show thalamic local field potentials highly coherent with tremor.[99,102] Moreover, phase-dependent closed-loop stimulation of the VL or VIM has shown high efficacy in ET, demonstrating that the thalamic oscillations are the key relay connecting tremor-generating brain areas to the motor cortices of corresponding body parts.[103] Notably, several recordings revealed that tremor onset can precede thalamo-muscular coherence, emphasizing the role of motor outputs and the contribution of thalamic-gated sensory feedback.[104]

Primary motor cortex

The primary motor cortex is the central controller of volitional movement. It receives inputs from the premotor cortex, the basal ganglia, and the cerebellum and sends motor outputs to the spinal cord. Strokes in the primary motor cortex not only abolish volitional movements, but also stop tremor.[4,105] Cortical stimulation using single-pulse transcranial magnetic stimulation can reset the action tremor in ET.[106] Cortico-EMG coherence was also observed during tremor in both EEG and MEG studies.[107,108]

While the motor cortex plays a necessary role in tremor generation, there are controversies regarding its role in tremor maintenance. EEG–EMG coherence studies in ET observed an intermittent loss of coherence between the primary motor cortex and muscles while the tremor remained[109,110]. More evidence is required to fully understand the precise role of the primary motor cortex in tremor circuits.

Basal ganglia circuits

As described above, the STN and the GPi are active players in rest tremor. STN or GPi lesioning has a reliable effect on rest-tremor suppression, confirming their critical roles. However, there is a paucity of information on rest tremor circuitry, frequency determination, and amplitude modulation. Current dimmer-switch models suggest that the basal ganglia determines tremor on-off switches, but the detailed mechanism remains largely unclear.

Summary

The cerebro-ponto-cerebello-thalamo-cortical circuit plays a key role in action tremor. The IO, PC, and DCN provide pacemaking properties and can be oscillation rhythm sources. Activation of the premotor cortex (SMA) via the pons as well as recruitment of the olivocerebellum further drive or augment IO-PC-DCN circuit oscillations. The thalamus serves as a critical relay to transmit cerebellar output from the DCN toward the premotor and primary motor cortices, which regulate spinal motor neurons via the corticospinal tracts and finally generate tremor in muscles.

Notably, while the IO-PC-DCN olivocerebellar circuit and the overlapping Guillain-Mollaret triangle have oscillatory capabilities and form closed loops, it remains unclear whether these circuits are sufficient to be the oscillatory generators of tremor by themselves. Instead, the cerebro-ponto-cerebello-thalamo-cortical circuit, given the evidence mentioned above, may be the oscillatory circuit to generate tremor. In the context of this proposed big oscillatory circuit, the main roles of the IO-PC-DCN and Guillain-Mollaret triangle circuits may be to augment oscillations and consolidate oscillatory frequencies.

Besides action tremor, rest tremor also requires the cerebro-ponto-cerebello-thalamo-cortical circuit to generate oscillations. Basal ganglia components, especially the STN and GPi, play essential roles in rest tremor.

PERIPHERAL NETWORKS OF RHYTHMIC MOVEMENTS

Besides central networks, oscillations and tremor can be generated in the system composed of *spinal cord and muscles*, commonly termed the "peripheral mechanism" for tremor generation. Oscillations in the peripheral system are the cause of *physiological tremor*. In contrast to the central network, which focuses on the pacemaking neurons generating electrical rhythmic activities, the peripheral system uses a different mechanism related to the mechanical properties of bones, elastic tissues and muscles to induce oscillations (Figure 3.1, right column). Also, in contrast to centrally generated tremors, physiological tremor is observed only as action tremor, and does not occur under resting conditions.

Mechanisms generating peripheral oscillations

The mechanical components of the peripheral system

Every rigid object attached to a spring-like elastic structure can have an intrinsic oscillatory frequency (Figure 3.1, right column). Taking a spring with hinged mass as an example, the oscillatory frequency is $1/(2\pi)*(k/m)^{1/2}$, where k is the elastic coefficient of the spring and m is the mass hinged to the spring. In the forelimb, our combined bone and soft tissue structures determine the mass that hinges to the joint. The elastic components include tendons and muscles that contribute to the elastic coefficient and force generation. Therefore, our limb can have an intrinsic oscillatory frequency that is prone to tremor. Muscle contractions that coincide with the oscillatory frequency can augment the oscillations to build up tremor. Evidence

suggests that hand tremor oscillatory frequency is determined by hand volume and by additional weight added on to the hand, consistent with the prediction that increased mass leads to decrement of oscillatory frequency.[111]

The spinal reflex circuit

Needle EMG provides clear evidence that spinal motor neurons activate each muscle fiber or motor unit to the maximal firing rate, around 10 Hz.[96] Generating additional muscle strength requires muscle fiber recruitment, which leads to more muscle fibers activated at the 10 Hz frequency. The cumulative effect of the muscle fiber activity, recorded by surface EMG, generates an 8–12 Hz activity that correlates well with tremor detected by accelerometry.[112] In addition, feedback control mechanisms are mediated through Renshaw cells. Spinal motor neurons send monosynaptic collateral outputs to Renshaw cells, which send GABAergic inhibition back to the same spinal motor neuron. This feedback inhibition dampens the 10 Hz oscillations[113] and maintains the 20 Hz M1-EMG coupling. In addition, gamma-motor neurons increase tremor amplitude during muscle shortening by increasing proprioceptive sensory feedback.[114]

The corticospinal projection

The motor cortex provides 10 Hz and 20 Hz inputs into the spinal cord via corticospinal transmission.[115-117]

Spino-cerebellar feedback

The cerebellum has abundant reciprocal interactions with the spinal cord. In addition to indirect communication via cerebral cortex, the cerebellum sends direct outputs to spinal cord via rubrospinal and interpositospinal pathways, and receives sensory feedback inputs via spino-reticular pathways. Moreover, the cerebral cortex also sends a motor command copy to the cerebellum via the propriospinal pathways.[118] In cats with harmaline-induced tremor, lateral reticular neurons receive spinoreticular input, fire at the tremor frequency, and send axonal outputs to the cerebellar cortex.[119]

The peripheral components (intrinsic mechanical properties and the spinal reflex) and their interaction with central networks (corticospinal projections and spino-cerebellar feedback) work together to generate peripheral oscillations. Notably, the base frequencies of these properties either align to the same frequency range, around 8–12 Hz, or its harmonic frequency, around 20 Hz, allowing them to work collaboratively instead of canceling each other. It is unclear whether this frequency tuning is related to developmental adaptation or evolution. Interestingly, physiological tremor in mice also falls in the range of 8–12 Hz.[5,26]

Physiological and enhanced physiological tremor

By understanding the oscillatory properties in the peripheral system, it is clear that healthy people often have mild, unnoticed tremor. This normal type of tremor is called *physiological tremor*, an 8–12 Hz action tremor predominantly contributed by the mechanical components of the peripheral system described above. Physiological tremor frequency tends to decrease with aging. Physiological tremor can be augmented by physiological factors such as fatigue, or iatrogenic factors such as medications. Peripherally, these provoking factors recruit the spinomuscular feedback system to oscillate at the frequency of the peripheral mechanical system, and augment physiological tremor amplitudes. Physiological tremor augmentation is common, and is termed *enhanced physiological tremor*. Other common provoking factors of *enhanced physiological tremor* include alcohol withdrawal, hypoglycemia, caffeine intake, hyperthyroidism, and toxin exposure. Notably, these provoking factors also have central targets. For example, HCN channels can be modulated by beta-adrenergic stimulation or caffeine exposure (see also the "Inferior Olive" section, above). Therefore, enhanced physiological tremor can have central components. The same centrally acting provoking factors can enhance pathological central tremor such as ET.

Neurophysiological characteristics

Clinical electrophysiology is useful in detecting physiological and enhanced physiological tremor.[120,121] Tremor frequency, amplitude, and neuromuscular recruitment can be studied by simultaneous recording of tremor acceleration (accelerometer) and EMG activities (surface EMG). The mechanical oscillations of the peripheral system are the universal components in human body parts. Therefore, all people will have subtle tremor during posturing, detectable by sensitive accelerometer. In *physiological tremor*, subtle posture tremor can be detected by accelerometer without consistent EMG activities at the tremor frequency. In *enhanced physiological tremor*, rhythmic EMG activities are detected at the tremor frequency, suggesting additional

recruitment of the neuromuscular system on top of the mechanical components. In order to distinguish the peripheral and central components of tremor, *weight loading* is applied during posturing of body parts. As mentioned above, the mechanical oscillatory properties of the peripheral system are sensitive to mass (inertia) changes. Therefore, frequency of peripheral tremor decreases with increased weight loading.[111,122,123] The frequency-drift phenomenon can be applied to both physiological and enhanced physiological tremor. In enhanced physiological tremor, the frequency of EMG activities is also shifted with tremor frequency, indicating the contribution of peripheral spinal reflex components.[120,121] In contrast, central tremors, whose tremor frequency is determined by the abnormal oscillations in the cerebro-ponto-cerebello-thalamo-cortical circuit, do not react to the weight-loading changes in the peripheral system.[122,123] Notably, people with enhanced physiological tremor could have additional central components. With central components, some of the tremor and EMG signal remains in the original tremor frequency during the weight-loading test. In this context, there can be two tremor frequencies occurring simultaneously during the weight-loading test.

Mechanism of provoking peripheral tremor

While there are many provoking factors that cause enhanced physiological tremor, only a few of them have been studied. Stress, sympathomimetics, and acute fatigue are those with the clearest peripheral mechanisms; they are described below. Notably, these three provoking factors also have additional central mechanisms, described either previously or in the later section titled "Interaction between central and peripheral networks."

It is a common experience that *anxiety and stress* may lead to enhanced physiological tremor, presenting as increased tremor amplitudes but with no change in the tremor frequency. This is caused, at least partially, by stimulating the beta-adrenergic receptors in the peripheral nervous system. Activation of beta-adrenergic receptors on skeletal muscle leads to stronger contraction.[124] *Sympathomimetics* also act on muscle spindles and synchronize motor outflows via the modulation of spinal reflex.[125] In alcohol withdrawal and hypoglycemia, sympathetic tone is increased, which may partially explain the tremor enhancement.

Acute fatigue is related to intensive use of certain muscle groups and is usually accompanied by increased beta-adrenergic tone. There are additional factors for fatigue to enhance tremor. During prolonged muscle usage, needle EMG data shows recruitment of additional motor units and increased synchrony among motor units.[126] Both factors enhance the intrinsic motor unit ~10 Hz oscillations.

Sensory feedback impacting physiological tremor

Subtle, physiological oscillations of limbs during movements may be required to enrich the proprioceptive sensory feedback, yet these occur in a predictive pattern (frequency-specific oscillations) that facilitates the cerebellar calculation for motor coordination[127]. In mice, disturbing proprioceptive sensory information to the cerebellum causes impaired skilled movements and tremor-like phenomena.[118,128] Clinically, diminished sensory feedback in neuropathic patients leads to neuropathic tremor, which can be considered a compensatory rhythmic movement for the attenuated sensory inputs.[129,130] These observations highlight an area of rhythm control in the sensorimotor system that requires further investigation.

Summary

Physiological and enhanced physiological tremor reflect the physiological characteristics of the motor system, expressing its intrinsic oscillatory components. Frequency shift during weight loading is the key feature to identify physiological tremor and distinguish it from centrally driven, pathological tremor. More work is required on the importance of physiological tremor in fine-tuning the motor control system.

INTERACTION BETWEEN CENTRAL AND PERIPHERAL TREMOR NETWORKS

As laid out in this chapter, the mechanical properties of the musculoskeletal system and spinal reflex loops contribute to the generation of physiological tremor at its own oscillatory frequency. The tremor can be tamed or modified by cortical or cerebellar inputs to the spinal cord. In parkinsonian rest tremor, two tremor frequencies can be recorded in the limbs, reflecting the 4–5 Hz rest tremor and the 8–12 Hz physiological tremor, respectively[63]. In ET, physiological tremor is usually embedded in the pathological central tremor. Weigh-loading technique, which shifts physiological tremor to a lower frequency, can separate the peripheral and central tremor in enhanced physiological tremor[120,121] and sometimes in ET.[122]

Many provoking factors of physiological tremor have mixed central and peripheral mechanisms. Increased sympathetic tone, alcohol withdrawal, or sympathomimetic drugs not only increase conductance of HCN channels via the cGMP pathway in the central pacemaking neurons, but also increase motor unit synchrony via the stretch reflex in the peripheral system.

Another mechanism worth noting is the potential role of the cerebellum in communicating to both the central and peripheral pathways. The cerebellum is involved in inertia (mass) calculation[131,132], emphasizing that motor coordination does require adequate estimation of the limb momentum. With weight-loading postures, the cerebellum adequately adapts the motor system to a shifted physiological tremor frequency. In pathological centrally generated tremors, this mechanism no longer works well due to the frequency entrapment in the cerebro-ponto-cerebello-thalamo-cortical circuit. In some patients, weight-loading leads to tremor with two frequencies, including the unchanged central mechanism tremor frequency and the reduced peripheral mechanism frequency[122]. With diminished sensory feedback to the cerebellum, mouse models can show tremor-like abnormal behaviors[118,128] that may explain the pathophysiology of neuropathic tremor.

FUTURE DIRECTIONS

Despite the depth of information around tremor mechanisms, many important areas remain to be explored. For example, why does action tremor diminish in rest and vice versa? What is the role of the primary motor cortex in tremor regulation? How does the basal ganglia regulate or gate tremor? What is the core loop for tremor generation: the smaller olivocerebellar circuit/Guillain-Mollaret triangle, or the large cerebro-ponto-cerebello-thalamo-cortical circuit? What are the factors that determine the final frequency of tremor? These are only a fraction of the open questions concerning tremor. Animal models have been critical to advance understanding of central and peripheral tremor networks. Optogenetic technologies provide precise modulation of neuronal activities in millisecond precision, allowing iatrogenic generation of oscillations in specific neurons. In-vivo calcium or voltage imaging facilitates the observation of neuronal activities with detailed spatial information, therefore allowing the investigation of spatial synchrony between nearby neurons. At the same time, animal work opens up many questions, such as how these models connect to pathological tremors in humans, and why some phenomena such as rest tremors are difficult to reproduce in model systems. In this context, computational modeling can potentially bridge animal-derived findings to human pathophysiology. Of note, studying rhythmic movement and tremor, a relatively stable-in-time, stereotypic, and predictable version of movement, provides a more reliable readout compared to other brisk movements, and could be a window to investigate highly complicated normal motor coordination.

REFERENCES

1. Bhatia KP et al. Consensus Statement on the classification of tremors. From the task force on tremor of the International Parkinson and Movement Disorder Society. *Mov Disord.* 2018;33:75–87. doi: 10.1002/mds.27121
2. Dupuis MJ, Delwaide PJ, Boucquey D, Gonsette RE. Homolateral disappearance of essential tremor after cerebellar stroke. *Mov Disord.* 1989;4:183–187. doi: 10.1002/mds.870040210
3. Urushitani M et al. Disappearance of essential neck tremor after pontine base infarction. *No To Shinkei Brain Nerve.* 1996;48:753–756.
4. Dupuis MJ, Evrard FL, Jacquerye PG, Picard GR, Lermen OG. Disappearance of essential tremor after stroke. *Mov Disord.* 2010;25:2884–2887. doi: 10.1002/mds.23328.
5. Brown AM et al. Purkinje cell misfiring generates high-amplitude action tremors that are corrected by cerebellar deep brain stimulation. *Elife.* 2020;9:e51928. doi: 10.7554/eLife.51928.
6. Long MA, Deans MR, Paul DL, Connors BW. Rhythmicity without synchrony in the electrically uncoupled inferior olive. *J Neurosci.* 2002;22:10898–10905. doi: 22/24/10898 [pii].
7. Llinas R, Yarom Y. Properties and distribution of ionic conductances generating electroresponsiveness of mammalian inferior olivary neurones in vitro. *J Physiol.* 1981;315:569–584. doi: 10.1113/jphysiol.1981.sp013764.
8. Llinas R, Yarom Y. Oscillatory properties of guinea-pig inferior olivary neurones and their pharmacological modulation: an in vitro study. *J Physiol.* 1986;376:163–182. doi: 10.1113/jphysiol.1986.sp016147
9. Park YG et al. Ca(V)3.1 is a tremor rhythm pacemaker in the inferior olive. *Proc Natl Acad Sci U S A.* 2010;107:10731–10736. doi: 10.1073/pnas.1002995107
10. Zolles G et al. Association with the auxiliary subunit PEX5R/Trip8b controls responsiveness of HCN channels to cAMP and adrenergic stimulation. *Neuron.* 2009;62:814–825. doi: 10.1016/j.neuron.2009.05.008
11. Matsumoto-Makidono Y et al. Ionic basis for membrane potential resonance in neurons of the inferior olive. *Cell Rep.* 2016;16:994–1004. doi: 10.1016/j.celrep.2016.06.053
12. Garden DLF et al. Inferior olive HCN1 channels coordinate synaptic integration and complex spike timing. *Cell Rep.* 2018;22:1722–1733. doi: 10.1016/j.celrep.2018.01.069
13. McKay BE et al. Ca(V)3 T-type calcium channel isoforms differentially distribute to somatic and dendritic compartments in rat central neurons. *Eur J Neurosci.* 2006;24:2581–2594. doi: 10.1111/j.1460-9568.2006.05136.x
14. Chemin J et al. Specific contribution of human T-type calcium channel isotypes (alpha(1G), alpha(1H) and alpha(1I)) to neuronal excitability. *J Physiol.* 2002;540:3–14. doi: 10.1113/jphysiol.2001.013269
15. Beurrier C, Congar P, Bioulac B, Hammond C. Subthalamic nucleus neurons switch from single-spike activity to burst-firing mode. *J Neurosci.* 1999;19:599–609.
16. Mathy A et al. Encoding of oscillations by axonal bursts in inferior olive neurons. *Neuron.* 2009;62:388–399. doi: 10.1016/j.neuron.2009.03.023
17. Shaikh AG et al. Oculopalatal tremor explained by a model of inferior olivary hypertrophy and cerebellar plasticity. *Brain.* 2010;133:923–940. doi: 10.1093/brain/awp323
18. Borruat FX. Oculopalatal tremor: current concepts and new observations. *Curr Opin Neurol.* 2013;26:67–73. doi: 10.1097/WCO.0b013e32835c60e6
19. Jun B. The development of hypertrophic inferior olivary nucleus in oculopalatal tremor. *Neuro-Ophthalmology (Aeolus Press).* 2016;40:297–299. doi: 10.1080/01658107.2016.1226903
20. Tilikete C, Desestret V. Hypertrophic olivary degeneration and palatal or oculopalatal tremor. *Front Neurol.* 2017;8:302. doi: 10.3389/fneur.2017.00302
21. Kuo SH et al. Climbing fiber-Purkinje cell synaptic pathology in tremor and cerebellar degenerative diseases. *Acta Neuropathol.* 2017;133:121–138. doi: 10.1007/s00401-016-1626-1
22. Lin CY et al. Abnormal climbing fibre-Purkinje cell synaptic connections in the essential tremor cerebellum. *Brain.* 2014;137:3149–3159. doi: 10.1093/brain/awu281
23. Kattah JC, Elble RJ, De Santo J, Shaikh AG. Oculopalatal tremor following sequential medullary infarcts that did not cause hypertrophic olivary degeneration. *Cerebellum Ataxias.* 2020;7:3. doi: 10.1186/s40673-020-00112-2
24. Louis ED, Lenka A. The olivary hypothesis of essential tremor: time to lay this model to rest? *Tremor Other Hyperkinet Mov.* 2017;7:473. doi: 10.7916/d8ff40rx
25. Saranza G, Fasano A. Excessive cerebellar oscillations in essential tremor: insights into disease mechanism and treatment. *Mov Disord.* 2020;35:758. doi: 10.1002/mds.28040
26. Pan MK et al. Cerebellar oscillations driven by synaptic pruning deficits of cerebellar climbing fibers contribute to tremor pathophysiology. *Sci*

Transl Med. 2020;12. doi: 10.1126/scitranslmed.aay1769

27. Yan H, Pablo JL, Wang C, Pitt GS. FGF14 modulates resurgent sodium current in mouse cerebellar Purkinje neurons. *Elife.* 2014;3:e04193. doi: 10.7554/eLife.04193

28. Raman IM, Sprunger LK, Meisler MH, Bean BP. Altered subthreshold sodium currents and disrupted firing patterns in Purkinje neurons of Scn8a mutant mice. *Neuron.* 1997;19:881–891. doi: 10.1016/S0896-6273(00)80969-1

29. Grieco TM, Malhotra JD, Chen C, Isom LL, Raman IM. Open-channel block by the cytoplasmic tail of sodium channel beta4 as a mechanism for resurgent sodium current. *Neuron.* 2005;45:233–244. doi: 10.1016/j.neuron.2004.12.035

30. Best AR, Regehr WG. Inhibitory regulation of electrically coupled neurons in the inferior olive is mediated by asynchronous release of GABA. *Neuron.* 2009;62:555–565. doi: 10.1016/j.neuron.2009.04.018

31. Canto CB, Witter L, De Zeeuw CI. Whole-cell properties of cerebellar nuclei neurons in vivo. *PLoS One.* 2016;11:e0165887. doi: 10.1371/journal.pone.0165887

32. Molineux ML et al. Specific T-type calcium channel isoforms are associated with distinct burst phenotypes in deep cerebellar nuclear neurons. *Proc Natl Acad Sci U S A.* 2006;103:5555–5560. doi: 10.1073/pnas.0601261103

33. Zhang X, Santaniello S. Role of cerebellar GABAergic dysfunctions in the origins of essential tremor. *Proc Natl Acad Sci U S A.* 2019;116:13592–13601. doi: 10.1073/pnas.1817689116

34. Sugihara I, Shinoda Y. Molecular, topographic, and functional organization of the cerebellar nuclei: analysis by three-dimensional mapping of the olivonuclear projection and aldolase C labeling. *J Neurosci.* 2007;27:9696–9710. doi: 10.1523/jneurosci.1579-07.2007

35. Lin F et al. Comparison of efficacy of deep brain stimulation and focused ultrasound in parkinsonian tremor: a systematic review and network meta-analysis. *J Neurol Neurosurg Psychiatry.* 2021. doi: 10.1136/jnnp-2020-323656

36. Do MT, Bean BP. Sodium currents in subthalamic nucleus neurons from Nav1.6-null mice. *J Neurophysiol.* 2004;92:726–733. doi: 10.1152/jn.00186.2004

37. Sharott A et al. Dopamine depletion increases the power and coherence of beta-oscillations in the cerebral cortex and subthalamic nucleus of the awake rat. *Eur J Neurosci.* 2005;21:1413–1422. doi: 10.1111/j.1460-9568.2005.03973.x

38. Moran RJ et al. Alterations in brain connectivity underlying beta oscillations in parkinsonism. *PLoS Comput Biol.* 2011;7:e1002124. doi: 10.1371/journal.pcbi.1002124

39. Cassidy M et al. Movement-related changes in synchronization in the human basal ganglia. *Brain.* 2002;125:1235–1246. doi: 10.1093/brain/awf135

40. Kühn AA et al. Event-related beta desynchronization in human subthalamic nucleus correlates with motor performance. *Brain.* 2004;127:735–746. doi: 10.1093/brain/awh106

41. de Hemptinne C et al. Therapeutic deep brain stimulation reduces cortical phase-amplitude coupling in Parkinson's disease. *Nat Neurosci.* 2015;18:779–786. doi: 10.1038/nn.3997

42. Pogosyan A et al. Parkinsonian impairment correlates with spatially extensive subthalamic oscillatory synchronization. *Neuroscience.* 2010;171:245–257. doi: 10.1016/j.neuroscience.2010.08.068

43. Williams D et al. The relationship between oscillatory activity and motor reaction time in the parkinsonian subthalamic nucleus. *Eur J Neurosci.* 2005;21:249–258. doi: 10.1111/j.1460-9568.2004.03817.x

44. Chen CC et al. Complexity of subthalamic 13–35 Hz oscillatory activity directly correlates with clinical impairment in patients with Parkinson's disease. *Exp Neurol.* 2010;224:234–240. doi: 10.1016/j.expneurol.2010.03.015

45. Loukas C, Brown P. Online prediction of self-paced hand-movements from subthalamic activity using neural networks in Parkinson's disease. *J Neurosci Methods.* 2004;137:193–205. doi: 10.1016/j.jneumeth.2004.02.017

46. Pan MK et al. Neuronal firing patterns outweigh circuitry oscillations in parkinsonian motor control. *J Clin Investig.* 2016;126:4516–4526. doi: 10.1172/jci88170

47. Pan MK et al. Deranged NMDAergic cortico-subthalamic transmission underlies parkinsonian motor deficits. *J Clin Investig.* 2014;124:4629–4641. doi: 10.1172/JCI75587

48. Elias S, Ritov Y, Bergman H. Balance of increases and decreases in firing rate of the spontaneous activity of basal ganglia high-frequency discharge neurons. *J Neurophysiol.* 2008;100:3086–3104. doi: 10.1152/jn.90714.2008

49. Raz A, Vaadia E, Bergman H. Firing patterns and correlations of spontaneous discharge of pallidal neurons in the normal and the tremulous 1-methyl-4-phenyl-1,2,3,6-tetrahydropyridine vervet model of parkinsonism. *J Neurosci.* 2000;20:8559–8571. doi: 10.1523/jneurosci.20-22-08559.2000

50. Chen L et al. Hyperpolarization-activated cyclic nucleotide-gated (HCN) channels regulate firing of globus pallidus neurons in vivo. *Mol Cell Neurosci.* 2015;68:46–55. doi: 10.1016/j.mcn.2015.04.001

51. Asch N et al. Independently together: subthalamic theta and beta opposite roles in predicting Parkinson's tremor. *Brain Commun.*

2020;2:fcaa074. doi: 10.1093/braincomms/fcaa074

52. Godinho F et al. Spectral characteristics of subthalamic nucleus local field potentials in Parkinson's disease: Phenotype and movement matter. *Eur J Neurosci.* 2021;53:2804–2818. doi: 10.1111/ejn.15103

53. Hirschmann J, Schoffelen JM, Schnitzler A, van Gerven MAJ. Parkinsonian rest tremor can be detected accurately based on neuronal oscillations recorded from the subthalamic nucleus. *Clin Neurophysiol.* 2017;128:2029–2036. doi: 10.1016/j.clinph.2017.07.419

54. Shi X, Du D, Wang Y. Interaction of indirect and hyperdirect pathways on synchrony and tremor-related oscillation in the basal ganglia. *Neural Plast.* 2021;2021:6640105. doi: 10.1155/2021/6640105

55. Hirschmann J et al. Parkinsonian rest tremor is associated with modulations of subthalamic high-frequency oscillations. *Mov Disord.* 2016;31:1551–1559. doi: 10.1002/mds.26663

56. Hirschmann J et al. A direct relationship between oscillatory subthalamic nucleus-cortex coupling and rest tremor in Parkinson's disease. *Brain.* 2013;136:3659–3670. doi: 10.1093/brain/awt271

57. Meng D et al. Characteristics of oscillatory pallidal neurons in patients with Parkinson's disease. *J Neurol Sci.* 2020;410:116661. doi: 10.1016/j.jns.2019.116661

58. Hurtado JM, Rubchinsky LL, Sigvardt KA, Wheelock VL, Pappas CT. Temporal evolution of oscillations and synchrony in Gpi/muscle pairs in Parkinson's disease. *J Neurophysiol.* 2005;93:1569–1584. doi: 10.1152/jn.00829.2004

59. Hutchison WD, Lozano AM, Tasker RR, Lang AE, Dostrovsky JO. Identification and characterization of neurons with tremor-frequency activity in human globus pallidus. *Exp Brain Res.* 1997;113:557–563. doi: 10.1007/pl00005606

60. Hurtado JM, Gray CM, Tamas LB, Sigvardt KA. Dynamics of tremor-related oscillations in the human globus pallidus: a single case study. *Proc Natl Acad Sci U S A.* 1999;96:1674–1679. doi: 10.1073/pnas.96.4.1674

61. Bergman H et al. Physiology of MPTP tremor. *Mov Disord.* 1998;13(Suppl 3):29–34. doi: 10.1002/mds.870131305

62. Bekar L et al. Adenosine is crucial for deep brain stimulation-mediated attenuation of tremor. *Nat Med.* 2008;14:75–80. doi: 10.1038/nm1693

63. Timmermann L et al. The cerebral oscillatory network of parkinsonian resting tremor. *Brain.* 2003;126:199–212.

64. Hallett M. Parkinson's disease tremor: pathophysiology. *Parkinsonism Relat Disord.* 2012;18(Suppl 1):S85–S86. doi: 10.1016/s1353-8020(11)70027-x

65. Milosevic L et al. Physiological mechanisms of thalamic ventral intermediate nucleus stimulation for tremor suppression. *Brain.* 2018;141:2142–2155. doi: 10.1093/brain/awy139

66. Helmich RC, Hallett M, Deuschl G, Toni I, Bloem BR. Cerebral causes and consequences of parkinsonian resting tremor: a tale of two circuits? *Brain.* 2012;135:3206–3226. doi: 10.1093/brain/aws023

67. Helmich RC. The cerebral basis of Parkinsonian tremor: a network perspective. *Mov Disord.* 2018;33:219–231. doi: 10.1002/mds.27224

68. Kuo SH et al. Current opinions and consensus for studying tremor in animal models. *Cerebellum.* 2019. doi: 10.1007/s12311-019-01037-1

69. Louis ED, Zheng W, Mao X, Shungu DC. Blood harmane is correlated with cerebellar metabolism in essential tremor: a pilot study. *Neurology.* 2007;69:515–520.

70. Louis ED et al. Blood harmane (1-methyl-9H-pyrido[3,4-b]indole) concentration in essential tremor cases in Spain. *Neurotoxicology.* 2013;34:264–268. doi: 10.1016/j.neuro.2012.09.004

71. Kunisawa N et al. Pharmacological characterization of nicotine-induced tremor: responses to anti-tremor and anti-epileptic agents. *J Pharmacol Sci.* 2018;137:162–169. doi: 10.1016/j.jphs.2018.05.007

72. Kralic JE et al. Genetic essential tremor in gamma-aminobutyric acid A receptor alpha1 subunit knockout mice. *J Clin Investig.* 2005;115:774–779.

73. Nietz A et al. Selective loss of the GABA(Aα1) subunit from Purkinje cells is sufficient to induce a tremor phenotype. *J Neurophysiol.* 2020;124:1183–1197. doi: 10.1152/jn.00100.2020

74. Luo J. Effects of ethanol on the cerebellum: advances and prospects. *Cerebellum.* 2015;14:383–385. doi: 10.1007/s12311-015-0674-8

75. Paris-Robidas S et al. Defective dentate nucleus GABA receptors in essential tremor. *Brain.* 2012;135:105–116. doi: 10.1093/brain/awr301

76. Boecker H et al. GABAergic dysfunction in essential tremor: an 11C-flumazenil PET study. *J Nucl Med.* 2010;51:1030–1035. doi: 10.2967/jnumed.109.074120

77. Morgan JC, Sethi KD. Drug-induced tremors. *Lancet Neurol.* 2005;4:866–876.

78. Young RR, Growdon JH, Shahani BT. Beta-adrenergic mechanisms in action tremor. *N Engl J Med.* 1975;293:950–953. doi: 10.1056/nejm197511062931902

79. Ohno Y et al. Hcn1 is a tremorgenic genetic component in a rat model of essential tremor. *PLoS One.* 2015;10:e0123529. doi: 10.1371/journal.pone.0123529

80. Odgerel Z et al. Whole genome sequencing and rare variant analysis in essential tremor families.

PLoS One. 2019;14:e0220512. doi: 10.1371/journal.pone.0220512

81. Bergareche A et al. SCN4A pore mutation pathogenetically contributes to autosomal dominant essential tremor and may increase susceptibility to epilepsy. *Hum Mol Genet.* 2015;24:7111–7120. doi: 10.1093/hmg/ddv410

82. Leng XR, Qi XH, Zhou YT, Wang YP. Gain-of-function mutation p.Arg225Cys in SCN11A causes familial episodic pain and contributes to essential tremor. *J Hum Genet.* 2017;62:641–646. doi: 10.1038/jhg.2017.21

83. Dirkx MF et al. Cerebral differences between dopamine-resistant and dopamine-responsive Parkinson's tremor. *Brain.* 2019;142:3144–3157. doi: 10.1093/brain/awz261

84. Muthuraman M et al. Cerebello-cortical network fingerprints differ between essential, Parkinson's and mimicked tremors. *Brain.* 2018;141:1770–1781. doi: 10.1093/brain/awy098

85. Akkal D, Dum RP, Strick PL. Supplementary motor area and presupplementary motor area: targets of basal ganglia and cerebellar output. *J Neurosci.* 2007;27:10659–10673. doi: 10.1523/jneurosci.3134-07.2007

86. Bostan AC, Dum RP, Strick PL. Cerebellar networks with the cerebral cortex and basal ganglia. *Trends Cogn Sci.* 2013;17:241–254. doi: 10.1016/j.tics.2013.03.003

87. Maier MA et al. Differences in the corticospinal projection from primary motor cortex and supplementary motor area to macaque upper limb motoneurons: an anatomical and electrophysiological study. *Cereb Cortex.* 2002;12:281–296. doi: 10.1093/cercor/12.3.281

88. Gallea C et al. Intrinsic signature of essential tremor in the cerebello-frontal network. *Brain.* 2015;138:2920–2933. doi: 10.1093/brain/awv171

89. Williams D et al. Dopamine-dependent changes in the functional connectivity between basal ganglia and cerebral cortex in humans. *Brain.* 2002;125:1558–1569.

90. Muthuraman M et al. Oscillating central motor networks in pathological tremors and voluntary movements. What makes the difference? *Neuroimage.* 2012;60:1331–1339. doi: 10.1016/j.neuroimage.2012.01.088

91. Çakar NE, Aksu Uzunhan T. A case of juvenile Canavan disease with distinct pons involvement. *Brain Dev.* 2020;42:222–225. doi: 10.1016/j.braindev.2019.11.009

92. Sharma P et al. Central pontine myelinolysis presenting with tremor in a child with celiac disease. *J Child Neurol.* 2014;29:381–384. doi: 10.1177/0883073812475086

93. Shakkottai VG et al. Current opinions and areas of consensus on the role of the cerebellum in dystonia. *Cerebellum.* 2017;16:577–594. doi: 10.1007/s12311-016-0825-6

94. Bologna M, Berardelli A. The cerebellum and dystonia. *Handb Clin Neurol.* 2018;155:259–272. doi: 10.1016/b978-0-444-64189-2.00017-2

95. Hoogland TM, De Gruijl JR, Witter L, Canto CB, De Zeeuw CI. Role of synchronous activation of cerebellar Purkinje cell ensembles in multi-joint movement control. *Curr Biol.* 2015;25:1157–1165. doi: 10.1016/j.cub.2015.03.009

96. McAuley JH, Marsden CD. Physiological and pathological tremors and rhythmic central motor control. *Brain.* 2015;123(Pt 8):1545–1567. doi: 10.1093/brain/123.8.1545 x

97. Deuschl G, Wilms H, Krack P, Würker M, Heiss WD. Function of the cerebellum in parkinsonian rest tremor and Holmes' tremor. *Ann Neurol.* 1999;46:126–128. doi: 10.1002/1531-8249(199907)46:1<126::aid-ana20>3.0.co;2-3

98. Bucher SF, Seelos KC, Dodel RC, Reiser M, Oertel WH. Activation mapping in essential tremor with functional magnetic resonance imaging. *Ann Neurol.* 1997;41:32–40.

99. Marsden JF, Ashby P, Limousin-Dowsey P, Rothwell JC, Brown P. Coherence between cerebellar thalamus, cortex and muscle in man: cerebellar thalamus interactions. *Brain.* 2000;123(Pt 7):1459–1470.

100. Joutsa J, Shih LC, Fox MD. Mapping Holmes tremor circuit using the human brain connectome. *Ann Neurol.* 2019;86:812–820. doi: 10.1002/ana.25618

101. Erickson-DiRenzo E, Sung CK, Ho AL, Halpern CH. Intraoperative evaluation of essential vocal tremor in deep brain stimulation surgery. *Am J Speech-Lang Path.* 2020;29:851–863. doi: 10.1044/2019_ajslp-19-00079

102. Pedrosa DJ et al. Essential tremor and tremor in Parkinson's disease are associated with distinct "tremor clusters" in the ventral thalamus. *Exp Neurol.* 2012;237:435–443. doi: 10.1016/j.expneurol.2012.07.002

103. Cagnan H et al. Phase dependent modulation of tremor amplitude in essential tremor through thalamic stimulation. *Brain.* 2013;136:3062–3075. doi: 10.1093/brain/awt239

104. Pedrosa DJ et al. Thalamomuscular coherence in essential tremor: hen or egg in the emergence of tremor? *J Neurosci.* 2014;34:14475–14483. doi: 10.1523/jneurosci.0087-14.2014

105. Kim JS et al. Disappearance of essential tremor after frontal cortical infarct. *Mov Disord.* 2006;21:1284–1285. doi: 10.1002/mds.20894

106. Lu MK et al. Resetting tremor by single and paired transcranial magnetic stimulation in Parkinson's disease and essential tremor. *Clin Neurophysiol.* 2015;126:2330–2336. doi: 10.1016/j.clinph.2015.02.010

107. Hellwig B et al. Tremor-correlated cortical activity in essential tremor. *Lancet.* 2001;357:519–523.

108. Govindan RB, Raethjen J, Arning K, Kopper F, Deuschl G. Time delay and partial coherence analyses to identify cortical connectivities. *Biol Cybern.* 2006;94:262–275. doi: 10.1007/s00422-005-0045-5

109. Raethjen J, Govindan RB, Kopper F, Muthuraman M, Deuschl G. Cortical involvement in the generation of essential tremor. *J Neurophysiol.* 2007;97:3219–3228.

110. Sharifi S et al. Intermittent cortical involvement in the preservation of tremor in essential tremor. *J Neurophysiol.* 2017;118:2628–2635. doi: 10.1152/jn.00848.2016

111. Raethjen J, Pawlas F, Lindemann M, Wenzelburger R, Deuschl G. Determinants of physiologic tremor in a large normal population. *Clin Neurophysiol.* 2000;111:1825–1837. doi: 10.1016/s1388-2457(00)00384-9

112. Elble RJ, Randall JE. Motor-unit activity responsible for 8- to 12-Hz component of human physiological finger tremor. *J Neurophysiol.* 1976;39:370–383. doi: 10.1152/jn.1976.39.2.370

113. Williams ER, Baker SN. Renshaw cell recurrent inhibition improves physiological tremor by reducing corticomuscular coupling at 10 Hz. *J Neurosci.* 2009;29:6616–6624. doi: 10.1523/jneurosci.0272-09.2009

114. Jalaleddini K et al. Physiological tremor increases when skeletal muscle is shortened: implications for fusimotor control. *J Physiol.* 2017;595:7331–7346. doi: 10.1113/jp274899

115. Conway BA et al. Synchronization between motor cortex and spinal motoneuronal pool during the performance of a maintained motor task in man. *J Physiol.* 1995;489(Pt 3):917–924. doi: 10.1113/jphysiol.1995.sp021104

116. Halliday DM, Conway BA, Farmer SF, Rosenberg JR. Using electroencephalography to study functional coupling between cortical activity and electromyograms during voluntary contractions in humans. *Neurosci Lett.* 1998;241:5–8. doi: 10.1016/s0304-3940(97)00964-6

117. Murthy VN, Fetz EE. Coherent 25- to 35-Hz oscillations in the sensorimotor cortex of awake behaving monkeys. *Proc Natl Acad Sci U S A.* 1992;89:5670–5674. doi: 10.1073/pnas.89.12.5670

118. Azim E, Jiang J, Alstermark B, Jessell TM. Skilled reaching relies on a V2a propriospinal internal copy circuit. *Nature.* 2014;508:357–363. doi: 10.1038/nature13021

119. Bernard JF, Horcholle-Bossavit G. Harmaline-induced rhythm in the lateral reticular nucleus. *Arch Ital Biol.*1983;121:139–150.

120. Haubenberger D, Hallett M. Essential tremor. *N Engl J Med.* 2018;378:1802–1810. doi: 10.1056/NEJMcp1707928

121. Vial F, Kassavetis P, Merchant S, Haubenberger D, Hallett M. How to do an electrophysiological study of tremor. *Clin Neurophysiol Pract* 2019;4:134–142. doi: 10.1016/j.cnp.2019.06.002

122. Cao H, Thompson-Westra J, Hallett M, Haubenberger D. The response of the central and peripheral tremor component to octanoic acid in patients with essential tremor. *Clin Neurophysiol.* 2018;129:1467–1471. doi: 10.1016/j.clinph.2018.03.016

123. Pan MK, Kuo SH. Tracking the central and peripheral origin of tremor. *Clin Neurophysiol.* 2018;129:1451–1452. doi: 10.1016/j.clinph.2018.04.607

124. Marsden CD, Foley TH, Owen DA, McAllister RG. Peripheral beta-adrenergic receptors concerned with tremor. *Clin Sci.* 1967;33:53–65.

125. Hagbarth KE, Young RR. Participation of the stretch reflex in human physiological tremor. *Brain.* 1979;102:509–526. doi: 10.1093/brain/102.3.509

126. Arihara M, Sakamoto K. Contribution of motor unit activity enhanced by acute fatigue to physiological tremor of finger. *Electromyogr Clin Neurophysiol.* 1999;39:235–247.

127. Hoellinger T et al. Biological oscillations for learning walking coordination: dynamic recurrent neural network functionally models physiological central pattern generator. *Front Comput Neurosci.* 2013;7:70. doi: 10.3389/fncom.2013.00070

128. Fink AJ et al. Presynaptic inhibition of spinal sensory feedback ensures smooth movement. *Nature.* 2014;509:43–48. doi: 10.1038/nature13276

129. Hallett M. Overview of human tremor physiology. *Mov Disord.* 1998;13(Suppl 3):43–48.

130. Saifee TA et al. Tremor in Charcot-Marie-Tooth disease: no evidence of cerebellar dysfunction. *Clin Neurophysiol.* 2015;126:1817–1824. doi: 10.1016/j.clinph.2014.12.023

131. Bhanpuri NH, Okamura AM, Bastian AJ. Predicting and correcting ataxia using a model of cerebellar function. *Brain.* 2014;137:1931–1944. doi: 10.1093/brain/awu115

132. Zimmet AM, Cowan NJ, Bastian AJ. Patients with cerebellar ataxia do not benefit from limb weights. *Cerebellum.* 2019;18:128–136. doi: 10.1007/s12311-018-0962-1

4

Neuropathology of Tremors

HOLLY SHILL

PATHOLOGY IN ESSENTIAL TREMOR

Postmortem studies in essential tremor (ET) were very sparse with only a handful of studies prior to 2004. No consistent pathology had been described. In 2004, a large series of 20 ET patients was published, again with no consistent pathology found. However, following that, there has been a relative explosion of papers examining the pathology of ET with a variety of findings. Despite the larger numbers of papers, most of the work has been done by only a small number of investigators. It is with this caveat that this literature is reviewed.

ET and Parkinson disease (PD) pathology

There are many clinical papers that support the idea that PD may arise in ET patients, reporting frequencies as high as 24% in specialized movement disorder clinics[18] and a four-fold incidence increase in a large Spanish epidemiological study.[1] The current Movement Disorders Society tremor classification system includes ET and ET-plus as ET with mild signs such as parkinsonism, dystonia, or gait ataxia but not enough for another syndromic diagnosis such as PD.[2] The extent to which ET and forms of ET-plus will share pathologies and etiologies is as yet unknown. Pathological studies can be critical in addressing these issues.

An early study published in 1991 reported a small series of ET patients studied pathologically, and included six subjects followed prospectively in a longitudinal brain donation program in Saskatchewan, Canada. Patients were followed in a movement disorder clinic prior to death, and none had clinical features of parkinsonism. None had PD findings pathologically, and the substantia nigra was examined specifically.[3] A follow-up pathological series of 20 ET cases in this same program confirms that there is no increase in Parkinson's pathology (e.g., Lewy bodies) in patients unless they had additional features of

parkinsonism sufficient for a PD diagnosis.[4] In this study, only one case had Lewy bodies (LBs), and this was an ET case who later developed PD. The other ET cases with clinical parkinsonism (N = 5), which may now have been classified as ET-plus, had alternate explanations for this parkinsonism, including cribiform changes of the basal ganglia and PSP pathology (N = 2). It is worth pointing out that these early studies did not use immunohistochemistry aging alpha-synuclein, which is a more sensitive way to ascertain LBs in the substantia nigra. In 2005, a case of a patient with severe, long-standing ET without clinical parkinsonism was reported, who had focal LBs in the locus coeruleus.[5] A year later, this same group published a pathological series of 10 subjects with ET.[6] Six had LBs, with four of the six having an atypical brainstem distribution with greater involvement of the locus coeruleus over the substantia nigra. One of these cases can likely be excluded from the series because of development of PD with dementia later in life. Only four of the ten of the cases were prospectively collected. These authors concluded from these studies that the ET might result from arrested development of LBs in the locus coeruleus. In subsequent larger series of 33 patients, only 8 of 33 cases (24%) had LBs.[3] One had a clinicopathological diagnosis of PD and another had a pathological diagnosis of PD (clinical parkinsonism is required for a pathological diagnosis of PD, although the authors state that the patients had no such features 2 years prior to death). Only 2 (9.5%) of the control brains had LBs. Controls meeting neuropathological criteria for AD or PD were excluded, as were those with clinical parkinsonism, making an argument that the controls were biased (more "clean"). In this larger series, 23 ET cases were prospectively collected and only two of these had LBs. Therefore, the percentage of LB cases in the ET (8.7%) and control groups (9.5%) was similar in the prospectively acquired sample of ET. The study's authors speculated that the pathological findings of PD might represent a LB variant of ET.

This finding of LBs in the LC, associated with ET, has not been replicated. In another pathological series[7] of ET subjects compared to controls, neither group having parkinsonism or dementia prior to death, 3 of 24 ET subjects (12.5%) had LBs, only one of these with the LC pattern reported previously. Two of 21 controls (9.5%) had LBs. This would argue that the control and ET cases with LBs should be considered incidental LBs (ILBD). ILBD is the pathological finding of LBs without clinical parkinsonism or dementia. There is some evidence to say that ILBD may be prodromal PD, with increased rate of hyposmia in this group, although there is lack of REM sleep behavioral disorder.[8,9] The frequency of LBs in both these series mimics the frequency of incidental Lewy body disease (ILBD) in large autopsy series (as high as 20–30% when looked for carefully).[10] Another way to look at this issue is to examine clinical findings in people who have come to autopsy and are found to have ILBD. In a series of control subjects who did not have parkinsonism or dementia during life, it has been demonstrated that ILBD does not have a higher frequency of action tremor disorder during life.[11] In this series, 277 autopsied subjects who had clinical evaluations within the previous 3 years, 76 did not have PD, a related disorder, or dementia of which 15 (20%) had ILBD. Minor extrapyramidal signs were common in subjects with and without ILBD. Action tremor of the hands was seen in 6/13 (46%) ILBD cases and 22/55 (40%) controls. Tyrosine hydroxylase is the rate limiting step for the conversion to dopamine and reduction of it in the striatum is known to be one of the earliest findings in PD pathology. Patients with ET do not have lower tyrosine hydroxylase levels compared with controls,[12] whereas those with ILBD have a 50% reduction, putting ILBD at an intermediate stage between control and PD.[13]

Most recently, the Saskatchewan group has published a series of ET cases in their brain bank who developed parkinsonism later in life and came to autopsy since the program started in 1968.[14] There were 21 subjects who were all followed at least annually by the same two movement disorder specialists. Median age of onset for ET was 51 years. Mean duration of ET prior to the diagnosis of parkinsonian syndrome was 30 years, and mean survival after ET diagnosis was 38 years. Pathologically, most cases met pathological criteria for PD (N = 13), although 3 of these cases had only rest tremor in addition to typical long-standing ET. These three would fit the ET-plus classification. PSP was seen in five cases

(missed clinically in all; diagnosed with idiopathic PD). One of each had PD plus cerebellar degeneration, MSA and Pick's disease. The MSA and Pick's disease were recognized clinically, as was the cerebellar ataxia. One case was felt to have PD clinically but had only ILBD pathologically (the LB pathology was not sufficient to warrant a diagnosis of PD). Some of the cases in this series would have had alpha-synuclein staining for LBs as it became available, but it is unclear how many.

Other clinical features, which, if seen in ET, might suggest the concurrent development of PD, have not been shown to be associated with PD pathologically. Up to 25–33% of ET patients will develop rest tremor.[4,15] This clinical finding is not associated with LB pathologically.[16] Likewise, jaw tremor in isolation or in the setting of ET does not predict LB pathology. Only jaw tremor with other typical clinical features of PD predicts PD pathologically.[17]

Taken together, this suggests that PD pathology is likely not responsible for a significant percentage of ET in the absence of overt, not subtle, features of parkinsonism. Nor does it appear that those who die with ET would have developed PD at a higher rate than control had they lived longer. Last, the parkinsonism, when seen, is not all idiopathic PD.

This discrepancy with the pathology literature remains challenging to resolve. It is possible that ET patients who are developing PD biologically are simply more likely to seek specialty care due to a change in their tremor symptoms after many years resulting in a biased impression in movement disorder clinics. Additionally, these clinical case series and epidemiological studies do not have pathological confirmation that PD is indeed present; Rajput et al. have demonstrated that even those ET patients who look like they may be developing PD clinically may have alternate explanations for the parkinsonism at autopsy (e.g., cribiform changes in the basal ganglia) or PSP.[4] There is a caveat with all of this. Pathology is typically done on relatively small groups of patients with advanced age, where there is often an accumulation of pathologies. Further, many of these types of small studies are biased toward the more interesting or confusing patients, which may lead to over-representing the overlap cases. Indeed, many of the early studies emphasized this.[4,7] Therefore, outside the setting of very large, prospective multi-institutional studies of ET with brain bank pathology done in a uniform manner, it is nearly impossible to exclude that there may be a small subset of ET patients who are at risk for both ET and PD and that they are indeed related. However, as has been shown above, there are those who look like they have PD clinically but do not pathologically, and vice versa. So, some caution should be used in interpreting the clinical literature supporting a link unless there has been pathological confirmation. At this point, it is difficult to know if having the ET-plus classification is useful in addressing this question. It will be important for the clinician to not just simply note whether it is ET or ET-plus, but also to carefully specify which clinical features are present or absent (e.g., rest tremor, reduced arm swing, slow gait). Over time, this should help us to better clarify the relationship between ET and PD.

ET and other degenerative disorders

Continuing with a theme of parkinsonism, it has been reported that 11 of 89 patients (12.4%) in a large ET brain bank repository had ET followed by the later clinical development of parkinsonism and/or dementia with pathological findings of progressive supranuclear palsy.[18] There was speculation that ET patients were at much greater risk for PSP, and that this might be responsible for the reported increased clinical findings of parkinsonism or dementia in ET patients. However, another group has examined this in an ET population without dementia or parkinsonism and found similar rates of PSP in their ET brains compared to controls. Two of 56 (3.4%) had PSP versus 4 of 62 (6.5%) controls. Overall rates of incidental PSP (without dementia or parkinsonism) in large brain banks may be close to 2%,[19] and there are much larger numbers in those with parkinsonism and/or dementia (often misdiagnosed as PD or AD during life or as having PSP as an additive pathology).[20] Therefore, this may be an incidental and not unexpected finding.

Alzheimer disease neuropathologic changes (ADNC) seems to be seen at the same rate and severity in ET and non-ET populations.[21] However, there is the confounding factor of the nearly universal appearance of at least low-grade ADNC seen at high frequency in the elderly. This makes it difficult to parse out where there might be more subtle changes in ET subjects compared with elderly controls.

ET and cerebellar pathology

The cerebellum has been implicated in ET for several decades. Early imaging studies support that the cerebellar hemispheres are overactive in ET,[22,23] and that this overactivity responds to treatment.[24] The underlying neuropathologic changes in the cerebellum began to be examined more systematically in the mid-2000s.

The first studies looked at standard assessments of brains of those with ET and compared them with controls. In a study published in 2006,[6] there were 10 ET cases compared with 12 controls. ET cases and controls were compiled from a variety of sources and included archived and prospectively acquired cases. In the 4 ET cases without pathological features of PD, there was evidence for gliosis in the cerebellum and torpedoes, both felt to be indicators of Purkinje cell loss. Bergmann cell gliosis occurs in the Purkinje cell layer and is thought to be an astrocytic reaction to damage to the cells there. It can be seen due to many types of insults to the cerebellum, including toxins and hypoxic/ischemic damage. Torpedoes are abnormal swellings seen on the proximal portion of the Purkinje cell axon that reflect neuronal dysfunction. They contain abnormally accumulated and disorganized phosphorylated neurofilaments and abundant organelles.[25]

In another early publication, another group studied 24 ET cases and compared them to 21 controls.[7] All subjects were prospectively followed in a longitudinal brain bank program and received identical, yearly in-person examinations, with the motor examination performed by a movement disorder specialist. ET was defined according to Consensus Criteria current at the time[26]; patients did not need to have functionally impairing tremor to be diagnosed. Cognitive impairment and parkinsonism were assessed prospectively, and all subjects were initially free of both. Control cases were defined based on clinical features alone. In this series, 7 of 21 ET cases had cerebellar findings; none of these had LBs. Three had Bergmann cell gliosis, and only one had identifiable cerebellar hemispheric atrophy. Torpedo formation was not notable in any case, although it was not specifically looked for in this sample. Notably, in this study, there were a variety of other pathologies seen in both ET and controls, underscoring the complexity of pathological assessment in the elderly even in the absence of overt clinical signs.

These preliminary studies, suggesting that a subset of ET patients may have cerebellar alterations, led to additional studies that were more hypothesis-driven in which both cerebellar Purkinje cells and torpedoes were quantified.

Thirty-three ET cases were compared with 21 controls by neuropathologic examination of the cerebellum.[27] Clinically, the ET patients were relatively severe: at least 5 years of tremor and disability related to tremor (defined as interference with two or more ADLs or requiring medication). Nearly 90% of this population required treatment, and one-third had rest tremor. Controls did not have a clinical diagnosis of ET or a degenerative disorder (e.g., AD or PD), nor did they have pathological findings of such. Nineteen of 21 controls were prospectively followed for aging-related research. Twenty of 33 of the ET patients were selectively recruited nationally for this pathological assessment, with clinical assessment done by a standardized videotaping protocol; the remainder came from previously banked specimens of patients who had been followed by a variety of mechanisms.

Purkinje cells were quantified in the cerebellar hemisphere by counting cells in five high power fields and averaging them. Torpedoes and Bergmann cells were similarly quantified. In the 25 patients without any evidence of abnormal alpha-synuclein accumulation to indicate PD, there was a decrease in Purkinje cells (6.6±2.4 vs. 9.2 + 2.1) and an increase in torpedoes (19.6± 14.5 vs. 5.5±4.8) and Bergmann cells (9.6±6.6 vs. 10.6 ± 5.9). While positive findings were statistically significant, there was substantial overlap between groups, particularly for Purkinje cells counts, where about 75% of patients and controls overlapped. Cases with LBs did not have these cerebellar findings, although one could argue that they should have been included as the LBs are almost certainly incidental and excluding them may bias the samples.

Given that the findings of axon torpedoes seem to be more discriminating between ET and controls, additional work was done on the subset of ET patients with cerebellar findings.[28] These ET subjects were compared to neurologic disease controls: established AD and PD/DLB cases. AD and PD/DLB cases came from a variety of sources. The mean numbers of torpedoes were 12 times higher in ET compared to controls and 2.5 times higher than either of the degenerative groups. ET patients were 5 years older than controls and PD/DLB, but were similar in age to the AD group. However, there is no correlation between age and torpedo counts. This finding of fairly high rates of cerebellar pathology in established PD and AD (albeit less than in ET) suggests that these pathologies should be accounted for in studies of the cerebellum and controlled for in any comparisons.

Additional studies were done to further quantify cerebellar Purkinje cells using a more accurate method. Because Purkinje cells form a layer in the cerebellum, they are amenable to quantification using linear cell density. Simply put, a line is drawn through the layer on the histological specimen, and then the number of cells intersecting the line divided by the line length is the linear density (see Figure 4.1). The first study using this method had 14 ET patients, and they were compared with 11 controls.[29] In the six without LBs, Purkinje cell linear density was 2.14±0.82 cells/mm versus 3.46±1.27 for controls (p = 0.04). The numbers of torpedoes were 10.8 ±6.3 versus 1.2±1.1 in cases versus controls. ET patient with LBs did not differ from controls in terms of Purkinje cell counts. Purkinje cell density correlated with age and number of torpedoes, but the differences between ET and controls remained significant (p = 0.03) after adjustment for age, gender, and postmortem interval. There was less overlap between groups using this method than was observed in the study described above. A larger study in this same brain bank confirmed the finding.[30] These same authors then looked at age and relationship to cerebellar degenerative pathology and found a correlation in the nine subjects with postmortem tissue.[31]

Other groups have not found cerebellar Purkinje cell loss. A study of 12 ET, 6 controls, and 41 PD controls showed no differences using the mean Purkinje cell (PC) count as measured by counting cells in five 100-power fields using three different counting methods (sectioned through the nucleus, nucleolus, or any part of the PC neuron).[32] ET subjects were followed annually in a movement disorder clinic and had a mean duration of tremor of 24 years. Another group studied

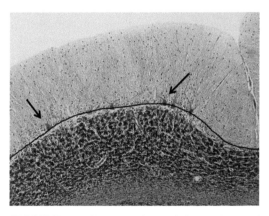

FIGURE 4.1: Hematoxylin and Eosin Stain of the Cerebellum with the Line Drawn through the Purkinje Cell Layer and the Arrows Indicating Individual Purkinje Cells.

56 ET cases and compared them to 62 controls using Purkinje linear cell density.[21] Mean duration of tremor at time of death in the ET group was 10.3 ± 12.6 years. All subjects were followed annually by movement disorder neurologists. PC linear density was 3.80 ± 0.81 cells per mm for the ET cases and 3.82 ± 0.91 cells per mm for controls. (Δ 0.02, 95% CI−0.30 to 0.34). A criticism of this paper was that ET subjects who did not have a clinical diagnosis of ET but only a research diagnosis were included. Therefore, those who had both clinical and research diagnoses of ET and a mean duration of tremor of 18.0 years were analyzed separately and found to have a slightly higher, though non-significant, increase, rather than a decrease, in PCs compared with controls. Further, PC counts did not correlate with tremor duration.

There are several other pathological findings reported in the cerebellums of ET patients. ET patients have three times as many heterotopic PCs,[33] a finding that is seen in spinocerebellar ataxia or neurodevelopmental disorders that affect the cerebellum. These heterotopias are found within the molecular layer of the cerebellum. Basket cells, which are GABAergic cells that synapse on the PC soma, are noted to be unusually dense and appear tangled, hence the term "hairy." The significance of this finding is unknown but is speculated to reflect loss of nearby Purkinje cells resulting in increased synapse formation around remaining cells.

Climbing-fiber-to-Purkinje-cell synaptic density is lower in ET and correlated with PC counts and torpedoes.[34] These climbing fibers seem to be pruned, synapsing instead on PC dendrites within the parallel fiber territory.[35,36] More recently, this has been shown to be associated with GluRδ2 protein reduction.[37] This in turn has prompted investigation into an animal model of GluRδ2 insufficiency that develops ET-like tremor. Increased activity at the climbing-fiber-to-Purkinje cell junction seems to be required for the excessive cerebellar activity.

Macroautophagy is the mechanism to clear damaged cellular proteins and organelles. It is impaired in neurodegenerative disorders. This pathway was investigated in ET patients using microtubule-associated protein light chain 3-II (LC3-II), S6K, phosphorylated S6K, beclin-1, and mitochondrial membrane proteins detected by Western blot.[38] LC3-II levels were reduced in ET and correlated with disease duration. Mitochondrial membrane proteins were accumulated in ET. Beclin-1 was deficient in ET. It was concluded that the abnormal findings supported the hypothesis of Purkinje cell degeneration in ET. There is a single report of isolated ubiquitin inclusions in the Purkinje cells in a childhood-onset ET patient, providing support for a theory of neurodegeneration given that many of the neurodegenerative processes are known for their various neuronal inclusions (e.g., LBs in Parkinson disease).

In addition to some of these positive findings, there are studies that report no difference in other cerebellar structures in ET patients. Cerebellar parallel fibers counts and density are similar in cases and controls.[39] This was studied in 20 ET cases and 19 controls. These ET cases had documented PC pathology. Therefore, this was interpreted to mean that the pathological changes seen in ET seem specific to the Purkinje cells. The inferior olivary nucleus (ION) was examined in ET.[40] This structure has relevance since the ION has inherent pacemaking properties, and, with its projections to the cerebellum, might be a logical source of tremor generation. However, this study of 14 ET cases and 15 controls showed no differences in olivary neuronal density or gliosis, making it unlikely that degeneration in this structure is the source or is involved in the degenerative pathology of ET.

With findings of PC loss and other changes in some studies of the cerebellum, it is tempting to conclude that ET may be a neurodegenerative process of the cerebellum. Indeed, this has been the source of some vibrant discussion over the years.[41,42] However, there are some difficulties with this concept. For a disease to be neurodegenerative, several criteria should be considered. The neuronal loss, synapse loss, or other pathological aberrancy should be related to the development of clinical symptoms (e.g., PC loss causes tremor). This loss should reach a certain threshold prior to development of clinical symptoms and, therefore, should be present in most, if not all, patients at death and be demonstrable in a single subject (not simply on average). Finally, the severity of pathological change should be correlated with disease duration and severity of symptoms. Unfortunately, this does not seem to be the case for most of the findings seen to date with ET and the cerebellum. In fact, a more recent study of childhood-onset ET and adult-onset ET showed no differences in PC counts, torpedo counts, heterotopic PC counts, and other cerebellar findings (Louis, 2017). It seems likely, therefore, that there may be alternate explanations for these cerebellar findings when present. Excitatory amino acid transporter expression is lower in the cerebellar cortex of ET but higher in the dentate.[43] These changes support that the cerebellar cortex and deep cerebellar nuclei are exposed to long-term excitatory stimulation. This is in keeping with imaging findings and in vivo recordings of tremor. The reduction in the cerebellar cortex may reflect inability of this area to "keep up" with this excitation over time, which in turn might lead to PC loss. Deep brain stimulation seems to reduce some of the pathology seen in ET.[44] Taken together, one could speculate that tremor itself might be responsible for some of these changes. Alternately, it is possible that there is substrate change that is minor and difficult to quantify but serves as the initiation of a network dysfunction leading to tremor. Another potential confound to consider remains treatment for ET. Patients with ET are often treated for years with anti-seizure medication for control of tremor. It is unknown whether these drugs might cause some of these subtle pathological findings in ET. This aspect of pathology needs to be further explored.

Biochemical changes in ET

The adrenergic system is a biochemical pathway that is often addressed as treatment for ET through the use of beta blockers. However, there have been surprisingly few pathophysiological studies done on the mechanisms underlying this clinical aspect. Due to often massive outpouring of adrenaline during the agonal process, combined with difficulties studying fresh tissue, these biochemical studies, when they are done, rely on enzymatic analysis, which should be more stable. As reviewed above, the dopaminergic system seems to be intact as measured by tyrosine hydroxylase.[12] Raput et al. did find higher levels of noradrenalin in ET in the cerebellar structures and locus coeruleus, the opposite of what is found in PD (Rajput, 2001). More work should be done alone these lines.

The GABAergic system has also been studied. Paris-Robidas et al. reported a decrease in GABA(A) and GABA(B) receptors of 20–30% in the dentate nucleus of the cerebellum from deceased individuals with ET, compared with controls or individuals with PD.[45] Concentrations of GABA(B) receptors in the dentate nucleus were inversely related to the duration of ET ($r(2) = 0.44$, $P < 0.05$). GABA(B(1a + b)) receptor messenger RNA was reduced in the dentate in ET by 27%. In contrast, no significant changes of GABA(A) and GABA(B) receptors (protein and messenger RNA), GluN2B receptors, cytochrome oxidase-1, or GABA concentrations were detected in molecular or granular layers of the cerebellar cortex. It was proposed that a decrease in GABA receptors in the dentate nucleus results in disinhibition of cerebellar pacemaker output activity, propagating along the cerebello-thalamo-cortical pathways to generate tremors.

OTHER TREMOR DISORDERS

There are many other tremor types that have definable pathology, but unfortunately, little work has been done on them with respect to tremor correlates. This would include tremors associated with inflammatory and hereditary demyelinating polyneuropathy, as well as action tremor seen with spinocerebellar degeneration. Among 315 SCA patients, postural tremor was most common in SCA2 patients (SCA1, 5.8%; SCA2, 27.5%; SCA3, 12.4%; SCA6, 16.9%).[46] Correlating pathology with tremor in these types of patients might teach us something about ET and tremor in general.

Intention tremor in MS

Multiple sclerosis can often have an intention tremor, and, indeed, imaging studies suggest that involvement of the cerebellar inflow and outflow pathways but not total lesion load correlate with tremor.[47,48] No pathology work has been done along these lines.

Fragile X tremor ataxia syndrome

Fragile X tremor ataxia syndrome is a neurodegenerative disorder that stems from the premutation (55–200) expansion of CGG repeat in carriers of the *FMR1* gene on the X chromosome. Intention tremor is a common finding in this condition. Significant cerebral and cerebellar white matter disease is seen in this disorder, with spongiform changes in the middle cerebellar peduncle seen in 7 of 8 cases in this series.[49] The tremor in FXTAS may very well stem from the specific involvement in the middle cerebellar peduncles in this condition.

Oculopalatal tremor

Symptomatic oculopalatal tremor occurs in the setting of a lesion, mostly vascular, in the dento-rubral olivary pathways. These tremors are associated with hypertrophic olivary degeneration. This was examined pathologically in 16 autopsied subjects with cerebrovascular lesions of the dentate-olivary tract,[50] and the pathological findings were correlated with clinical features. Palatal tremor was observed in eight patients. In 7 of 8 patients, the tremor appeared 1–2 months after interruption of the afferents, then progressed to reach a peak approximately 1–2 years from the onset. Tremor persisted for the rest of the subjects' lives without decreasing in severity. Neuronal hypertrophic change began radiologically 20–30 days after the onset of the causative lesions and reached maximum size 6–7 months later. Associated with the clinical findings were prominent olivary astrocytosis and synaptic and axonal remodeling pathologically. The number of olivary neurons decreased to <10% of that in controls in patients who survived more than 6 years. Despite the persistence of clinical tremor, both the myelin and the axons of efferent fibers from olivary neurons were severely degenerated in long-term surviving patients. Based on this, it was speculated that the persistence of tremor was probably due to both the disturbance of natural rhythmicity in the body (due to olivary disruption) and the lack of feedback from the abnormal movement.

CONCLUSION

According to pathological studies, there does not appear to be an increased risk for ET developing into Parkinson disease. There are many findings suggesting cerebellar degeneration affecting Purkinje cells in ET, but this is not seen in all patients or all studies; therefore, more work should be done on this to explore alternate hypothesis for these findings. The climbing fiber pathology is of interest, as it is associated with a biochemical abnormality, which, in turn could lead to treatments for ET. Last, while some work has been done in other tremor disorders besides ET, more exploration of these other tremor types might help us to understand tremor generation and propagation as a whole.

REFERENCES

1. Benito-Leon J, Louis ED, Bermejo-Pareja F. Neurological disorders in Central Spain Study G. Risk of incident Parkinson's disease and parkinsonism in essential tremor: a population-based study. *J Neurol Neurosurg Psychiatry*. 2009;80(4):423–425.
2. Bhatia KP, Bain P, Bajaj N, et al. Consensus statement on the classification of tremors. from the task force on tremor of the International Parkinson and Movement Disorder Society. *Mov Disord*. 2018;33(1):75–87.
3. Rajput AH, Rozdilsky B, Ang L, Rajput A. Clinicopathologic observations in essential tremor: report of six cases. *Neurology*. 1991;41(9):1422–1424.
4. Rajput A, Robinson CA, Rajput AH. Essential tremor course and disability: a clinicopathologic study of 20 cases. *Neurology*. 2004;62(6):932–936.
5. Louis ED, Honig LS, Vonsattel JP, Maraganore DM, Borden S, Moskowitz CB. Essential tremor associated with focal nonnigral Lewy bodies: a clinicopathologic study. *Neurol.* 2005;62(6):1004–1007.
6. Louis ED, Vonsattel JP, Honig LS, Ross GW, Lyons KE, Pahwa R. Neuropathologic findings in essential tremor. *Neurology*. 2006;66(11): 1756–1759.
7. Shill HA, Adler CH, Sabbagh MN, et al. Pathologic findings in prospectively ascertained essential tremor subjects. *Neurology*. 2008;70(16 Pt 2):1452–1455.
8. Driver-Dunckley E, Adler CH, Hentz JG, et al. Olfactory dysfunction in incidental Lewy body disease and Parkinson's disease. *Parkinsonism Relat Disord*. 2014;20(11):1260–1262.
9. Shprecher DR, Adler CH, Zhang N, et al. Predicting alpha-synuclein pathology by REM sleep behavior disorder diagnosis. *Parkinsonism Relat Disord*. 2018;55:92–96.
10. Saito Y, Ruberu NN, Sawabe M, et al. Lewy body-related alpha-synucleinopathy in aging. *J Neuropathol Exp Neurol*. 2004;63(7):742–749.
11. Adler CH, Connor DJ, Hentz JG, et al. Incidental Lewy body disease: clinical comparison to a control cohort. *Mov Disord*. 2010;25(5):642–646.
12. Shill HA, Adler CH, Beach TG, et al. Brain biochemistry in autopsied patients with essential tremor. *Mov Disord*. 2012;27(1):113–117.
13. Beach TG, Adler CH, Lue L, et al. Unified staging system for Lewy body disorders: correlation with nigrostriatal degeneration, cognitive impairment and motor dysfunction. *Acta Neuropathol*. 2009;117(6):613–634.
14. Rajput AH, Rajput EF, Bocking SM, Auer RN, Rajput A. Parkinsonism in essential tremor cases: a clinicopathological study. *Mov Disord*. 2019;34(7):1031–1040.
15. Louis ED, Borden S, Moskowitz CB. Essential tremor centralized brain repository: diagnostic validity and clinical characteristics of a highly selected group of essential tremor cases. *Mov Disord*. 2005;20(10):1361–1365.
16. Louis ED, Asabere N, Agnew A, et al. Rest tremor in advanced essential tremor: a postmortem study of nine cases. *J Neurol Neurosurg Psychiatry*. 2011;82(3):261–265.

17. Aslam S, Zhang N, Adler CH, Mehta S, Beach TG, Shill HA. The clinical role of jaw tremor in movement disorders. *Neurology.* 2020;94:2143.

18. Louis ED, Babij R, Ma K, Cortes E, Vonsattel JP. Essential tremor followed by progressive supranuclear palsy: postmortem reports of 11 patients. *J Neuropathol Exp Neurol.* 2013;72(1):8–17.

19. Evidente VG, Adler CH, Sabbagh MN, et al. Neuropathological findings of PSP in the elderly without clinical PSP: possible incidental PSP? *Parkinsonism Relat Disord.* 2011;17(5):365–371.

20. Rigby HB, Dugger BN, Hentz JG, et al. Clinical features of patients with concomitant Parkinson's disease and progressive supranuclear palsy pathology. *Mov Disord Clin Pract.* 2015;2(1):33–38.

21. Symanski C, Shill HA, Dugger B, et al. Essential tremor is not associated with cerebellar Purkinje cell loss. *Mov Disord.* 2014;29(4):496–500.

22. Jenkins IH, Bain PG, Colebatch JG, et al. A positron emission tomography study of essential tremor: evidence for overactivity of cerebellar connections. *Ann Neurol.* 1993;34(1):82–90.

23. Wills AJ, Jenkins IH, Thompson PD, Findley LJ, Brooks DJ. A positron emission tomography study of cerebral activation associated with essential and writing tremor. *Arch Neurol.* 1995;52(3):299–305.

24. Boecker H, Wills AJ, Ceballos-Baumann A, et al. The effect of ethanol on alcohol-responsive essential tremor: a positron emission tomography study. *Ann Neurol.* 1996;39(5):650–658.

25. Louis ED, Yi H, Erickson-Davis C, Vonsattel JP, Faust PL. Structural study of Purkinje cell axonal torpedoes in essential tremor. *Neurosci Lett.* 2009;450(3):287–291.

26. Deuschl G, Bain P, Brin M. Consensus statement of the Movement Disorder Society on Tremor. Ad Hoc Scientific Committee. *Mov Disord.* 1998;13(Suppl 3):2–23.

27. Louis ED, Faust PL, Vonsattel JP, et al. Neuropathological changes in essential tremor: 33 cases compared with 21 controls. *Brain.* 2007;130(Pt 12):3297–3307.

28. Louis ED, Faust PL, Vonsattel JP, et al. Torpedoes in Parkinson's disease, Alzheimer's disease, essential tremor, and control brains. *Mov Disord.* 2009;24(11):1600–1605.

29. Axelrad JE, Louis ED, Honig LS, et al. Reduced Purkinje cell number in essential tremor: a postmortem study. *Arch Neurol.* 2008;65(1):101–107.

30. Louis ED, Babij R, Lee M, Cortes E, Vonsattel JP. Quantification of cerebellar hemispheric Purkinje cell linear density: 32 ET cases versus 16 controls. *Mov Disord.* 2013;28(13):1854–1859.

31. Louis ED, Faust PL, Vonsattel JP, et al. Older onset essential tremor: more rapid progression and more degenerative pathology. *Mov Disord.* 2009;24(11):1606–1612.

32. Rajput AH, Robinson CA, Rajput ML, Robinson SL, Rajput A. Essential tremor is not dependent upon cerebellar Purkinje cell loss. *Parkinsonism Relat Disord.* 2012;18(5):626–628.

33. Kuo SH, Erickson-Davis C, Gillman A, Faust PL, Vonsattel JP, Louis ED. Increased number of heterotopic Purkinje cells in essential tremor. *J Neurol Neurosurg Psychiatry.* 2011;82(9):1038–1040.

34. Lee D, Gan SR, Faust PL, Louis ED, Kuo SH. Climbing fiber-Purkinje cell synaptic pathology across essential tremor subtypes. *Parkinsonism Relat Disord.* 2018;51:24–29.

35. Kuo SH, Lin CY, Wang J, et al. Climbing fiber-Purkinje cell synaptic pathology in tremor and cerebellar degenerative diseases. *Acta Neuropathol.* 2017;133(1):121–138.

36. Lin CY, Louis ED, Faust PL, Koeppen AH, Vonsattel JP, Kuo SH. Abnormal climbing fibre-Purkinje cell synaptic connections in the essential tremor cerebellum. *Brain.* 2014;137(Pt 12):3149–3159.

37. Pan MK, Li YS, Wong SB, et al. Cerebellar oscillations driven by synaptic pruning deficits of cerebellar climbing fibers contribute to tremor pathophysiology. *Sci Transl Med.* 2020;12(526). doi:10.1126/scitranslmed.aay1769

38. Kuo SH, Tang G, Ma K, et al. Macroautophagy abnormality in essential tremor. *PLoS One.* 2012;7(12):e53040.

39. Kuo SH, Faust PL, Vonsattel JP, Ma K, Louis ED. Parallel fiber counts and parallel fiber integrated density are similar in essential tremor cases and controls. *Acta Neuropathol.* 2011;121(2):287–289.

40. Louis ED, Babij R, Cortes E, Vonsattel JP, Faust PL. The inferior olivary nucleus: a postmortem study of essential tremor cases versus controls. *Mov Disord.* 2013;28(6):779–786.

41. Rajput AH, Robinson CA, Rajput A. Purkinje cell loss is neither pathological basis nor characteristic of essential tremor. *Parkinsonism Relat Disord.* 2013;19(4):490–491.

42. Deuschl G, Elble R. Essential tremor—neurodegenerative or nondegenerative disease towards a working definition of ET. *Mov Disord.* 2009;24(14):2033–2041.

43. Wang J, Kelly GC, Tate WJ, et al. Excitatory Amino acid transporter expression in the essential tremor dentate nucleus and cerebellar cortex: a postmortem study. *Parkinsonism Relat Disord.* 2016;32:87–93.

44. Kuo SH, Lin CY, Wang J, et al. Deep brain stimulation and climbing fiber synaptic pathology in essential tremor. *Ann Neurol.* 2016;80(3):461–465.

45. Paris-Robidas S, Brochu E, Sintes M, et al. Defective dentate nucleus GABA receptors in essential tremor. *Brain.* 2012;135(Pt 1): 105–116.

46. Gan SR, Wang J, Figueroa KP, et al. Postural tremor and ataxia progression in spinocerebellar ataxias. *Tremor Other Hyperkinet Movements (N Y).* 2017;7:492.

47. Boonstra F, Florescu G, Evans A, et al. Tremor in multiple sclerosis is associated with cerebello-thalamic pathology. *J Neural Transm.* 2017;124(12):1509–1514.

48. Feys P, Maes F, Nuttin B, et al. Relationship between multiple sclerosis intention tremor severity and lesion load in the brainstem. *Neuroreport.* 2005;16(12):1379–1382.

49. Greco CM, Berman RF, Martin RM, et al. Neuropathology of fragile X-associated tremor/ataxia syndrome (FXTAS). *Brain.* 2006;129(Pt 1):243–255.

50. Nishie M, Yoshida Y, Hirata Y, Matsunaga M. Generation of symptomatic palatal tremor is not correlated with inferior olivary hypertrophy. *Brain.* 2002;125(Pt 6):1348–1357.

Neuroimaging of Tremors

RICK C. HELMICH

INTRODUCTION

Most tremor syndromes are associated with changes in the central nervous system, and neuroimaging can help to make these changes visible. Neuroimaging is defined as the production of images of the human brain using non-invasive or minimally invasive (e.g., nuclear imaging) approaches. This can serve a clinical purpose, to investigate the etiology of a clinical tremor syndrome during the diagnostic workup. Neuroimaging is also increasingly used for scientific purposes, to address the pathophysiology of a clinical tremor syndrome. The current clinical tremor classification describes tremor along two independent axes: clinical tremor syndrome (Axis I) and etiology (Axis II).[1] Pathophysiology is not included in this classification. It is important to point out that etiology and pathophysiology are not the same thing, although they are sometimes used interchangeably.[2] Etiology refers to the study of the *causes* of a tremor, which directly *initiate* the disease process and are therefore *necessary* for the development of a tremor. For example, a microbleed near the red nucleus can cause Holmes tremor—therefore, this is an etiological factor. Pathophysiology refers to the processes and factors associated with the *perpetuation* and *maintenance* of tremor, and these factors do not necessarily have to precede the onset of disorder. For example, the cerebello-thalamo-cortical circuit is involved in Parkinson's rest tremor, but (altered) activity in this circuit is not the cause of Parkinson disease—therefore, this is a pathophysiological factor. In this chapter, different neuroimaging techniques will be discussed that can visualize various aspects of brain structure and function in tremor, both during clinical workup (to assess etiology) and in scientific research (to assess the pathophysiology of tremor). The primary focus will be on the four most common clinical tremor syndromes: essential tremor, Parkinson's rest tremor, dystonic tremor syndromes, and orthostatic tremor.

NEUROIMAGING DURING CLINICAL WORKUP

Structural imaging

In general, a cerebral magnetic resonance imaging (MRI) scan is worthwhile when the differential diagnosis includes an etiology that involves structural brain abnormalities. This deserves special consideration when there is a *combined* tremor syndrome that is (1) focal/unilateral, or (2) unusual in appearance (for example, very proximal, very low frequency, or jerky), or (3) in cases where there is a sudden onset or stepwise deterioration, or (4) a family history of movement disorders combined with cognitive or psychiatric symptoms.[3]

In tremor combined with parkinsonism (bradykinesia and rigidity), specific signs to look for include hummingbird sign, morning glory sign (both suggestive of progressive supranuclear palsy, PSP), hot cross bun sign, and middle cerebral peduncle (MCP) sign (suggestive of multiple system atrophy, MSA). In patients with tremor combined with dystonia, the "panda sign" in the mesencephalon may be suggestive of Wilson disease. In patients with tremor combined with ataxia, the MCP sign (T2 hyperintensity) and splenium sign may be suggestive of fragile X associated tremor ataxia syndrome (FXTAS), and cerebellar atrophy may be suggestive of spinocerebellar ataxia (SCA). Finally, look for acquired lesions in the brain stem (mesencephalon), cerebellum, or thalamus in patients who have (Holmes) tremor combined with dystonia or ataxia.[4,5] In (rare) patients with palatal tremor, hypertrophy of the inferior olive on T2-weighted images can sometimes be observed.[6]

Generally, patients with an *isolated* tremor syndrome will have normal MRI scans and thus structural imaging is not indicated. However, this rule of thumb should be abandoned in isolated tremor patients in case of either hints at an acquired cause (sudden onset or stepwise deterioration, unilateral tremor), or a family history of movement disorders combined with cognitive or psychiatric symptoms.

Nuclear imaging

Presynaptic dopamine transporter imaging (123I-FP-CIT single photon emission computed tomography, DAT-SPECT), or dopamine receptor imaging (such as F-DOPA positron emission tomography, PET) can be helpful in specific circumstances.[3] Because these techniques are aimed at assessing the presence of a presynaptic dopaminergic deficit, they are mainly relevant to differentiate tremor combined with parkinsonism from other tremor syndromes, particularly essential tremor and dystonic tremor syndromes. Clinically, dystonic tremor syndromes can mimic parkinsonian tremor, since hand dystonia can be mistaken for bradykinesia. Accordingly, many suspected Parkinson patients with SWEDDS (scans without evidence of dopaminergic deficit) are thought to have dystonic tremor.[7] Furthermore, presynaptic DAT imaging can be used to distinguish drug-induced parkinsonism (including tremor) from neurodegenerative forms of parkinsonism. However, DAT imaging is not suitable to distinguish between different forms of atypical parkinsonism, or between these atypical parkinsonism and Parkinson disease. Glucose PET has been used for this purpose, but that falls outside the scope of this chapter on tremor.[8] Finally, dopaminergic imaging can be abnormal in patients with Holmes tremor, since acquired lesions in the mesencephalon may disrupt nigrostriatal dopaminergic projections.[9,10] However, since acquired lesions in brain regions outside the dopaminergic system (thalamus, cerebellum) may also cause Holmes tremor,[5] this is not necessarily the case.

Structural connectivity mapping for stereotactic surgery

The most common stereotactic target for treating tremor is the dentato-rubro-thalamic tract (DRTT), which contains the efferent fibers from the cerebellum toward the contralateral motor cortex via the contralateral ventrolateral thalamus. Lesioning this tract at the level of the thalamus (ventral intermediate nucleus, VIM), or just below the thalamus (subthalamic zone) has been shown to be very effective for Parkinson's tremor, essential tremor, dystonic tremor syndromes, but also rare forms of tremor such as tremor associated with multiple sclerosis or Holmes tremor.[11,12]

Specifically, the success of deep brain stimulation on tremor has been linked to the distance of the target from the DRTT.[13] The difficulty is that the different nuclei of the thalamus or the DRTT cannot be seen on a conventional MRI. Therefore, some centers have started to use diffusion tensor imaging–based (DTI-based) tractography to visualize the DRTT during surgical planning.[14,15]

NEUROIMAGING APPROACHES TO STUDY THE PATHOPHYSIOLOGY OF TREMOR

Unlike the previous paragraph, this section focuses on neuroimaging of tremor in a research context. The most commonly used neuroimaging methods are MRI, PET, and SPECT. These methods can help to image structural and functional brain abnormalities in patients with tremor. Electrophysiological methods such as electro-encephalography (EEG) and magneto-encephalography (MEG) are sometimes mentioned under the umbrella of neuroimaging, but these techniques are focused on identifying neurophysiological properties of tremor, rather than generating brain images. Therefore, these findings will not be discussed here. This section will start with a general discussion of what neuroimaging can show. Then, an overview of different neuroimaging approaches to tremor will be given (see also Table 5.1), and the section will end with interpretational caveats. Afterward, a more in-depth discussion of neuroimaging findings for essential tremor, Parkinson's rest tremor, dystonic tremor syndromes, and orthostatic tremor will be provided.

Tremor trait and tremor state

Tremor has both trait and state characteristics. Trait refers to tremor as a property of an individual, and its cerebral mechanisms can be studied by comparing individuals with or without tremor (or individuals with different types of tremor). State refers to tremor as (also) a property of the prevailing context (e.g., motoric or cognitive). Examples of studies that regard tremor as a trait include structural imaging (MRI, diffusion tensor imaging, DTI), molecular imaging (PET or SPECT), and resting state functional connectivity (functional MRI). A caveat here is that group differences may be related to tremor, but also to other factors. For example, cerebral differences between tremor-dominant and non-tremor Parkinson disease could be driven by cognitive

TABLE 5.1: NEUROIMAGING APPROACHES TO TREMOR

Technique	Method	Tremor feature	Example	References
Structural MRI	VBM / cortical thickness	Trait	Gray matter atrophy in the cerebellum of ET patients	Gallea et al., *Brain* 2015
DWI / DTI	VBM, tractography, free water imaging	Trait	Decreased white matter integrity in all three cerebellar peduncles in ET	Juttukonda et al., *Neurology* 2019
Functional MRI	Concurrent fMRI–EMG / accelerometry	State	Activity in the cerebello-thalamo-cortical circuit correlates with fluctuations in tremor power in PD	Helmich et al., *Ann Neurol* 2011
	Task-related activity, which modulates tremor amplitude	State	Grip-force-related cerebellar activity is similar in dystonic tremor and ET; reduced grip-force-related functional connectivity in cortical, basal ganglia, and cerebellar regions in dystonic tremor	DeSimone et al., *Brain* 2019
	Resting state functional connectivity	Trait	Connectivity of the cerebellum is abnormal in ET	Fang et al., *HBM* 2016
	Task-related effective connectivity (DCM, PPI)	State	Effective connectivity between cerebellar cortex and dentate is increased as a function of tremor power in ET	Buijink et al., *Brain* 2015
	Regional homogeneity (ReHo)	Trait	ET patients show decreased ReHo in the bilateral cerebellar lobes, the bilateral thalamus, and the insular lobe, and increased ReHo in the bilateral prefrontal and parietal cortices, the left primary motor cortex, and the left SMA	Fang et al., *PLoS One* 2013
	Lesion network mapping	Trait	Lesions causing Holmes tremor map to a network consisting of red nucleus, GPi, thalamus (VOP and pulvinar nucleus), cerebellum (vermis, lateral cerebellar cortex, and flocculonodular), and the pontomedullary junction	Joutsa et al., *Ann Neurol* 2019
Metabolic PET	Spatial covariance pattern	State	VIM-DBS reduces activity in cerebellum, VIM, and motor cortex in PD tremor	Mure et al., *Neuroimage* 2011
Dopamine-PET/ SPECT	Voxel-wise or ROI-wise group comparisons	Trait	Tremor-dominant PD patients have more striatal dopamine transporter binding than non-tremor PD patients	Helmich et al., *Ann Neurol* 2011
GABA-PET (flumazenil)	Voxel-wise or ROI-wise group comparisons	Trait	ET patients have altered GABA receptor binding in motor cortex, thalamus, and cerebellum	Boecker et al., *J Nucl Med* 2010
Serotonin-PET	Voxel-wise or ROI-wise group comparisons	Trait	Tremor-dominant PD patients have less ^{123}I-DAT binding in the raphe compared to non-tremor PD patients	Qamhawi et al., *Brain* 2015

This table lists different neuroimaging approaches to tremor, and which aspect of tremor (trait or state) they measure, with an example. Please note that this table does not contain all available approaches to tremor. DTI = diffusion tensor imaging; DWI = diffusion-weighted imaging; DCM = dynamic causal modeling; EMG = electromyography; ET = essential tremor; MRI = magnetic resonance imaging; PD = Parkinson disease; PET = positron emission tomography; PPI = psychophysiological interaction; ReHo = regional homogeneity; ROI = region of interest; VBM = voxel-based morphometry.

dysfunction—which is often more pronounced in non-tremor Parkinson subtypes—instead of tremor. Correlations between a cerebral effect and measures of tremor severity may help support the idea that they are related.

Other studies focus on state characteristics of tremor. For example, essential tremor is present during posturing of the arms, but usually absent during rest, and Parkinson's rest tremor amplitude is increased by cognitive coactivation. Furthermore, tremor severity can be manipulated by specific treatments (pharmacological or stereotactic interventions). This tremor feature allows within-subject comparisons between high-versus low-severity tremor conditions, thereby controlling for inter-individual differences. In this way, tremor-related activity can be identified more reliably, and its anatomical distribution can be compared between groups. If the control group involves healthy subjects, sometimes mimicked tremor is chosen as a control condition, although obviously this involves a qualitatively different process (i.e., voluntary movement). Examples of studies that investigated tremor states are task-based fMRI or metabolic PET, studies that combined fMRI with electromyography (EMG) or accelerometry, and intervention studies.

Nuclear imaging of tremor

Historically, neuroimaging of tremor started in the 1990s, when metabolic PET was used to image brain regions showing abnormal brain metabolism in patients with essential tremor. For example, in 1990, a PET study measured cerebral blood flow during inhalation of carbon-15-labeled carbon dioxide in four patients with essential tremor and four normal controls. The authors found increased metabolism in the bilateral cerebellum during posturing (which evoked tremor) in essential tremor patients but not healthy controls (where posturing did not evoke tremor).[16] PET and SPECT can also be used to image the distribution of specific molecules in the brains of tremor patients. For example, several studies showed that dopamine transporter (DAT) imaging of the striatum was normal in patients with essential tremor.[17] In Parkinson disease, it was found that although striatal DAT binding is reduced, the severity of striatal dopamine depletion did not correlate with the severity of tremor.[18] This raised the question whether Parkinson's tremor has a dopaminergic basis. Other nuclear imaging studies have focused on the role of different molecules in tremor, such as serotonin[19,20] or GABA.[21]

Structural MRI

In the 2000s, when the technology of MRI took a leap forward, several studies tested for structural brain differences between tremor patients and healthy controls. The most widely used method to investigate this is voxel-based morphometry (VBM) on T1-weighted MRI images. VBM is a morphological approach that performs a voxel-wise statistical analysis of the brain volume related to the gray matter (GM) and white matter (WM) tissues. These are relative measures (statistical probabilities) rather than absolute volumes. For example, in 2001 a VBM study showed increased gray matter density in the thalamus (ventral intermediate nucleus; VIM) of 10 tremor-dominant Parkinson disease patients compared to controls.[22] In essential tremor, a first VBM study in 2006 showed no differences in cerebellar gray matter volume between 27 essential tremor patients and 27 healthy controls,[23] but several subsequent studies collectively provided evidence of cerebellar atrophy in essential tremor.[24]

Diffusion-weighed imaging (DWI) and DTI allow an investigation of white matter tracts. Although initial (smaller) studies showed no differences between essential tremor patients and controls,[25] later (larger) studies identified reductions in fractional anisotropy in the cerebellar peduncles.[26]

Specific MRI sequences (sensitive to R* relaxation rates) allow the investigation of iron deposition. For example, a comparison between different tremor disorders showed that nigral iron deposition was increased in tremor-dominant Parkinson disease, but normal in dystonic tremor and essential tremor.[27]

Functional MRI

Since the end of the 1990s, functional MRI has increasingly been used to study altered brain function in patients with tremor. Functional MRI uses blood-oxygen-level-dependent- (BOLD-) sensitive images to detect changes in the relative levels of oxyhemoglobin and deoxyhemoglobin (oxygenated and deoxygenated blood), based on their differential magnetic susceptibility. Whole-brain images with a relatively high resolution (isotropic voxels with a width of 2–5 mm) can be collected in the order of seconds, and technological advances have considerably increased both the spatial and temporal resolution. With fMRI, different task conditions can be compared to each other: this approach has been used to investigate differences between a tremor-evoking condition (e.g., posturing) and a non-tremor-evoking condition (e.g., rest, or passive movements) in patients with essential tremor versus healthy controls. In 1997, a first comparison of 12 essential tremor patients and 15 controls showed that essential tremor was associated with increased activity in the bilateral cerebellum and red nucleus.[28] Other studies focused on tasks that are independent of tremor, but can be used to assess different features in essential tremor patients, for example working memory.[29] Recently, a few studies have contrasted deep brain stimulation conditions (ON versus OFF) in the fMRI scanner.[30] This is more complicated given safety concerns about the electrical currents in a magnetic field.

Since the 2010s, fMRI has also been used in combination with neurophysiological measures, such as EMG and accelerometry, to identify brain regions where activity correlates with changes in tremor power during scanning. Since tremor is much faster (3–6 Hz) than the sampling rate of standard fMRI sequences (0.3–2 Hz), these fMRI studies focused on detecting brain activity associated with (much slower) changes in tremor power during scanning. To this end, accelerometry or EMG collected during fMRI scanning can be used to build a time course of tremor power during scanning. Given the very short neuromuscular delay times, it can be assumed that the tremor time course (derived from EMG) approximates fluctuations in neuronal activity. Thus, when down-sampled to the sampling rate of fMRI, this time course can be used as a covariate in a regression analysis to identify brain regions where activity follows the same time course. However, because fMRI is sensitive to BOLD activity instead of neuronal activity, a mathematical transformation has to be done first. This is necessary because there is a temporal delay between neuronal activity and changes in cerebral blood flow (which drive the BOLD signal). The BOLD signal has a consistent shape, peaking around six seconds after a change in neuronal activity and then falling back to baseline over the next several seconds. This shape can be modeled with a mathematical function called a gamma distribution, and is referred to as the canonical hemodynamic response function (HRF). Thus, when the tremor time course is multiplied (convolved) with the HRF, a regressor results that models the expected BOLD time course of a brain region with tremor-related activity. This approach, which is illustrated in Figure 5.1, has been applied to essential tremor and to Parkinson's rest tremor. In 2011, a first study in Parkinson's rest tremor showed that

activity in the cerebello-thalamo-cortical circuit was correlated with spontaneous fluctuations in rest tremor amplitude during scanning.[31] In 2015, a similar study in essential tremor patients showed that bilateral cerebellar activity was correlated to fluctuations in postural tremor amplitude, independent of posturing itself. Furthermore, this correlation was observed to a larger extent in patients with essential tremor as compared to healthy controls who mimicked postural tremor[32] (Figures 5.2A and 5.2B).

Network approaches to tremor

Since the 2010s, fMRI studies have focused more on the role of network parameters in tremor. A rather simple example is seed-based functional connectivity between two (or more) regions, for example the thalamus and motor cortex.[33] More complex techniques involve graph theory, which examines the overall connectivity pattern among tens to hundreds of brain regions, and which can test local or global network properties such as efficiency, modularity, or "hubs".[34] While these approaches are usually rather exploratory in nature, other network analyses allow very specific hypothesis testing, such as dynamic causal modeling (DCM).

DCM is a Bayesian method of inference where one defines one or more cerebral model(s) based on predefined hypotheses, to test for causal influences that one neural system may exert over the other.[35] Specifically, one defines a cerebral model by including brain regions that can be influenced by (i) fixed connections between included nodes (DCM.A); (ii) modulation of these fixed connections by exogenous inputs (DCM.B); and (iii) exogenous inputs that drive network activity (DCM.C). To set up models that are relevant for tremor, a priori knowledge is required to select brain regions that are expected to play a role in tremor. An advantage of DCM is that it allows the researcher to statistically compare different models with different network architectures in order to identify which pattern of (directional) connections best fits the data. DCM can be applied to resting state data, but also allows the incorporation of tremor-specific data such as EMG recordings collected during scanning, which provide information on fluctuations in tremor amplitude. These regressors can then be entered as exogenous inputs (DCM.B or DCM.C) into the network, to investigate which nodes or functional connections are sensitive to tremor power and changes in tremor power. This approach has been applied to Parkinson's tremor[36] and to

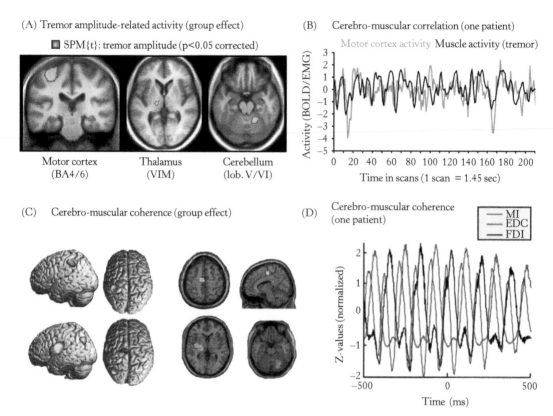

FIGURE 5.1: The Role of the Cerebello-Thalamo-Cortical Circuit in Parkinson's Rest Tremor. This figure shows two different ways of looking at tremor. In panels A and B, fMRI was used to test for cerebral activity correlated with slow fluctuations in muscular activity at tremor frequency (i.e., tremor power). Taken from [31], with permission. The temporal resolution is in the order of seconds. In panels C and D, MEG was used to test for cerebral oscillatory activity coherent with muscular activity at double tremor frequency. Here the temporal resolution is in the order of milliseconds. Taken from [92], with permission. Both methods show the involvement of the cerebello-thalamo-cortical circuit in Parkinson's rest tremor. Abbreviations: BA = Brodmann Area; EDC = extensor digitorum communis muscle; FDI = first dorsal interosseus muscle; M1 = primary motor cortex; SPM = statistical parametric map; VIM = ventral intermediate nucleus of the thalamus.

essential tremor.[37] These studies have revealed new knowledge about the underlying networks: in Parkinson disease, tremor-related activity first starts in the basal ganglia (globus pallidus) and is then relayed to the cerebello-thalamo-cortical circuit through the pallido-thalamo-cortical connection.[36] In contrast, essential tremor is associated with increased connectivity between cerebellum and the thalamus (VIM), which contributes to variations in tremor power.[37] Dynamic causal models of tremor can be further enriched by incorporating manipulations ("states") of the network (and of tremor), to investigate how, for example, deep brain stimulation,[30] dopaminergic medication,[38,39] or a cognitive task[40] influence the flow of information in the brain network, as well as its output (tremor).

Lesion mapping

Although neuroimaging usually does not allow inferences on causality, this has been approached by localizing brain regions where an acquired lesion reduces or even removes tremor (in essential tremor), or where an acquired brain lesion evokes tremor (in Holmes tremor). An interesting study has brought together all the case reports where a stroke reduced essential tremor. It was found that all of the "curative strokes" interrupted the connecting pathways between the cerebellum and the primary sensorimotor cortex, or the pyramidal tract.[41] These findings provide further support for the causal role of the cerebello-thalamo-cortical circuit in essential tremor. In Parkinson's tremor, there are only a few case studies available. In two

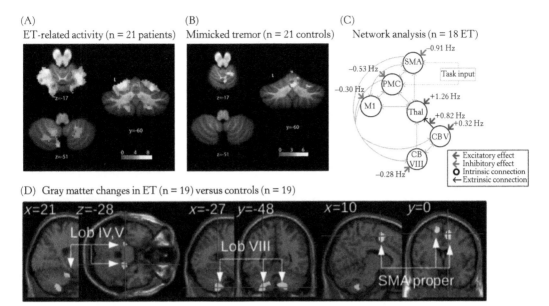

(A)
ET-related activity (n = 21 patients)

(B)
Mimicked tremor (n = 21 controls)

(C)
Network analysis (n = 18 ET)

(D) Gray matter changes in ET (n = 19) versus controls (n = 19)

FIGURE 5.2: Cerebral Changes in Essential Tremor. Panel A shows the pattern of tremor-related activity, identified using combined EMG-fMRI mapping. Brain activity is independent from activity related to posturing. Panel B shows the same effect during mimicked tremor in healthy controls. Taken from [32], with permission. Panel C shows the result of network analysis, using dynamic causal modeling (DCM) on combined EMG-fMRI data from the same group of essential tremor patients. Graphical representation of the significant estimated connectivity parameters resulting from Bayesian Model Averaging in essential tremor. Only modulatory influences (of tremor power, derived from EMG) are depicted. Coupling parameter strength is depicted in red (excitatory effect) and blue (inhibitory effect). Significant modulatory input is depicted in Hz. In essential tremor, there is a significant excitatory modulating effect of tremor variation on the cerebello-dentato-thalamic connection and on intrinsic thalamic and cerebellar lobule V activity. Taken from [37], with permission. Panel D shows the statistical parametric maps of the comparison between essential tremor patients (n = 19) and healthy volunteers (n = 19), showing decreased gray matter (GM) volume in the cerebellum (blue) and increased gray matter volume in both SMAs (yellow). Clusters are significant at p < 0.05, corrected for multiple comparisons. Taken from [66], with permission. Abbreviations: CB lob V = right cerebellar lobule V; CB lob VIII = right cerebellar lobule VIII; Lob = cerebellar lobule; M1 = primary motor cortex; PMC = premotor cortex; SMA = supplementary motor area; Thal = left thalamus.

cases, a (small) stroke in the thalamus removed the tremor, mimicking the effect of a thalamotomy.[42,42] Interestingly, in another case removal of the cerebellum did not remove Parkinson's rest tremor, but altered its appearance: the frequency was lowered, and the tremor became more pronounced during posturing.[44] This phenotype resembles Holmes tremor. These findings, although based on only case reports, suggest that the cerebellum may play a different role in the pathophysiology of essential tremor versus Parkinson's tremor.

A more recent and systematic approach bundled 36 case studies where an acquired brain lesion led to Holmes tremor[45] (Figure 5.3). Using a technique called "lesion network mapping",[46] the authors showed that, in a group of healthy

individuals, all these lesions are functionally connected to a common network. This lesion connectome includes the red nucleus, internal globus pallidus (GPi), thalamus (ventral oralis posterior nucleus, VOP), pontomedullary junction, and cerebellum. In a subset of cases, stereotactic surgery was applied to the VIM, the VOP, or the GPi, with different success rates. It was found that those targets with the highest success rates (in terms of tremor reduction) were located closest to the lesion connectome: the GPi and VOP. A recent case report in a patient with Holmes tremor due to a peri-rubral microbleed investigated the relationship between tremor-related activity (assessed with combined accelerometry and fMRI) and the lesion connectome.[9] It was found that Holmes tremor was associated

(A)   Lesions causing Holmes tremor   (B)   Lesion network mapping

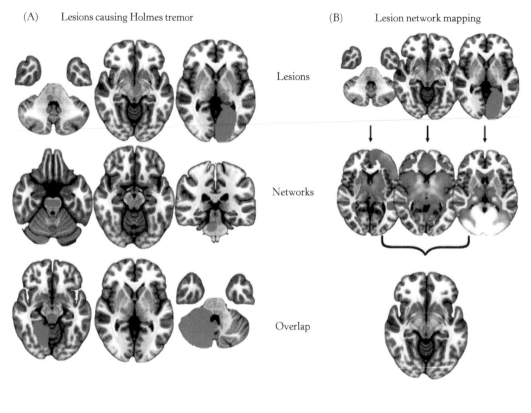

Lesions

Networks

Overlap

(C)   Holmes tremor circuit (using lesion network mapping)

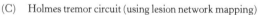

| Red nucleus | GPi | VOP | Pulvinar nucleus | Vermis, lateral cerebellum | Flocculonodular, Ponto-medullary |

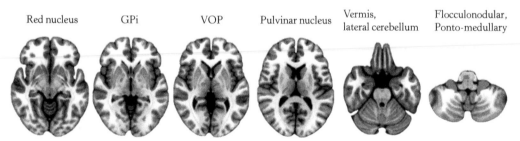

FIGURE 5.3: Lesion Network Mapping in Holmes Tremor. Panel A: Nine representative lesions causing Holmes tremor (selected from n = 36). Panel B: lesion mapping approach. Lesions from the literature are traced onto a standard brain atlas (upper row). The set of voxels functionally connected to each lesion location (in n = 1000 healthy volunteers from the Human Connectome Project) are identified ("lesion networks," middle row). Finally, lesion networks are overlapped to identify regions connected to all lesion locations (bottom row). Panel C: The resultant lesion network for Holmes tremor. Taken from [45], with permission. Abbreviations: GPi = internal globus pallidus; VOP = ventralis oralis posterior nucleus of the thalamus.

with tremor-related activity in the cerebellum and sensorimotor cortex. These regions were distinct from, but functionally connected to, the Holmes lesion connectome.[45] This suggests that Holmes tremor may involves three distinct cerebral mechanisms: a structural brain lesion, an intermediate lesion connectome, and a brain network that produces tremor-related activity. Taken together, lesion mapping and lesion network mapping allow more causal inferences with respect to tremor. It should be kept in mind that these lesions, or the interconnected network (lesion connectome), may not be directly involved in the generation of tremor itself.

Interpretational caveats: cause or consequence

A disadvantage of many neuroimaging approaches is that it is often not possible to distinguish cause from consequence. For example, tremor-related activity may reflect both efferent (tremor oscillator) and afferent processes (tremor-related somatosensory feedback). In a similar vein, abnormal GABAergic binding in essential tremor, as assessed with flumazenil-PET, may be the cause or consequence of long-standing tremor.[21] The same may even hold for structural imaging, given evidence that motor training can induce neuroplastic changes that can be detected with structural MRI.[47] Having said that, the interplay between afferents and efferents in the central nervous system is also a key pathophysiological component of tremor, and separating them (if possible) would ignore the reality. For example, in Parkinson's rest tremor, somatosensory afferents are thought to stabilize the tremor rhythm within the cerebello-thalamo-cortical circuit, likely through the ascending fibers to the cerebellum.[48] Evidence for this idea comes from studies showing that manipulation of somatosensory input (e.g., denervation, electrical stimulation, passive movements) can influence tremor amplitude, without removing the tremor.[49] To disentangle afferent from efferent contributions of a particular brain region, intervention studies are needed, such as non-invasive brain stimulation.[50] The following paragraphs summarize the insights that neuroimaging findings have provided into the pathophysiology of the four most common clinical tremor syndromes: essential tremor, Parkinson's rest tremor, dystonic tremor syndromes, and orthostatic tremor. The section focuses mainly on the most specific approaches: studies that demonstrated tremor-related activity using PET or fMRI.

NEUROIMAGING OF ESSENTIAL TREMOR

Essential tremor is an *isolated* tremor syndrome (Axis 1), which is defined as a bilateral action tremor of the upper limbs with a duration of at least three years, with or without tremor in other body areas, and without other neurological signs.[1] It is recognized that the essential tremor syndrome is clinically variable (for example in age at onset, location of symptoms, family history, response to treatment).[51,52] Furthermore, "essential tremor plus" is a new clinical entity, where tremor with the characteristics of essential

tremor is combined with additional neurological signs of unknown significance (such as questionable dystonic posturing). This may represent a temporary label, concerning patients on their way to a more definite clinical diagnosis.[53] This clinical variability is not always considered, which may explain some of the differences between the studies reviewed later.

Tremor-related activity in essential tremor

In patients with essential tremor, metabolic PET imaging has been used to identify increased tremor-related activity in the cerebellum[16] and the red nucleus.[28] In these studies, specificity was achieved by adding control conditions such as passive movements and mimicked tremor (in the controls). Furthermore, an intervention design (metabolic PET before and after gamma knife VIM thalamotomy) showed stimulation-related decreases of metabolic activity in the left thalamus, and remote metabolic decreases in the right cerebellum, left temporal gyri, and bilateral frontal gyri.[54] In a similar vein, the influence of deep brain stimulation (DBS) of the caudal zona incerta on the cerebello-thalamo-cortical circuit was investigated during postural holding and rest in essential tremor, comparing two conditions in the fMRI scanner: DBS-ON versus OFF.[55] This unique ON/OFF design allows the investigation of both pathological activity and its response to treatment. During tremor-inducing postural holding, DBS was associated with decreased cerebral activity in the primary sensorimotor cortex and cerebellar lobule III, and with increased cerebral activity in the supplementary motor area and cerebellar lobule V during rest. These effects of DBS onto the cerebellum were located within the sensorimotor cerebellar lobules (IV/V and VIII) where previous studies have shown increased tremor-related activity. This can be taken as normalization of cerebellar overactivity through treatment.

Another approach has been to use combined EMG and fMRI during voluntary posturing, to quantify brain activity associated with spontaneous fluctuations in essential tremor during posturing of the upper limbs. This revealed increased tremor-related activity in the cerebellum when compared to mimicked tremor in healthy individuals[32] (Figures 5.2A + 5.2B). In an extension of that approach, a study used effective connectivity analyses (DCM) to understand the role of interregional connectivity in essential tremor.[37] In this study, tremor variations (derived from the EMG regressor) were added as an exogenous modulatory input onto several nodes and functional connections of the cerebello-thalamo-cortical circuit in essential tremor patients. DCM was then used to test which cerebral model was most likely, given the data. The authors found a significant excitatory modulating effect of tremor variation on the cerebello-dentato-thalamic connection and on intrinsic thalamic and cerebellar lobule V activity[37] (Figure 5.2C). This finding provides support for the cerebellar oscillation hypothesis of essential tremor, which states that pathophysiological changes in the cerebellum actively drive the thalamo-cortical circuit into tremor.[2,56]

Finally, a set of studies assessed tremor-related activity by using a task that evokes tremor or modulates tremor amplitude. Specifically, a precision grip-force task can induce action tremor in patients with essential and dystonic tremor, and online visual feedback related to force ("gain") can further modulate tremor amplitude (such that a high visual gain increases tremor amplitude)[57] (Figure 5.4). A comparison of high versus low visual gain conditions observed increased task-related brain activity in the primary motor cortex, the superior parietal lobe, and the cerebellum (lobule VI) in essential tremor versus healthy controls.[58] This provides further support for the idea that cerebellar dysfunction has a role in the pathophysiology of essential tremor, since cerebellar tremors are known to worsen under visual guidance.[59] Furthermore, a direct comparison of task-related brain activity in essential tremor and dystonic tremor patients revealed differences in several nodes of the cortical motor network, but not the cerebellum[60] (Figure 5.4).

Resting state functional connectivity in essential tremor

Taken together, the studies discussed previously show that essential tremor is associated with tremor-related activity in the cerebellum, thalamus, and motor cortex. This activity is larger than that seen in voluntary movements (such as mimicked tremor), and it is reduced after effective stereotactic treatment. These findings suggest that a hyperactive cerebellum may be involved in essential tremor (cerebellar oscillator hypothesis).[2] Other studies, primarily based on resting state fMRI data, provide a different view on the role of the cerebellum, suggesting that cerebellar decoupling from the motor circuit may be involved in essential tremor (cerebellar decoupling hypothesis). For example, one study used seed-based functional connectivity in 25 essential tremor patients versus 26 healthy controls.[61] They observed decreased functional connectivity between the dentate nucleus and cortical, subcortical, and cerebellar areas in essential tremor patients. More specifically, dentate nucleus functional connectivity with the supplementary motor area, pre- and post-central gyri and prefrontal cortex negatively correlated with tremor severity and disease duration. Furthermore, dentate nucleus functional connectivity with the cerebellar cortex correlated positively with tremor amplitude, while dentate-thalamus connectivity correlated negatively with tremor amplitude. Another resting state fMRI study showed a suppression of general connectivity of the cerebellum in essential tremor patients versus controls, in line with the idea that essential tremor is a disorder with cerebellar damage.[62] Other resting state fMRI studies have shown similar effects,[33,63,64] as well as reduced regional homogeneity in the cerebellum of essential tremor patients.[65]

Structural imaging in essential tremor

In essential tremor, an MRI study showed that, relative to the healthy controls, the cerebellum in essential tremor patients exhibited reduced gray matter in lobule VIII, but increased gray matter volume in the supplementary motor area (SMA), as well as increased fractional anisotropy (FA) within the cortico-cortical tract departing from the SMA[66] (Figure 5.2D). This would suggest that the SMA compensates for cerebellar dysfunction in essential tremor. Further support for cerebellar dysfunction in essential tremor comes from a white matter microstructural integrity study.[26] The study investigated a cohort of 57 essential tremor and 99 Parkinson disease patients, who were sedated for the implantation of DBS devices, indicating that they had clinically severe motor symptoms. The greatest distinctions in essential tremor versus Parkinson disease encompassed decreased integrity in all three cerebellar peduncles, which are densely packed with afferent and efferent cerebellar projections, mediating the dentate-rubro-thalamic and cortico-ponto-cerebellar tracts. The authors hypothesized that a myelin-related process disrupts the cerebello-thalamo-cortical network, ultimately leading to the manifestation of action tremor. The white matter changes in the cerebellar peduncles were also reported by another DTI study[67] that compared 19 ET patients to 15 healthy subjects, and by a DTI study showing diffusion abnormalities

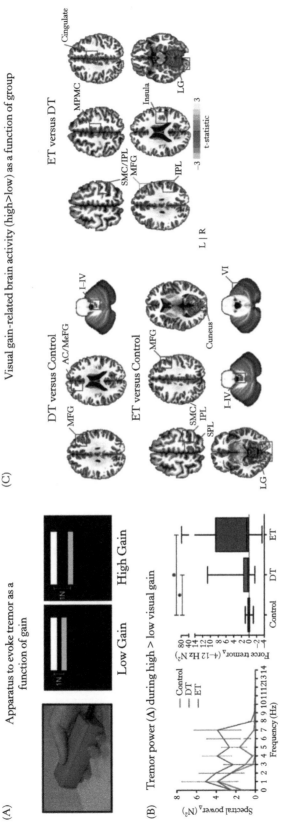

FIGURE 5.4: Task-Related Brain Activity in Dystonic Tremor (DT), Essential Tremor (ET), and Controls. Panel A shows that subjects performed a precision grip-force task wherein online visual feedback related to force was manipulated across high and low spatial feedback levels. Panel B shows that tremor power was influenced by the task (y-axis, differential spectral power during high > low gain; Δ), and more so in patients with DT and ET. This shows that the task evoked tremor. Panel C shows the pattern of brain activity evoked by the task (the difference for high>low gain is shown, which is contrasted between groups). Blue voxels represent a reduced gain-related activity in patients versus controls (on the left), and reduced gain-related activity in ET versus DT patients (on the right), while orange voxels represent the opposite. Taken from [60], with permission.

in all three cerebellar peduncles.[61] For a more complete review of structural abnormalities in the cerebellum of essential tremor, see Ref [24].

Taken together, the studies reviewed previously suggest that the cerebellum plays a key role in the pathophysiology of essential tremor, while other regions (such as the SMA) may have a compensatory role. Some studies point to cerebellar *hyperactivity*, supporting the idea that the cerebellum may act as an oscillator in essential tremor.[56] Other studies indicate structural and functional cerebellar *disconnection* from the motor network, supporting the idea that cerebellar decoupling contributes to essential tremor.[2] Whether or not both phenomena play a role in (different patients with) essential tremor remains to be investigated.

NEUROIMAGING OF TREMOR IN PARKINSON DISEASE

Parkinson's tremor falls into the category of the *combined* tremor syndromes (Axis 1) and is clinically defined as tremor accompanied by parkinsonism (bradykinesia and rigidity).[1] Classical parkinsonian tremor is characterized by a 4- to 7-Hz rest tremor of the hand ("pill-rolling" tremor), lower limb, jaw, tongue, or foot. It is well-known that other types of tremor also exist in Parkinson disease.[68] The most common postural tremor, occurring in approximately two-thirds of patients, is re-emergent tremor: rest tremor that diminishes after a rapid movement of the trembling limb, but returns to a stable postural position after a variable amount of time (usually seconds, but may take up to several minutes), at approximately the same frequency as rest tremor. Another subtype of parkinsonian postural tremor is pure postural tremor, which is seen in a smaller proportion of patients and starts immediately upon change from a resting to a postural position of the hand, displays a clearly higher frequency than rest tremor (>1.5 Hz) and smaller amplitude, and does not respond to dopaminergic medication.[68] Finally, kinetic tremors and (more rarely) orthostatic tremor can occur in PD.[69] Most of the studies reviewed later focused on the classical parkinsonian rest tremor.

Tremor-related brain activity in Parkinson's rest tremor

One of the first neuroimaging studies that mapped the cerebral tremor network in Parkinson disease used 15-O-labeled water ($H_2^{15}O$) PET in eight patients that had received unilateral ventral intermediate (VIM) thalamic nucleus DBS

for severe tremor.[70] Decreased regional cerebral blood flow during stimulation was observed in the contralateral motor cortex, the SMA, and the ipsilateral cerebellum. In another study, the same researchers compared brain activity OFF versus ON DBS of the VIM, which is homologous to the posterior ventrolateral nucleus of the thalamus (VLp) according to Jones,[71] and of the subthalamic nucleus (STN) in two separate groups of Parkinson disease patients[72] (Figure 5.5). This study showed a consistent metabolic pattern associated with stimulation-mediated tremor suppression, characterized by covarying increases in the activity of the cerebellum/dentate nucleus and primary motor cortex, and, to a lesser degree, the caudate/putamen. While DBS of both the STN and the VIM reduced brain activity in this tremor-related network, only STN stimulation reduced activity in a distinct, Parkinson's Disease Related Pattern (PDRP), which has been associated with bradykinesia and rigidity.[8]

Other studies investigated Parkinson's tremor by combining resting state fMRI with EMG recordings, to quantify brain activity associated with spontaneous fluctuations in rest tremor. More specifically, in these studies the EMG regressor was used to capture two different aspects of the spontaneous tremor dynamics: tremor amplitude (scan-by-scan EMG power at tremor frequency) and tremor on/offset (first temporal derivative of the tremor amplitude regressor, which peaks whenever tremor amplitude increases)[31,36] (Figure 5.1). In this way, tremor amplitude-related activity was identified in the cerebello-thalamo-cortical circuit, and tremor on/offset related activity was identified in the basal ganglia. These findings are robust, and have been consistently shown across multiple different cohorts.[38,39] This distinction formed the basis for the dimmer-switch hypothesis of rest tremor in Parkinson disease, which states that the basal ganglia trigger tremor episodes, while the cerebello-thalamo-cortical circuit maintains and amplifies the tremor.[73]

Further studies tested the effect of dopaminergic medication and cognitive task conditions on tremor-related activity. Specifically, a pharmacological imaging study in Parkinson disease patients showed that there was stronger tremor-related activity in the thalamus (VIM) and internal globus pallidus (GPi) during an untreated (OFF-state) session as compared to a session where patients had taken their dopaminergic medication (ON-state).[38] Effective connectivity analyses (DCM) showed that the main target of dopamine was the VIM rather than the GPi, and

Cerebral perfusion on vs. off VLp stimulation (PET)

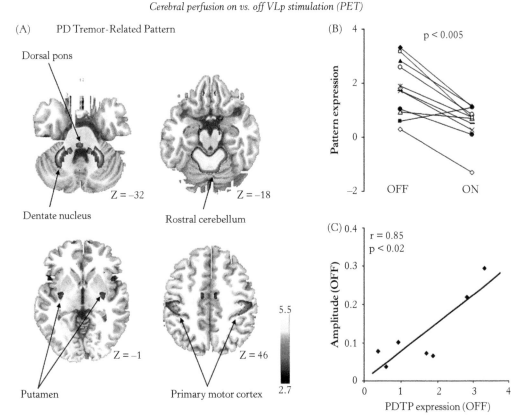

FIGURE 5.5: Metabolic Correlates of Parkinson's Rest Tremor **(PET).** (A) Spatial covariance pattern identified by ordinal trends canonical variate analysis of FDG PET data from 11 hemispheres of nine tremor-dominant PD patients scanned on and off VLp stimulation (labeled VIM in the original manuscript). VLp (which is homologous to VIM) stimulation improved tremor severity and reduced metabolic activity in the primary motor cortex, anterior cerebellum / dorsal pons, and the caudate / putamen. (B) The expression of this PD tremor-related metabolic pattern (PDTP) was reduced by VLp stimulation in 10 of the 11 treated hemispheres. (C) Baseline PDTP expression (i.e., off-stimulation pattern scores) correlated (r = 0.85, p<0.02) with tremor amplitude, measured with concurrent accelerometry. These data show that metabolic activity in both the cortico-cerebellar circuit and the basal ganglia is related to tremor severity. Reprinted from [72], with permission. Abbreviations: VLp = ventral lateral nucleus, posterior part; PD = Parkinson's disease; PDTP = Parkinson's disease tremor-related pattern; PET = positron emission tomography.

that the effect in the VIM was not a downstream consequence of dopamine acting on the basal ganglia (Figure 5.6C). Thus, dopaminergic projections to the thalamus, which are present both in non-human primates and in humans,[74,75] may have a role in the pathophysiology of rest tremor in Parkinson disease.

Another study compared different Parkinson subgroups with each other, i.e., Parkinson disease patients with a (clinically) dopamine-responsive or dopamine-resistant rest tremor.[39] Clinical studies suggest that ± 40% of Parkinson disease patients with rest tremor do not respond

to a levodopa challenge (200/50 mg levodopa benserazide + 10 mg domperidone), even though other motor symptoms (bradykinesia and rigidity) respond well to levodopa.[76] Using combined EMG and fMRI, it was found that patients with a dopamine-resistant tremor had more tremor-related activity in the cerebellum (including the interposed nuclei), while patients with a dopamine-responsive tremor had more tremor-related activity in the thalamus (VIM) and somatosensory cortex (Figures 5.6A and 5.6B).[39] Thus, regional differences in the dysfunction of nodes within the cerebello-thalamo-cortical may

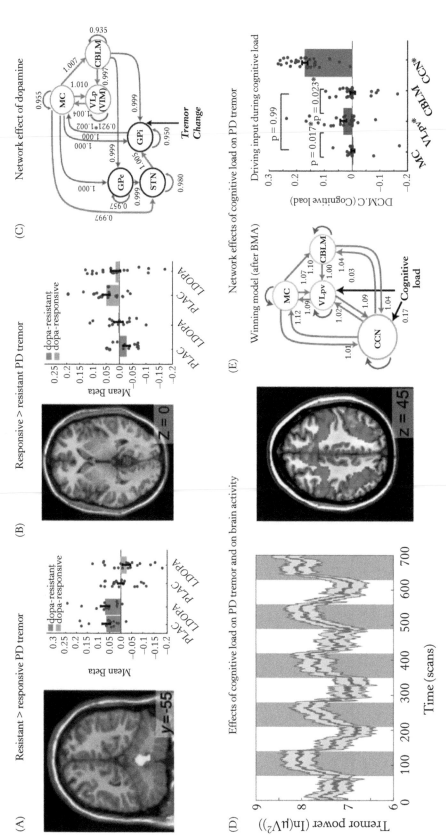

FIGURE 5.6: The Effects of Dopamine and Noradrenaline on Parkinson's Rest Tremor.

FIGURE 5.6 CONTINUED

Panels A and B show differences in tremor-related activity (using concurrent EMG-fMRI; mean beta on the y-axis) in PD patients with a dopamine-resistant (blue bars) versus dopamine-responsive (orange bars) tremor. All patients were measured twice: during placebo and during 200/50 mg levodopa-benserazide (x-axis). Taken from [39], with permission. Panel C shows the winning model in a model comparison of how dopaminergic medication (two sessions: OFF versus ON the patients' own medication) influenced the basal ganglia-cerebello-thalamo-cortical circuit, using dynamic causal modeling. In the winning model, dopaminergic medication influenced the circuit by acting on the ventrolateral thalamus (ventral intermediate nucleus; VIM, indicated in yellow). Taken from [38], with permission. Panel D shows how cognitive load (mental arithmetic) influences tremor power (measured with EMG, y-axis). The x-axis shows the time in scans; rest (white columns) and mental arithmetic (gray columns) conditions (60 seconds per block) alternated. The image on the right shows brain activity that increased as a function of cognitive load (in red), which overlapped with brain regions where activity correlated with changes in pupil diameter (in yellow) during scanning (SPM{t}, shown at a threshold of p<0.001 uncorrected, for graphical purposes). Panel E shows the winning model of how cognitive load influenced the cerebello-thalamo-cortical network, using dynamic causal modeling (DCM): by acting on the ventrolateral thalamus (VLpv) and by connecting, through the cognitive control network (CCN, see panel D) with the different regions of the cerebello-thalamo-cortical network (red arrows). The posterior ventrolateral nucleus of the thalamus (VLp according to Jones), especially the ventral portion (VLpv), is analogous to the VIM [71]. Taken from [40], with permission. Abbreviations: CBLM = cerebellum, CCN = cognitive control network; GPe = external globus pallidus, GPi = internal globus pallidus, LDOPA = levodopa; MC = motor cortex; PD = Parkinson's disease, PLAC = placebo, STN = subthalamic nucleus, VIM = ventral intermediate nucleus, VLp = ventral lateral nucleus of the thalamus, posterior part.

explain the response of rest tremor to dopaminergic medication in Parkinson disease.

Finally, a related study addressed the well-known clinical observation that cognitive effort and stress can increase Parkinson's rest tremor.[77,78] Using a block-wise alternation of rest versus cognitive load (mental arithmetic) while measuring tremor-related brain activity with concurrent EMG and fMRI, it was shown that Parkinson disease patients had stronger tremor-related activity in the thalamus (VIM) and secondary somatosensory cortex during cognitive load as compared to the rest condition, while tremor-related activity in the cerebello-thalamo-cortical circuit was present across both conditions.[40] Furthermore, cognitive load was associated with facilitatory network effects onto the thalamus, and these effects correlated with inter-individual differences in increased pupil diameter during cognitive load. Taken together, this suggests that ascending noradrenergic projections toward the thalamus may have a role in increasing tremor during cognitive stress (Figures 5.6D and 5.6E).

Structural imaging in Parkinson's rest tremor

Several studies compared regional gray matter volume between Parkinson disease patients with and without rest tremor, using VBM of T1-weighted MRI scans. A comparison of tremor-dominant PD patients to matched healthy controls revealed increased gray matter volume in the thalamus (VIM) contralateral to the tremor side, and increased volume correlated positively with tremor amplitude.[22] The positive correlation with tremor amplitude suggests that the finding is specific to tremor. Another study compared 14 Parkinson disease patients with rest tremor to 10 non-tremor patients, and reported reduced gray matter volume in the right cerebellum (posterior part of the right quadrangular lobe and the declive) in the tremor-dominant group.[79] A comparison of Parkinson disease patients with the postural instability and gait disorder subtype (PIGD) versus tremor-dominant patients showed widespread reductions in gray matter volume in the PIGD group, compared with the tremor-dominant group, in brain areas that involve motor, cognitive, limbic, and associative functions.[80] A subsequent study from the same group of researchers demonstrated also lower amygdala and globus pallidus gray matter volume in the PIGD group.[81] These studies show that it is difficult to attribute cerebral differences between clinical subtypes of Parkinson disease to a particular symptom (such as tremor). Instead, the findings fit with the notion that the PIGD subtype has a more widespread pathophysiology than is found in patients with a tremor-dominant phenotype.

Resting state fMRI in Parkinson's rest tremor

A number of studies have used resting state fMRI in Parkinson disease patients with and without tremor to identify cerebral "traits" that differ between subgroups, for example a higher amplitude of low-frequency fluctuations (ALFF) in the cerebellum,[82] increased functional connectivity of the VIM with the cerebellum and motor cortex, among other regions,[83] and increased functional connectivity between the dentate nucleus and the cerebellar cortex.[84]

Taken together, the studies reviewed previously suggest that the cerebello-thalamo-cortical circuit plays a key role in the pathophysiology of Parkinson's rest tremor, likely in concert with the basal ganglia, and under influence of both dopaminergic and noradrenergic projections primarily to the thalamus (VIM). The pathophysiology of other types of tremor in Parkinson disease, such as re-emergent tremor, "pure postural tremor," and kinetic tremor, is less clear.

NEUROIMAGING OF DYSTONIC TREMOR SYNDROMES

Dystonic tremor syndromes are tremor syndromes combining tremor and dystonia as the leading neurological signs.[1] Tremor in a body part affected by dystonia is called "dystonic tremor." Common examples include tremulous cervical dystonia (dystonic head tremor) and segmental tremulous dystonia affecting the head and upper limbs. If the tremor is located in a different body part than the dystonia, this is called "tremor associated with dystonia." Dystonic tremor syndromes are perhaps even more variable, clinically, than essential tremor. Unlike essential tremor, which by definition occurs during actions of both arms, dystonic tremor syndromes can occur in the head, the voice, the arms, or (rarely) the legs. This clinical variability, together with the small number of available imaging studies, makes it more difficult to clarify the cerebral mechanisms involved in dystonic tremor syndromes. The available evidence is summarized later.

A structural MRI study compared gray matter volume and white matter integrity (using DTI) in 10 patients with primary writing tremor versus 10 heathy controls. It was found that patients with primary writing tremor had predominant gray matter atrophy in parts of cerebellum and frontal lobe, along with white matter changes of the cingulum and frontal lobe connections.[85] Another study used MRI to compare 12 dystonic tremor patients to 14 essential tremor patients and 23 healthy controls. Patients with dystonic tremor showed a thickening and increased gray matter volume of the left sensorimotor cortex when compared to the other groups.[86]

Patients with spasmodic dysphonia with and without voice tremor were compared using fMR during sentence production, which evokes dystonia in these patients. A group comparison showed that patients with voice tremor had increased task-related activity in the right cerebellum (lobule VIIa) and the right middle frontal gyrus.[87] The same research group reported that spasmodic dysphonia patients with and without voice tremor both show reduced functional connectivity in left inferior parietal cortex, putamen, and bilateral premotor cortices compared to healthy controls. This finding was not tremor specific, but rather a characteristic of dystonia. In the subsequent effective connectivity analysis, patients with voice tremor showed decreased self-inhibitory influences in the left inferior parietal cortex, right premotor cortex and the left putamen compared to patients without tremor. This tremor-specific finding argues for involvement of a basal-ganglia-cortical loop in voice tremor.[88]

Finally, patients with essential tremor and dystonic tremor were compared used fMRI during a grip-force-task (sensitive to grip-force tremor).[60] The dystonic tremor group included primarily cervical dystonia patients with dystonic head tremor (19/20) and the majority of these (13/19) had additional upper-limb tremor. The essential tremor group was unfortunately not further specified. Cerebellar activity did not differ between patients with dystonic tremor and patients with essential tremor. Although cerebral activity in this task is only a proxy of actual tremor-related activity, this finding supports the notion that tremor in dystonia might emerge from similar cerebellar mechanisms as essential tremor. Also, widespread reduced functional connectivity was found in cortical, basal ganglia and cerebellar regions in patients with dystonic tremor compared to essential tremor (Figure 5.4). It remains unclear whether this is characteristic of dystonia, dystonic tremor, or a combination.

Taken together, the studies reviewed previously suggest that dystonic tremor syndromes are linked to abnormal brain activity in the cerebellum, basal ganglia, and more widespread cortical regions.[2] Given the large inter-individual differences in tremor phenotype, it is possible that there are different pathophysiological subgroups that fall under the umbrella of dystonic tremor syndromes, each with their own neuroimaging characteristics.

NEUROIMAGING OF ORTHOSTATIC TREMOR

Primary orthostatic tremor (OT) is defined as a generalized high-frequency (13–18 Hz) isolated tremor syndrome that occurs when standing.[1] Confirmation of the tremor frequency is needed, typically with EMG. Patients typically complain of instability when standing, and the tremor itself is often not observed. OT is a rare disorder, and therefore neuroimaging studies are scarce.

A comparison of 17 OT patients with 17 healthy controls revealed reduced gray matter volume in the lateral cerebellum (lobule VI) and SMA, and increased gray matter volume in the cerebellar vermis. The latter was interpreted as compensatory, given a positive correlation with the duration of standing position.[89] Another study used DTI to investigate white matter tracts in OT. White matter changes (both increases and decreases in OT versus controls) were preferentially located in the cerebellum, its efferent pathways, and in the pontine tegmentum and elements of the frontal-thalamic-cerebellar circuit.[90] Finally, a PET study investigated cerebral metabolism (using 18-FDG PET) in 10 OT patients and 10 healthy controls during standing and lying. While lying, patients had an increased regional cerebral glucose metabolism in the pontine tegmentum, posterior cerebellum (including the dentate nuclei), ventral intermediate and ventral posterolateral nucleus of the thalamus, and the bilateral primary motor cortex, compared to controls. Similar glucose metabolism changes occurred with clinical manifestation of the tremor during standing. The glucose metabolism was relatively decreased in medial frontal cortical areas, and this effect correlated with increased body sway.[91]

Taken together, these findings point to the key role of the cerebellum in the pathophysiology of OT, but also to the role of the medial frontal cortex (including the SMA) in balance disorders in OT patients.

CONCLUSION

Neuroimaging can be used during the clinical workup of a patient with tremor to identify the etiology. Specifically, structural MRI is useful to search for underlying brain lesions especially if the tremor is combined with other signs or symptoms, is unilateral or focal, started abruptly, and/or is unusual in appearance. Nuclear imaging of the dopaminergic system (e.g., DAT-SPECT) is useful to distinguish tremor combined with parkinsonism (Parkinson disease or atypical parkinsonism) from other tremor syndromes (dystonic tremor syndrome, essential tremor syndrome).

Furthermore, neuroimaging is also increasingly used in research contexts to assess the pathophysiology of tremor. Different approaches have assessed the cerebral mechanisms of tremor as a trait (a comparison of groups with different expressions of tremor) or as a state (a comparison of different conditions associated with more or less tremor). Most evidence is available for essential tremor and Parkinson's rest tremor. In essential tremor, neuroimaging studies suggest that individuals with essential tremor have reduced gray matter volume in the cerebellum and reduced structural and functional connectivity of the cerebellum. At the same time, activity in the cerebello-thalamo-cortical circuit is increased during conditions that evoke postural or kinetic tremor. This suggest that essential tremor patients have a structurally impaired, "decoupled" cerebellum, which at the same time is actively involved in tremor generation ("cerebellar oscillation hypothesis"). It remains unclear whether these effects may vary between individuals. In Parkinson's rest tremor, tremor-related activity has been found both in the basal ganglia and in the cerebello-thalamo-cortical circuit. Dopaminergic medication reduces tremor by acting on the thalamus (VIM), while cognitive load increases tremor by exciting the VIM, likely through ascending noradrenergic projections. Parkinson disease patients with a dopamine-resistant tremor have increased tremor-related activity in the cerebellum as compared to dopamine-responsive patients. In patients with dystonic tremor and OT syndromes, the available empirical evidence is limited. Future studies may focus on the role of cerebral network properties in the pathophysiology of tremor, and on inter-individual differences between patients with tremor.

REFERENCES

1. Bhatia KP, Bain P, Bajaj N, et al. Consensus statement on the classification of tremors. from the task force on tremor of the International Parkinson and Movement Disorder Society. *Mov Disord.* 2017;33(1):75–87.

2. Madelein van der Stouwe AM, Nieuwhof F, Helmich RC. Tremor pathophysiology: lessons from neuroimaging. *Curr Opin Neurol.* 2020;33(4):474–481.

3. van de Wardt J, van der Stouwe AMM, Dirkx M, et al. Systematic clinical approach for diagnosing upper limb tremor. *J Neurol Neurosurg Psychiatr.* 2020;91(8):822–830. doi: 10.1136/jnnp-2019-322676

4. Cho C, Samkoff LM. A lesion of the anterior thalamus producing dystonic tremor of the hand. *Arch Neurol.* 2000;57(9):1353–1355.

5. Raina GB, Cersosimo MG, Folgar SS, et al. Holmes tremor: clinical description, lesion localization, and treatment in a series of 29 cases. *Neurology.* 2016;86(10):931–938. doi: 10.1212/WNL.0000000000002440

6. Tilikete C, Desestret V. Hypertrophic olivary degeneration and palatal or oculopalatal tremor. *Front Neurol.* 2017;8:302.

7. Schneider SA, Edwards MJ, Mir P, et al. Patients with adult-onset dystonic tremor resembling parkinsonian tremor have scans without evidence of dopaminergic deficit (SWEDDs). *Mov Disord.* 2007;22(15):2210–2215.

8. Schindlbeck KA, Eidelberg D. Network imaging biomarkers: insights and clinical applications in Parkinson's disease. *Lancet Neurol.* 2018;17(7):629–640.

9. Nieuwhof F, de Bie RMA, Praamstra P, et al. The cerebral tremor circuit in a patient with Holmes tremor. *Ann Clin Transl Neurol.* 2020;7(8):1453–1458. doi: 10.1002/acn3.51143

10. Seidel S, Kasprian G, Leutmezer F, et al. Disruption of nigrostriatal and cerebello-thalamic pathways in dopamine responsive Holmes' tremor. *J Neurol Neurosurg Psychiatr.* 2009;80(8):921–923.

11. Fasano A, Helmich RC. Tremor habituation to deep brain stimulation: underlying mechanisms and solutions. *Mov Disord.* 2019;13(3):2–13.

12. Fasano A, Lozano AM, Cubo E. New neurosurgical approaches for tremor and Parkinson's disease. *Curr Opin Neurol.* 2017;30(4):435–446.

13. Coenen VA, Allert N, Paus S, et al. Modulation of the cerebello-thalamo-cortical network in thalamic deep brain stimulation for tremor. *Neurosurgery.* 2014;75(6):657–670.

14. Nowacki A, Schlaier J, Debove I, Pollo C. Validation of diffusion tensor imaging tractography to visualize the dentatorubrothalamic tract for surgical planning. *J Neurosurg.* 2018;130(1):99–108.

15. Sajonz BEA, Amtage F, Reinacher PC, et al. Deep brain stimulation for tremor tractographic versus traditional (distinct): study protocol of a randomized controlled feasibility trial. *JMIR Res Protoc.* 2016;5(4):e244.

16. Colebatch JG, Findley LJ, Frackowiak RS, et al. Preliminary report: activation of the cerebellum in essential tremor. *Lancet.* 1990;336(8722):1028–1030.

17. Isaias IU, Marotta G, Hirano S, et al. Imaging essential tremor. *Mov Disord.* 2010;25(6):679–686.

18. Pirker W. Correlation of dopamine transporter imaging with parkinsonian motor handicap: how close is it? *Mov Disord.* 2003;18(S7):S43–S51.

19. Qamhawi Z, Towey D, Shah B, et al. Clinical correlates of raphe serotonergic dysfunction in early Parkinson's disease. *Brain.* 2015;138(Pt 10):2964–2973.

20. Doder M, Rabiner EA, Turjanski N, et al. Tremor in Parkinson's disease and serotonergic dysfunction: an 11C-WAY 100635 PET study. *Neurology.* 2003;60(4):601–605.

21. Boecker H, Weindl A, Brooks DJ, et al. GABAergic dysfunction in essential tremor: an 11C-Flumazenil PET study. *J Nucl Med.* 2010;51(7):1030–1035.

22. Kassubek J, Juengling FD, Hellwig B, et al. Thalamic gray matter changes in unilateral Parkinsonian resting tremor: a voxel-based morphometric analysis of 3-dimensional magnetic resonance imaging. *Neurosci Lett.* 2002;323(1):29–32.

23. Daniels C, Peller M, Wolff S, et al. Voxel-based morphometry shows no decreases in cerebellar gray matter volume in essential tremor. *Neurology.* 2006;67(8):1452–1456.

24. Cerasa A, Quattrone A. Linking essential tremor to the cerebellum—neuroimaging evidence. *Cerebellum.* 2015;15(3):263–275.

25. Martinelli P, Rizzo G, Manners D, et al. Diffusion-weighted imaging study of patients with essential tremor. *Mov Disord.* 2007;22(8):1182–1185.

26. Juttukonda MR, Franco G, Englot DJ, et al. White matter differences between essential tremor and Parkinson disease. *Neurology.* 2019;92(1):e30–e39.

27. Homayoon N, Pirpamer L, Franthal S, et al. Nigral iron deposition in common tremor disorders. *Mov Disord.* 2019;34(1):129–132. doi: 10.1002/mds.27549

28. Bucher SF, Seelos KC, Dodel RC, et al. Activation mapping in essential tremor with functional magnetic resonance imaging. *Ann Neurol.* 1997;41(1):32–40.

29. Passamonti L, Novellino F, Cerasa A, et al. Altered cortical-cerebellar circuits during verbal working memory in essential tremor. *Brain.* 2011;134(Pt 8):2274–2286. doi: 10.1093/brain/awr164

30. Kahan J, Urner M, Moran R, et al. Resting state functional MRI in Parkinson's disease: the

impact of deep brain stimulation on "effective" connectivity. *Brain*. 2014;137(4):1130–1144.

31. Helmich RC, Janssen MJR, Oyen WJG, et al. Pallidal dysfunction drives a cerebellothalamic circuit into Parkinson tremor. *Ann Neurol*. 2011;69(2):269–281.

32. Broersma M, van der Stouwe AMM, Buijink AWG, et al. Bilateral cerebellar activation in uni-laterally challenged essential tremor. *Neuroimage Clin*. 2016;11:1–9.

33. Fang W, Chen H, Wang H, et al. Essential tremor is associated with disruption of functional con-nectivity in the ventral intermediate Nucleus–Motor Cortex–Cerebellum circuit. *Hum Brain Mapp*. 2016;37(1):165–178.

34. Benito-León J, Sanz Morales E, Melero H, et al. Graph theory analysis of resting-state functional magnetic resonance imaging in essential tremor. *Hum Brain Mapp*. 2019;40(16):4686–4702.

35. Friston KJ, Harrison L, Penny W. Dynamic causal modelling. *NeuroImage*. 2003;19(4):1273–1302.

36. Dirkx MF, Ouden den H, Aarts E, et al. The cerebral network of Parkinson's tremor: an effective connectivity fMRI study. *J Neurosci*. 2016;36(19):5362–5372.

37. Buijink AWG, van der Stouwe AMM, Broersma M, et al. Motor network disruption in essential tremor: a functional and effective connectivity study. *Brain*. 2015;138(Pt 10):2934–2947.

38. Dirkx MF, Ouden den HEM, Aarts E, et al. Dopamine controls Parkinson's tremor by inhibiting the cerebellar thalamus. *Brain*. 2017;140(3):721–734.

39. Dirkx MF, Zach H, Van Nuland A, et al. Cerebral differences between dopamine-resistant and dopamine-responsive Parkinson's tremor. *Brain*. 2019;16:197–114.

40. Dirkx MF, Zach H, van Nuland AJ, et al. Cognitive load amplifies Parkinson's tremor through excitatory network influences onto the thalamus. *Brain*. 2020;143(5):1498–1511.

41. Dupuis MJ-M, Evrard FL, Jacquerye PG, et al. Disappearance of essential tremor after stroke. *Mov Disord*. 2010;25(16):2884–2887.

42. Choi S-M, Lee S-H, Park M-S, et al. Disappearance of resting tremor after thalamic stroke involv-ing the territory of the tuberothalamic artery. *Parkinsonism Relat Disord*. 2008;14(4):373–375.

43. Probst-Cousin S, Druschky A, Neundörfer B. Disappearance of resting tremor after "stereotaxic" thalamic stroke. *Neurology*. 2003;61(7):1013–1014.

44. Deuschl G, Wilms H, Krack P, et al. Function of the cerebellum in Parkinsonian rest tremor and Holmes' tremor. *Ann Neurol*. 1999;46(1):126–128.

45. Joutsa J, Shih LC, Fox MD. Mapping Holmes tremor circuit using the human brain connec-tome. *Ann Neurol*. 2019;27(3):327–9.

46. Fox MD. Mapping symptoms to brain networks with the human connectome. *N Engl J Med*. 2018;379(23):2237–2245.

47. Draganski B, Gaser C, Busch V, et al. Neuroplasticity: changes in grey matter induced by training. *Nature*. 2004;427(6972):311–312.

48. Volkmann J, Joliot M, Mogilner A, et al. Central motor loop oscillations in parkinsonian resting tremor revealed by magnetoencephalography. *Neurology*. 1996;46(5):1359–1370.

49. Helmich RC. The cerebral basis of Parkinsonian tremor: a network perspective. *Mov Disord*. 2018;33(2):219–231.

50. Ni Z, Pinto AD, Lang AE, Chen R. Involvement of the cerebellothalamocorti-cal pathway in Parkinson disease. *Ann Neurol*. 2010;68(6):816–824.

51. Hopfner F, Ahlf A, Lorenz D, et al. Early- and late-onset essential tremor patients repre-sent clinically distinct subgroups. *Mov Disord*. 2016;31(10):1560–1566.

52. Louis ED. Essential tremors: a family of neu-rodegenerative disorders? *Arch Neurol*. 2009;66(10):1202–1208.

53. Vidailhet M. Essential tremor-plus: a temporary label. *Lancet Neurol*. 2020;19(3):202–203. doi: 10.1016/S1474-4422(19)30442-9

54. Verger A, Witjas T, Carron R, et al. Metabolic pos-itron emission tomography response to gamma knife of the ventral intermediate nucleus in essen-tial tremor. *Neurosurgery*. 2019;84(6):E294–E303.

55. Awad A, Blomstedt P, Westling G, Eriksson J. Deep brain stimulation in the caudal zona incerta modulates the sensorimotor cerebello-cerebral circuit in essential tremor. *NeuroImage*. 2020;209:116511.

56. Pan M-K, Li Y-S, Wong S-B, et al. Cerebellar oscillations driven by synaptic pruning defi-cits of cerebellar climbing fibers contribute to tremor pathophysiology. *Sci Transl Med*. 2020;12(526):1–14.

57. Neely KA, Kurani AS, Shukla P, et al. Functional brain activity relates to 0–3 and 3–8 Hz force oscillations in essential tremor. *Cereb Cortex*. 2015;25(11):4191–4202.

58. Archer DB, Coombes SA, Chu WT, et al. A wide-spread visually-sensitive functional network relates to symptoms in essential tremor. *Brain*. 2017;141(2):472–485.

59. Sanes JN, LeWitt PA, Mauritz KH. Visual and mechanical control of postural and kinetic tremor in cerebellar system disorders. *J Neurol Neurosurg Psychiatr*. 1988;51(7):934–943.

60. DeSimone JC, Archer DB, Vaillancourt DE, Wagle Shukla A. Network-level connectiv-ity is a critical feature distinguishing dystonic tremor and essential tremor. *Brain*. 2019;28(Pt 1):863–816.

61. Tikoo S, Pietracupa S, Tommasin S, et al. Functional disconnection of the dentate nucleus in essential tremor. *J Neurol*. 2020;267(5):1358–1367. doi: 10.1007/s00415-020-09711-9

62. Mueller K, Jech R, Hoskovcová M, et al. General and selective brain connectivity alterations in essential tremor: a resting state fMRI study. *NeuroImage: Clinical*. 2017;16:468–476.

63. Benito-León J, Louis ED, Romero JP, et al. Altered functional connectivity in essential tremor. *Medicine*. 2015;94(49):e1936–e1939.

64. Fang W, Chen H, Wang H, et al. Multiple resting-state networks are associated with tremors and cognitive features in essential tremor. *Mov Disord*. 2015;30(14):1926–1936.

65. Fang W, Lv F, Luo T, et al. Abnormal regional homogeneity in patients with essential tremor revealed by resting-state functional MRI. *PLoS ONE*. 2013;8(7):e69199–e69111.

66. Gallea C, Popa T, Garcia-Lorenzo D, et al. Intrinsic signature of essential tremor in the cerebello-frontal network. *Brain*. 2015;138(Pt 10):2920–2933.

67. Pietracupa S, Bologna M, Bharti K, et al. White matter rather than gray matter damage characterizes essential tremor. *Eur Radiol*. 2019;29(12):6634–6642. doi: 10.1007/s00330-019-06267-9

68. Dirkx MF, Zach H, Bloem BR, et al. The nature of postural tremor in Parkinson disease. *Neurology*. 2018;90(13):e1095–e1103.

69. Louis ED, Levy G, Côte LJ, et al. Clinical correlates of action tremor in Parkinson disease. *Arch Neurol*. 2001;58(10):1630–1634.

70. Fukuda M. Thalamic stimulation for parkinsonian tremor: correlation between regional cerebral blood flow and physiological tremor characteristics. *NeuroImage*. 2004;21(2):608–615.

71. Percheron G, François C, Talbi B, et al. The primate motor thalamus. *Brain Res Brain Res Rev*. 1996;22(2):93–181.

72. Mure H, Hirano S, Tang CC, et al. Parkinson's disease tremor-related metabolic network: characterization, progression, and treatment effects. *NeuroImage*. 2011;54(2):1244–1253.

73. Helmich RC, Hallett M, Deuschl G, et al. Cerebral causes and consequences of parkinsonian resting tremor: a tale of two circuits? *Brain*. 2012;135(Pt 11):3206–3226.

74. García-Cabezas MA, Rico B, Sánchez-González MA, Cavada C. Distribution of the dopamine innervation in the macaque and human thalamus. *NeuroImage*. 2007;34(3):965–984.

75. Sánchez-González MA, García-Cabezas MA, Rico B, Cavada C. The primate thalamus is a key target for brain dopamine. *J Neurosci*. 2005;25(26):6076–6083.

76. Zach H, Dirkx MF, Roth D, et al. Dopamine-responsive and dopamine-resistant resting tremor in Parkinson disease. *Neurology*. 2020;95(11):e1461–e1470.

77. Berlot R, Rothwell JC, Bhatia KP, Kojovic M. Variability of movement disorders: the influence of sensation, action, cognition, and emotions. *Mov Disord*. 2020;75(2):1132–1133.

78. Zach H, Dirkx M, Bloem BR, Helmich RC. The clinical evaluation of Parkinson's tremor. *J Parkinsons Dis*. 2015;5(3):471–474.

79. Benninger DH, Thees S, Kollias SS, et al. Morphological differences in Parkinson's disease with and without rest tremor. *J Neurol*. 2009;256(2):256–263.

80. Rosenberg-Katz K, Herman T, Jacob Y, et al. Gray matter atrophy distinguishes between Parkinson disease motor subtypes. *Neurology*. 2013;80(16):1476–1484. doi: 10.1212/WNL.0b013e31828cfaa4

81. Rosenberg-Katz K, Herman T, Jacob Y, et al. Subcortical volumes differ in Parkinson's disease motor subtypes: new insights into the pathophysiology of disparate symptoms. *Front Hum Neurosci*. 2016;10:387–389.

82. Chen H-M, Wang Z-J, Fang J-P, et al. Different patterns of spontaneous brain activity between tremor-dominant and postural instability/gait difficulty subtypes of Parkinson's disease: a resting-state fMRI study. *CNS Neurosci Ther*. 2015;21(10):855–866.

83. Zhang J-R, Feng T, Hou Y-N, et al. Functional connectivity of vim nucleus in tremor- and akinetic-/rigid-dominant Parkinson's disease. *CNS Neurosci Ther*. 2016;22(5):378–386.

84. Ma H, Chen H, Fang J, et al. Resting-state functional connectivity of dentate nucleus is associated with tremor in Parkinson's disease. *J Neurol*. 2015;262(10):2247–2256.

85. Jhunjhunwala K, George L, Kotikalapudi R, et al. A preliminary study of the neuroanatomical correlates of primary writing tremor: role of cerebellum. *Neuroradiology*. 2016;58(8):827–836. doi: 10.1007/s00234-016-1700-3

86. Cerasa A, Nisticò R, Salsone M, et al. Neuroanatomical correlates of dystonic tremor: a cross-sectional study. *Parkinsonism Relat Disord*. 2014;20(3):314–317.

87. Kirke DN, Battistella G, Kumar V, et al. Neural correlates of dystonic tremor: a multimodal study of voice tremor in spasmodic dysphonia. *Brain Imaging Behav*. 2017;11:166–175. doi:10.1007/s11682-016-9513-x

88. Battistella G, Simonyan K. Top-down alteration of funct ional connectivity within the sensorimotor network in focal dystonia. *Neurology*. 2019;92(16):e1843–e1851.

89. Gallea C, Popa T, Garcia-Lorenzo D, et al. Orthostatic tremor: a cerebellar pathology? *Brain*. 2016;139(8):2182–2197.

90. Benito-León J, Romero JP, Louis ED, et al. Diffusion tensor imaging in orthostatic tremor: a tract-based spatial statistics study. *Ann Clin Transl Neurol*. 2019;6(11):2212–2222.

91. Schöberl F, Feil K, Xiong G, et al. Pathological ponto-cerebello-thalamo-cortical activations in primary orthostatic tremor during lying and stance. *Brain*. 2016;140(1):83–97.

92. Timmermann L, Gross J, Dirks M, et al. The cerebral oscillatory network of parkinsonian resting tremor. *Brain*. 2003;126(Pt 1):199–212.

6

Genetics of Tremors

KRISTOFFER HAUGARVOLL AND OWEN A. ROSS

INTRODUCTION

According to revised consensus criteria for classifying tremor disorders published by the International Parkinson and Movement Disorder Society in 2018, tremor is defined as *an involuntary, rhythmic, oscillatory movement of a body part*.[1] Importantly, slight tremor of the limbs and head when unsupported is a physiological phenomenon, termed physiological tremor. Physiological tremor is generally not visible or symptomatic unless it is enhanced by fatigue or anxiety, whereas pathological tremor is usually visible and persistent.

Tremor is classified along two axes: Axis 1—clinical characteristics, including historical features (age at onset, family history, and temporal evolution), tremor characteristics (body distribution, activation condition), associated signs (systemic, neurological), and laboratory tests (electrophysiology, imaging); and Axis 2—etiology (acquired, genetic, or idiopathic). Tremor syndromes, consisting of either isolated tremor or tremor combined with other clinical features, are defined within Axis 1.[1] Two broad categories of tremor syndromes are proposed in Axis 1: isolated tremor in which tremor is the only abnormal sign and combined tremor in which other abnormal signs are present. Combined tremor may occur with other neurological signs (e.g., dystonic postures, parkinsonism, ataxia, or myoclonus) or with relevant systemic signs (e.g., Kayser-Fleischer ring, hepatosplenomegaly, or exophthalmos). Importantly, the very same genetic etiology may be associated with multiple Axis 1 tremor syndromes and/or other phenotypes.

The role of genetics in the etiology of tremor has been highlighted since the nineteenth century, particularly in ET.[2–4] The genetic contribution to tremors can be either casual mutations (i.e., mutations that usually segregate with disease in families) that directly cause tremor syndromes in individual patients or genetic risk factors that are associated with increased risk of disease at the population level. Herein, we review the genetics of tremors both in isolated tremor syndromes and tremor syndromes with prominent additional signs.

ESSENTIAL TREMOR

Essential tremor (ET) is the most common movement disorder, and about 1 percent of the population is affected globally.[5,6] The recent task force of the International Parkinson and Movement Disorder Society defines ET as an isolated tremor syndrome of bilateral upper-limb action tremor.[1,5] A symptom duration of at least 3 years is required, with or without tremor in other locations, such as head, larynx (voice tremor), or lower limbs. Other neurological signs, such as dystonia, ataxia, or parkinsonism, must be absent.[1]

Furthermore, the task force defined the term ET-plus to clearly label ET with additional neurological signs of uncertain significance such as impaired tandem gait, questionable dystonic posturing, memory impairment, or other mild neurologic signs of unknown significance. These signs are not sufficient to make an additional syndrome classification or diagnosis. Exclusion criteria for a diagnosis of ET and ET-plus have been identified,[1] and it remains unresolved what the etiological overlap is between these phenotypic entities.

About 50% of ET patients have a positive family history, and transmission is consistent with an autosomal-dominant trait with variable penetrance.[2,7–10] The additive genetic variance was recently estimated to be at least 75%.[11] Given the heritability estimates for ET, genetic variation is likely to play an important role in the etiology of the disease and influence susceptibility to more complex genetic forms of the disorder. Historically, twin studies have helped define the estimates of the genetic contribution, but there are a number of caveats, among them that this can be difficult to interpret in a common adult-onset disease with reduced penetrance such as

ET.[12–14] Genetic linkage approaches have identified loci linked to ET in large families with an apparent autosomal-dominant mode of transmission (*ETM1*[15]; *ETM2*[16]; *ETM3*[17]). However, no pathogenic mutations causing ET have been found within these loci (Figure 6.1), and many large ET kindreds remain unexplained.

Genome-wide association studies (GWAS) are performed under the assumption that common genetic variation influences the susceptibility to disease. The basic principle is that linkage disequilibrium (LD; the non-random association of alleles at two or more loci in a general population) will be able to detect an association signal due to the difference in allele frequency between affected subjects and healthy controls.[18] In 2009, the first GWAS in ET was performed in the Icelandic population by deCODE genetics, utilizing about 300,000 single-nucleotide polymorphisms (SNPs), and nominated a single variant (rs9652490) within the *LINGO1* gene that reached genome-wide significance (p<1 x 10⁻⁸).[19] Independent replication studies have shown inconsistent results,[20] and, as yet, no variant has been identified that can be specifically pinpointed as functionally driving the association (Deng et al., 2012). Thier and colleagues reported a second GWAS in 2012, examining the frequency of over 600K SNPs in 436 patients with ET, as well as in 928 healthy subjects (Stage I) from the German population.[21] No SNPs reached a genome-wide significance in Stage 1; however, after replication (Stage II), a combined analysis of both Stages I and II identified a single variant in the solute

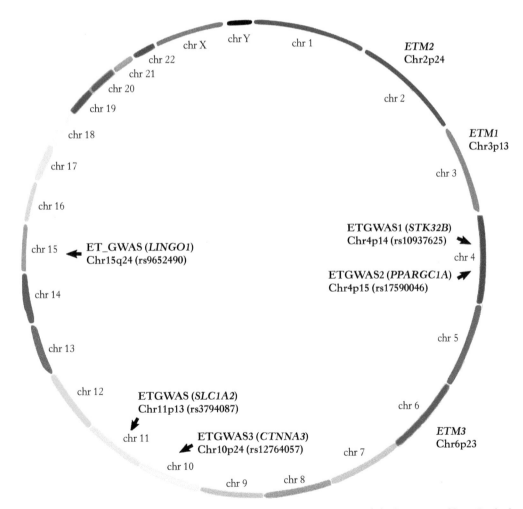

FIGURE 6.1: A Circos Plot Representing the Human Chromosomes and the Location of Loci Linked to Essential Tremor (Outside the Circle) and Hits from Genome-Wide Association Studies (Inside the Circle).

carrier family 1 (rs3794087; glial high-affinity glutamate transporter), member 2 (*SLC1A2*) gene. However, independent replication is lacking, as with *LINGO1* in the first GWAS, and neither GWAS supports the others results.

In 2016, Müller and colleagues conducted a relatively large GWAS in patients and controls of European descent, containing 1778 patients and 5376 controls.[22] Although no variants reached genome-wide significance in the initial discovery stage (GWAS), a number of suggestive loci ($p<1x10^{-5}$) were genotyped in a replication phase (1029 patients and 1065 controls), and in the combined analysis three loci showed significant association with susceptibility to ET (*STK32B*, *PPARGC1A* and *CTNNA3*; $p<1x10^{-8}$). As with any association study pinpointing the specific gene/variant driving the association is not straightforward and thus one must be cautious in determining functionality or assigning pathogenicity to any specific gene in the region. The latest ET GWAS of over 7000 patients with ET has reported five independent genome-wide significant loci.[23] The variants are located across chromosomes 1, 4, 5, 18 and 21 with again unfortunately no clear gene or pathway highlighted. Notably, variants in the *LINGO1* and *SLC1A2* that had previously been associated with ET in GWAS efforts did not demonstrate any association in this study,[19,21] thus highlighting the critical need of replication for any of the variants/loci nominated in disease risk.

Beyond simple replication, attempts have been made to validate the GWAS-generated gene association signals. Given the heritability of ET, one possibility is that genes, nominated through GWAS, would not only have common variation that drives disease risk but also may harbor rare, more penetrant mutations that cause disease manifestation in families. Houle et al. (2017), using a combined next-generation sequencing approach using whole-exome, whole-genome, and targeted capture of these three genes in 14 multiplex families and 269 unrelated patients (and, importantly, 287 ethnically matched controls), assessed the role of potential pathogenic mutations.[24] The investigators did not observe any common coding variants that were driving the GWAS signal; however, a small number of rare variants were observed. They then applied a gene burden analysis. Given the low frequency of rare variants, which precludes single variant analysis, a gene burden approach allows the combined number of rare variants in cases and controls to be examined for excess rare variants in cases (or controls). Although no burden of rare variants

was associated with disease, there are a number of caveats to these approaches, especially in smaller sample sizes; as usual, much larger patient series (and more multi-incident families) are needed to assess the potential role of rare variants in these loci. Indeed, a set of research recommendations that were published the same year as the Müller et al. GWAS noted the need for large patient-focused collections (n>10,000) to truly facilitate well-powered studies.[25] This collaborative group effort also called for the development and use of a set of common data elements that can be employed across studies to promote large genetic efforts and allow detailed phenotype-genotype approaches that may get at the heart of the clinical-genetic heterogeneity of ET that has hindered genetic discovery.

In an effort to expand beyond the classical genetic approaches (familial and population) to elucidate ET-disease pathophysiology, a number of groups have moved toward integrating other-omic approaches. The most widely used to date is transcriptomics (the use of large unbiased RNA sequencing efforts), which can be combined with genetic and epigenetic datasets.[26–28] These approaches allow for resolution of dysfunction at the pathway level as well identifying key differentially expressed genes (DEGs) that may define the underlying phenotypic determinants and nominate potential therapeutic targets. Candidate pathways include calcium-related, axon guidance, and synaptic transmission; however, it should be noted that heterogeneity across age, gender, tissue integrity, and cellular content, for example, means that replication is likely even more critical than in genetic studies, and samples sizes to date have been much smaller compared to classical genetics studies (e.g., n<50 for studies of ET brain tissue).

The current status of ET genetics reveals there is so much more to learn. We still eagerly await the first confirmed ET gene that harbors high penetrant mutations that cause inherited disease. A number of candidate loci and genes have been nominated by screening in a single family or a small cluster of patients and have yet to be confirmed (e.g., *FUS*,[25–27] *HTRA2*[29–31] and *TENM4*[32–34]), and this trend is likely to continue as the cost of whole-genome sequencing is further reduced. Given our current understanding of rare variants and assigning of pathogenicity, replication/validation is critical to our interpretation of these possible candidate genes. In addition, further large-scale GWAS and population efforts may provide some exciting insights into the common genetic drivers of disease suscepti-bility. Recently, GGC repeat expansions in the 5' region of the human-specific *NOTCH2NLC* gene were found to cosegregate with disease in 11 out of 197 Chinese ET families (5.6%).[35] The number of GGC repeats in ET patients ranged from 60 to 250, compared with 7 to 23 repeats in unaffected family members. Notably, GGC repeat expan-sions in *NOTCH2NLC* have also been associ-ated with neuronal intranuclear inclusion body disease (NIID),[36–39] a neurodegenerative disease characterized by eosinophilic intranuclear inclu-sions in neuronal and glial cells. Clinical features in NIID include dementia, urinary incontinence, and neuropathy; tremor and ataxia have also been observed.[40] A recent replication study detected expanded *NOTCH2NLC* GGC repeats (>80 units) in 4 (0.86%) sporadic ET patients out of a total of 462 ET patients from Singapore.[39] These are intriguing findings, but further replication stud-ies are needed to clarify the role of *NOTCH2NLC* GGC repeats in ET. It is likely that large-scale col-laborative efforts will help decipher the underly-ing genetic etiology of ET and aid in integration across multiple data sets, the defining of common clinical data elements, and the use of multi-omic approaches that will drive our understanding of ET and direct therapeutic intervention strategies.

ISOLATED FOCAL TREMORS

Hereditary Geniospasm

Hereditary geniospasm (HG) is an isolated tremor syndrome causing episodes of involuntary tremor of the chin and the lower lip due to due to rhyth-mic mentalis muscle contractions at frequen-cies between 4 and 30 Hz.[41,42] Episodes typically start in early childhood and may be precipitated by stress and may last seconds to hours. HG is inherited as an autosomal-dominant trait, but no genetic mutation has been identified, probably due to genetic heterogeneity.[41]

TREMOR SYNDROMES WITH PROMINENT ADDITIONAL SIGNS

Dystonic tremor syndromes

Dystonic movements may be tremulous and, therefore all genes linked to dystonia may exhibit isolated or combined tremor syndromes.[43] Tremor may occur before dystonia in dystonic tremor syndrome.[42,43] Recent reviews on the genetics of dystonia are available elsewhere.[44–46] Herein, we

will discuss tremor associated with some genetic forms of dystonia. Mutations in the *ANO3* gene (anoctamin 3) were originally reported in patients with predominantly craniocervical dystonia with both early and late disease onset.[47] Mutations were detected in about 1% of dystonia patients, and segregation was shown in small families with *ANO3* variants. Notably, *ANO3* missense variants can be found in variant databases and in healthy individuals, thus making the pathogenicity of *ANO3* variants uncertain.[48] A pathogenic role of *ANO3* mutations has recently been supported by the identification of additional families and a de novo mutation in a patient with dystonia and myoclonic jerks.[44,49] Tremor may involve the head, voice, and upper limbs in various combinations and may be the sole initial manifestation in some individuals with DYT-*ANO3*, leading to misdiag-nosis as ET.[50]

Dopa-responsive dystonia caused by hetero-zygous mutations in the *GCH1* gene (DYT/PARK-*GCH1*) has been associated with upper-limb postural tremor and with voice, head, chin, and parkinsonian rest tremor. The tremor is dopa-responsive and shows diurnal fluctuation, which is typical for dopa-responsive dystonia.[51,52] Resting tremor associated with dystonia and parkinson-ism has also been reported in dopa-responsive dystonia due to recessive mutations in the tyro-sine hydroxylase (*TH*) gene.[53–55] Importantly, a levodopa trial should be carried out in all chil-dren with an unexplained movement disorder, especially when tremor or dystonia is present.

There is a substantial overlap between focal dystonia (especially cervical dystonia) and ET. Focal dystonia has been found in about one-third of ET family members.[56] Both tremor with focal dystonia or pure tremor was linked to a region on chromosome 6p23.[57]

Tremor combined with Parkinson disease (PD)

Rest tremor is a cardinal feature of PD and all monogenic forms of PD may exhibit rest tremor. Rest tremor in PD normally affects the upper limbs asymmetrically, but may also start in a lower limb. Postural and action tremor are rare, but have been reported in all the three autosomal-dominant monogenic PD forms: *SNCA*, *LRRK2*, and *VPS35*.[58] Patients with recessive forms of monogenic PD (*PRKN*, *PINK1* and *PARK7*) also often have resting tremor.[59–61] Importantly, *PRKN* may often display isolated foot dystonia as the ini-tial symptom.[59]

Intention tremor syndromes—hereditary cerebellar ataxias

Postural and intention tremor are well-known features in hereditary cerebellar ataxias (HCAs), hereditary spastic paraplegias,[56–58] and mitochondrial spinocerebellar ataxia caused by *POLG1* mutations.[62] These syndromes can also comprise progressive ataxia with palatal tremor.[42,63,64] Palatal tremor is associated with hypertrophic olivary degeneration (HOD); however, HOD leads only to palatal tremor in some cases.[63] Spinocerebellar ataxias (SCAs) can present with parkinsonism, including rest tremor, e.g., SCA2 (*ATXN2*),[65,66] SCA3 (*ATXN3*)[67] and SCA17 (*TBP*).[68]

Fragile X-associated tremor/ataxia syndrome (FXTAS)

Intention tremor is an important feature in fragile X-associated tremor/ataxia syndrome (FXTAS).[69,70] Additional core features are progressive cerebellar ataxia and later development of cognitive impairment. Psychiatric symptoms are common. Age at onset is commonly between 60 and 65 years. Symmetrical regions of increased T2 signal intensity on MRI in the middle cerebellar peduncles (MCP sign) and adjacent cerebellar white matter are considered highly sensitive for this syndrome.[69] FXTAS is caused by premutation-sized CGG trinucleotide repeat expansion (55–200 CGG repeats) in the 5' UTR of the *FMR1* gene. The *FMR1* gene is located on the X chromosome. Consequently, FXTAS affects males, who are hemizygous for the premutation, more often than women, who are heterozygous for the premutation. Examining the family history, including instances of mental retardation and premature ovarian failure (which has been observed in 20% of women who carry a premutation allele compared to 1% in the general population[71]), is of particular importance in the diagnostic workup.

Wilson's disease

Wilson's disease (WD) is a treatable autosomal recessive disorder of copper metabolism leading to excess copper deposition due to mutations in the *ATP7B* gene. Neurologic symptoms generally manifest in the second or third decade, but age of onset can range from childhood to after 70 years.[72] WD can present with a tremor, parkinsonism, dystonia, chorea, dysarthria, and dysphagia.[73] Tremor is of particular importance as it is the first symptom in up to 55% of WD patients

with neurologic symptoms.[73–75] WD can manifest with any type of tremor, including resting, postural, or kinetic. Thus, tremor in WD in can look like ET, dystonic tremor, Holmes tremor, or parkinsonian resting tremor.[73,76,77] The diagnostic workup includes biochemical findings (low serum copper and ceruloplasmin concentrations, and increased urinary copper excretion), MRI findings, Kayser-Fleischer corneal ring, or genetic testing for biallelic *ATP7B* mutations. Liver biopsy may sometimes be necessary.

Other rare genetic syndromes associated with tremor

Combined tremor syndromes can be caused by a range of genetic disorders, including neurodegeneration with brain iron accumulation (NBIA),[78] autosomal recessive metabolic disorders,[42,79] and other complex syndromes. Thorough workup of family history and comprehensive clinical evaluation is paramount, but genetics often play an important role in order to reach a final diagnosis in rare complex syndromes.

CHALLENGES, OPPORTUNITIES, AND FUTURE PERSPECTIVES

The recent consensus statement on the classification of tremors[1] provides an applicable guide to address the challenge of phenotypic heterogeneity that can inhibit genetic discovery in common disorders. By identifying key phenotypic traits and detailed clinical evaluations, we can hopefully derive more homogenous patient groups/subtypes for genetic analysis. Furthermore, continuous or ordinal phenotype traits can be used to test against genetic variants, an approach that could take us beyond a binary (yes/no) disease phenotype. A challenge has always been pinpointing genetic variants that may be causative in families or driving association signals in population-based studies.[80] However, with what is now a readily accepted revolution in terms of genetic sequencing technologies, whole-genome sequencing (and in particular the long-read approaches) have allowed researchers to assess not only single-nucleotide variants or rare point mutations but also copy number and structural alterations, and to assess the understudied role of simple expansion of repeat sequences that we recognize as a major contributor to ataxias and other neurodegenerative disorders such as FTD/ALS.[81–83]

These genomic sequencing approaches allow for full, detailed characterization of patients and families for less than $2000 per sample, and for regular whole-genome sequencing we are well under the $1000 genome. This will create a paradigm in terms of the way we consider clinical genetics as a field, in the sense that genomic variation will become a part of the standard health workup and will likely be available to use in conjunction with large-scale electronic medical health records. Thus, given the commonality of ET, for example, the hope would be that large data sets for genetic discovery and with specific phenotypic traits will become available in the relatively near future. Until then, we will rely on the global efforts of researchers to establish large, ethnically diverse consortia and the collection/banking of biospecimens.

Determining biomarkers and understanding genetic risk will likely be driven by multi-omic approaches across different tissue types. For drug discovery the use of pathway-based analysis and integration of transcriptomics/epigenetics from disease relevant tissue will be critical. Access to brains from tremor patients will play an important role in these endeavors, and the development of novel transcriptomic technologies has opened up new avenues of research. Currently, single nuclei (or cell) transcriptome sequencing (snRNA-Seq) provides a platform for examining transcript changes in specific cell types and will allow the integration of GWAS and sequencing data to identify cell-specific expression quantitative loci (eQTL) that may nominate the underlying functional genes that are influenced by GWAS association signals. A further step is the use of long-read sequencing applications to identify specific transcript isoforms and determine how they may also be influenced by genetic variation (splice QTLs). These genetic approaches, coupled with the blossoming field of large-scale unbiased proteomics, lipidomics, and metabolomics, to name a few, means that the future is bright as regards our ability to understand the pathogenesis of tremor disorders and to address the need for diagnostics/prognostics and the development of therapeutics.

REFERENCES

1. Bhatia KP, Bain P, Bajaj N, et al. Consensus Statement on the classification of tremors. From the task force on tremor of the International Parkinson and Movement Disorder Society. *Mov Disord*. 2018;33(1):75–87. doi: 10.1002/mds.27121
2. Dana CL. Hereditary tremor, a hitherto undescribed form of motor neurosis. *Am J Med Sci*. 1887;94:386–393.
3. Louis ED, Broussolle E, Goetz CG, Krack P, Kaufmann P, Mazzoni P. Historical underpinnings of the term essential tremor in the late 19th century. *Neurology*. 2008;71(11):856–859. doi: 10.1212/01.wnl.0000325564.38165.d1
4. Burresi P. Sopra un caso di tremore essenziale. Memore originali. Conferenza raccolta dallo studente Alfredo Rubini (22 febbraio 1874, Siena). *Lo Sper*. 1874;33:475–481.
5. Haubenberger D, Hallett M. Essential tremor. Solomon CG, ed. *N Engl J Med*. 2018;378(19):1802–1810. doi: 10.1056/NEJMcp1707928
6. Louis ED, Ferreira JJ. How common is the most common adult movement disorder? Update on the worldwide prevalence of essential tremor. *Mov Disord*. 2010;25(5):534–541. doi: 10.1002/mds.22838
7. Larsson T, Sjogren T. Essential tremor: a clinical and genetic population study. *Acta Psychiatr Scand Suppl*. 1960;36(144):1–176.
8. Busenbark K, Barnes P, Lyons K, Ince D, Villagra F, Koller WC. Accuracy of reported family histories of essential tremor. *Neurology*. 1996;47(1):264–265. doi: 10.1212/wnl.47.1.264
9. Brin MF, Koller W. Epidemiology and genetics of essential tremor. *Mov Disord*. 1998;13(Suppl 3):55–63. doi: 10.1002/mds.870131310
10. Jasinska-Myga B, Wider C. Genetics of essential tremor. *Parkinsonism Relat Disord*. 2012;18(Suppl 1):S138–S139. doi: 10.1016/S1353-8020(11)70043-8
11. Diez-Fairen M, Bandres-Ciga S, Houle G, et al. Genome-wide estimates of heritability and genetic correlations in essential tremor. *Parkinsonism Relat Disord*. 2019;64:262–267. doi: 10.1016/j.parkreldis.2019.05.002
12. Tanner CM, Goldman SM, Lyons KE, et al. Essential tremor in twins: an assessment of genetic vs environmental determinants of etiology. *Neurology*. 2001;57(8):1389–1391. doi: 10.1212/wnl.57.8.1389
13. Goldman SM, Marek K, Ottman R, et al. Concordance for Parkinson's disease in twins: a 20-year update. *Ann Neurol*. 2019;85(4):600–605. doi: 10.1002/ana.25441
14. Mayhew AJ, Meyre D. Assessing the heritability of complex traits in humans: methodological challenges and opportunities. *Curr Genomics*. 2017;18(4):332–340. doi: 10.2174/1389202918666170307161450
15. Gulcher JR, Jónsson P, Kong A, et al. Mapping of a familial essential tremor gene, FET1, to chromosome 3q13. *Nat Genet*. 1997;17(1):84–87. doi: 10.1038/ng0997-84
16. Higgins JJ, Pho LT, Nee LE. A gene (ETM) for essential tremor maps to chromosome 2p22-p25. *Mov Disord*. 1997;12(6):859–864. doi: 10.1002/mds.870120605

17. Shatunov A, Sambuughin N, Jankovic J, et al. Genomewide scans in North American families reveal genetic linkage of essential tremor to a region on chromosome 6p23. *Brain*. 2006;129(Pt 9):2318–2331. doi: 10.1093/brain/awl120

18. Manolio TA. Genomewide association studies and assessment of the risk of disease. *N Engl J Med*. 2010;363(2):166–176. doi: 10.1056/NEJMra0905980

19. Stefansson H, Steinberg S, Petursson H, et al. Variant in the sequence of the LINGO1 gene confers risk of essential tremor. *Nat Genet*. 2009;41(3):277–279. doi: 10.1038/ng.299

20. Deng H, Gu S, Jankovic J. LINGO1 variants in essential tremor and Parkinson's disease. *Acta Neurol Scand*. 2012;125(1):1–7. doi: 10.1111/j.1600-0404.2011.01516.x

21. Thier S, Lorenz D, Nothnagel M, et al. Polymorphisms in the glial glutamate transporter SLC1A2 are associated with essential tremor. *Neurology*. 2012;79(3):243–248. doi: 10.1212/WNL.0b013e31825fdeed

22. Müller SH, Girard SL, Hopfner F, et al. Genomewide association study in essential tremor identifies three new loci. *Brain*. 2016;139(Pt 12):3163–3169. doi: 10.1093/brain/aww242

23. Liao C, Castonguay C-E, Heilbron K, et al. Association of Essential Tremor With Novel Risk Loci: A Genome-Wide Association Study and Meta-analysis. *JAMA Neurol*. 2022;79(2):185–193. doi:10.1001/jamaneurol.2021.4781.

24. Houle G, Ambalavanan A, Schmouth J-F, et al. No rare deleterious variants from STK32B, PPARGC1A, and CTNNA3 are associated with essential tremor. *Neurol Genet*. 2017;3(5):e195. doi: 10.1212/NXG.0000000000000195

25. Hopfner F, Haubenberger D, Galpern WR, et al. Knowledge gaps and research recommendations for essential tremor. *Parkinsonism Relat Disord*. 2016;33:27–35. doi: 10.1016/j.parkreldis.2016.10.002

26. Liao C, Sarayloo F, Rochefort D, et al. Multiomics analyses identify genes and pathways relevant to essential tremor. *Mov Disord*. 2020;35(7):1153–1162. doi: 10.1002/mds.28031

27. Martuscello RT, Kerridge CA, Chatterjee D, et al. Gene expression analysis of the cerebellar cortex in essential tremor. *Neurosci Lett*. 2020;721:134540. doi: 10.1016/j.neulet.2019.134540

28. Paul JL, Dashtipour K, Chen Z, Wang C. DNA methylome study of human cerebellar tissues identified genes and pathways possibly involved in essential tremor. *Precis Clin Med*. 2019;2(4):221–234. doi: 10.1093/pcmedi/pbz028

29. Unal Gulsuner H, Gulsuner S, Mercan FN, et al. Mitochondrial serine protease HTRA2 p.G399S in kindred with essential tremor and Parkinson disease. *Proc Natl Acad Sci USA*. 2014;111(51):18285–18290. doi: 10.1073/pnas.1419581111

30. Tzoulis C, Zayats T, Knappskog PM, et al. HTRA2 p.G399S in Parkinson disease, essential tremor, and tremulous cervical dystonia. *Proc Natl Acad Sci USA*. 2015;112(18):E2268. doi: 10.1073/pnas.1503105112

31. Hopfner F, Müller SH, Lorenz D, et al. Mutations in HTRA2 are not a common cause of familial classic ET. *Mov Disord*. 2015;30(8):1149–1150. doi: 10.1002/mds.26252

32. Hor H, Francescatto L, Bartesaghi L, et al. Missense mutations in TENM4, a regulator of axon guidance and central myelination, cause essential tremor. *Hum Mol Genet*. 2015;24(20):5677–5686. doi: 10.1093/hmg/ddv281

33. Chao YX, Lin Ng EY, Tio M, et al. Essential tremor linked TENM4 mutation found in healthy Chinese individuals. *Parkinsonism Relat Disord*. 2016;31:139–140. doi: 10.1016/j.parkreldis.2016.05.003

34. Houle G, Schmouth J-F, Leblond CS, et al. Teneurin transmembrane protein 4 is not a cause for essential tremor in a Canadian population. *Mov Disord*. 2017;32(2):292–295. doi: 10.1002/mds.26753

35. Sun Q-Y, Xu Q, Tian Y, et al. Expansion of GGC repeat in the human-specific NOTCH2NLC gene is associated with essential tremor. *Brain*. 2020;143(1):222–233. doi: 10.1093/brain/awz372

36. Ishiura H, Shibata S, Yoshimura J, et al. Noncoding CGG repeat expansions in neuronal intranuclear inclusion disease, oculopharyngodistal myopathy and an overlapping disease. *Nat Genet*. 2019;51(8):1222–1232. doi: 10.1038/s41588-019-0458-z

37. Sone J, Mitsuhashi S, Fujita A, et al. Long-read sequencing identifies GGC repeat expansions in NOTCH2NLC associated with neuronal intranuclear inclusion disease. *Nat Genet*. 2019;51(8):1215–1221. doi: 10.1038/s41588-019-0459-y

38. Tian Y, Wang J-L, Huang W, et al. Expansion of human-specific GGC repeat in neuronal intranuclear inclusion disease-related disorders. *Am J Hum Genet*. 2019;105(1):166–176. doi: 10.1016/j.ajhg.2019.05.013

39. Ng ASL, Lim WK, Xu Z, et al. NOTCH2NLC GGC repeat expansions are associated with sporadic essential tremor: variable disease expressivity on long-term follow-up. *Ann Neurol*. 2020;88(3):614–618. doi: 10.1002/ana.25803

40. Sone J, Mori K, Inagaki T, et al. Clinicopathological features of adult-onset neuronal intranuclear inclusion disease. *Brain*. 2016;139(Pt 12):3170–3186. doi: 10.1093/brain/aww249

41. Jarman PR, Wood NW, Davis MT, et al. Hereditary geniospasm: linkage to chromosome

9q13-q21 and evidence for genetic heterogeneity. *Am J Hum Genet*. 1997;61(4):928–933. doi: 10.1086/514883

42. Magrinelli F, Latorre A, Balint B, et al. Isolated and combined genetic tremor syndromes: a critical appraisal based on the 2018 MDS criteria. *Parkinsonism Relat Disord*. 2020;77:121–140. doi: 10.1016/j.parkreldis.2020.04.010

43. Albanese A, Bhatia K, Bressman SB, et al. Phenomenology and classification of dystonia: a consensus update. *Mov Disord*. 2013;28(7):863–873. doi: 10.1002/mds.25475

44. Lohmann K, Klein C. Update on the genetics of dystonia. *Curr Neurol Neurosci Rep*. 2017;17(3):26. doi: 10.1007/s11910-017-0735-0

45. Jinnah HA, Sun YV. Dystonia genes and their biological pathways. *Neurobiol Dis*. 2019;129:159–168. doi: 10.1016/j.nbd.2019.05.014

46. Weisheit CE, Pappas SS, Dauer WT. Chapter 16—Inherited dystonias: clinical features and molecular pathways. In: Geschwind DH, Paulson HL, Klein C, eds. *Handbook of Clinical Neurology*. Vol 147. Neurogenetics, Part I. Elsevier; 2018: 241–254. doi: 10.1016/B978-0-444-63233-3.00016-6

47. Charlesworth G, Plagnol V, Holmström KM, et al. Mutations in ANO3 cause dominant craniocervical dystonia: ion channel implicated in pathogenesis. *Am J Hum Genet*. 2012;91(6):1041–1050. doi: 10.1016/j.ajhg.2012.10.024

48. Zech M, Gross N, Jochim A, et al. Rare sequence variants in ANO3 and GNAL in a primary torsion dystonia series and controls. *Mov Disord*. 2014;29(1):143–147. doi: 10.1002/mds.25715

49. Zech M, Boesch S, Jochim A, et al. Clinical exome sequencing in early-onset generalized dystonia and large-scale resequencing follow-up. *Mov Disord*. 2017;32(4):549–559. doi: 10.1002/mds.26808

50. Stamelou M, Charlesworth G, Cordivari C, et al. The phenotypic spectrum of DYT24 due to ANO3 mutations. *Mov Disord*. 2014;29(7):928–934. doi: 10.1002/mds.25802

51. Segawa M, Hosaka A, Miyagawa F, Nomura Y, Imai H. Hereditary progressive dystonia with marked diurnal fluctuation. *Adv Neurol*. 1976;14:215–233.

52. Trender-Gerhard I, Sweeney MG, Schwingenschuh P, et al. Autosomal-dominant GTPCH1-deficient DRD: clinical characteristics and long-term outcome of 34 patients. *J Neurol Neurosurg Psychiatry*. 2009;80(8):839–845. doi: 10.1136/jnnp.2008.155861

53. Willemsen MA, Verbeek MM, Kamsteeg E-J, et al. Tyrosine hydroxylase deficiency: a treatable disorder of brain catecholamine biosynthesis. *Brain*. 2010;133(Pt 6):1810–1822. doi: 10.1093/brain/awq087

54. Clot F, Grabli D, Cazeneuve C, et al. Exhaustive analysis of BH4 and dopamine biosynthesis genes in patients with Dopa-responsive dystonia. *Brain*. 2009;132(7):1753–1763. doi: 10.1093/brain/awp084

55. Haugarvoll K, Bindoff LA. A novel compound heterozygous tyrosine hydroxylase mutation (p.R441P) with complex phenotype. *J Park Dis*. 2011;1(1):119–122. doi: 10.3233/JPD-2011-11006

56. Louis ED, Hernandez N, Alcalay RN, Tirri DJ, Ottman R, Clark LN. Prevalence and features of unreported dystonia in a family study of "pure" essential tremor. *Parkinsonism Relat Disord*. 2013;19(3):359–362. doi: 10.1016/j.parkreldis.2012.09.015

57. Shatunov A, Sambuughin N, Jankovic J, et al. Genomewide scans in North American families reveal genetic linkage of essential tremor to a region on chromosome 6p23. *Brain*. 2006;129(Pt 9):2318–2331. doi: 10.1093/brain/awl120

58. Trinh J, Zeldenrust FMJ, Huang J, et al. Genotype-phenotype relations for the Parkinson's disease genes SNCA, LRRK2, VPS35: MDSgene systematic review. *Mov Disord*. 2018;33(12):1857–1870. doi: 10.1002/mds.27527

59. Kitada T, Asakawa S, Hattori N, et al. Mutations in the parkin gene cause autosomal recessive juvenile parkinsonism. *Nature*. 1998;392(6676):605–608.

60. Bonifati V, Rizzu P, van Baren MJ, et al. Mutations in the DJ-1 gene associated with autosomal recessive early-onset parkinsonism. *Science*. 2003;299(5604):256–259.

61. Valente EM, Abou-Sleiman PM, Caputo V, et al. Hereditary early-onset Parkinson's disease caused by mutations in PINK1. *Science*. 2004;304(5674):1158–1160.

62. Tzoulis C, Engelsen BA, Telstad W, et al. The spectrum of clinical disease caused by the A467T and W748S POLG mutations: a study of 26 cases. *Brain*. 2006;129(Pt 7):1685–1692. doi: 10.1093/brain/awl097

63. Tzoulis C, Neckelmann G, Mork SJ, et al. Localized cerebral energy failure in DNA polymerase gamma-associated encephalopathy syndromes. *Brain*. 2010;133(Pt 5):1428–1437. doi: 10.1093/brain/awq067

64. Gass J, Blackburn PR, Jackson J, Macklin S, van Gerpen J, Atwal PS. Expanded phenotype in a patient with spastic paraplegia 7. *Clin Case Rep*. 2017;5(10):1620–1622. doi: 10.1002/ccr3.1109

65. Charles P, Camuzat A, Benammar N, et al. Are interrupted SCA2 CAG repeat expansions responsible for parkinsonism? *Neurology*. 2007;69(21):1970–1975. doi: 10.1212/01.wnl.0000269323.21969.db

66. Modoni A, Contarino MF, Bentivoglio AR, et al. Prevalence of spinocerebellar ataxia type 2 mutation among Italian Parkinsonian patients. *Mov Disord*. 2007;22(3):324–327. doi: 10.1002/mds.21228

67. Gwinn-Hardy K, Singleton A, O'Suilleabhain P, et al. Spinocerebellar ataxia type 3 phenotypically resembling Parkinson disease in a black family. *Arch Neurol.* 2001;58(2):296–299.

68. Kim J-Y, Kim SY, Kim J-M, et al. Spinocerebellar ataxia type 17 mutation as a causative and susceptibility gene in parkinsonism. *Neurology.* 2009;72(16):1385–1389. doi: 10.1212/WNL.0b013e3181a18876

69. Jacquemont S, Hagerman RJ, Leehey M, et al. Fragile X premutation tremor/ataxia syndrome: molecular, clinical, and neuroimaging correlates. *Am J Hum Genet.* 2003;72(4):869–878. doi: 10.1086/374321

70. Hunter JE, Berry-Kravis E, Hipp H, Todd PK. FMR1 disorders. In: Adam MP, Ardinger HH, Pagon RA, et al., eds. *GeneReviews®.* University of Washington, Seattle; 1993. Accessed June 19, 2020. http://www.ncbi.nlm.nih.gov/books/NBK1384/

71. Fink DA, Nelson LM, Pyeritz R, et al. Fragile X Associated Primary Ovarian Insufficiency (FXPOI): case report and literature review. *Front Genet.* 2018;9:529. doi: 10.3389/fgene.2018.00529

72. Mulligan C, Bronstein JM. Wilson Disease: An overview and approach to management. *Neurol Clin.* 2020;38(2):417–432. doi: 10.1016/j.ncl.2020.01.005

73. Członkowska A, Litwin T, Chabik G. Wilson disease: neurologic features. *Handb Clin Neurol.* 2017;142:101–119. doi: 10.1016/B978-0-444-63625-6.00010-0

74. Oder W, Grimm G, Kollegger H, Ferenci P, Schneider B, Deecke L. Neurological and neuropsychiatric spectrum of Wilson's disease: a prospective study of 45 cases. *J Neurol.* 1991;238(5):281–287. doi: 10.1007/BF00319740

75. Oder W, Prayer L, Grimm G, et al. Wilson's disease: evidence of subgroups derived from clinical findings and brain lesions. *Neurology.* 1993;43(1):120–124. doi: 10.1212/wnl.43.1_part_1.120

76. Compston A. Progressive lenticular degeneration: a familial nervous disease associated with cirrhosis of the liver, by S. A. Kinnier Wilson (From the National Hospital, and the Laboratory of the National Hospital, Queen Square, London) Brain 1912: 34; 295–509. *Brain.* 2009;132(Pt 8):1997–2001. doi: 10.1093/brain/awp193

77. Marsden CD. Wilson's disease. *Q J Med.* 1987;65(248):959–966.

78. Hayflick SJ, Kurian MA, Hogarth P. Neurodegeneration with brain iron accumulation. *Handb Clin Neurol.* 2018;147:293–305. doi: 10.1016/B978-0-444-63233-3.00019-1

79. Haugarvoll K, Johansson S, Tzoulis C, et al. MRI characterisation of adult-onset alpha-methylacyl-coa racemase deficiency diagnosed by exome sequencing. *Orphanet J Rare Dis.* 2013;8:1. doi: 10.1186/1750-1172-8-1

80. Testa CM. Key issues in essential tremor genetics research: Where are we now and how can we move forward? *Tremor Other Hyperkinet Mov (N Y).* 2013;3:1–19. doi: 10.7916/D8Q23Z0Z

81. Klockgether T, Mariotti C, Paulson HL. Spinocerebellar ataxia. *Nat Rev Dis Primer.* 2019;5(1):24. doi: 10.1038/s41572-019-0074-3

82. Dejesus-Hernandez M, Mackenzie IR, Boeve BF, et al. Expanded GGGGCC hexanucleotide repeat in noncoding region of C9ORF72 causes chromosome 9p-linked FTD and ALS. *Neuron.,* 2011;72(2):245–256. doi: 10.1016/j.neuron.2011.09.011

83. Dejesus-Hernandez M, Rayaprolu S, Soto-Ortolaza AI, et al. Analysis of the c9orf72 repeat in Parkinson's disease, essential tremor and restless legs syndrome. *Parkinsonism Relat Disord.* 2013;19(2):198–201. doi: 10.1016/j.parkreldis.2012.09.013

7

Tremor in Medicine and Other Secondary Tremors

MARGI PATEL, CHRISTOPHER Y. CAUGHMAN,
AND STEWART A. FACTOR

DEFINITION AND CLASSIFICATION OF TREMOR

The Tremor Task Force of the International Parkinson and Movement Disorder Society defines "tremor" as an involuntary, rhythmic, oscillatory movement of a body part.[1] The classification system[1] comprises two axes, one on clinical phenomenology and the second on acquired, genetic, or idiopathic etiology. This chapter will specifically cover Axis 2–acquired etiologies of tremor, associated with drugs, metabolic disorders, toxins, lesions, and systemic diseases. The tremors resulting from all these are grouped into a category called "symptomatic" or "secondary" or "acquired" tremors. However, we would first like to consider the Axis 1 classification based on activation conditions and tremor frequency, as they relate to our topic. Briefly, tremor is broadly divided into rest and action types. *Rest* tremor (e.g., tremor of Parkinson disease) is present, as the name suggests, at rest, with the body part being completely in repose, supported against gravity, without any voluntary muscle activation of the body part in which tremor is present. It increases with distraction and diminishes, at least transiently, with initiation of goal-directed voluntary activity of the tremor-affected part. On the other hand, *action* tremor appears in a specific body part when that body part is voluntarily activated, either maintaining a position against gravity (*postural and orthostatic*) or performing a movement (*kinetic*). Kinetic tremor can be further divided into *simple kinetic*, in which tremor remains roughly the same amplitude throughout the movement, and *intention tremor*, where the amplitude of the tremor in the affected body part increases in a crescendo fashion upon reaching a target. Other forms of action tremor include *task-specific* (occurs during a specific task, such as writing), *position-specific* (occurs while holding a specific position), *isometric* (occurs when there is

sustained muscle contraction against a rigid stationary object), and *re-emergent* (re-emerges after a certain delay upon holding a posture and has waveform similarities with rest tremor).[1] When unsupported, the head and limbs exhibit slight tremor, referred to as *physiologic tremor*, which is not generally visible or dysfunctional unless exaggerated by anxiety, fatigue, or stress.[2] The tremor disorders we discuss can fall into any of these clinical phenomenological categories.

DRUG-INDUCED TREMOR

Tremor characteristics and proposed mechanism of action

Many classes and types of drugs cause tremor of different clinical characteristics. The most common are listed in Table 7.1.[3-15] As new drugs are being developed, this list continues to grow. Drug-induced tremor is usually an *isolated tremor syndrome* (under Axis 1 classification)[1]; however, it can be associated with other neurological signs and symptoms in some cases as Axis 1 *combined tremor syndrome*—for example, drug-induced parkinsonism and tremor caused by antipsychotics and antiemetics. Drug-induced tremor also mainly affects limbs and very rarely, if at all, the head. The mechanism of action has been debated upon and varies, but literature suggests that drug-induced tremor, in most cases, represents an *enhanced physiologic tremor* (8–12 Hz). This tremor mostly has an action component, postural and kinetic included.[12,16] It is often a low-amplitude and high-frequency tremor, although, in severe cases, the amplitude can be moderate to severe. The enhanced physiologic tremor has two major components: peripheral reflex mechanical oscillation and an 8–12 Hz central component.[17] The former can be amplified by sympathomimetics. The inferior olive or thalamus have been thought to be the origin of the central oscillator, with the transmission occurring through the corticospinal tract.[17,18] Additional

TABLE 7.1: COMMON DRUGS CAUSING TREMOR AND THE MOST COMMON TREMOR CHARACTERISTICS

Drug class	Drug examples	Tremor characteristics (most common)	Tremor syndrome(s) (most common)
Dopamine receptor–blocking agents	Antipsychotics (e.g., risperidone, haloperidol) antiemetics/prokinetics (e.g., metoclopramide)	Rest tremor Re-emergent postural tremor Mixture of rest, postural and action (mainly intention) tremor	Parkinsonian tremor Tardive tremor
Dopamine-depleting drugs	VMAT2 inhibitors (e.g., tetrabenazine) Reserpine	Rest tremor Re-emergent postural tremor	Parkinsonian tremor
Antidepressants/mood stabilizers	Lithium SSRIs (e.g., citalopram, fluoxetine, fluvoxamine, sertraline) TCAs (e.g., amitriptyline)	Postural and kinetic tremor (8–12Hz) Postural tremor (6–12 Hz) Rest tremor	Enhanced physiologic tremor For lithium, parkinsonian syndromes with tremor
Antiepileptics	Valproic acid Lamotrigine	Postural and kinetic tremor (8–12 Hz) Rest tremor	Enhanced physiologic tremor For valproic acid, parkinsonian tremor
Chemotherapy/immunosuppressants	Tacrolimus, cyclosporine, ifosfamide Interferons, tamoxifen Cytarabine, 5-fluorouracil Vincristine, cisplatin, paclitaxel Methotrexate, doxorubicin	Postural and kinetic tremor (8–12 Hz) Intention tremor, especially with cerebellum toxicity caused by drugs like cytarabine	Enhanced physiologic tremor
Antiarrhythmics	Amiodarone Procainamide	Rest tremor Postural and kinetic tremor (8–12 Hz) Intention tremor	Parkinsonian tremor Enhanced physiologic tremor
Bronchodilators/beta-2 agonists	Salbutamol, albuterol Xanthine derivatives: caffeine, theophylline	Postural and kinetic tremor (8–12 Hz)	Enhanced physiologic tremor
Hormones	Adrenaline, medroxyprogesterone	Postural and kinetic tremor (8–12 Hz)	Enhanced physiologic tremor
Sympathomimetics	Amphetamine, dextroamphetamine, ephedrine	Postural and kinetic tremor (8–12 Hz)	Enhanced physiologic tremor
Abused drugs	Cocaine, alcohol, MDMA	Postural and kinetic tremor (8–12 Hz) Intention tremor	Enhanced physiologic tremor
Antibiotics/antifungals	Trimethoprim-sulfamethoxazole, amphotericin-B	Postural and kinetic tremor (8–12 Hz)	Enhanced physiologic tremor

mechanisms of action for causing tremor have been proposed for some drugs; for example, cytarabine and alcohol could cause direct cerebellar toxicity and thus result in a cerebellar-type tremor.[19] Some drugs, like dopamine-depleting drugs (e.g., antipsychotics, antiemetics), cause dopamine blockade and a subsequent rest tremor. Overall, literature suggests that the mechanism of drug-induced tremor remains largely unknown and is variable from drug to drug.

Common drugs causing tremor

Cardiovascular drugs (e.g., amiodarone, other antiarrhythmics), antidepressants (e.g., tricyclics [TCAs] and selective serotonin reuptake inhibitors [SSRIs]), anti-manic drugs (e.g., lithium, valproic acid), chemotherapy drugs (e.g., tacrolimus, vincristine), and sympathomimetics (e.g., amphetamines, bronchodilators) are the most notorious for causing drug-induced enhanced physiological action tremor. It is worth mentioning that amiodarone not only causes tremor, but can also cause various other neurological disorders including parkinsonism, ataxia, neuropathy, and vestibular dysfunction.[20] Tremor with a predominantly rest component is caused by anti-dopaminergic drugs: neuroleptics, gastrointestinal antiemetic/prokinetics, VMAT2 (vesicular monoamine transporter2) inhibitors, methyldopa, and reserpine. These drugs often cause concomitant bradykinesia and rigidity, and the rest tremor seen with these drugs may be symmetric or asymmetric. *Tardive tremor* is a separate form of tremor caused by dopamine receptor–blocking drugs (DRBAs). This tremor typically occurs after prolonged use of such drugs and, similar to tardive dyskinesia, can persist or worsen after their discontinuation. Tardive tremor has mainly a postural component of 3–5 Hz frequency and can also be accompanied by intention and rest components. Other parkinsonian features are usually absent, but hyperkinetic movement disorders such as orolingual dyskinesia can accompany tardive tremor.[21]

Among the drugs most likely to cause drug-induced tremor are lithium and valproic acid, which are worth mentioning in more detail. Video 7.1 shows an example of lithium-induced tremor. According to a review, the pooled percentage of lithium-induced tremor prevalence was about 27% of treated patients, but there has been a wide variability, ranging from 4 to 65% of the treated patients and occurring more frequently in older men.[10] Out of the affected patients, about 18 to 53% have to discontinue taking lithium because of bothersome tremor.[22,23] However, in most cases, lithium-induced tremor is often mild and non-disabling, and patients grow tolerant to it. Furthermore, the tremor improves over time, even with continuation of lithium in some cases.[12] Likewise, valproic acid causes tremor in about 80% of treated patients, and about half of those patients are disabled by it.[24] There is a clear dose–severity relationship, and tremor amplitude is higher with immediate release formulation (possibly related to the greater peak-to-trough variation in drug levels).[25] Just as with lithium, the tremor may improve over time even with the continuation of the drug.[24] With both agents, the tremor can occur with therapeutic blood levels; one does not have to have toxic levels to have tremor. It would also be worthwhile to note that toxic serum levels of lithium could potentially result in myoclonus, which is an important differential diagnosis for tremor. Among other movement disorders caused by lithium toxicity, notable are chorea and ataxia.[26] In addition to the commonly known drug-induced enhanced physiological type of tremor (with action and postural components), lithium and valproic acid can alternatively cause either true parkinsonism, with the characteristic parkinsonian rest tremor, or akinetic rigid parkinsonism.[14,27] In the past, this was controversial, as the presence of tremor led some to overdiagnose parkinsonism. But true parkinsonism does occur rarely, is subacute in onset, is disabling, and is reversible with discontinuation of the inciting agent. Valproate-induced parkinsonism is levodopa responsive, and many such patients may even develop dyskinesia.[14]

SSRIs, including sertraline, fluvoxamine, fluoxetine, and citalopram, also commonly cause tremor, impacting about 20% of treated patients. The tremor is typically bilateral, postural type, and the frequency ranges between 6 and 12 Hz.[28]

Although it is well known that alcohol improves essential tremor,[29] chronic consumption of alcohol can also cause tremor through direct cerebellar toxicity. The chronic alcohol-induced tremor is characterized mainly by an intention component in the upper and lower extremities; it may also have an action tremor component. Another mechanism by which alcohol can induce tremor is through hepatic failure; it is well known that alcohol can cause hepatic insufficiency, and this metabolic derangement can induce a tremor with a predominantly action component. Alcohol-induced tremor often occurs on a background of encephalopathy and often in association with other hyperkinetic movement disorders including asterixis, tics, and myoclonus, but may also occur in isolation.[29,30] Alcohol withdrawal after chronic consumption can also lead to tremor; this has been thought to be a variant of enhanced physiologic tremor precipitated by stress.[3]

Caffeine has been known to enhance the action tremor component of essential tremor and to cause an enhanced physiological tremor independently. Its specific mechanism of action has been debated upon: whether it is through a direct effect on muscle or through inhibition of phosphodiesterase and stimulation of catecholamine.[31]

Additionally, tremor can be a symptom of withdrawal from chronically used drugs, such as benzodiazepines and opiates. Therefore, reduction of dose and abrupt discontinuation of such drugs should be asked for in the history.

Diagnosis

As with other drug-induced adverse effects, some features in clinical history may be telltale for drug-induced tremor, specifically a temporal relationship between the drug initiation and tremor onset (although there might be some delay in onset of tremor in some cases), as well as a dose–tremor severity relationship. There is often an absence of tremor progression over time if the culprit drug dose is stable. In addition, drug-induced tremor usually maintains relative symmetry (upper extremities, in most cases) of involvement, but it can be asymmetrical, especially the drug-induced parkinsonian rest tremor. It is also important to exclude other common medical and neurological causes of tremor before reaching the diagnosis of a drug-induced tremor.[32] In certain cases, like lithium or valproic acid exposure, drug levels can also be checked in the serum (although tremor can be present despite therapeutic levels). Other factors to consider as contributory are anxiety and stress, use of caffeine, hyper/hypothermia, hyperthyroidism, and polypharmacy.[7]

Treatment

As with general treatment rules, the side-effect-to-benefit ratio should be considered. If the tremor is minimal and not bothersome to the patient and the medication causing the tremor is essential, one may elect to maintain the drug and not treat the tremor. This strategy often involves an interdisciplinary discussion with the patient's clinicians; for example, their cardiologists, pulmonologists, primary care doctors, psychiatrists, and others involved in patient care. If the tremor is bothersome, one may choose a dose reduction and/or discontinuation of the causative agent. For example, valproic acid may be changed over to other antiepileptics like topiramate, gabapentin, or primidone, which have been additionally shown to be effective in treating essential tremor in patients who are treated for seizure suppression. For patients who are on valproic acid for mood stabilization, alternatives like carbamazepine and lamotrigine can be considered. In psychiatric disease, dose reduction is often helpful in valproic acid–induced tremor without

making the underlying mood disorder worse. After discontinuation of the offending drug, the tremor resolution may be delayed for some time depending on the tremor characteristic and the drug. Generally speaking, action tremors resolve quickly within days; rest tremors may take weeks to months; whereas some, like tardive tremors, may never resolve. Valproate-induced tremors may also take months to resolve.

Anecdotally, medications including propranolol, acetazolamide, and amantadine have been used to address drug-induced tremors if discontinuation is not possible or if bothersome tremor persists after discontinuation of the offending drug.[32] Tardive tremor, like tardive dyskinesia, can be treated with clozapine, tetrabenazine, deutetrabenazine, or valbenazine.[15]

TREMOR ASSOCIATED WITH METABOLIC DYSFUNCTION

Common metabolic conditions causing tremor and proposed mechanisms of action

Metabolic disorders are well established as causes of tremor in the medical and neurological literature. Box 7.1[3,5,6,16,31,33–39] lists some of the most common metabolic conditions. Clinically, the tremor is primarily the enhanced physiological type.

BOX 7.1
COMMON METABOLIC DYSFUNCTIONS CAUSING TREMOR

- Electrolyte disturbances:
  - Hyponatremia
  - Hypomagnesemia
  - Hypocalcemia
- Hormonal disturbances:
  - Hypoglycemia
  - Hyperthyroidism
  - Hyperparathyroidism
- Vitamin deficiencies:
  - Vitamin B12
  - Vitamin B6
- Liver disorders:
  - Hyperammonemia
  - Hepatic encephalopathy
  - Chronic hepatocerebral degeneration
- Renal disturbances

Severe hyponatremia causes tremor in 1% of affected individuals. It is less common than other manifestations of hyponatremia and is often accompanied by seizures and encephalopathy.[36]

Tremor due to hypoglycemic episodes is very well described in patients with diabetes, insulin-secreting tumors, and other causes of hypoglycemia including alcoholism and starvation. The pathophysiology is unknown, but there has been speculation that both central and peripheral mechanisms may play a role. Central mechanisms include ischemia/anoxia topographically selective for the basal ganglia and thus causing disruption to pallidal inhibition of the thalamus, resulting in an increased thalamocortical outflow. Peripheral mechanisms for hypoglycemic tremor include changes in the sympathetico-adrenal pathway due to activation of catecholamines, which also includes shivering, hunger, and diaphoresis.[37,40]

Hyperthyroidism causes enhanced physiologic tremor and is generally present in the upper extremities more than in the lower extremities, with rare occurrence of a head tremor. The mechanism is unclear but could be a mixture of the direct effect of the thyroid hormone as well as through the adrenergic system both peripherally and centrally (intraspinal and supraspinal mechanisms, as previously described for enhanced physiologic tremor).[41] There have been reports of correlation between thyroid hormone levels and tremor frequency and amplitude; the tremor has also been shown to dissipate when the hyperthyroidism is treated.[38,42] Generally, thyroid function studies should be examined even when essential tremor is suspected, as hyperthyroidism can worsen most tremors.

Asterixis (previously referred to as "flapping tremor," an old term that is no longer used) is characterized by jerking movements of the hands when the wrist is extended; it may also be present in the arms when they are held up against gravity (the movement often looks like a bird flapping its wings, hence the old name). It occurs because of a loss of muscle activity—a negative phenomenon—and thus is not truly classified as a tremor. It is now more commonly known as negative myoclonus. Asterixis is most commonly associated with hepatic and renal disorders.[6] It is, in fact, a very sensitive sign for hepatic encephalopathy, although not very specific, as other metabolic conditions like renal disorders and drugs including valproic acid and lithium toxicity can induce it. Asterixis is often used to grade the severity of the hepatic involvement, as

it has a severity-dependent relationship.[6] There have also been case reports demonstrating association of asterixis with hypercalcemia caused by hyperparathyroidism.[33]

Vitamin B12 deficiency causes several neurological symptoms; most notable are encephalopathy and subacute combined degeneration. Movement disorders due to vitamin B12 deficiency are less well known, but the literature suggests causation of hyperkinetic movement disorders including tremor, myoclonus, and chorea.[43] Postulated pathophysiology for tremor in such cases include elevated levels of homocysteine and methyl tetrahydrofolate causing basal ganglia dysfunction and non-specific interference of cleavage of glycine, which then acts as an NMDA agonist at a spinal level causing involuntary movements.[43] This type of tremor usually affects the limbs, can be asymmetric, and can persist in sleep; it is often accompanied by myoclonus, chorea, or dystonia, thus presenting as a combined tremor syndrome. Interestingly, tremor can also occur during rapid parenteral replacement of vitamin B12 in a chronically deficient patient. The mechanism for this phenomenon is not clear but includes theories of denervation super-sensitivity, hyperglycinemia, and imbalance of excitatory versus inhibitory activity.[39,43] In this setting, tremor may be more severe and often involves the tongue. Such a tremor can become even more intense with tactile stimulation. It usually remits when the stores are replete.[43]

Diagnosis and treatment

Tremor associated with metabolic syndromes is often not isolated. The clues to diagnosis can thus be based on accompanying symptoms. Examples include adrenergic symptoms of tachycardia, sweating, and increased blood pressure, all of which are associated with thyrotoxic tremor. Cognitive dysfunction, megaloblastic anemia, and paresis are associated with vitamin B12 deficiency tremor. It is therefore important to rule out such metabolic causes of tremor, as they are often completely reversible by addressing the underlying etiology. Laboratory studies including thyroid and parathyroid hormones, vitamin levels, hepatic and renal function tests, and electrolyte and glucose levels are often necessary.

Usually, treating the underlying cause will reduce and/or dissipate the tremor. Sometimes, medications such as beta blockers are needed as adjunctive therapy. For example, in thyrotoxicosis, propranolol may work by reducing the sympathetic drive.[38]

TOXIN-INDUCED TREMORS

Toxic exposures resulting in tremor can occur in a variety of settings. Toxicities associated with different occupations or environmental settings are most commonly seen in relation to heavy metal exposures. Heavy metals, including lead, mercury, arsenic, manganese, and bismuth, can cause a variety of types of tremor. The neurotoxic effects of these heavy metals are generally the result of chronic exposure, rather than acute intoxication, leading to chronic ataxia and postural tremors.[3] These forms of tremor can be difficult to manage, as the hallmark of treatment is to avoid further exposure; tremors may also persist following the period of exposure. However, there are limited reports that suggest that the use of typical drugs for essential tremor (propranolol, primidone) may be helpful.[3]

Manganese differs from other heavy metals in that overexposure presents as a parkinsonian and dystonic syndrome. Exposures to toxic levels of manganese are associated with a number of occupations, including welding, mining, and using certain fungicides.[44] With recurrent, high-level exposure, manganese is deposited in the putamen, globus pallidus, and substantia nigra, leading to loss of dopaminergic and striatal neurons. The resultant parkinsonian syndrome includes bradykinesia, rigidity, and dystonia. While the typical parkinsonian rest tremor is not seen in manganism, dystonic tremor has been reported. Avoiding further exposure to manganese is paramount, as the neurologic manifestations are not responsive to levodopa or any other treatment.

Drugs of abuse have also been associated with tremor. Cocaine, methamphetamine, and nicotine have all been associated with enhanced physiologic tremor as well as other types of tremor.[3] Toluene, which is often found in solvents but can be inhaled as a drug of abuse, has also been associated with the development of tremor. Solvents are frequently found in different forms of adhesives, paints, and fuels. The tremor in toluene toxicity is typically a postural tremor and seen in conjunction with loss of vision, nystagmus, and other pyramidal signs.[45]

A number of additional neurotoxic agents, including, but not limited to, carbon monoxide, naphthalene, DDT, lindane, kepone, cyanide, dioxins, trimethyltin, and radiation, are also associated with new onset postural tremor.[3,46,47] Again, the mainstay of treatment in these instances is to further avoid the offending agent. If there are any chronic effects and persistent tremor, a treatment approach using drugs offered for management of essential tremor is favored.

LESIONAL TREMOR

Structural lesions in neurology have historically served as launch points for neuropathologists and neurophysiologists to determine localization and etiology of neurologic disease. The understanding of the mechanisms of various forms of tremor has similarly benefited by studying the presentation of tremor and the underlying lesions associated with it.

One prime example of this is the well-described Holmes tremor. This tremor was first described in 1904 by Gordon Holmes as the presence of unilateral resting, intentional, and postural tremor associated with lesions involving the red nucleus.[48] The involvement of the red nucleus has also led to the term "rubral" tremor, but the tremor has become better understood over the years with other localizations being reported. Hence, it has also been referred to as thalamic tremor or midbrain tremor.[3] Further investigation into the pathophysiology of this tremor has shown that disruption of the dopaminergic, cerebello-thalamic, and cerebello-olivary systems results in the development of a slow (less than 4.5 Hz), irregular tremor.[47] The tremor is generally delayed in onset and can appear anywhere between 1 month and 2 years after the lesion occurs. Holmes tremor is most frequently the result of stroke or traumatic brain injury, but it can also be seen with infectious lesions (tuberculosis, toxoplasmosis), midbrain neoplasms, and demyelinating disease, and as part of a paraneoplastic syndrome.[49,50] Video 7.2 shows the resultant tremor from a midbrain germ cell tumor. The same patient's brain MRI is seen in Figure 7.1, which shows T2-weighted MRI brain with germ cell tumor visualized in the right midbrain.

Given the involvement of the dopaminergic system, there are cases in which the tremor is responsive to dopaminergic medications.[51] However, some patients remain refractory to levodopa; there have been case reports of benefit from levetiracetam, carbamazepine, and anticholinergics.[52,53] Of note, tremors resulting from infectious or neoplastic lesions may benefit from removal and treatment of the underlying lesion. Thalamic ventral intermediate nucleus deep brain stimulation remains an alternative to selected refractory Holmes tremors, although the benefit is not as robust as is seen in essential tremor due

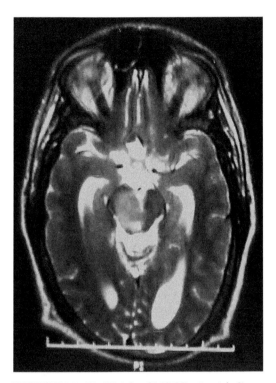

FIGURE 7.1: T2-Weighted MRI Brain with Germ Cell Tumor Visualized in the Right Midbrain of Patient with Holmes Tremor.

to the inability to adequately control proximal tremor and tremor recurrence.[54]

Lesions to the dentate nucleus of the cerebellum and cerebellar outflow tract within the superior cerebellar peduncle often present with an intention tremor.[47] Unlike Holmes tremor, this form of tremor is classically seen with lesions secondary to demyelinating disease, with symptoms occurring ipsilateral to the lesion.[50] Historically, this tremor is described as a 3–5 Hz tremor, but this can vary depending on the affected body part. Tremor in the upper extremities can be as fast as 8 Hz, while those that affect the head, trunk, or lower extremities typically have a tremor that oscillates closer to 3 Hz.[3] Rest and postural tremors have likewise been reported in cerebellar strokes and trauma, as well as paraneoplastic cerebellar degeneration.[55] Tremor secondary to lesions of the dentate nucleus or cerebellar outflow tracts is difficult to manage, often with little response to the medications typically used for essential tremor. Low-dose benzodiazepines and deep brain stimulation of the ventral intermediate nucleus of the thalamus have been shown to be helpful in some cases.[3]

Palatal tremor can be seen in settings both with lesions (symptomatic; Axis 2 acquired etiology) and without (essential; Axis 2 idiopathic etiology). Lesions within the Guillain-Mollaret triangle, connecting the red nucleus, inferior olivary nucleus, and dentate nucleus, result in symptomatic palatal tremor of the levator veli palatini muscle, as seen in Video 7.3.[56] This patient's symptomatic palatal tremor was caused by a hemorrhage as shown, in the CAT scan (Figure 7.2).

Lesions are typically secondary to stroke or hemorrhage, but they have also been reported in demyelinating disease and trauma.[47] These lesions typically result in hypertrophy of the inferior olive.[57] Palatal tremor can also be seen in the setting of anti-GAD65 syndrome.[58] While the etiology of acquired palatal tremor is well established, the mechanism of essential (idiopathic) palatal tremor is not well understood. Essential palatal tremor, which some consider to be a functional neurologic disorder, presents as an ear click with tensor veli palatini contraction, as seen in Video 7.4.[3] While the etiology remains unknown, it is responsive to injections with botulinum toxin.

While stroke can cause any of the above forms of tremor, stroke as a tremor etiology is rare. Dystonia secondary to stroke can lead to dystonic tremor, and tremor has been reported following strokes to the subthalamic nucleus, although ballism and chorea are more common.[47]

Traumatic injuries have also been known to cause tremor. Diffuse axonal injury, associated with sudden and abrupt deceleration injuries, often causes midbrain injury. This midbrain injury has been reported to result in tremor and parkinsonism.[47,59] Cerebellar trauma has also

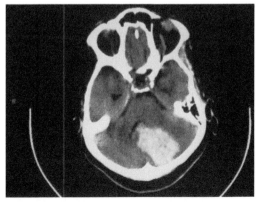

FIGURE 7.2: Cerebral Hemorrhage in the CT Scan of a Patient with Symptomatic Palatal Tremor.

been reported to cause postural, rest, axial, and intention tremor.[55]

Tremor can also be secondary to neoplasms and subsequent treatment of the underlying tumor. Specifically, brainstem and cerebellar astrocytomas have rarely caused isolated tongue tremor.[60] This has also been reported following treatment of acoustic schwannomas. Tremors with these tumors can present as a 3–5 Hz protrusion and retraction tremor of the tongue without any other findings of tremor. Outside of removing the lesion, treatment with anticholinergics and valproate has been shown to be effective.

TREMOR SECONDARY TO SYSTEMIC DISEASE

As previously discussed under "Tremor associated with metabolic dysfunction," tremor is highly associated with thyroid disease. However, thyroid disease is far from the only systemic illness that is known to cause tremor.

Wilson disease, an autosomal recessive systemic disease primarily affecting the central nervous system and liver, is classically taught to present as a postural "wing beating tremor"; however, this is typically a late presentation of the disease. Patients who initially report tremor in the setting of Wilson disease can present with many forms of tremor, including rest, action, postural, intention, and isolated tongue tremor,[47] as well as parkinsonism, dystonia, and chorea. New onset tremor in a young patient should trigger a workup for Wilson disease. Serum ceruloplasmin can be checked, although a normal value does not rule out Wilson's. If there is a significant index of suspicion, a 24-hour urine copper level is recommended, as it is much more sensitive. Chelation therapy should be initiated in the setting of a positive screen.[61]

Chronic liver failure is likewise associated with new onset tremor. In this setting, there can be increased deposition of manganese in the basal ganglia. As discussed in the toxicity section of this chapter, manganese deposition in the brain can lead to a parkinsonian presentation. This deposition and subsequent neurologic sequelae, including cognitive impairment, chorea, dystonia, asterixis, and behavioral changes in the setting of chronic liver disease, are known as acquired hepatocerebral degeneration.[62] Similar to manganese toxicity, the degree of rest tremor is typically reduced when compared to other parkinsonian findings, but tremors have been noted. MRI will typically show T1-weighted hyperintensities in the basal ganglia, which is secondary to manganese deposition.[62]

Metabolic diseases are not alone in causing tremor. Infectious disease has also been associated with new onset tremor. Human Immunodeficiency Virus (HIV) primary infection can occasionally present with a new onset postural tremor, which is often bilateral and mild.[3] Tremor in HIV becomes more common if the disease is left untreated, as patients with HIV-associated neurocognitive disorder have a higher incidence of tremor. HIV can also cause Holmes tremor.[63] Furthermore, the lesions associated with opportunistic infections like tuberculosis or toxoplasmosis, as well as central nervous system (CNS) lymphoma, can cause a variety of the tremors discussed in the previous section.[64]

Peripheral neuropathy is a common feature of many forms of systemic disease, and some forms of peripheral neuropathy, including monogenetic forms, have been associated with neuropathic tremor. Specifically, IgM neuropathy, chronic inflammatory demyelinating polyneuropathy, and Charcot-Marie-Tooth disorder have been known to have subacute development of tremor.[3] This tremor is often bilateral, involving the hands, and has a more profound postural component. In Charcot-Marie-Tooth, this is known as Roussy-Levy syndrome. In a patient who presents with physical signs of peripheral neuropathy as well as tremor, a serum protein electrophoresis should be obtained to check for monoclonal gammopathy of undetermined significance. Further consideration can be given to EMG, lumbar puncture, and nerve biopsy.[47] The mechanism for neuropathic tremor is unclear, but it is possible that weakness causes an enhancement of physiological tremor through loss of dampening of movements due to central oscillatory output; abnormal sensory input may lead to tremulous movements. Other neuromuscular disorders, including certain forms of myopathy, have also been associated with tremor.[65]

CONCLUSION

Tremor can present in a wide variety of clinical scenarios. Medications, metabolic disturbances, toxins, systemic illness, and structural lesions can all cause a new onset of tremor or worsen tremor that is already present. The phenomenology of these acquired or secondary tremors can vary widely, and can occur at rest, with action, or with maintaining posture, or they may be intention tremors. The overlap and variety of presentations can make it difficult to identify the etiology.

Therefore, a thorough history and proper workup are paramount. In any patient that presents with new onset tremor, an exhaustive review of medications, both past and current, is necessary. Occupational history should also be obtained to rule out any possible toxic exposures that can also cause tremor. Equally important is reviewing the patient's past medical history, as a number of systemic illnesses and metabolic derangements can also present with tremor. However, in some instances, tremor can be the first known manifestation. Metabolic and toxic evaluation, including checking serum for thyroid panel, metabolic panel, levels of vitamins B12 and B6, ammonia, ceruloplasmin, and heavy metal screen (when appropriate), should be considered for new onset tremor evaluation. In the setting of focal deficits or a known history of focal neurologic disease, imaging of the brain with MRI can be useful if a lesional tremor is suspected. In addition, MRI can often give other clues based on T1- and T2-weighted hyperintensities, for example in manganese toxicity. Once identified, a strategy can be put in place to remove an offending drug or toxin exposure, treat the underlying systemic disease, correct the metabolic abnormality, or remove the lesion in the brain wherever possible. If the above strategy does not result in improvement, or if removal of an inciting agent cannot be considered, a trial of therapeutic agents often used for primary tremor disorders such as essential tremor and Parkinson disease can be tried. In summary, there is a wide variety of Axis 2–acquired causes of tremor. A methodical approach is necessary to find the proper etiology, but a comprehensive evaluation can lead to appropriate therapy.

REFERENCES

1. Bhatia KP, et al. Consensus statement on the classification of tremors. From the task force on tremor of the International Parkinson and Movement Disorder Society. *Mov Disord.* 2018;33(1):75–87.

2. Schnitzler A, Gross J, Normal and pathological oscillatory communication in the brain. *Nat Rev Neurosci.* 2005;6(4):285–296.

3. Pont-Sunyer C, Tolosa E, Navarro-Otano J. Other tremors. In: Albanese A, Jankovic J, eds. *Hyperkinetic Movement Disorders.* Blackwell; 2012: 95–111.

4. Basden C. Medication- and toxin-induced neurologic syndromes. *Prim Care.* 2015;42(2):259–265.

5. Crawford P, Zimmerman EE. Tremor: sorting through the differential diagnosis. *Am Fam Physician.* 2018;97(3):180–186.

6. Ellul MA, Cross TJ, Larner AJ. Asterixis. *Pract Neurol.* 2017;17(1):60–62.

7. Factor SA et al. Recent developments in drug-induced movement disorders: a mixed picture. *Lancet Neurol.* 2019;18(9):880–890.

8. Farouk SS, Rein JL. The many faces of calcineurin inhibitor toxicity: what the FK? *Adv Chronic Kidney Dis.* 2020;27(1):56–66.

9. Fitzgerald KT, Bronstein AC. Adderall® (amphetamine-dextroamphetamine) toxicity. *Top Companion Anim Med.* 2013;28(1):2–7.

10. Gelenberg AJ, Jefferson JW. Lithium tremor. *J Clin Psychiatry.* 1995;56(7):283–287.

11. Kovács A, et al. Lamotrigine induces tremor among epilepsy patients probably via cerebellar pathways. *Tohoku J Exp Med.* 2019;248(4):273–284.

12. Morgan JC, Sethi KD. Drug-induced tremors. *Lancet Neurol.* 2005;4(12):866–876.

13. Robottom BJ, Shulman LM, Weiner WJ. Drug-induced movement disorders: emergencies and management. *Neurol Clin.* 2012;30(1):309–320, x.

14. Silver M, Factor SA. Valproic acid-induced parkinsonism: levodopa responsiveness with dyskinesia. *Parkinsonism Relat Disord.* 2013;19(8):758–760.

15. Stacy M, Jankovic J. Tardive tremor. *Mov Disord.* 1992;7(1):53–57.

16. Louis ED. Tremor. *Continuum (Minneap Minn).* 2019;25(4):959–975.

17. Deuschl G, et al. Treatment of patients with essential tremor. *Lancet Neurol.* 2011;10(2):148–161.

18. Elble RJ. Central mechanisms of tremor. *J Clin Neurophysiol.* 1996;13(2):133–144.

19. Morgan JC, et al. Insights into pathophysiology from medication-induced tremor. *Tremor Other Hyperkinet Mov (N Y).* 2017;7:442.

20. Charness ME, Morady F, Scheinman MM. Frequent neurologic toxicity associated with amiodarone therapy. *Neurology.* 1984;34(5):669–671.

21. Savitt D, Jankovic J. Tardive syndromes. *J Neurol Sci.* 2018;389:35–42.

22. Burgess S, Geddes J, Hawton K, Townsend E, Jamison K, Goodwin G. Lithium for maintenance treatment of mood disorders. *Cochrane Database Syst Rev.* 2001;(3):CD003013. doi:10.1002/14651858.CD003013. PMID: 11687035.

23. Baek JH, Kinrys G, Nierenberg AA. Lithium tremor revisited: pathophysiology and treatment. *Acta Psychiatr Scand.* 2014;129(1):17–23.

24. Alonso-Juarez M, et al. The clinical features and functional impact of valproate-induced tremor. *Parkinsonism Relat Disord.* 2017;44:147–150.

25. Rinnerthaler M, et al. Computerized tremor analysis of valproate-induced tremor: a comparative study of controlled-release versus conventional valproate. *Epilepsia.* 2005;46(2):320–323.

26. Podskalny GD, Factor SA. Chorea caused by lithium intoxication: a case report and literature review. *Mov Disord.* 1996;11(6):733–737.

27. Hermida AP, et al. A case of lithium-induced parkinsonism presenting with typical motor symptoms of Parkinson's disease in a bipolar patient. *Int Psychogeriatr.* 2016;28(12):2101–2104.

28. Wernicke JF. Safety and side effect profile of fluoxetine. *Expert Opin Drug Saf.* 2004;3(5):495–504.

29. Mostile G, Jankovic J. Alcohol in essential tremor and other movement disorders. *Mov Disord.* 2010;25(14):2274–2284.

30. Koller W, et al. Tremor in chronic alcoholism. *Neurology.* 1985;35(11):1660–1662.

31. Jankovic J, Fahn S. Physiologic and pathologic tremors. Diagnosis, mechanism, and management. *Ann Intern Med.* 1980;93(3):460–465.

32. Burkhard PR. Acute and subacute drug-induced movement disorders. *Parkinsonism Relat Disord.* 2014;20(Suppl 1):S108–S112.

33. Argov Z, Melamed E, Katz S. Hyperparathyroidism presenting with unusual neurological features. *Eur Neurol.* 1979;18(5):338–340.

34. Becktepe JS, Goevert F, Deuschl G. [Rare tremor syndromes]. *Nervenarzt.* 2018;89(4):386–393.

35. Elias WJ, Shah BB. Tremor. *JAMA.* 2014;311(9):948–954.

36. Ellis SJ. Severe hyponatraemia: complications and treatment. *QJM.* 1995;88(12):905–909.

37. Guerrero WR, Okun MS, McFarland NR. Encephalopathy, hypoglycemia, and flailing extremities: a case of bilateral chorea-ballism associated with diabetic ketoacidosis. *Tremor Other Hyperkinet Mov (N Y).* 2012;2:tre-02-58-235-1. doi:10.7916/D8RX99T2.

38. Lazarus S, Bell GH. Tremor in hyperthyroidism. its value in the diagnosis and assessment of the condition. *Glasgow Med J.* 1943;140(3):77–86.

39. Zanus C, et al. Involuntary movements after correction of vitamin B12 deficiency: a video-case report. *Epileptic Disord.* 2012;14(2):174–180.

40. Valente LG, et al. Clinical presentation of 54 patients with endogenous hyperinsulinaemic hypoglycaemia: a neurological chameleon (observational study). *Swiss Med Wkly.* 2018;148:w14682.

41. Abila B, et al. Tremor: an alternative approach for investigating adrenergic mechanisms in thyrotoxicosis? *Clin Sci (Lond).* 1985;69(4):459–463.

42. Milanov I, Sheinkova G. Clinical and electromyographic examination of tremor in patients with thyrotoxicosis. *Int J Clin Pract.* 2000;54(6):364–367.

43. de Souza A, Moloi MW. Involuntary movements due to vitamin B12 deficiency. *Neurol Res.* 2014;36(12):1121–1128.

44. Peres TV, et al. Manganese-induced neurotoxicity: a review of its behavioral consequences and neuroprotective strategies. *BMC Pharmacol Toxicol.* 2016;17(1):57.

45. Dick F, et al. Neurological deficits in solvent-exposed painters: a syndrome including impaired colour vision, cognitive defects, tremor and loss of vibration sensation. *QJM.* 2000;93(10):655–661.

46. Caito S, Aschner M. Neurotoxicity of metals. *Handb Clin Neurol.* 2015;131:169–189.

47. Puschmann A, Wszolek ZK. Diagnosis and treatment of common forms of tremor. *Semin Neurol.* 2011;31(1):65–77.

48. Holmes G. On certain tremors in organic cerebral lesions. *Brain.* 1904;27(3):327–375.

49. Tan H, et al. Rubral tremor after thalamic infarction in childhood. *Pediatr Neurol.* 2001;25(5):409–412.

50. Koch M, et al. Tremor in multiple sclerosis. *J Neurol.* 2007;254(2):133–145.

51. Findley LJ, Gresty MA. Suppression of "rubral" tremor with levodopa. *Br Med J.* 1980;281(6247):1043.

52. Ferlazzo E, et al. Successful treatment of Holmes tremor by levetiracetam. *Mov Disord.* 2008;23(14):2101–2103.

53. Harmon RL, Long DF, Shirtz J. Treatment of post-traumatic midbrain resting-kinetic tremor with combined levodopa/carbidopa and carbamazepine. *Brain Inj.* 1991;5(2):213–218.

54. Ramirez-Zamora A, Okun MS. Deep brain stimulation for the treatment of uncommon tremor syndromes. *Expert Rev Neurother.* 2016;16(8):983–997.

55. Lenka A, Louis ED. Revisiting the clinical phenomenology of "cerebellar tremor": beyond the intention tremor. *Cerebellum.* 2019;18(3):565–574.

56. Zadikoff C, Lang AE, Klein C. The "essentials" of essential palatal tremor: a reappraisal of the nosology. *Brain.* 2006;129(Pt 4):832–840.

57. Pearce JM. Palatal myoclonus (syn. palatal tremor). *Eur Neurol.* 2008;60(6):312–315.

58. Pittock SJ, Palace J. Paraneoplastic and idiopathic autoimmune neurologic disorders: approach to diagnosis and treatment. *Handb Clin Neurol.* 2016;133:165–183.

59. Krauss JK, Tränkle R, Kopp KH. Post-traumatic movement disorders in survivors of severe head injury. *Neurology.* 1996;47(6):1488–1492.

60. Ure RJ, et al. Unusual tremor syndromes: know in order to recognise. *J Neurol Neurosur PS.* 2016;87(11):1191–1203.

61. Aggarwal A, Bhatt M. Advances in treatment of Wilson disease. *Tremor Other Hyperkinet Mov (N Y).* 2018;8:525.

62. Sureka B, et al. Neurologic manifestations of chronic liver disease and liver cirrhosis. *Curr Probl Diagn Radiol.* 2015;44(5):449–461.

63. Mattos JP, et al. Movement disorders in 28 HIV-infected patients. *Arq Neuropsiquiatr.* 2002;60(3-a):525–530.

64. De Mattos JP, et al. Involuntary movements and AIDS: report of seven cases and review of the literature. *Arq Neuropsiquiatr.* 1993;51(4):491–497.

65. Stavusis J, et al. Novel mutations in MYBPC1 are associated with myogenic tremor and mild myopathy. *Ann Neurol.* 2019;86(1):129–142.

SECTION 2

The Family of Tremors

Like many families, the family of tremors is diverse, sometimes messy, and ever changing. This section presents the full extended family, spanning isolated tremors, tremor as one of several features of a neurological disorder, and hyperkinetic movement phenotypes commonly referred to, mimicking, and framed as tremors. Chapters center around distinct tremor syndromes, whether idiopathic or of known etiology.

The section starts with disorders classically considered tremor, including isolated tremor syndromes. Next, complex tremor syndromes are presented, shading into areas of phenotypic overlap. The language in these chapters reflects the level of active investigation in the field, and will undoubtedly continue to evolve. Of note, there is a long literature predating the 2018 International Parkinson Disease and Movement Disorder Society classification of tremor, considering task-specific tremors and isolated head/neck and vocal tremors as forms of essential tremor. Chapter 10 illustrates the importance of continuing to tie action-based limb tremors and vocal tremor together to further pathophysiology and new therapeutic development work, and of utilizing the 2018 classification system as a flexible framework rather than dogma. Chapter 11 breaks down ways to consider tremor, dystonia, and their combinations to generate empiric evidence that advances etiologic understanding of both, especially within currently purely clinically defined entities. As work advances, the Axis 1 definition of essential tremor will inevitably change again, perhaps breaking into syndromes closer to dystonia versus limb and vocal essential tremors.

Finally, entities some consider tremor "cousins" are presented: ataxia, myoclonus, myorhythmia, and functional tremors. All have phenotypic, etiological, or treatment intersections with classic tremors, and are important to fully understand the family of tremors.

8

Orthostatic Tremor

PETER G. BAIN

THE DEFINITION OF ORTHOSTATIC TREMOR

OT has been defined by the International Parkinson's and Movement Disorder Society Task Force on Tremor as follows:[1]

Different forms of orthostatic tremor share the core symptom of tremor during standing. Primary orthostatic tremor (POT) is defined as an isolated tremor syndrome, and its accurate diagnosis requires electrophysiological testing.[2] Primary orthostatic tremor is a generalized high-frequency (13–18 Hz) isolated tremor syndrome that occurs when standing. Confirmation of the tremor frequency is needed, typically with an electromyography (EMG). OT with the electrophysiological properties of POT has occurred in combination with other neurological conditions (e.g., dementia, PD, and spinocerebellar ataxia), and it should then be labeled as primary orthostatic tremor plus.[3] The pathophysiological relation of POT and the other conditions is unclear and may be coincidental. POT may be palpable but not visible, and the diagnosis needs confirmation with EMG recordings that reveal a 13- to 18-Hz tremor that is uniquely highly coherent among affected body parts.[2-4]

An audible rhythm called the "helicopter sign" may be detected by auscultation of the lower leg muscles or by listening to EMG.[5]

There are additional clinical syndromes with tremor during standing that have a lower frequency than 13 Hz and have been labeled as slow OT, tremor in orthostatism, and pseudo-orthostatic tremor. We propose the term pseudo-orthostatic tremor.[6] These slower orthostatic tremors (frequency less than 13 Hz) are frequently associated with other neurological signs. Cases with various forms of parkinsonism, ataxia, and dystonia have been described. A rare differential diagnosis (which is not tremor) with a similar clinical picture is orthostatic myoclonus syndrome.[6]

CLINICAL FEATURES OF PRIMARY ORTHOSTATIC TREMOR

Demographics

The incidence and prevalence of primary orthostatic tremor are unknown, and it is likely underrecognized given the long delays from the onset of POT to diagnosis (Table 8.1).

TABLE 8.1: PRIMARY ORTHOSTATIC TREMOR: SEX DISTRIBUTION, AGE OF ONSET, AND YEARS FROM ONSET TO DIAGNOSIS

Study	Number of patients	Percentage who were female	Age of onset, years Mean (range or SD)	Years from OT onset to diagnosis Mean (range or SD)
Hassan et al. (2016)[3]	184	63.3%	59.3 (Range: 13–85)	7.2 (Range: 0–44)
Colmenares et al. (2019)[7]	82	62.2%	50.3 (SD + 16.2)	8.1 (SD ± 9.7)
Ganos et al. (2016)[8]	68	76.5%	54.0 (SD ± 12.8)	4.5 (Range 0–44)
Yaltho and Ondo (2014)[9]	45	49.0%	59.5 (SD ± 10.5)	6.7 (SD ± 4.3)
Gerschlager et al. (2004)[10]	31	70.1%	50.4 (SD ± 15.1)	5.7 (SD ± 4.3)
Piboolnurak et al. (2001)[11]	26	80.7%	57.1 (Range: 34–81)	NS

Key: NS: not specified

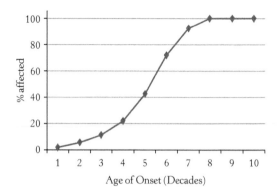

FIGURE 8.1: Cumulative Age of Orthostatic Tremor Onset Plot.

Most major studies indicate that primary orthostatic tremor afflicts women more commonly than men, with a ratio of approximately 2 to 1 (Table 8.1).[3,7–11] The mean age at onset of POT is in the sixth decade (Table 8.1), with an age of onset ranging from the first to the tenth decade (Figure 8.1).[3,7–11]

There is conflicting evidence about whether women have a later age of onset and presentation of POT than men. (Table 8.2 and Figures 8.2 and 8.3).[8,10–12]

Symptoms of primary orthostatic tremor

Presenting complaint

The two most common presenting complaints of patients with POT are tremor in the legs while standing and a feeling of unsteadiness on standing that improves on walking (Table 8.3).[3,9–13] However, there are also other less frequent presentations, including tremor in the hands (12.5%), pain and numbness in the legs (5.4%), gait disturbance (3.6%), and trunk tremor (1.8%).[12]

Thus, in the majority of cases the diagnosis of POT can be strongly suspected from the patient's initial description of their symptoms.

Standing in queues and at social gatherings is often problematic for those afflicted by POT. Furthermore, performing a manual task becomes more difficult while the patient is standing. For example, patients compensate by leaning against the sink to facilitate brushing their teeth.

Intriguingly, patients with POT describe how their standing time is greatly prolonged when standing in chest-high water in a swimming pool, to the extent that it is no longer an issue. This effect is likely to be the result of buoyancy, which reduces the weight borne on the legs, thus decreasing the severity of POT. This finding suggests that POT would not be apparent in space, which might be a potential future therapy.

Types of tremor reported by patients

Patients with POT report tremor affecting various body parts: Piboolnurak and colleagues (2005) noted that 18 (69.2%) of their patients complained of tremor elsewhere, including in the lips, jaw, hands, and the "whole body," in addition to the legs.[11] Similarly, Bain and Jones (2010) described tremor affecting the hands, head, trunk, voice, and tongue.[12] It is noteworthy that occasionally patients are aware of the tremor in only one leg (Table 8.4).

Clinical course

Patients with long-standing POT may describe gradual deterioration of their "standing time" over several years, indicating progression of the condition. However, the conflicting information about progression in the literature is probably because the condition may plateau for a few years but then deteriorates. Progression was noted by Mestre et al. (2012) in 72%, Ganos et al. (2016)

TABLE 8.2: MEAN AGE OF ONSET AND MEAN AGE AT PRESENTATION FOR MALES AND FEMALES WITH ORTHOSTATIC TREMOR

Study	Number of patients	Mean age of onset in males (years)	Mean age of onset in females (years)	Mean age at presentation in males (years)	Mean age at presentation in females (years)
Ganos et al. (2016)[8]	68	57.0	53.1	NS	NS
Bain and Jones (2010)[12]	56	46.3	54.5	56.0	64.3
Gerschlager et al. (2004)[10]	41	60.0	50.4	NS	NS
Piboolnurak et al. (2005)[11]	26	55.4	58.7	NS	NS

Key: NS: not specified

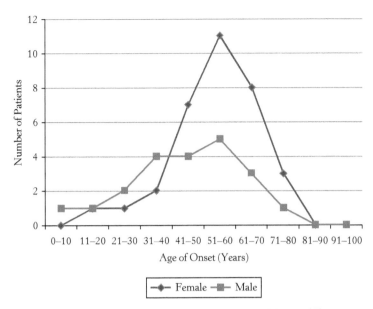

FIGURE 8.2: Age of Onset Plot for Primary Orthostatic Tremor in Men and Women.

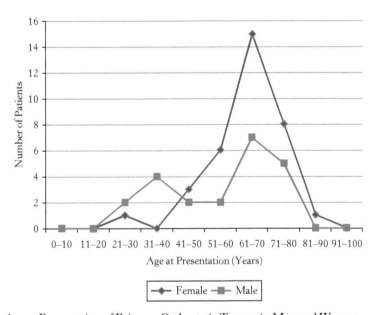

FIGURE 8.3: Age at Presentation of Primary Orthostatic Tremor in Men and Women.

TABLE 8.3: PRESENTATIONS OF PRIMARY ORTHOSTATIC TREMOR

Study	Number of patients	Presentation with leg tremor number (%)	Presentation with unsteadiness number (%)	Other presentation number (%)
Bain and Jones (2010)[12]	56	31 (55.4%)	12 (21.4%)	13 (23.2%)
Mestre et al. (2012)[13]	26	18 (69.2%)	8 (30.8%)	0 (0%)
Hassan et al. (2016)[3]	184	NS	NS	NS
Gerschlager et al. (2004)[10]	41	NS	NS	NS
Yaltho and Ondo (2014)[9]	30	NS	NS	NS
Piboolnurak et al. (2005)[11]	26	NS	NS	NS

TABLE 8.4: PARTS OF THE BODY REPORTED BY PATIENTS WITH PRIMARY ORTHOSTATIC TREMOR TO BE AFFECTED BY TREMOR

Type of tremor	Number (/56)	Percentage (%)
RLL tremor	55	98.2
LLL tremor	55	98.2
RUL tremor	28	50.0
LUL tremor	25	44.6
Head tremor	11	19.6
Trunk tremor	9	16
Voice tremor	4	7.1
Tongue tremor	4	7.1

Note that two patients were aware of OT in one leg only (i.e., symptomatically unilateral POT).[12]
Key: RLL: right lower limb, RUL: right upper limb, LLL: left lower limb, LUL: left upper limb

in 79.4%, and Hassan et al. (2016) in 91% of their patients, respectively.[3,8,13]

Falls

The percentage of patients with POT who reported having fallen is shown in Table 8.5. Although falls occur in about 16.1% to 26.4% of people with POT, the frequency of falls is usually deemed as "rare," although this may not be the case in severe cases.[3,8,11,12]

The types of aid used by patients with POT indoors and outdoors are shown in Table 8.6.[12] In addition, many patients with POT tend to "furniture walk" indoors.

Social history

Seven percent of patients with POT either had a stair lift fitted or had to move from a house to a bungalow because of difficulty managing stairs.[12]

Smoking tobacco was documented in 43.5% of 184 patients in the study by Hassan and colleagues (2016); Bain and Jones (2010) found that

TABLE 8.6: WALKING AIDS USED BY PEOPLE WITH PRIMARY ORTHOSTATIC TREMOR[12]

Type of aid utilized	Indoors number of patients using aid	Outdoors number of patients using aid
Stick	6	7
Wheelchair	1	5
Stool	2	2
Zimmer frame	1	2
Trolley	2	1
Total number (%)	12(21.4%)	17(30.4%)

29.5% of POT patients currently smoked, while a further 20.5% had smoked in the past.[3,12] The proportion of patients with orthostatic tremor who drank alcohol at the time of consultation and whose OT responded are shown in Table 8.7.[3, 10–13]

Family history

A family history of OT is unusual (Table 8.8). Intriguingly, an affected pair of homozygous twins with OT has been reported.[8,14]

Patients with POT may also report having a family history of Parkinson's or essential tremor, although the frequency with which these are reported varies between studies. Furthermore, some caution should be exercised in interpreting this data, as the relatives were not examined (Table 8.9).

Affective disorders and quality of life

Gerschlager and colleagues (2003) used self-administered questionnaires, the Beck Depression Inventory (BDI) and the Medical Outcomes Short Form 36 Health Survey (SF-36), to assess depression and quality of life (QoL) of 20 people with POT.[15] They found that 6 (30%) had "moderate

TABLE 8.5: PERCENTAGE OF PATIENTS WITH PRIMARY ORTHOSTATIC TREMOR REPORTING HAVING FALLEN

Study	Number of patients questioned about falls	Percentage of patients reporting having fallen
Hassan et al. (2016)[3]	133	24.1%
Ganos et al. (2016)[8]	68	26.4%
Bain and Jones (2010)[12]	56	16.1%
Piboolnurak et al. (2005)[11]	19	21.1%
Range across studies		**16.1%–26.4%**

TABLE 8.7: PROPORTION OF PATIENTS WITH ORTHOSTATIC TREMOR WHO DRANK ALCOHOL AT THE TIME OF CONSULTATION, AND THE PROPORTION WHOSE TREMOR RESPONDED TO ALCOHOL

Study	Proportion of patients (%) drinking alcohol	Proportion of patients (%) whose OT responded to alcohol
Hassan et al. (2016)[3]	102/171 (59.6%)	10/23 (43.5%)
Bain and Jones (2010)[12]	35/43 (81.4%)	15/28 (51.7%)
Mestre et al. (2012)[13]	3/7 (42.8%)	NS
Gerschlager et al. (2004)[10]	NS	8/31 (25.8%)
Piboolnurak et al. (2005)[11]	NS	3/11 (27.3%)
Range in the above studies	**42.8%–81.4%**	**25.8%–51.7%**

TABLE 8.8: FAMILY HISTORY OF ORTHOSTATIC TREMOR

Study	Number of patients in study	Number (%) of patients reporting a FH of OT	Number (%) of patients reporting a 1st-degree relative with OT
Hassan et al. (2016)[3]	184	9 (4.9%)	8 (4.3%)
Ganos et al. (2016)[8]	68	1 (1.5%)	1 (1.5%)
Bain and Jones (2010)[12]	56	3 (5.4%)	3 (5.4%)
Yaltho and Ondo (2014)[9]	40*	3 (6.7%)	NS
Mestre et al. (2012)[13]	26	0 (0%)	0 (0%)
Gerschlager et al. (2004)[10]	26*	5 (19.2%)	2 (7.7%)
Piboolnurak et al. (2005)[11]	26	1 (3.8%)	1 (3.8%)
Range in above studies		**0%–19.2%**	**0%–5.4%**

Key: *Including POT ($\pm$ upper limb tremor) only. NS: not specified

TABLE 8.9: SHOWS THE PERCENTAGE OF PATIENTS WITH ORTHOSTATIC TREMOR IN VARIOUS STUDIES WITH A FAMILY HISTORY OF ESSENTIAL TREMOR, UNSPECIFIED TREMOR*, OR PARKINSON DISEASE

Study	Number in study	Number (%) of patients with a FH of 'Parkinson'	Number (%) of patients with a FH of 'ET'
Hassan et al. (2016)[3]	184	17 (9.2%)	22 (12.0%)
Ganos et al. (2016)[8]	68	3 (4.4%)	6 (8.8%)
Bain and Jones (2010)[10]	56	3 (5.4%)	10.7% (1st degree) 8.9% (2nd degree)
Gerschlager et al. (2004)[10]	41	NS	NS
Mestre et al. (2012)[13]	26	0 (0%)	3 (11.5%) UST*
Piboolnurak et al. (2005)[11]	26	3 (11.5%)	3 (15.4%)
Range in above studies		**0%–11.5%**	**8.8%–15.40%**

Key: *The patients had a family history of hand $\pm$ head tremor. UST: unspecified tremor.

TABLE 8.10: AFFECTIVE DISORDERS
REPORTED BY OT PATIENTS[12]

Affective disorder	Bain and Jones 2010 number (/56) (%)	Gerschlager et al. 2003 number (/20) (%)
Depression	11 (19.6%)	11 (55%)*
Fatigue	8 (14.3%)	NR
Frustration	6 (10.7%)	NR
Anxiety	5 (8.9%)	NR

Key: *Includes mild-moderate and moderate-severe depression cases. NR: not reported.

to severe" and 5 had (20%) "mild to moderate" depression on the BDI. There was a weak correlation between the BDI scores with the duration but not the severity of OT; the latter was estimated from standing times.[15] Fatigue, frustration, and anxiety have also been reported by patients with POT (Table 8.10).[12]

The mean QoL scores on the SF-36 by the patients with OT were significantly worse than those of UK population norms for the group aged 65–74 years, with the scores for physical and social functioning and physical and social role limitations being most affected.[15]

The clinical examination
Leg tremor

Examination typically reveals a fine tremor of the patient's legs while stance is maintained; this is sometimes better appreciated as a fine ripple in the patient's trousers or dress. However, as stance is continued, a visible and palpable tremor usually becomes apparent in the legs, which typically increases in severity as stance is prolonged and may spread to affect the trunk. Auscultation of the gastrocnemius or quadriceps while the patient is standing may reveal a noise similar to a helicopter's rotor blades, termed the "helicopter sign."[5] In rare instances, when the patient reports unilateral POT, a slight tremor can also be detected in the apparently unaffected leg if stance is prolonged (i.e., the POT is markedly asymmetric). (PGB: personal observation). POT disappears if the patient is lifted off their feet. The leg tremor may be apparent while the feet are pushing against a rigid object (isometric tremor).[16] Rarely, POT persists on walking; Mestre et al. (2012) detected it in 2 of 26 (7.7%), when it was associated with a "wobbly gait," and Piboolnurak et al. (2005) in 1 of 26 (3.8%) of their cases, respectively.[11,13]

Rest tremor in the legs is not usually present when the patient is seated, although there are rare exceptions. Mild postural tremor of the legs was observed in 56% of cases by Bain and Jones (2010) and was invariably mild (mean: 1/10, range 0–2 on the Bain and Findley (1993) tremor scale).[12,17]

The patients may often be observed adopting a broad-based stance and may appear unsteady, shuffling to maintain balance. They may also stiffen their legs, claw the ground with their toes, and hold onto a nearby object to prevent falling.[18]

Upper limb tremor

Tremor is frequently detected in parts of the body other than the legs in patients with POT: Hassan and colleagues (2016) found that 60.3% of their 184 patients with OT had tremor in their arms.[3] Several different types of upper limb tremor have been documented in patients with POT, including rest, postural, kinetic, and intention tremor, as well as tremor when engaged in handwriting and spiral drawings.[3,8,10–13] These forms of tremor may be present while the patient is sitting, standing, or both, with the upper limb postural tremor tending to be more severe while patients are standing.[9,11] In addition, tremor can be detected in the patients' arms while standing with their arms hanging by their sides and when leaning with their arms against a wall (isometric tremor).[10,11] The prevalence of the rest, postural, and intention tremors in the upper limbs of patients with POT are shown in Table 8.11, from which it can be seen that a rest component is rare (less than 5% of cases), whereas postural tremor is common, and intention tremor is apparent in about one-third of cases.[3,8–13,19]

When collected systematically (Table 8.12),[3,8–13] tremor was detected in the handwriting of over one-quarter of patients and the spiral drawings of over half of patients.[12] The severity of tremor in the spiral drawings, assessed using the Bain and Findley Spiral rating scale, was mild in 70.7%, moderate in 7.3%, and severe in 2.4% of patients.[12,17] Examples are shown in Figures 8.4A and 8.4B.

Head, jaw, and lip tremor

Tremor of the head can be detected in a minority of patients, with jaw and lip tremor rarely present (Table 8.13).[3,8,12,11]

Gait abnormalities

Gait abnormalities are frequently present in patients with POT (Table 8.14), with the majority of patients (83.9%) having an abnormal gait.[12] Over half the patients have a broad-based gait, and one-third have a reduced arm swing while

TABLE 8.11: PREVALENCE OF THE REST, POSTURAL (ARMS HELD OUTSTRETCHED) AND INTENTION TREMOR OF UPPER LIMBS DETECTED ON EXAMINATION IN PATIENTS WITH PRIMARY ORTHOSTATIC TREMOR

Study	Number in study	Rest tremor in arms N (%)	Postural tremor in arms N (%)	Intention tremor in arms N (%)
Hassan et al. (2016)[3]	184	5 (2.7%)	42 (22.8%)	NS
Ganos et al. (2016)[8]	59*	NS	30 (50.8%)	NS
Bain and Jones (2010)[12]	56	2 (3.6%)	50 (89.3%)	33 (58.9%)
Yaltho and Ondo (2014)[9]	40*	NS	30 (75.0%)	NS
Mestre et al. (2012)[13]	24	NS	NS	NS
Gerschlager et al. (2004)[10]	31*	NS	24 (77.4%)	NS
Piboolnurak et al. (2005)[11]	26	NS	NS	NS
McManis and Sharborough (1993)[19]	30	NS	9 (30%)	NS
Range in above studies		**2.7%–3.6%**	**22.8%–89.3%**	**33.0%**

Key: *Including POT (± upper limb tremor) only. NS: not specified

TABLE 8.12: TREMOR IN HANDWRITING AND SPIRAL DRAWINGS

Study	Number in study	Tremor in handwriting	Tremor in spiral drawings
Hassan et al. (2016)[3]	184	1 (0.5%)	NS
Ganos et al. (2016)[8]	59*	NS	NS
Bain and Jones (2010)[12]	56	15 (26.8%)	33 (58.9%)
Yaltho and Ondo (2014)[9]	40*	NS	NS
Mestre et al. (2012)[13]	26	NS	NS
Gerschlager et al. (2004)[10]	26*	NS	NS
Piboolnurak et al. (2005)[11]	26	NS	NS
Range in above studies		**0.5%–26.8%**	**58.9%**

Key: *Including POT (± upper limb tremor) only. NS: not specified

walking (but not when the shoulders are passively shrugged). A combination of an unsteady gait with small steps is also seen.[12]

Eye movements

Careful clinical examination of 18 patients with OT revealed mild faults in the saccadic smooth pursuit eye movements of all of them, with many also having various types of nystagmus and ataxia in at least one limb.[20] These finding support the notion that OT is associated with faults with the cerebellum or cerebellar system.

Other physical signs found in patients with POT

Various physical signs have been found in patients with POT that are insufficient to classify the patient

as having "primary orthostatic tremor plus" (i.e., POT and another neurological condition). These include subtle features of parkinsonism that are insufficient to diagnose a parkinsonian disorder, for example facial or vocal impassivity, which were apparent in 37.5% and 8.9% of patients, respectively. A decreased blink rate was observed in 15% of cases.[12]

Cognitive function

Benito-Leon et al. (2016) examined the cognitive function and personality of 16 patients with OT and compared the results to 32 age-matched controls using a neuropsychological battery and the Personality Assessment. Their results, adjusted for various factors, showed that patients with OT performed worse on tests of executive function,

(A)

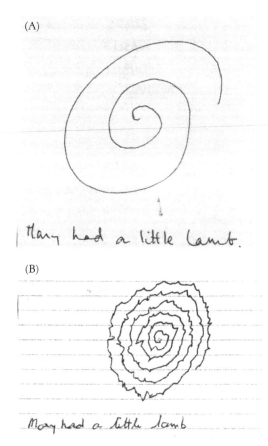

(B)

FIGURE 8.4: Examples of Spirals Drawn by Two Different Patients With: **(A)** Mild Orthostatic Tremor and **(B)** Severe Orthostatic Tremor. Both spirals were drawn while the patients were sitting. Note the changes in tremor axis and jerky nature of the tremor in spiral B. [The spirals in OT tend to be worse when drawn while the patient is standing].

visuo-spatial ability, visual memory, verbal memory, and language tests. In addition, patients had increased scores on somatic concerns, anxiety related disorders, depression, and antisocial features than the control subjects. The authors conclude that OT patients have specific neuropsychological profiles that suggest dysfunction in the fronto-cerebellar circuity, which is intriguing given interest in the role of the cerebellum in cognitive function.[20,22]

Differential diagnosis

The differential diagnosis of POT is very limited because of its characteristic history and the presence of a fast leg tremor on standing that improves on walking. The main alternatives are pseudo-orthostatic tremor ("slow OT") (see section on pseudo-OT below) and orthostatic myoclonus

(OM). The latter differs from POT in that there is invariably a coexistent neurological condition in about one-third of patients with parkinsonism.[23] Unlike POT, the leg shake in OM does not improve on walking. Severe small vessel cerebrovascular disease is also a common finding on MR imaging of patients with OM. OM can also be distinguished from POT, as it has a slower frequency (3–7 Hz) and a shorter burst duration (30–100ms).[23]

INVESTIGATIONS

Blood tests

Routine laboratory investigations are usually normal in patients with POT unless the patient has concomitant medical conditions. However, a raised (abnormal) gamma glutamyl transferase was present in 47% of 23 patients tested in one study, suggesting that high alcohol intake is common in patients with orthostatic tremor.[12] Furthermore, hyperthyroidism could exacerbate OT; in three patients with Grave's disease, two with pseudo-orthostatic 8–9 Hz tremor, and one with 14–16 Hz POT, remission was obtained after treatment with methimazole.[24–26]

Neuro-imaging
Magnetic resonance imaging

Cerebral MR imaging should be considered, although the result is normal in 76% of cases if involutional changes are included. The most common abnormality detected is small vessel white matter disease (SVWMD), which was apparent in 24% of the patients scanned by Bain and Jones (2010) and 15.4% of those scanned by Piboolnurak et al. (2005).[11,12] SVWMD typically causes unsteadiness on walking, and a slow gait with small steps and a broad-based stance ("ataxia-parkinsonism"). However, although there are similarities, the gait and stance of SVWMD are subtly different from those in POT, in which stance is characteristically more unsteady than gait, which is often quick. Structural lesions in the pons and cerebellar atrophy are also rarely detected in patients with OT.[27–29]

Spinal MR imaging is warranted if the neurological signs indicate that a possible spinal lesion might be present, and a spinal cord generator for OT has even been proposed.[30,31] However, Bain and Jones (2010) found no cord lesions on MRI scans performed on 16 patients with OT in whom no signs of spinal cord disease were evident, although degenerative changes in the spine were commonplace.[12]

TABLE 8.13: SITES OF TREMOR DETECTED BY EXAMINATION OF THE HEAD OR NECK IN THE LARGER STUDIES OF ORTHOSTATIC TREMOR

Study	Number in study	Head tremor	Jaw tremor	Lip tremor
Hassan et al. (2016)[3]	184	1 (0.5%)	1 (0.5%)	NS
Ganos et al. (2016)[8]	59*	4 (6.7%)	0 (0%)	NS
Bain and Jones (2010)[12]	56	11 (19.6%)	0 (0%)	0 (0%)
Yaltho and Ondo (2014)[9]	40*	NS	NS	NS
Mestre et al. (2012)[13]	26	NS	NS	NS
Gerschlager et al. (2004)[10]	31*	NS	NS	NS
Piboolnurak et al. (2005)[11]	26	NS	≥1	≥1 (≥3.8%)**
Range in above studies		0.5%–19.6%	0.0%–0.5%	0–(>3.8%)**

Key: *Including Primary OT (POT) (± upper limb tremor) only. **Piboolnurak et al. (2005) reported "at least one patient as having jaw and lip tremor." NS: not specified.

Benito-Leon and colleagues (2016) used proton magnetic resonance spectroscopy to probe in vivo metabolic profiling on 14 patients with OT and 14 matched healthy controls.[32] They detected a decrease in the absolute concentrations of N-acetylaspartate + N-acetylaspartyl glutamate (NAA) in the mid-parietal gray matter, cerebellar vermis, and cerebellar white matter, but no differences in the choline-containing compounds, myoinositol, and glutamate + glutamine tocreatine levels. The authors speculated whether these data might indicate that OT has a neurodegenerative basis.[32]

Single-photon emission tomography dopamine transporter imaging

Dopamine transporter imaging using 123IFP-CIT ([123I]-2b-carbomethoxy-3b-(-4-iodophenyl)-N-(3-fluoropropyl)-nortropane) has shown conflicting results. An initial report suggested that the tracer uptake was subtly decreased symmetrically in the putamen and caudate, but to a milder degree

TABLE 8.14: GAIT ABNORMALITIES DETECTED IN PATIENTS WITH PRIMARY ORTHOSTATIC TREMOR

Gait abnormality	Number (/56)	Percentage (%)
Broad base	30	53.6
Reduced arm swing	21	37.5
Small steps	8	14.3
Unsteady	7	12.5
Normal	9	16.1

than in Parkinson disease.[33] However, subsequent studies demonstrated that the dopaminergic and serotonergic systems were intact.[12,4–36]

Transcranial Sonography

Typically, studies involving transcranial sonography have shown an increased area of echogenicity of the substantia nigra (SN) in patients with Parkinson disease, which is considered to be the result of increased iron concentrations.[37] Spiegel et al. (2005) examined the SN in four patients with OT, finding increased echogenicity, unilateral in three and bilateral in one case.[38] These findings suggest that there are mild deficits in the substantia nigra. However, this data awaits confirmation, as initially there had been some methodological issues concerning the reliability of this technique.[37]

Functional imaging

H_2 ^{15}O Positron emission tomography (PET) has been used to assess the cerebral activation pattern associated with postural upper limb tremor in four patients with 14–16 Hz POT.[39] Regional cerebral blood flow was measured during involuntary postural tremor in the right arm and again while the arm was at rest. Analysis of the data showed that postural right arm tremor was associated with abnormal bilateral cerebellar, contralateral lentiform, and thalamic activation. Furthermore, even at rest, cerebellar blood flow was significantly greater than in matched healthy control subjects. These findings are similar to those detected in similar studies of essential tremor and primary writing tremor and support the notion of cerebellar involvement in the pathophysiology of OT.[39]

Schobert and colleagues (2016) used fluorode-oxy glucose (FDG) PET to demonstrate increased glucose metabolism in the pontine tegmentum, posterior cerebellum, ventral intermediate and ventroposterolateral nuclei of the thalamus, and the bilateral primary motor cortex in 10 patients with OT compared to 10 healthy controls while standing and lying down.[40] Relative inactivity of the mesiofrontal cortical areas and bilateral anterior insula was also found.[40]

Thirteen patients with OT and thirteen healthy matched control subjects underwent cognitive function tests and resting state functional magnetic resonance imaging (fMRI) to identify differences in several resting state networks (RSNs) between the groups.[41] The data indicated that patients with OT had increased connectivity in the default mode network and fronto-parietal network, which are involved in cognitive function, but diminished connectivity in the cerebellum and sensori-motor networks compared to controls. The changes in these networks were associated with the duration of OT and, in at least two of the networks, with worse cognitive performance with respect to attention, executive function, visuospatial ability, visual memory, and language.[41]

In a similar study, Gallea et al. (2016) used multimodal MR imaging to compare 17 patients with OT with 17 matched healthy control subjects.[42] The results revealed increased functional connectivity between the lateral cerebellum and the supplementary motor area (SMA) in the OT patients compared to the controls, which correlated positively with OT severity. In addition, the gray matter volumes in the cerebellar vermis (CV) and SMA of the OT patients was increased, whereas in the lateral cerebellum (LC) was decreased compared to controls. The changes in the CV positively correlated with patients' stance times, while those in the SMA and LC correlated with the disease duration. Furthermore, the authors were able to decrease the functional connectivity between the LC and the SMA using repetitive transcranial stimulation.[42]

Neurophysiology

The crucial clinical point when requesting EMG studies for patients with suspected POT is to state that recordings *must* be done from the leg muscles while the patient is *standing*, so that the "hallmark" 13–18 Hz tremor can be identified.

Given that surface EMGs may not be readily available, it is reasonable to use an accelerometer instead (including those found in smart phones), although occasionally an 8-Hz sub-harmonic rather than a 16-Hz OT is recorded, so care is needed in interpreting the results.[16,43] The frequency of POT appears to remain constant over several years.[8]

The 13–18 Hz tremor has also been recorded in the cranial, cervical, thoracic, and lumbar paraspinal muscles, as well as in the arms when they are weight bearing, for example leaning against a wall [Figure 8.5]. Postural arm tremor is more often in the 6–11 Hz frequency range but can be between 13–18 Hz.[16] Both co-contracting and alternating EMG patterns may occur, although phase variability, which is dependent on the posture adopted and varies between patients, was found to be constant for the same patient adopting the same posture.[44]

High coherence has been demonstrated in EMG bursts in the right and left leg, the ipsilateral arm and leg, and the cranial muscles.[2,45] The strength of coherence is dependent on the context of the postural task; for example, it may be greater in the arm muscles while the patient is leaning on them compared to when they are outstretched and lifting a weight.[44] Characteristic of an action tremor, POT consists of abnormal insertions of silence into EMG activity, creating a 13–18 Hz tremor. The burst durations are between 10 to 80 ms and can be biphasic or short and polyphasic.[46,47] Single motor unit recordings show that within the EMG bursts the motor units fire at 8 Hz.[46]

Resetting studies have shown that POT cannot be reset by peripheral nerve stimulation of either the tibial or peroneal nerves nor by magnetic stimulation of the lumbar spine[45,46,48] However, there has been some success with transcranial magnetic stimulation of the motor cortex and cerebellum, supporting the notion that the neural circuitry that generates POT is more accessible centrally.[42,49–52]

Simultaneous recordings of EEG (primary leg area) and EMG (tibialis anterior) showed high coherence between them, which was transient bilaterally and decreased considerably for the ipsilateral side after 15 seconds. In one patient, thalamic field potentials were also recorded and showed the same behavior with the source signal, suggesting that the thalamus was unlikely to be the generator of POT.[53]

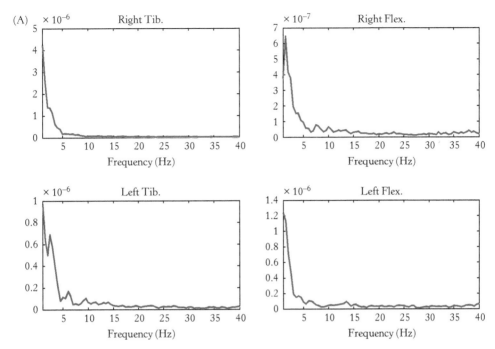

FIGURE 8.5A: Power spectra from EMG of bilateral tibialis anterior and forearm flexor muscles obtained while the patient is seated with their arms resting, showing no 13–18Hz tremor peak.

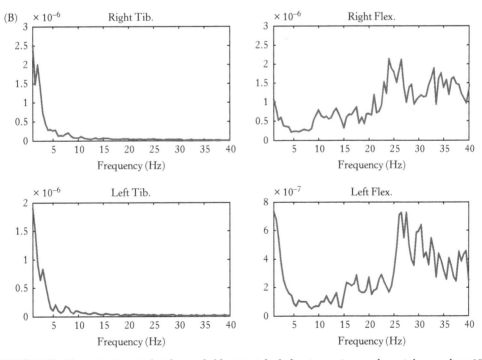

FIGURE 8.5B: The patient is seated with arms held outstretched, showing various peaks mainly at or above 25Hz.

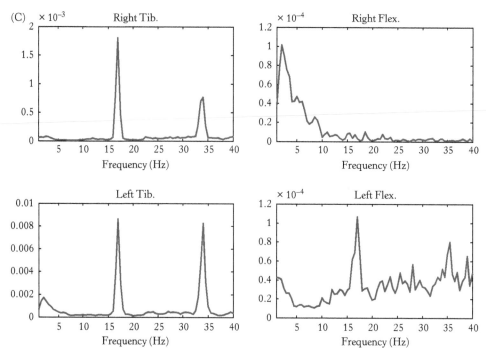

FIGURE 8.5C: The patient is standing with their arms by their sides, showing a clear peak at about 16–17Hz with harmonics at about 33–34Hz in the tibialis anterior muscles bilaterally, with a slightly broader peak and harmonic at the above frequencies in the left forearm flexors.

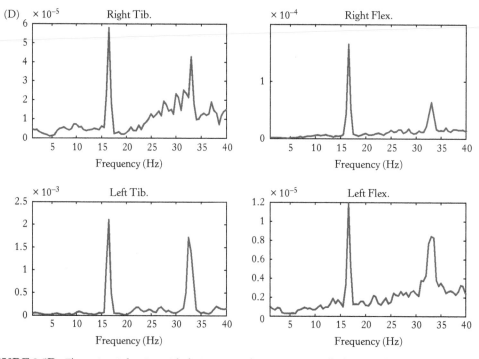

FIGURE 8.5D: The patient is leaning with their arms pushing against a wall, showing clear 16–17Hz peaks in all four muscle groups and harmonics at about 33–34Hz.

ORTHOSTATIC TREMOR PLUS AND PSEUDO-ORTHOSTATIC TREMOR

Orthostatic tremor plus

"OT plus" is the term recommended by the International Parkinson's and Movement Disorder Society Task force on tremor to describe 13–18 Hz OT found in combination with other neurological conditions.[1] These include various forms of parkinsonism (Parkinson disease, cerebrovascular parkinsonism, primary gait ignition failure, progressive supranuclear palsy), cerebellar degeneration, dementia with Lewy bodies, and restless legs syndrome.[13,51,54,55] However, it is noteworthy that Mestre and colleagues (2012) found no difference in any of the demographic variables, the clinical features, the neurophysiology, or patients' responses to treatment between patients with OT and OT plus.[13]

In addition, 13–18 Hz OT has been reported in patients with spinocerebellar ataxia type 2, stiff person syndrome, mitochondrial C10orf2 TWINKLE mutation, female carriers of a REEP 1 mutation (spastic paraparesis SPG31), focal dystonia, oro-facial dyskinesia, (minor) head injury, a pontine tuberculoma, and a midbrain lesion.[13,29,56–59] Single patients with Graves disease, biclonal (IgG and IgA) gammopathy of uncertain significance, vitamin B12 deficiency, and solvent misuse also had 13–17 Hz OT.[13,60–63] Intriguingly, dopamine-blocking agents have been recorded to cause OT in four patients, which resolved or improved following medication withdrawal.[64]

Pseudo-OT

There are clinical syndromes termed pseudo-orthostatic tremor that consist of a slower tremor (frequencies below 13 Hz) that occurs during standing, usually within the context of a neurological disorder.[1,6,65] The patient demographics of 70 patients with pseudo-OT were similar to those of primary (13–18 Hz) OT in that two-thirds were female, with a mean age 60 years (range 26–86), and mean disease duration of 6 years (range 0–32). One-third of patients had isolated pseudo-OT, while coexistent disorders, including various forms of parkinsonism (30%), ataxia (12%), and dystonia (10%), were found in two-thirds, and postural arm tremor was present in 34% of cases. Rarer causes of pseudo-OT are listed in Table 8.15.[25,29,64,68–73]

These patients had a median tremor frequency of 6–7 Hz (range 3–12). Tremor bursts ranged from 50 to 150 ms duration, and were alternating or synchronous in antagonistic and/or analogous muscles. Low and high coherences were reported.[65] Clonazepam was the most effective medication across all frequencies, and levodopa was effective for 4–7 Hz OT with coexistent parkinsonism. Two cases resolved with the treatment of Graves' disease.[65] There is also a case report describing successful intravenous immunoglobulin for a patient with pseudo-OT.[66]

However, care needs to be taken to distinguish low-frequency pseudo-OT from possible subharmonic oscillations of typical 13–18 Hz POT. This is important clinically because lower oscillation frequencies induce more conspicuous and symptomatic tremor due to less attenuation by the low-pass filtering properties of skeletal muscle.[67]

OT AND ESSENTIAL TREMOR

POT is by definition different from essential tremor (ET). The hallmark of POT is a 13–18 Hz tremor in the legs on standing, while that of ET is a slower (6–8 Hz) bilateral upper limb action tremor; which is clearly different. Furthermore, the age of onset profile of ET is bimodal, with peaks in the second and sixth decade, whereas that of OT has a single peak between 50.3 and 59.5 years (Table 8.1).[74] Furthermore, the sequence of spread of tremor to other parts of the body reported by most patients with ET is from the arms, if at all, whereas it is from the legs in nearly every patient with OT.

However, there is some evidence of an overlap: first, between 8.8% and 15.4% of patients in the larger case series concerning OT had a family history of ET (Table 8.9). Second, between 22.8% and 89.3% of patients with OT had postural arm tremor, 33% intention tremor, and 59% tremor in spiral drawings (Tables 8.11 and 5.12). In addition, head tremor is not infrequent in OT, having been detected in up to 19.6% of patients (Table 8.13). Furthermore, both OT and ET commonly respond to alcohol, although response is affected by the dose of alcohol and the duration and severity of tremor. Patients with either condition regularly state in my clinic that their OT or ET used to respond to alcohol but no longer does so, or that over time they have required more alcohol to suppress tremor. Alcohol responsiveness is present in about 50% of patients with familial ET, whereas 25.8%–51.7% with OT are responsive (Table 8.7).[74]

TABLE 8.15: SINGLE CASES OF NEUROLOGICAL CONDITIONS IN WHICH PSEUDO-ORTHOSTATIC TREMOR WAS PRESENT

Condition	Number of cases with pseudo-OT	Frequency (Hz) of pseudo-orthostatic tremor	Reference
Peripheral nervous system:			
Chronic relapsing polyneuropathy	1	6–7 Hz	*Gabellini et al. (1990)[68]*
Peripheral neuropathy	1	10–13 Hz	*Rigby et al. (2015)[69]*
Central nervous system:			
Myelopathy	2	10–13 Hz	*Rigby et al. (2015)[69]*
		12–13 Hz	*Lin et al. (2013)[25]*
Spinal dural arteriovenous fistula	1	10–13 Hz	*Rigby et al. (2015)[69]*
Multiple sclerosis	1	4 Hz	*Baker et al. (2009)[70]*
Alexander disease	1	4–4.5 Hz	*Stitt et al. (2018)[71]*
Pontine cavernoma	1	7–8 Hz	*Benito-Leon et al. (1997)[29]*
Hydrocephalus (aqueduct stenosis, parkinsonism)	1	6–7 Hz	*Gabellini et al.[68]*
Systemic medical conditions:			
Graves' disease	2	8–9 Hz	*Lin et al. (2013)[25]*
			Mazzuchi et al. (2014)[72]
Anti-Hu antibody (small cell lung cancer)	1	3–5 Hz	*Gelhaus et al. (2005)[73]*
PQ calcium channel antibodies	1	10–13 Hz	*Rigby et al. (2015)[69]*
Medications:			
Metoclopramide	1	5–6 Hz	*Alonso Navarro et al. (2004)[64]*
Sulpiride and thyethylperazine	1	6–7 Hz	*Alonso Navarro et al. (2004)[64]*

MONITORING RESPONSE AND CHANGE IN OT

A clinical rating scale for OT

Currently there is one clinical rating scale that has been developed for OT: the 10-item OT Severity and Disability Scale.[75] The scale performed well on test-retest reliability and on individual item test-retest reliability, and correlated well with the Clinical Global Impression, indicating good validity.[75]

QoL scales used for OT

The Short Form 36-item instrument (SF-36) was deployed by Gerschlager and colleagues (2003) and showed that all domains of the SF-36 were worse in 20 patients with OT compared to age-matched population norms.[15] Similarly, Rodrigues and colleagues (2005) adapted the 39-item Parkinson's Disease Questionnaire (PDQ-39) and were able to detect that the domains of activities of daily living, mobility, bodily discomfort, emotional wellbeing, and cognition were negatively affected and that the scale was sensitive to change; a mild improvement was detected with gabapentin.[76]

MANAGEMENT

Simple measures

Patients with OT should be given an information card to explain that they cannot stand still, so as to be excused from queuing, and the contact details for their national tremor charity. An occupational therapy assessment should be performed, as they may need aids (Table 8.6). OT patients with a raised BMI may benefit from losing weight, as this is likely to increase their standing time.

Medical therapy

The medical treatment of OT is unsatisfactory, and all current medications are currently deployed "off label." For those patients with alcohol-responsive OT (Table 8.7), judicious use of alcohol prior to important social occasions can be helpful. Similarly, for milder cases of OT, my preference is for the "as required" use of low doses of a benzodiazepine (usually clonazepam 0.25–0.5mg or alprazolam 250–500 micrograms), but the patient should be advised to take alprazolam or clonazepam infrequently (e.g., 2 to 3 times per week) and warned about the possibility of dependency and drowsiness that may affect driving.

Once regular treatment is necessary, clonazepam is the most popular first line agent for both OT and OT plus and can decrease and, rarely, temporarily stop OT (Table 8.16).[3,8,10,12,13] The response to clonazepam diminishes over time, perhaps because of tolerance or the progression of OT.[3,13] Furthermore, patients whose OT does not respond to clonazepam rarely do so to other medications.[3,13]

Small studies have reported on the benefits of gabapentin and levodopa for OT, although in clinical practice the effectiveness of either agent is not as impressive (Table 8.16).[77,78] Primidone, propranolol, and valproate are also regularly prescribed, but, judging from the larger studies of OT patients, self-reported response rates are lower than those for clonazepam (Table 8.16). In a double blind placebo crossover study, levetiracetam was shown to be ineffective for OT.[79]

Several other medications, predominantly benzodiazepines and anticonvulsants, have been utilized for treating patients with OT, some of which are shown in Table 8.16. Botulinum toxin administered into the tibialis anterior muscles of seven OT patients was unhelpful.[80]

TABLE 8.16: MEDICATIONS TAKEN BY PATIENTS FOR OT IN MAJOR STUDIES

Medication	Study: Number of patients treated and response rate (%)					
	Ganos et al. (2016)[8]	Mestre et al. (2014)[13]	Hassan et al. (2016)[3]	Gerschlager et al. (2004)[10]	Bain and Jones (2010)[12]	Total number of patients treated (Range in % response rate)
Clonazepam	38 (NS)	26 (30.8%)	124 (57.3%)	19 (38.3%)	28 (17.2%)	**235 (17.2–57.3%)**
Gabapentin	24 (NS)	14 (15.4%)	45 (33.0%)	1 (100%)*	14 (7.1%)	**98 (7.1–33.0%)**
Primidone	5 (NS)	12 (NS)	31 (22.6%)	7 (42.3%)	15 (26.7%)	**70 (22.6%–42.3%)**
Propranolol	2 (NS)	10 (10.0%)	38 (28.9%)	8 (12.5%)	19 (21.1%)	**77 (10.0–28.9%)**
Levodopa	4 (NS)	9 (22.3%)	33 (3%)	15 (13.3%)	13 (23.1%)	**54 (3.0–23.1%)**
Valproate	0 (NS)	1 (100%)*	37 (18.9%)	0	0	**37 (18.9%)**
Less utilized medications:						
Diazepam	0	0	9	0	4	**13**
Topiramate	1	0	6	0	4	**11**
Baclofen	0	0	8	2	0	**10**
Mirtazepine	0	4	3	0	2	**9**
Trihexyphenidyl	0	0	7	0	0	**7**
Pregabalin	2	0	4	0	0	**6**
Acetazolamide	0	2	3	0	0	**5**
Alprazolam	0	0	5	0	0	**5**
Lorazepam	0	0	5	0	0	**5**
Clozapate	0	0	5	0	0	**5**
Amitriptyline	0	0	3	0	2	**5**
Leviteracetam	0	0	3	0	0	**3**

Note: A medication was only included in this table if at least three patients were treated with that agent in a minimum of one of the above studies.

*Percentage not included in cumulative totals because only single cases were treated.

Surgery

Ventralis intermedius nucleus deep brain stimulation

Merola et al. (2017) created an international registry and reviewed the effects of deep brain stimulation (DBS) of the ventralis intermedius nucleus (VIM) of the thalamus on 17 patients with POT.[81] Their primary end point was a composite activities of daily living/instrumental activities of daily living (ADL/iADL) score assessed over the short (6–48 months) and long (≥48 months) term.[82,83] The authors reported modest 21.6% and 12.5% improvements in the ADL/iADL over the short and long term, respectively. Although the frequency of POT was unchanged, the amplitude of OT decreased and most patients felt steadier: the time from standing to onset of POT increased from a mean of 22 seconds pre-operatively to 196 seconds at 6–48 months but declined to 92 seconds over the longer term (≥48 months). It is noteworthy that the POT onset latency significantly correlated with the ADL/iADL composite score. A single patient treated with unilateral VIM stimulation had transient benefits only.[81] Three patients had DBS failure, and complications included lead misplacement requiring surgical revision and infection necessitating removal of the DBS system.[81]

A significant issue with DBS for POT is that the leg area is situated laterally in the homunculus in the VIM nucleus, which narrows the therapeutic window for stimulation because of the proximity to the internal capsule.[81] The study had limitations, as it was retrospective with no control arm. In addition, the optimal intra-cerebral target for treating POT with DBS has yet to be defined. Given the rarity with which patients with POT undergo DBS, there is a case for using "N of 1" studies, where the OT amplitude and patient's stance time are recorded by assessors blinded to different stimulation parameters.

Dorsal column spinal cord stimulation

A pioneering study involving chronic spinal cord stimulation (CSCS) was performed on two patients with 14–16 Hz OT, one of whom also had a painful diabetic neuropathy.[84] A quadripolar plate electrode was inserted into the epidural space at T11/T12. Chronic stimulation in the range of 50–150 Hz produced subjective and objective improvements in both patients. The optimal stimulation frequency was about 100 Hz, and effective stimulation invariably produced parasthesiae in the legs. At one year post-operatively, the duration for which each patient could maintain a stance increased from means of 10 seconds and 2 minutes to 102 seconds and 5 minutes, respectively. Although the amplitude of OT decreased, the frequency remained unchanged, leading the authors to suggest that CSCS influenced sensory feedback instead of acting as a tremor generator.[84]

A long-term follow-up study (34–133 months post-surgery) of four OT patients showed that CSCS resulted in an increased stance time from a mean of 51 (range 4–120) to a mean of 220 (range 10–480) seconds. This was associated with improved patient ratings and a 30–60% decrease in EMG activity in the tibialis anterior when stimulation was turned on compared to off.[85]

CONCLUSION

POT is a physical sign: a highly coherent 13–18 Hz tremor of the legs on standing. Since its early description by Pazzaglia and colleagues in 1970 and Heilmaan in 1984, its unique character has excited neurologists.[86,87] The same frequency tremor may occur in the legs during isometric and other maneuvers. It is often associated with a 13–18 Hz coherent tremor in the arms (particularly when leaning on them) and less commonly in other parts of the body. It can be a solitary finding or occur in the presence of numerous neurological and medical conditions. There are strong associations of POT with other tremulous conditions, particularly ET, various forms of parkinsonism, and cerebellar disease. POT is a progressive condition and has a negative impact on quality of life.

Medical therapy can be useful, particularly initially, but is often disappointing in the long run. Lateral VIM nucleus stimulation and, more recently, CSCS have shown some benefit but need further study. The circuitry involved in the expression of POT can be impacted by the effects of VIM and CSCS stimulation and repetitive magnetic stimulation over the cerebellum. Functional imaging studies incriminate the pons, cerebellum, thalamus, primary motor cortex, and SMA in the circuitry involved in POT. A specific generator for OT has not been identified. It may be that multiple influences that reduce damping or increase excitation at different points in the above circuitry are involved, and that once OT begins, it could slowly progress by a process of reiteration.

ACKNOWLEDGMENT

I would like to thank David Marsden, Philip Thompson, John Rothwell, and Leah Jones for their contributions to my understanding of OT.

REFERENCES

1. Bhatia KP, Bain P, Bajaj N, et al. Consensus statement on the classification of tremors, from the task force on tremor of the International Parkinson and Movement Disorder Society. *Mov Disord*. 2018;33(1):75–87. doi: 10.1002/mds.27121

2. Koster B, Lauk M, Timmer J, et al. Involvement of cranial muscles and high intermuscular coherence in orthostatic tremor. *Ann Neurol*. 1999;45:384–388. doi: 10.1002/1531-8249(199903)45:3<384

3. Hassan A, Ahlskog JE, Matsumoto JY, Milber JM, Bower JH, Wilkinson JR. Orthostatic tremor: clinical, electrophysiologic, and treatment findings in 184 patients. *Neurology*. 2016;86:458–464. doi: 101212/WNL.0000000000002328

4. Elble R, Deuschl G. Milestones in tremor research. *Mov Disord*. 2011;26:1096–1105. doi: 10.1002/MDS23579

5. DeOrchis VS, Geyer HL, Herskovitz S. Teaching video neuroimages: orthostatic tremor: the helicopter sign. *Neurology*. 2013;80:e161. doi: 101212/WNL.0b013e31828ab301

6. Erro R, Bhatia K, Cordivari C. Shaking on standing: a critical review. *Mov Disord Clin Pract*. 2014;1:173–179. doi: 10.1002/mdc3,12053

7. Colmenares M, Jones L, Tai Y, Bain P. Orthostatic tremor—a case series [abstract 1398]. *Mov Disord*. 2019;34(suppl 2). https://www.mdsabstracts.org/abstract/orthostatic-tremor-a-case-series/

8. Ganos C, Maugest L, Apartis E, et al. The long-term outcome of orthostatic tremor. *J Neurol Neurosurg Psychiatry*. 2016;87:167–172. doi: 10.1136/jnnp-2014-309942

9. Yaltho TC, Ondo WG. Orthostatic tremor: a review of 45 cases. *Parkinsonism Relat Disord*. 2014;20:723–725. doi: 10.1016/j.parkreldis.2014.013

10. Gerschlager W, Munchau A, Katzenschlager R, et al. Natural history and syndromic associations of orthostatic tremor: a review of 41 patients. *Mov Disord*. 2004;19:788–795.

11. Piboolnurak P, Yu QP, Pullman SL. Clinical and neurophysiologic spectrum of orthostatic tremor: case series of 26 subjects. *Mov Disord*. 2005 Nov;20:1455–1461.

12. Bain P, Jones L. Characterising orthostatic tremor: a study of 56 patients. *J Neurol Neurosurg Psychiatry* 2010;81:S536 [Jones L. BSc thesis: Imperial College London 2010].

13. Mestre TA, Lang AE, Ferreira JJ, et al. Associated movement disorders in orthostatic tremor. *J Neurol Neurosurg Psychiatry* 2012;83:725–729. doi: 10.1136/jnnp-2012-302436

14. Contarino MF, Welter ML, Agid Y, Hartmann A. Orthostatic tremor in monozygotic twins. *Neurology*. 2006;66:1600–1601. doi: 10.1212/01.wnl.000216263.23642.db

15. Gerschlager W, Katzenschlager R, Schrag A, et al. Quality of life in patients with orthostatic tremor. *J Neurol*. 2003;250:212–215. doi: 10.1007/s00415-003-0980-9

16. Lucking CH, Hellwig B. Uncommon tremors. In: Hallett M, ed. *The Handbook of Clinical Neurophysiology (Vol. 1)*. Elsevier B.V.; 2003: 397–399.

17. Bain PG, Findley LJ. *Assessing Tremor Severity: A Clinical Handbook*. Smith-Gordon; 1993.

18. Tinazzi M, Gerschlager W, Bhatia KP. Orthostatic tremor. In: Lyons KE, Pahwa R, eds. *Handbook of Essential Tremor and Other Movement Disorders*. Taylor & Francis; 2005: 251–261.

19. McManis PG, Sharbrough FW. Orthostatic tremor: clinical and electrophysiologic characteristics. *Muscle Nerve*. 1993;16(11):1254–1260. doi: 10.1002/mus.880161117

20. Feil K, Bottcher N, Guri F, et al. Long-term course of orthostatic tremor in serial posturographic measurement. *Parkinsonism Relat Disord*. 2015;21:905–910. doi: 10.1016/j.parkreldis.2015.05.021

21. Benito-Léon J, Louis ED, Puertas-Martín V, et al. Cognitive and neuropsychiatric features of orthostatic tremor: a case-control comparison. *J Neurolog Sci*. 2016;361:137–143. doi: 10.1016/j.jns.2015.12.031

22. Schmahmann JD. From movement to thought: anatomic substrates of the cerebellar contribution to cognitive processing. *Hum Brain Mapp*. 1996;4:174–198. doi: 10.1002/(SICI)1097-0193(1996)4:3,174::AID-HBM3.3.0.CO;2-0

23. Hassan A, van Gerpen JA. Orthostatic tremor and orthostatic myoclonus: weight bearing hyperkinetic disorders: a systematic review, new insights and unresolved question. *Tremor Other Hyperkinet Mov*. 2016;6:417. doi: 10.7916/D84X584K

24. Tan EK, Lo YL, Chan LL. Graves' disease and isolated OT. *Neurology*. 2008;70(Pt 2):1497–1498. doi: 10.1212/01.wnl.0000310405.36026.92

25. Lin FC, Wu MN, Chen CH, Huang P. Slow orthostatic tremor as the first manifestation of Grave's disease. *Mov Disord*. 2013;28:1158–1159. doi: 10.1002/mds.25313

26. Mazzucchi S, Frosini D, Calabrese R, Bonuccelli U, Ceravolo R. Symptomatic orthostatic tremor associated with Graves' disease. *Neurolog Sci*. 2014;35:929–931. doi: 0.1007/s10072-014-1672-1

27. Setta F, Jacquy J, Hildebrand J, Manto MU. Orthostatic tremor associated with cerebellar ataxia. *J Neurol*. 1998;245(5):299–302. doi: 10.1007/s004150050222

28. Manto MU, Setta F, Legros B, Jacquy J, Godaux E. Resetting of orthostatic tremor associated with cerebellar cortical atrophy by transcranial magnetic stimulation. *Arch Neurol*. 1999;56(12):1497–1500. doi: 10.1001/1rchneur.56.12.1497

29. Benito-Leon J, Rodriguez J, Orti-Pareja M, Ayuso-Peralta L, Jimenez-Jimenez FJ, Molina

JA. Symptomatic orthostatic tremor in pontine lesions. *Neurology*. 1997;49:1439–1441. doi: 10.1212/WNL.49.5.1439

30. Norton JA, Wood DE, Day BL. Is the spinal cord the generator of 16-Hz orthostatic tremor? *Neurology*. 2004;62(4):632–634. doi: 10.1212/WNL.62.4.632

31. Lee HM, Kwon DY, Park MH, Koh SB, Kim SH. Symptomatic orthostatic tremor with progressive cognitive impairment in spinal cord lesions. *Clin Neurol Neurosurg*. 2012;114:1329–1331. doi: 10.1016/j.clineuro.2012.03.021

32. Benito-León J, Louis ED, Mato-Abad V, et al. In vivo neurometabolic profiling in orthostatic tremor. *Medicine (Baltimore)*. 2016;95(37):e4848. doi: 10.1097/MD.0000000000004848

33. Katzenschlager R, Costa D, Gerschlager W, et al. [123I]-FP-CITSPECT demonstrates dopaminergic deficit in orthostatic tremor. *Ann Neurol*. 2003;53:489–496. doi: 10.1002/ana.10475

34. Vaamonde J, García A, Flores JM, Ibáñez R, Gargallo L. Study of presynaptic nigrostriatal pathway by 123-I-FD-CIT-SPECT (DatSCAN SPECT) in primary orthostatic tremor. *Neurologia*. 2006;21:37–39.

35. Trocello JM, Zanotti-Fregonara P, Roze E, et al. Dopaminergic deficit is not the rule in orthostatic tremor. *Mov Disord*. 2008;23:1733–1738. doi: 10.1002/mds.22224

36. Wegner F, Strecker K, Boeckler D, et al. Intact serotonergic and dopaminergic systems in two cases of orthostatic tremor. *J Neurol*. 2008;255:1840–1842. doi: 10.1007/s00415-008-0023-7

37. Mehnert S, Reuter I, Schepp K, Maaser P, Stolz E. Transcranial sonography for diagnosis of Parkinson's disease. BMC *Neurol*. 2010;10:9. doi: 10.1186/1471-2377-10-9

38. Spiegel J, Behnke S, Fuss G, Becker G, Dillmann U. Echogenic substantia nigra in patients with orthostatic tremor. *J Neural Trans*. 2005;112:915–920. doi: 10.1007/s00702-004-0236-6

39. Wills AJ, Thompson PD, Findley LJ, Brooks DJ. A positron emission tomography study of primary orthostatic tremor. *Neurology*. 1996;46:747–752. doi: 10.1212/WNL.46.3.747

40. Schöberl F, Feil K, Xiong G, et al. Pathological ponto-cerebello-thalamo-cortical activations in primary orthostatic tremor during lying and stance. *Brain*. 2017;140:83–97. doi: 10.1093/brain/aww268

41. Benito-Leon J, Louis ED, Manzanedo E, et al. Resting state functional MRI reveals abnormal network connectivity in orthostatic tremor. *Medicine*. 2016;95:e4310. doi: 10.1097/MD.0000000000004310

42. Gallea C, Popa T, Garcia-Lorenzo D, et al. Orthostatic tremor: a cerebellar pathology? *Brain*. 2016;139:2182–2197. doi: 10.1093/brain/aww140

43. Bhatti D, Thompson R, Hellman A, Penke C, Bertoni JM, Torres-Russotto D. Smartphone apps provide a simple, accurate bedside screening tool for orthostatic tremor. *Mov Disord Clin Pract*. 2017;4:852–857. doi: 10.1002/mdc3.12547

44. McAuley JH, Britton TC, Rothwell JC, Findley LJ, Marsden CD. The timing of primary orthostatic tremor bursts has a task-specific plasticity. *Brain*. 2000;123(Pt 2):254–266. doi: 10.1093/brain/123.2.254

45. Britton TC, Thompson PD, van der Kamp W, et al. Primary orthostatic tremor: further observations on six cases. *J Neurol*. 1992;239:209–217. doi: 10.1007/BF00839142

46. Deuschl G, Lucking CH, Quintern J. Orthostatischer tremor. Clinical signs, pathophysiology and therapy. *Klin Neurophysiol*. 1987;18:13–19. doi: 10.1055/s-2008-1060891

47. Wu YR, Ashby F, Lang AE. Orthostatic tremor arises from an oscillator in the posterior fossa. *Mov Disord*. 2001;16:272–279. doi: 10.1002/mds.1045

48. Munhoz RP, Hanajima R, Ashby P, Lang AE. Acute effect of transcutaneous electrical nerve stimulation on tremor. *Mov Disord*. 2003;18:191–194. doi: 10.1002/mds.10311

49. Tsai CS, Semmler JG, Kimber TE, et al. Resetting of orthostatic tremor by magnetic stimulation of the motor cortex. *J Neurol Neurosurg Psychiatry*. 1998;64:33–36. doi: 10.1136/jnnp64.1.33

50. Sander HW, Masdeu JC, Tavoulareas G, Walters A, Zimmerman T, Chokrverty S. Orthostatic tremor: an electrophysiological analysis. *Mov Disord*. 1998;13:735–738. doi: mds.870130422

51. Manto MU, Setta F, Legros B, Jacquy J, Godaux E. Resetting of orthostatic tremor associated with cerebellar cortical atrophy by transcranial magnetic stimulation. *Arch Neurol*. 1999;56:1497–1500. doi: 10.1001/archneur.56.12.1497

52. Pfeiffer G, Hinse P, Humbert T, Riemer G. Neurophysiology of orthostatic tremor. Influence of transcranial magnetic stimulation. *Electromyogr Clin Neurophysiol*. 1999;39:49–53.

53. Muthuraman M, Hellriegel H, Paschen S, et al. The central oscillatory network of orthostatic tremor. *Mov Disord*. 2013;28:142–1230. doi: 10.1002/mds.25616

54. Setta F, Jacquy J, Hildebrand J, Manto MU. Orthostatic tremor associated with cerebellar ataxia. *J Neurol*. 1998;245:299–302. doi: 10.1007/s004150050222

55. Sarva H, Severt WL, Jacoby N, Pullman SL, Saunders-Pullman R. Secondary orthostatic tremor in the setting of cerebellar degeneration. *J Clin Neurosci*. 2016;27:173–178. doi: 10.1016/j.jocn.2015.10.027

56. Milone M, Klassen BT, Landsverk ML, Haas RH, Wong LJ. Orthostatic tremor, progressive external ophthalmoplegia, and Twinkle.

JAMA Neurol. 2013;70:1429–1431. doi: 10.1001/jamaneurol.2013.3521

57. Sanitate SS, Meerschaert JR. Orthostatic tremor: delayed onset following head trauma. *Arch Phys Med Rehabil.* 1993;74:886–889. doi: 10.1016/0003-9993(93)90017-5

58. Vetrugno R, D'Angelo R, Alessandria M, Mascalchi M, Montagna P. Orthostatic tremor in a left midbrain lesion. *Mov Disord.* 2010;25:793–795. doi: 10.1002/mds.23018

59. Erro R, Cordivari C, Bhatia KP. SPG31 presenting with orthostatic tremor. *Eur J Neurol.* 2014;21:e34–35. doi: 10.1111/ene.12360

60. Tan EK, Lo YL, Chan LL. Graves' disease and isolated orthostatic tremor. *Neurology.* 2008;70:1497–1498. doi: 10.1212/01.wnl.0000310405.36026.92

61. Stich O, Fritzsch C, Heimbach B, Rijntjes M. Orthostatic tremor associated with biclonal IgG and IgA lambda gammopathy of undetermined significance. *Mov Disord.* 2009;24:154–155. doi: 10.1002/mds.22200

62. Benito-Leo´n J, Porta-Etessam J. Shaky-leg syndrome and vitamin B12 deficiency. *N Engl J Med.* 2000;342:981. doi: 10.1056/NEJM200003303421318

63. Cruz Tabuenca H, Camacho Velasquez JL, Rivero Sanz E, Sánchez Valiente S, López Del Val J. Orthostatic tremor secondary to recreational use of solvents. *Neurologia.* 2015;32(6):401–403. doi: 10.1016/j.nrl.2015.10.007

64. Alonso-Navarro H, Orti-Pareja M, Jiménez-Jiménez FJ, Zurdo-Hernández JM, de Toledo M, Puertas-Muñoz I. Orthostatic tremor induced by pharmaceuticals. *Rev Neurol.* 2004;39:834–836.

65. Hassan A, Caviness J. Slow orthostatic tremor–review of the current evidence. *Tremor Other Hyperkinet Mov.* 2019;9. doi: 10.7916/tohm.v0.721

66. Hegde M, Glass GA, Dalmau J, Christine CW. A case of slow orthostatic tremor, responsive to intravenous immunoglobulin. *Mov Disord.* 2011;26:1563–1565. doi: 10.1002/mds.23610

67. Torres-Russotto D, Elble RJ. Slow orthostatic tremor and the case for routine electrophysiological evaluation of all tremors. *Tremor Other Hyperkinet Mov.* 2019;9. doi: 10.7916/tohm.v0.740

68. Gabellini AS, Martinelli P, Gulli MR, Ambrosetto G, Ciucci G, Lugaresi E. Orthostatic tremor: essential and symptomatic cases. *Acta Neurolog Scand.* 1990;81:113–117. doi: 10.1111/j.1600-0404.1990.tb00944.x

69. Rigby HB, Rigby MH, Caviness JN. Orthostatic tremor: a spectrum of fast and slow frequencies or distinct entities? *Tremor Other Hyperkinet Mov.* 2015;5:324. doi: 10.7916/D8575FHK

70. Baker M, Fisher K, Lai M, Duddy M, Baker S. Slow orthostatic tremor in multiple sclerosis. *Mov Disord.* 2009;24:1550–1553. doi: 10.1002/mds.22630

71. Stitt DW, Gavrilova R, Watson R, Hassan A. An unusual presentation of late-onset Alexander's disease with slow orthostatic tremor and a novel GFAP variant. *Neurocase.* 2018;24:266–268. doi: 10.1080/13554794.2019.1580749

72. Mazzucchi S, Frosini D, Calabrese R, Bonuccelli U, Ceravolo R. Symptomatic orthostatic tremor associated with Graves' disease. *Neurolog Sci.* 2014;35:929–931. doi: 0.1007/s10072-014-1672-1

73. Gilhuis HJ, van Ommen HJ, Pannekoek BJ, Sillevis Smitt PA. Paraneoplastic orthostatic tremor associated with small cell lung cancer. *Eur Neurol.* 2005;54:225–226. doi: 10.1159/000090715

74. Bain PG, Findley LJ, Thompson PD, et al. A study of hereditary essential tremor. *Brain.* 1994;117:805–824. doi: 10.1093/brain/117.4.805

75. Merola A, Torres-Russotto DR, Stebbins GT, et al. Development and validation of the Orthostatic Tremor Severity and Disability Scale (OT -10). *Mov Disord.* 2020. doi: 10.1002/mds.28142

76. Rodrigues JP, Edwards DJ, Walters SE, et al. Gabapentin can improve postural stability and quality of life in primary orthostatic tremor. *Mov Disord.* 2005;20:865–870. doi: 10.1002/mds.20392

77. Onofrj M, Thomas A, Paci C, D'Andreamatteo G. Gabapentin in orthostatic tremor: results of a double-blind crossover with placebo in four patients. *Neurology.* 1998;51:80–882. doi: 10.1212/WNL.51.3.880

78. Wills AJ, Brusa L, Wang HC, Brown P, Marsden CD. Levodopa may improve orthostatic tremor: case report and trial of treatment. *J Neurol Neurosurg Psychiatry.* 1999;66:681–684. doi: 10.1136/jnnp.66.5.681

79. Hellriegel H, Raethjen J, Deuschl G, Volkmann J. Levetiracetam in primary orthostatic tremor: a double-blind placebo-controlled crossover study. *Mov Disord.* 2011;26:2431–2434. doi: 10.1002/mds.23881

80. Bertram K, Sirisena D, Cowey M, Hill A, Williams DR. Safety and efficacy of botulinum toxin in primary orthostatic tremor. *J Clin Neurosci.* 2013;20:1503–1505. doi: 10.1016/j.jocn.2012.12.025

81. Merola A, Fasano A, Hassan A, et al. Thalamic deep brain stimulation for orthostatic tremor: a multicenter international registry. *Mov Disord.* 2017;32:1240–1242. doi: 10.1002/mds.27082

82. Katz S, Ford AB, Moskowitz RW, Jackson BA, Jaffe MW. Studies of illness in the aged. The index of ADL: a standardized measure of biological and psychosocial function. *JAMA.* 1963;185:914–919. doi: jama.1963.03060120024016

83. Lawton MP, Brody EM. Assessment of older people: self-maintaining and instrumental activities of daily living. *Gerontologist.* 1969;9:179–186.

84. Krauss JK, Weigel R, Blahak C, et al. Chronic spinal cord stimulation in medically intractable orthostatic tremor. *J Neurol Neurosurg*

Psychiatry. 2006;77:1013–1016. doi: 10.1136/jnnp.2005.086132

85. Blahak C, Sauer T, Baezner H, et al. Long-term follow-up of chronic spinal cord stimulation for medically intractable orthostatic tremor. *J Neurol.* 2016;263:2024–2028. doi: 10.1007/s00415-016-8239-4

86. Pazzaglia P, Sabattini L, Lugaresi E. On an unusual disorder of erect standing position (observation of 3 cases). *Riv Sper Freniatr Med Leg Alien Ment.* 1970;94:450–457.

87. Heilman KM. Orthostatic tremor. *Arch Neurol.* 1984;41:880–881. doi: 10.1001/archneur.1984.04050190086020

Essential Tremor

RODGER J. ELBLE

DEFINITION OF ESSENTIAL TREMOR

Essential tremor (ET) was originally viewed as a tremor diathesis in which tremor occurs in the absence of other neurological signs and is frequently associated with a family history of tremor.[1] However, early twentieth-century writers such as Critchley[2] noted that patients presenting predominantly with tremor often have other neurologic signs. A task force of the International Parkinson a Movement Disorder Society (MDS) recently published a new classification scheme for tremor disorders that is based on two axes of classification.[3] Axis 1 is clinical phenomenology and includes definable tremor syndromes in which tremor occurs in isolation or in combination with other neurologic signs (isolated and combined tremor syndromes). Axis 2 is etiology. ET is defined as an isolated tremor syndrome of bilateral upper extremity action tremor of at least three years' duration, with or without tremor in other locations (e.g., head, voice, or lower limbs), and in the absence of other neurological signs, such as dystonia, ataxia, or parkinsonism. Thus, by definition, ET affects the upper limbs. It also commonly affects the head (at least 30%) and voice (at least 10%), and less commonly the lower limbs (approximately 30%) and trunk (approximately 5%).[4,5]

The MDS definition of ET emphasizes the important fact that ET is a syndrome, not a specific disease. Focal (e.g., isolated head or voice tremor) and task-specific (e.g., primary writing tremor) are classified as separate tremor syndromes, not ET. The 3-year duration is stipulated in order to increase the odds of a stable tremor syndrome. Tremor of less than three years duration that otherwise fulfills criteria for ET is classified as indeterminate tremor.[3] With time, a person with ET may develop additional signs (e.g., dystonia or ataxia) that define a combined tremor syndrome (e.g., dystonic tremor or tremor-ataxia syndrome), and these people are then reclassified with the new syndrome and are said to have antecedent ET. Similarly, focal and task-specific tremors could conceivably evolve into ET.

The MDS Task Force was concerned that ET was often viewed as a specific disease, rather than a clinical syndrome, and that ET was not defined and diagnosed consistently in the clinic or in research.[6] The new MDS classification scheme clearly distinguishes causality (Axis 2 etiologies) from clinical phenotypes (Axis 1) and emphasizes the importance of careful clinical phenotyping in pursuit of underlying etiologies. The revised MDS definition of ET differs from the widely used TRIG (Tremor Investigation Group) definition only in the required duration of tremor (3 years versus 5 years) and differs from the old MDS consensus criteria only in the exclusion of isolated head tremor and the required 3-year history of tremor.[7] The new classification ET-plus was introduced to accommodate the very common clinical situation in which a patient meets all criteria for ET but has one or more neurological signs of questionable relevance to tremor or questionable abnormality.

DEFINITION OF ET-PLUS

The MDS Task Force defined ET-plus as tremor with the characteristics of ET but with "additional neurological signs of uncertain significance such as impaired tandem gait, questionable dystonic posturing, memory impairment, or other mild neurologic signs of unknown significance that do not suffice to make an additional syndrome classification or diagnosis. ET with tremor at rest should be classified here." True rest tremor occurs in less than 15% of clinic patients[4] and in less than 5% of people in the general population who otherwise fulfill criteria for ET.[8]

Some experts believe that this new classification is ill-advised because ET-plus has no specific pathology and is merely a "state condition" that can evolve into a different clinical phenotype.[9,10] However, these concerns are also true for ET. The MDS Task Force felt strongly that Axis 1 tremor

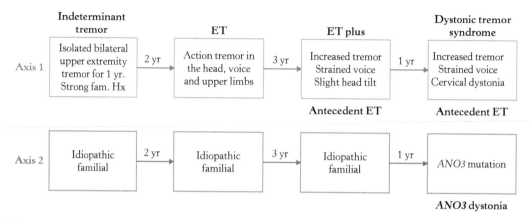

FIGURE 9.1: An Example of How Axis 1 and 2 Classifications Can Evolve en Route to a Final Diagnosis.

syndromes must be defined consistently to be useful in finding effective treatments and Axis 2 etiologies, and the Task Force chose to retain the original concept of ET being an isolated tremor syndrome. In so doing, the classification ET-plus became necessary for classifying patients with additional "soft" or questionable signs.[11]

Any Axis 1 syndrome may evolve into another, with the development of additional clinical signs. Clinicians encounter this problem every day, especially in psychiatry in which most diagnoses are syndromic with no known etiologies. Figure 9.1 illustrates how Axis 1 and Axis 2 classifications can change en route to a final diagnosis (i.e., the discovery of a specific etiology). In this example, a patient initially exhibits isolated bilateral upper extremity tremor of one year's duration. There is a strong family history. This patient is classified as having an indeterminate tremor, not ET, because the duration is only one year. The Axis 2 classification is idiopathic familial. Two years later, the patient still exhibits action tremor in the upper limbs, and she also exhibits action tremor in the head and voice. The tremor classification is now ET because she now has a three-year history of tremor. The Axis 2 classification is still idiopathic familial. Three years later, she exhibits increased tremor but now has a strained voice and slight head tilt. The presence of dystonia is uncertain. She is therefore classified as ET-plus, and she is said to have antecedent ET. The Axis 2 classification is still idiopathic familial. One year later, her tremor is increased, and she has definite cervical dystonia. Her Axis 1 classification becomes dystonic tremor syndrome with antecedent ET. Genetic testing reveals an *ANO3* (Anoctamin 3 gene) mutation. This patient now has a dystonic syndrome with antecedent ET (Axis 1) produced by an *ANO3* mutation (Axis 2), as described by Stamelou and coworkers.[12]

There is already growing evidence that the classification ET-plus is needed and useful. First, many patients previously classified as ET actually had other neurologic signs of potential significance. In one study of patients with action tremor in the lower limbs, 110 of 133 patients originally classified as ET were reclassified as ET-plus.[13] In the author's own practice, 20 of 34 consecutive patients that underwent thalamic deep brain stimulation surgery for ET were reclassified as ET-plus due to the soft signs summarized in Table 9.1. It is clear that ET, strictly defined, is far less common than generally believed, especially in clinic-based cohorts. The classification ET-plus encourages a deeper phenotyping and documentation of the clinical heterogeneity in patients previously and loosely classified as ET. Most of the soft signs pertain to rest tremor or questionable parkinsonism,

TABLE 9.1: SOFT SIGNS IN 20 OF 34 PATIENTS WHO UNDERWENT DBS SURGERY FOR ET

Signs	Number
Rest tremor or questionable rest tremor	9
Posturing/athetoid movement	14
Jerky tremor	5
Asymmetric upper limb action tremor*	8
Rapid progression	6
Raspy/strained voice	3
Mini-jerks	2
Impaired tandem gait	7
Wide-based gait	3

* ≥ 1-point asymmetry on the Essential Tremor Rating Assessment Scale (0–4 rating)

imbalance or subtle ataxia, and questionable dystonia.

The main limitation of ET-plus is that the documentation and interpretation of soft or questionable signs is dependent on the training and clinical focus of the clinician.[14-17] This problem requires further study.[16-18] It is unlikely that any soft sign will have sufficient sensitivity and specificity to be diagnostically useful in isolation, but combinations of soft signs may prove very useful diagnostically. ET-plus brings the documentation and interpretation of soft signs to the forefront of discussion, whereas these diagnostic uncertainties were previously "swept under the carpet" of loosely defined ET.

There is growing evidence that the classification ET-plus is clinically relevant from a therapeutic standpoint. One study found that subtle upper limb ataxia in quantitative spirography was a predictor of early tolerance to thalamic DBS.[19] There is anecdotal evidence that subtle or questionable signs of dystonia might predict the complication of disabling dystonia following thalamic DBS surgery and thalamotomy,[20] while in some cases these signs improve.[14] There is clearly much to be learned, and prospective studies with deep phenotyping of tremor patients are needed. The use of ET and ET-plus allows for varied hypothesis testing. For example, people with ET and ET-plus could be included in a genetic association study or epidemiologic study, and post hoc analyses of data from more specific subtypes of ET or ET-plus could be used for additional hypothesis generation. Such subtypes are discussed later in this chapter.

EPIDEMIOLOGY AND NATURAL HISTORY

It is virtually certain that people with ET and ET-plus have been grouped together in all published epidemiologic studies of ET. Therefore, epidemiologic studies should be interpreted with this limitation in mind and with the acknowledgment that ET, however defined, is a syndrome, not a specific disease. Furthermore, epidemiologic studies have not used consistent criteria in the diagnosis of ET.

These limitations notwithstanding, ET-like tremor may begin in the first decade of life,[21] but the prevalence and incidence of ET increase exponentially with age. The overall prevalence is estimated to be 0.4%, but the estimated prevalence is roughly 5% in people 65 and older in most populations.[22] The prevalence may be less in some populations,[23,24] and nearly all of the highest estimates are from studies featuring direct examination of all subjects by a neurologist.[25-27] The one exception is a recent study documenting a 0.47% to 1.89% prevalence of ET (age 65 or greater) in Arabic villages in Israel, a lower prevalence than PD in that population.[23] Consistent gender differences in ET prevalence have not been found.

The MDS definition of ET characterizes the vast majority of people with ET.[22,28] Community-based studies have consistently shown that at least 80% of people with ET have not seen a physician for their tremor, even though more than half of these patients have disability from tremor.[22,29-31] These people have a long-standing, relatively mild ET syndrome[32,33] with strong heritability.[34] Long-standing ET often seems to accelerate late in life, possibly due to age-associated comorbidities. Patients with tremor onset after age 65 tend to progress more rapidly, have a family history of tremor less commonly, and have greater comorbidity and mortality.[35-37]

CONSENSUS AND CONTROVERSIES

ET is often discussed as a specific disease rather than a clinical syndrome. This has led to illogical questions such as "Does ET *cause* Parkinson disease or dystonia?" ET is not a specific etiology that can cause other Axis 1 syndromes. However, patients presenting with ET or ET-plus can evolve into other syndromes of parkinsonism, dystonia, or ataxia.[12,38,39]

A syndrome is a group of signs or symptoms that occur together more commonly than can be attributed to chance. ET has never been defined consistently, and this has made the interpretation and comparison of research studies unnecessarily difficult. Similar difficulties have occurred with other clinical syndromes consisting of common nonspecific signs and symptoms, such as irritable bowel syndrome.[40] ET and other clinical syndromes are useful only if they are defined and used consistently.[41]

Subtypes of essential tremor

The main purpose of defining any syndrome is to find the underlying etiologies and pathophysiology and to identify effective treatments. The MDS definition of ET is very similar to the Tremor Investigation Group (TRIG) criteria,[7] which have been used frequently but not universally in clinical research since 1996. Nevertheless, little progress has been made in finding new treatments and etiologies. While some experts view the strict monosymptomatic definition of ET as too restrictive,[42] others believe that more restrictive definitions (i.e., subtypes) are needed to find new treatments and etiologies.[41]

Four ET subtypes were proposed by David Marsden and colleagues in 1983.[43] These four subtypes are summarized in Table 9.2. Type IV ET is an action tremor in the upper limbs that occurs in the context of other neurological conditions such as acquired and hereditary neuropathies, Parkinson disease and dystonias. The rationale for calling this action tremor a form of ET is that the action tremor in these conditions appeared to have the same electrophysiologic properties as isolated ET. It is now known that the electrophysiologic properties of ET are largely nonspecific, and type IV tremor is incompatible with the MDS consensus definition of ET. Nevertheless, patients with the syndrome of ET can eventually develop other signs and symptoms, indicative of a more complex tremor syndrome such as Parkinson disease. These patients are classified based on their current signs and symptoms and are said to have antecedent ET.

In the 1970s and early 1980s, a popular hypothesis was that ET emerged from oscillation in stretch reflex loops. However, subsequent electrophysiologic studies revealed properties that are incompatible with this hypothesis,[44] and there is now indisputable evidence that ET emerges from oscillation in central neural networks ("central neurogenic tremor"). These characteristics of ET clearly differ from enhanced physiologic tremor, in which the frequency of oscillation is strongly dependent on the mechanical properties of the limb and reflex loop time. Thus, Marsden's type I ET is no longer a legitimate subtype.

Marsden's type II and type III ET are still valid subtypes (Video 9.1). Type II ET consists of relatively mild action tremor in the upper limbs that is often associated with action tremor in the head and voice.[5] This condition is usually associated with a family history of tremor. Type II ET progresses slowly over decades,[45,46] and most people with this subtype have not seen a physician for their condition.[5] Nevertheless, type II ET produces significant disability and embarrassment.[31] Type III ET has a similar anatomical distribution but is far more severe. People with this subtype clearly need and desire treatment, and they are the type of patient referred for stereotactic surgery. Their tremor is so severe that a 50% reduction in tremor amplitude, typically achieved with available medications,[47] leaves the patient with persistent disability. Some people with type III ET have a long history of tremor with accelerating disability late in life. Others have a short history of only a few years, so their rate of progression clearly exceeds that of most ET patients.[45] It was Marsden's impression that type III ET was less commonly hereditary, but this impression has never been confirmed by proper epidemiologic studies.

ET type II and type III are completely compatible with the current MDS definition of ET syndrome, and other compatible subtypes are illustrated in Figure 9.2. However, studies of one subtype may not be applicable to other subtypes or to the general population of ET patients. For example, one epidemiologic study found people with ET are more likely to develop dementia if their tremor started after age 64 but not if tremor began earlier in life.[48] Other research provides additional justification for regarding late-onset ET and early-onset ET as distinct subtypes.[35-37,49-51]

TABLE 9.2: MARSDEN'S SUBTYPES OF ET[43]

Type I	**Mild ET of the hands**
	Indistinguishable from enhanced physiologic tremor
	Mechanical-reflex oscillation
Type II	**Benign pathological ET**
	Involvement of the hands ± head ± face ± tongue ± voice ± lower limbs
	Central neurogenic oscillation at 5–7 Hz
Type III	**Severe pathological ET**
	Involvement of the hands ± head ± face ± tongue ± voice ± lower limbs
	Central neurogenic oscillation at 4–6 Hz
Type IV	**Symptomatic ET**
	Associated with other neurologic conditions such as dystonia, peripheral neuropathy, and Parkinson disease

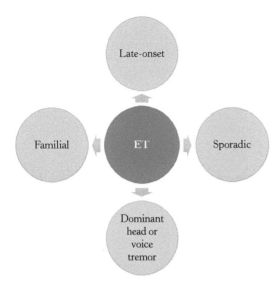

FIGURE 9.2: Essential Tremor Subtypes are Permissible in the New MDS Tremor Classification Scheme. However, data obtained from one subtype (e.g., late-onset) cannot be assumed to be relevant to other subtypes (e.g., greatest tremor in the head or voice).

Further separation of ET patients into familial (family history suggesting high likelihood of primarily genetic etiology) and sporadic (no family history) subtypes is also justifiable.[37]

Subtypes of ET-plus are also possible and even encouraged. One can envision ET-plus questionable rigidity, bradykinesia, ataxia, dystonic posturing, or myoclonus. ET-plus rest tremor is another subtype. The MDS Task Force excluded rest tremor from the definition of essential tremor because rest tremor is frequently a sign of dystonia or Parkinson disease, and true rest tremor occurs in less than 15% of ET clinic patients[4] and in less than 5% of people in the general population who otherwise fulfill criteria for ET.[8] Rest tremor in Parkinson disease has the unique characteristic of being suppressed by voluntary initiation of a new posture or movement (Video 9.2).[52] It may then re-emerge during a sustained posture.[53] Rest tremor in ET-plus does not diminish in this manner; instead, the voluntary activation of muscles typically makes tremor increase without delay (Video 9.3). Patients with ET-plus rest tremor usually have severe action tremor, and their lower limbs rarely, if ever, exhibit rest tremor. Head tremor persisting at rest is believed to be more compatible with dystonic tremor than ET.[54]

The high prevalence of ET-plus relative to ET and the uncertain significance of an isolated soft sign must be acknowledged in clinical studies, and the inclusion criteria for a study must be defined accordingly. One soft sign (e.g., unsteady tandem gait or spooning posture of the hands[55]) should not necessarily exclude a patient's participation in a clinical trial for ET. However, multiple soft signs might justify a patient's exclusion.

Genetics

The hereditary nature of ET is not included in its definition, but heritability estimates range from 45% to 90%, with a current best estimate of additive genetic variance being at least 75%.[56,57] Many large families with an autosomal pattern of inheritance have been studied, but nearly all of these studies have revealed candidate loci but no causal mutations.[57] Only rare monogenic etiologies of ET have been reported: fused in sarcoma gene (*FUS*),[58,59] GGC repeat expansion in the *NOTCH2NLC* gene,[60] and HTRA2 p.G399S.[61] Genome-wide association studies have revealed several possible risk genes, but they account for only a small fraction of ET heritability and have not been consistently replicated.[62] Thus, available evidence suggests that ET is genetically complex and is probably produced in most patients by the cumulative effect of various risk genes that individually make only a small contribution to the tremor diathesis.[57]

This genetic complexity was actually predicted by investigators in the late nineteenth and early twentieth centuries.[2] These investigators reasoned that multiple genetic abnormalities could produce tremor, and some of the same genetic abnormalities, in combination with others, could produce other clinical syndromes such as tremor with dystonia or with parkinsonism. It remains to be seen whether ET and ET-plus subtyping will aid in the search for ET genes. Very large patient cohorts will be needed to sort this out.[63]

Genetic relationship to other movement disorders

Genetic studies have conclusively shown that ET and ET-plus can be phenotypes of specific diseases that ordinarily produce more complex tremor syndromes. For example, ET-plus unusually jerky action tremor of the upper limbs can be the presenting phenotype of *PRKN* and *ANO3* mutations.[12,38] Action tremor of the head and upper limbs can be the presenting phenotype of spinocerebellar ataxia type 12.[39] These rare examples illustrate the need for careful, deep phenotyping of every patient being evaluated for ET.

KNOWLEDGE GAPS

Many knowledge gaps in ET and ET-plus are discussed in the preceding paragraphs. The genetic etiologies are largely unknown, and the mechanisms by which genetic abnormalities produce tremor are unclear. This should not deter researchers from investigating new treatments, and indeed has not.

ET is a disorder of rhythmic neuronal oscillation in the corticobulbocerebellothalamocortical loop (Figure 9.3).[64,65] Interruption of this loop in the ventrolateral thalamus or in the cerebellothalamic tract suppresses all forms of tremor. The pathophysiology of oscillation in the corticobulbocerebellothalamocortical loop is poorly understood. Louis and colleagues have described a loss of Purkinje cells and other microscopic abnormalities in the cerebellar cortex of most but not all patients with ET,[66,67] but Purkinje cell loss in ET has not been replicated by other investigators.[68,69] Furthermore, the microscopic changes reported by Louis et al. are not specific for ET. There is also a relative redistribution of climbing fiber synapses to the outer 20% of the Purkinje cell dendritic arbor,[66,70] but the pathophysiologic significance of these changes in cerebellar cortex is unclear. It should be emphasized that no one has demonstrated the cerebellum or other components of the Guillain-Mollaret triangle[64] to be the primary source of oscillation in ET or any other form of human pathologic tremor.

WORKUP

The most common conditions in the differential diagnosis are summarized in Table 9.3. The diagnosis of ET is based largely on the clinical exam. Parkinson disease and dystonic tremor (or tremor associated with dystonia) are commonly misdiagnosed as ET.[71,72] Upper extremity action tremor associated with tremulous dystonia in the voice or neck is particularly difficult to distinguish from ET. Head and voice tremors are generally mild in ET, and a dystonia syndrome should be suspected when head or voice tremor is the most severe aspect of a patient's tremor. Parkinson disease should be suspected when a patient exhibits micrographia or has a rest tremor that subsides with action, with or without re-emergence when a new posture is sustained. Rest tremor that is much greater in amplitude than action tremor is also a red flag for possible Parkinson disease. Abnormal dopamine transporter imaging is helpful in

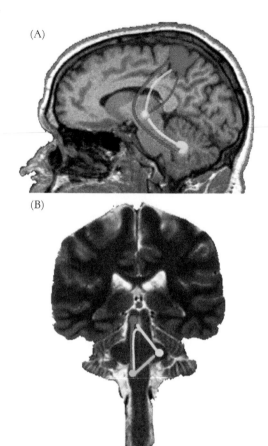

(A)

(B)

FIGURE 9.3: Corticobulbocerebellothalamocortical Loop (3A) and Guillain-Mollaret Triangle (3B). The dentate and interposed nuclei (Figure 3A; aqua) project to contralateral ventralis intermedius of the thalamus (yellow), which projects to the sensorimotor cortex (red). The cerebral cortex projects back to the thalamus and to the ipsilateral red nucleus and the precerebellar nuclei (pontine nuclei and inferior olive), which project to the cerebellum. All of these pathways are excitatory and prone to oscillation. The red nucleus and inferior olive receive input from cerebral cortex. The red nucleus (Figure 3B, red) projects to the inferior olive (green), which projects to the cerebellum (aqua), and both projections are excitatory. The deep cerebellar nuclei (dentate and interposed) send excitatory fibers to the contralateral red nucleus and inhibitory fibers to the contralateral inferior olive, forming the Guillain-Mollaret triangle.

confirming a diagnosis of Parkinson disease, but false negative scans have been reported, and a normal scan is not helpful in distinguishing ET from dystonic tremor.[73,74]

Enhanced physiologic tremor was more common than ET in two community-based studies[28,30]

TABLE 9.3: DISTINGUISHING CLINICAL FEATURES IN THE DIFFERENTIAL DIAGNOSIS OF ESSENTIAL TREMOR

Clinical feature	Essential tremor	Dystonia	Parkinson disease	Rhythmic cortical myoclonus	Enhanced physiologic tremor
Greatest in the head, face or voice		xx			
Focal or very asymmetric upper extremity action tremor*		xx	x		
Rest tremor > action tremor in upper limbs		x	xx		
Micrographia			xx		
Isolated head or voice tremor		xx			
Rest tremor in the head		x			
Suppression of rest tremor by voluntary muscle activation			xx		
Rest tremor in the lower limbs			xx		
Jerky 7–14 Hz uniform tremulousness from head to toe				xx	
Jerky tremor		x		x	
Negative myoclonus				xx	
> 1-Hz reduction in tremor frequency with inertial loading					x
Mild symmetrical action tremor in the hands only	x				xx

* ≥ 1-point asymmetry on the Essential Tremor Rating Assessment Scale (0–4 rating)
x = suggestive and xx = strongly suggestive

and should be high in the differential diagnosis when a patient exhibits relatively mild hand tremor of short (< 1 year) duration. The frequency of enhanced physiologic wrist tremor decreases more than 1 Hz when a 0.5–1Kg inertial load is attached to the hand, but this does not occur with central neurogenic tremors such as ET.[75,76] These phenomena can be demonstrated with electromyography, accelerometry or both.[75,76]

Electromyography is also helpful in distinguishing ET from rhythmic cortical myoclonus (a.k.a. cortical tremor, polymyoclonus).[77,78] Mild rhythmic cortical myoclonus can be difficult or impossible to distinguish from enhanced physiologic tremor in the hands. Regardless, there is frequently an underlying drug or systemic illness (e.g., thyrotoxicosis, renal failure, liver failure) that is responsible, and the laboratory evaluation of these patients often includes a thyroid function battery and complete metabolic panel.[78,79]

TREATMENT

Pharmacologic treatment

The pharmacologic treatment of ET has been reviewed extensively and is discussed elsewhere in this book.[47,80,81] Studies published prior to the multicenter topiramate trial generally would not meet the standards for publication today, and no new pharmacologic treatment for ET has been found since topiramate.[80] The efficacy of propranolol, primidone and topiramate has been demonstrated in double-blind placebo-controlled trials. These drugs are usually titrated over a period of weeks to reduce side effects, and they are generally administered on a twice—or thrice-daily dosing schedule, as summarized in Table 9.4. However, extended-release formulations of propranolol and topiramate are available. The choice of drug often depends on a patient's comorbidities. Propranolol and topiramate are also useful for migraine prophylaxis, and primidone is an effective anticonvulsant although the dosage required is typically greater than the dosage for ET.

Primidone occasionally produces a first-dose toxic reaction consisting of alarming drowsiness, nausea, ataxia, dizziness, or confusion. This is why primidone is usually started at 25mg at bedtime, but there is no evidence that even lower initial dosages reduce side effects in the first 48 hours.[82] Therefore, patients should be

TABLE 9.4: SUMMARY OF WELL-ESTABLISHED DRUGS FOR ESSENTIAL TREMOR

Drug	Initial dosage	Daily dose range	Average improvement	Cautions	Common side effects
Propranolol	10mg tid	60–240mg	50–60%	Must be tapered slowly in patients with coronary disease. Avoid in patients with bradycardia, heart block, asthma, sick sinus syndrome and heart failure.	Fatigue Bradycardia
Primidone	25mg hs	25–750mg	60%	Avoid abrupt withdrawal if there is a history of seizures. Caution in patients with history of depression, taking warfarin or renal or hepatic impairment.	First-dose acute toxic reaction Drowsiness Nausea Ataxia Dizziness Confusion
Topiramate	25mg bid	50–400mg	39%	Caution in patients with renal insufficiency or history of nephrolithiasis.	Reduced appetite Weight loss Cognitive impairment Paresthesia

warned of this problem and informed that the side effects resolve within 24 hours of stopping the drug.

On average, propranolol and primidone produce roughly a 50% reduction in tremor amplitude. Topiramate may be somewhat less effective, but the studies of propranolol and primidone were limited by small patient cohorts and limited assessments of tremor.[47,80] There are occasional dramatic responders to each of these drugs, but the dramatic response rarely, if ever, lasts more than a few weeks. This phenomenon and the lack of dose-response relationships are not understood. The average therapeutic effect of these drugs will provide satisfactory symptom relief in many patients with mild to moderate tremor (≤ grade 2 tremor, which is ≤ 3cm amplitude on a 0–4 rating[83]), but it will not be adequate for most patients with severe tremor (≥ grade 3, which is ≥ 5cm amplitude).

Chemodenervation
Botulinum toxin is strongly advocated by some experts, but its efficacy is modest and depends strongly on the skills of the clinician.[84–86] This approach is generally recommended in patients who fail to respond adequately to oral medications. The influence of diagnosis (e.g., ET vs. ET-plus vs. dystonic tremor) on clinical response has not been studied adequately.

All advocates of this therapy emphasize the need to tailor injections to the needs of the patient.[84] This is typically based on clinical exam, with or without electromyography.[84] Highly personalized injections of upper limb muscles and cervical muscles dictated by computerized algorithms using multiple goniometers are proposed but have not been studied in double-blind placebo-controlled trials.[87,88] Tremor in the fingers is particularly difficult to treat with botulinum toxin. The finger and wrist extensors are often avoided to prevent disabling finger and wrist drop. Muscle weakness is a common side effect, which makes blinding in clinical trials very difficult.[80]

Surgical treatment
Stereotactic deep brain stimulation (DBS) and ablative surgery are capable of reducing upper extremity tremor by more than 80% and are far more effective than any available drug.[47,89] Stereotactic ablations are performed with magnetic resonance-guided focused ultrasound (MRgFUS),[90] radiosurgery (e.g., Gamma Knife®)[91] and radiofrequency lesioning.[92] The preferred target for these procedures has been the thalamic nucleus ventralis intermedius (VIM; a.k.a.

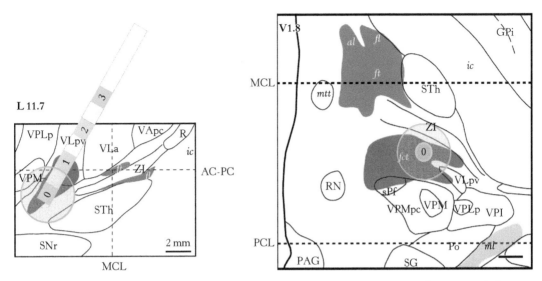

FIGURE 9.4: Posterior Subthalamic Area and Thalamic Stereotactic Targets for Essential Tremor. Sagittal section 11.7 mm lateral to the midline (left) and horizontal section of the subthalamic area 1.8 mm below the plane of the anterior and posterior commissures (right) are shown with a typical quadripolar electrode trajectory extending through VLpv (a.k.a., Ventralis intermedius, VIM) into the posterior subthalamic area. The volume of tissue activation (light blue) extends 1–3 mm from the cathode electrode contact(s), depending on the voltage/current and width of the electrical pulses. The midcommissural line (MCL) is midway between the anterior commissure (AC) and posterior commissure (PC). Adapted from the Morel stereotactic atlas. Abbreviations: Al = Ansa lenticularis, fct = Cerebellothalamic tract, fl = Fasciculus lenticularis, ft = Fasciculus thalamicus, GPi = Globus pallidus interna, ic = Internal capsule, mL = Medial lemniscus, mtt = Mammillothalamic tract, PAG = Periaqueductal gray, PCL = posterior commissure line, Po = Posterior nucleus, R = Reticular thalamic nucleus, RN = Red nucleus, SG = Suprageniculate nucleus, SNr = Substantia nigra pars reticulata, sPf = Subparafascicular nucleus, STh = Subthalamic nucleus, VApc = Ventralis anterior parvocellularis, VLa = Ventralis lateralis anterior, VLpv = Ventralis lateralis posterior ventral, VPI = Ventralis posterior inferior, VPLp = Ventralis posterior lateralis posterior, VPM = Ventral posterior medial nucleus, VPMpc = Ventralis posterior medialis parvocellular division, ZI = Zona incerta.

ventralis lateralis posterior) or posterior subthalamic area (PSA) immediately beneath the ventral border of VIM.[89] The PSA is lateral to the red nucleus and posteromedial to the subthalamic nucleus, and it contains the cerebellothalamic tract and caudal zona incerta.[93,94] The medial lemniscus is located posteriorly (Figure 9.4). Recent studies found that targeting the cerebellothalamic tract as it enters the ventral border of VIM produces comparable efficacy with lower adverse effects, compared with VIM.[95-97] This is true for DBS[98] and ablative surgery.[99] Other surgical teams favor the caudal zona incerta as the optimum target.[100,101]

VIM and PSA constitute a very small anatomical region (Figure 9.4). The anteroposterior thickness of VIM at its inferior border is about 3 mm.[94,102] The thickness of the cerebellothalamic tract as it enters VIM is 2–3 mm, and the thickness of the caudal zona incerta is less than 2 mm.

By comparison, DBS electrodes have a diameter of approximately 1.27–1.4 mm, depending on the manufacturer,[103] and a typical spherical volume of tissue activation around an active electrode has a radius of 2–4mm, depending on the stimulus voltage, pulse width, and tissue impedance.[104,105] Therefore, it is not surprising that the trauma produced by inserting a well-placed electrode usually produces significant reduction in tremor ("microlesion effect"),[106,107] and the stimulating electrode and surrounding volume of tissue activation will nearly always affect more than one structure.

Therefore, the key structure being stimulated or lesioned is difficult to determine.[108] The reported efficacy is similar for VIM and PSA, so it would take an unattainably large sample size to prove one target more effective than another.[89] Furthermore, the best target may differ among the underlying etiologies of ET and ET-plus, and the best target cannot be defined simply in terms of tremor suppression. Side effects, tolerance,[109] and maladaptive responses must also be considered, and these factors have never been systematically investigated in a large controlled prospective study. The only published controlled study failed to show a significant difference.[110]

The most common side effects of stereotactic DBS and ablative surgery in VIM and PSA stem from disruption of the cerebellothalamocortical pathway and neighboring thalamic and subthalamic structures. The cerebellothalamocortical pathway is critical for feedforward (i.e., anticipatory, based on prior motor learning) motor control by the cerebellum, and excessive stimulation or ablation of this pathway produces dysarthria, dysphagia, disequilibrium, and extremity ataxia.[89] Electrodes/ablations that are too posterior will produce paresthesia/sensory loss, and those that are too lateral will produce dysarthria and muscle contractions/weakness. These adverse sensorimotor events are common immediately after focused ultrasound or radiofrequency ablations because these procedures are designed to destroy brain parenchyma. They are less common and generally mild after DBS electrode insertion unless there is hemorrhage ($\approx$2%), which remains symptomatic in less than 1%.[89,111-113] These perioperative lesion-induced adverse events improve or resolve in most patients over 3–12 months.[89,112,114,115]

The incidence and severity of lesion/stimulation-induced sensorimotor side effects are impossible to compare among DBS and the three ablative procedures because there is only one well-designed comparison study using randomized treatment allocation and prospective documentation of adverse events (N = only 13 ET patients).[116] Furthermore, there are few studies in which adverse events were documented prospectively, and recall bias probably underlies the substantial variability in reported incidence of adverse events.[89,95,115] The adverse effects (and benefits) of radiosurgery do not appear until three or more months after surgery, and 2–10% of patients develop unexpectedly large lesions that may appear more than a year after treatment.[91,117,118] The reversibility of stimulation-induced side effects from DBS is widely acknowledged, but stimulation-induced side effects may be a necessary compromise when programming a pulse generator to achieve adequate tremor control. Even optimally placed electrodes will produce sensorimotor side effects if the pulse width and amplitude are increased enough to produce a volume of tissue activation that includes the medial

lemniscus, corticospinal tract, or red nucleus or that completely disables the cerebellothalamocortical pathway. As ET progresses, stronger stimulation is usually needed to control tremor, and side effects become more likely (20–50%).[89] Therefore, the reported long-term incidence of speech, motor, and somatosensory side effects from DBS is comparable to or greater than the incidence of these side effects from MRgFUS and radiosurgery thalamotomy.[115,119,120]

Since MRgFUS and radiosurgery are closed, incisionless procedures, the perioperative risks of infection and bleeding are avoided, as are the lifelong risks and expense of infection, pulse generator programming, and hardware replacement (e.g., for battery failure and lead breakage).[118,121,122] The risk of infection related to DBS surgery and hardware replacement is about 5%.[89,123] Radiosurgery[117,124] and MRgFUS have their advocates, but most centers prefer DBS, with MRgFUS reserved for patients with a contraindication to DBS or a preference for a closed, incisionless procedure. DBS has the distinct advantage of being adaptable to disease progression. Radiofrequency ablation is now performed uncommonly.[95] The main drawbacks of radiosurgery are 1) the effect of surgery occurs weeks or months after the procedure, so there is no way to judge efficacy and side effects during the procedure; and 2) some lesions continue to expand far beyond the intended size of the thalamotomy.[91,124,125] However, unilateral radiosurgery and MRgFUS were recommended as safe and effective, based on recent systematic reviews of the literature.[118,122]

The safety of bilateral ablative surgery is still debated. Ablative surgery is now performed more precisely and with less perioperative morbidity than in the early years of stereotactic radiofrequency ablations.[124,126,127] However, a recent position statement of the American Society for Stereotactic and Functional Neurosurgery concluded that bilateral thalamotomy with MRgFUS is contraindicated,[122] and a practice guideline from the International Stereotactic Radiosurgery Society offered no recommendation on this issue.[118] Bilateral DBS is viewed as being relatively safe even though the long-term adverse effects are more than double,[89,115] and quality of life may not be better than with unilateral DBS.[128] An aggressively programmed ET patient with bilateral DBS may have balance and speech problems comparable to those in patients with bilateral ablative lesions.[115,127] Furthermore, irreversible dysarthria and imbalance following uncomplicated bilateral thalamic DBS for advanced ET occurs in 25%

and 10% or more, even after unilateral surgery.[129-131] Consequently, most surgeons in the United States perform bilateral DBS for ET as a staged procedure,[132] separated by at least a few months, and bilateral ablative procedures should always be performed as staged procedures, if at all. The second surgery is generally avoided if the first surgery affects speech, swallowing, or balance adversely or if the patient has baseline speech or balance impairment.[127]

Head and voice tremor are relatively mild in most ET patients but are a concern to some. Improvement in these aspects of ET is largely fortuitous because intraoperative targeting is optimized on the basis of upper limb tremor. The reported response to ablation and DBS is generally better with bilateral surgery, but significant benefit may occur with unilateral surgery.[129,133-135]

The benefits of DBS may diminish over several weeks, only to return after re-optimization of stimulation parameters and electrode configuration in another programming session.[109] This rapid loss of efficacy cannot be explained by disease progression, declining microlesion effect, or poorly placed electrode. Instead, there appears to be an undesirable adaptation of the tremor network to DBS. Patients can be provided with two or more predefined stimulation programs that they can switch between to control side effects or loss of efficacy.[136, 137] Tolerance may be unappreciated in some studies because patients were evaluated in clinic with stimulators having been off for several hours before being turned on again to assess clinical benefit.[89,129] The benefit from DBS decreases significantly over the years following surgery,[138] and the contribution and treatment of short- and long-term tolerance to DBS require further study.[89,139]

Patients may also develop additional neurologic signs (e.g., ataxia and dystonia), raising the concern of maladaptation to an ablative lesion or DBS. Ataxia due to cerebellar maladaptation to thalamic DBS has been convincingly demonstrated,[140] and dystonia has occurred following DBS and thalamotomy.[20] ET generally progresses slowly over decades, but patients undergoing surgery do not have typical ET.[141] Therefore, rapid progression and the advent of additional signs are difficult to interpret pathophysiologically after surgery.

Another area of controversy is the need for microelectrode recording to localize the stereotactic target. VIM is not visible with MRI or CT,[142] but there are visible landmarks (red nucleus and subthalamic nucleus) that guide electrode placement in the posterior subthalamic area.[93] The incidence of intraoperative hemorrhage is less when surgery is performed without microelectrode recording[112] because the risk of hemorrhage increases with each penetration of the brain.[113] However, the added risk is small, especially in patients with ET,[89] and an international survey of stereotactic surgeons in 2010–2011 revealed that 83% of DBS surgeries for Parkinson disease, ET, and dystonia were performed with electrophysiologic confirmation of the target.[132] Thus, most experts view microelectrode recording as being helpful in target localization. There is a move to imaging-guided surgery under general anesthesia, made possible by ever-improving imaging technology.[143] The cost is lower,[144] and the overall improvement in quality of life may be the same.[145] More study is needed. Most patients have no significant complaints about the awake procedure with rigid stereotactic frame and microelectrode target mapping.[146]

The advantages of newer directional leads in ET are still being defined. Preliminary evidence suggests that directional leads and circumferential leads produce comparable benefit, but the threshold for side effects is increased with directional programming.[147,148] The newer pulse generators that come with directional leads are capable of pulse widths less than 60 microseconds, and there is evidence that lower pulse widths (e.g., 30 microseconds) produce less ataxia and paresthesia.[149-151]

Ultimately, the selected procedure and surgical outcome depends largely on the skills and resources of the surgical team and treating neurologist and on the characteristics of the patient being treated. Surgery for ET is recommended only when the anticipated benefits justify the risks. Patients must therefore have a clear understanding of the risks and potential benefits. The preferred procedure may be dictated by comorbidities such as cochlear implants, which preclude MRI and DBS. MRgFUS is not possible in patients who cannot undergo MRI and in patients with very dense skulls (ratio of cortical to cancellous bone < 0.4).[122] Unilateral thalamotomy is best suited for patients with very asymmetric upper extremity tremor.

Assistive technology and occupational therapy

There is a growing number of assistive devices for patients with tremor. Weighted eating utensils and sippy cups are used by many patients. There is also a growing number of commercially-available technologically-sophisticated devices for suppressing or counteracting hand tremor. The International Essential Tremor Foundation website is an excellent resource for these devices and other information about ET (https://essentialtremor.org/resource/assistive-devices/). Patients vary greatly in their satisfaction with these devices, and many patients do not find these devices useful. Randomized placebo-controlled clinical trials for efficacy are lacking for all devices. These devices are not cheap, and it is advisable to try them before purchasing. Many devices have an appropriate return policy. A knowledgeable occupational therapist can be a valuable resource in finding ways to better cope with ET.

Psychosocial

The impact of psychosocial factors on disability due to ET is an important and frequently overlooked phenomenon. It is important to determine each patient's expectations, which may not be realistic given the available treatment options, and patients should be counseled accordingly. Depression and anxiety are major determinants of quality of life in ET, so it is important to diagnose and treat these and any other psychosocial comorbidities.[31,32]

CLINICAL SCALES AND WEARABLE TRANSDUCERS

There are now several validated rating scales for the clinical assessment of ET and its impact on activities of daily living and quality of life.[152] There is also a growing number of motion transducers for the assessment of tremor amplitude.[153,154] Most of these transducers are wireless, and many are wearable. Furthermore, most smartphones contain motion transducers, most commonly a triaxial accelerometer, capable of recording pathologic tremor.[155] Here we will focus on the interpretation of scales vis-à-vis transducers and summarize their relative strengths and limitations in routine clinical assessments versus research applications.

Most tremor rating scales are ordinal scales in which various aspects of tremor are rated 0 to 4. The ratings of various aspects of tremor are summed to provide the total score. For most scales, particularly ADL and quality of life scales, a change in rating for a particular item or a change in total score is difficult to interpret in terms of change in actual tremor amplitude, even when numerical anchors are used, as in the Fahn-Tolosa-Marín (FTM) scale[156] and the Essential Tremor Rating Assessment Scale (TETRAS).[83]

Several research groups have examined the mathematical relationship between tremor severity ratings and actual tremor amplitude, measured with linear motion transducers, and all have found a logarithmic relationship between tremor amplitude and ratings.[157,158] This relationship is predicted by the Weber-Fechner law of psychophysics, which states that the perceptible change in a physical quantity (e.g., tremor amplitude) depends on its initial value, and because of this relationship, increments in perceptible change (i.e., increments in ratings) are associated with logarithmic changes in the physical quantity.[157] This relationship holds, regardless of the number of increments in the rating (e.g., 0–4, 0–10, etc.) and regardless of the total number of points in the scale.[157] The Weber-Fechner relationship for tremor is expressed mathematically in equation 1, where T is tremor amplitude, R is tremor rating, and α and β are the slope and y-intercept. From this equation, one can derive the percentage change in tremor amplitude for a given change in tremor rating (equation 2). Note that the percentage change in tremor amplitude is a function of the change in tremor rating, not the percentage change in rating.

$$\log_{10} T = \alpha R + \beta \qquad 1$$

$$\left(\frac{T_f - T_i}{T_i}\right)100 = \left[10^{\alpha(R_f - R_i)} - 1\right]100 \qquad 2$$

Using data from multiple labs, a best estimate of the coefficient α is 0.5 for a 0–4 scale, with a range of 0.4–0.6. Therefore, 0.4 can be used for conservative estimates, as in a recent review of surgery for ET.[89] For a scale with a maximum score of S, the coefficient $\alpha_s = \alpha \cdot 4/S$. For example, the estimated α for the 0–10 Bain and Findley spirography scale is $0.5 \cdot 4/10 = 0.2$, which is statistically equal to the value obtained empirically in a study that used the Bain and Findley scale and a digitizing tablet to assess tremor in spiral drawings.[159] The slope α can also be computed for subscales. For example, α for the 32-point subscale of the FTM scale used in the pivotal trial of MRgFUS is $0.5 \cdot 4/32 = 0.0625$.

The use of equation 2 to compute percentage change in tremor severity avoids misleading computations with clinical ratings.[157] It is incorrect and misleading to compute percentage changes in ordinal scales. For example, the pivotal trial of MRgFUS thalamotomy reported a 47% reduction in tremor, measured with a 32-point upper extremity subscale of the FTM. Few patients would undergo a risky surgical procedure for a 47% reduction in tremor, and few clinicians would recommend surgery with this benefit. However, the percentage reduction in tremor amplitude is actually much larger than 42%. Using the mean baseline and 3-month subscale scores (18.1 and 9.6),[160] the average percentage change in tremor amplitude is actually 71%, as shown in equation 3.

$$\left(\frac{T_f - T_i}{T_i}\right)100 = \left[10^{0.0625(9.6-18.1)} - 1\right]$$
$$\times 100 = -71\% \qquad 3$$

The TETRAS and FTM scales are the most widely used scales for ET. The FTM scale was introduced in 1988[161] and was revised in 1993.[156] FTM was the first scale for the comprehensive assessment of tremor and was used in most clinical trials until the introduction of TETRAS. FTM and TETRAS are comparable scales for patients with mild to moderate tremor. However, FTM has a significant ceiling effect for moderate-severe tremor because grade 4 upper limb tremor is any tremor greater than 4cm. Most surgical candidates have tremor that far exceeds 4 cm. TETRAS does not have a ceiling effect because grade 4 upper limb tremor is >20cm. TETRAS was developed specifically for the assessment of ET,[83] so its performance and ADL scores are predominantly influenced by upper extremity action tremor; TETRAS, in contrast to FTM, has no assessment of rest tremor. FTM might therefore be a better choice for patients with mild to moderate ET-plus rest tremor, but it should be noted that reliability of assessing rest tremor in this patient population is very poor.[162]

The precision and linearity of motion transducers have a strong allure because rating scales provide crude nonlinear estimates of tremor severity. Many motion transducers are now small, wireless and affordable, and free software for data analysis is available on the internet.[154,159,163] Motion transducers have been used to measure head tremor,[164] hand tremor,[165,166] tremor in writing and drawings,[159,167] and tremor at individual joints.[165,168] Accelerometers measure linear acceleration including earth's gravitational force, gyroscopic transducers measure angular rotation, goniometers measure angular rotation, and digitizing tablets measure motion of a pen on the tablet surface.[153] Digitized motion can be analyzed by methods of signal analysis (e.g., Fourier spectral analysis) to compute amplitude and frequency of motion during the time of recording.[154]

However, it would take several transducers and considerable time to perform a comprehensive assessment of tremor comparable to the FTM or TETRAS, and several studies have shown that transducers are no better than scales in detecting change that exceeds random variation in tremor amplitude (i.e., minimum detectable change).[154,164,167,169] In other words, the advantages of the precision and accuracy of transducers are mitigated by the large random variability in tremor, such that the minimum detectable change with transducers is comparable to that with a good rating scale.[152,153]

Accelerometers have three important limitations in the clinical assessment of tremor: 1) accelerometers cannot distinguish inertial acceleration from earth's gravity; 2) accelerometers measure linear acceleration, and tremor is predominately angular rotation in space; and 3) accelerometers sense angular rotation in proportion to their distance from the axis of rotation.[170] Consequently, an accelerometer spinning or oscillating about a point in space will detect only the fluctuating relationship of earth's gravity with the accelerometer axes of sensitivity. To get consistent recordings of inertial acceleration, an accelerometer must be mounted a consistent distance from the axis of rotation, but the axis of rotation may fluctuate greatly in the upper and lower limbs if all joints are free to rotate. Consequently, gyroscopic transducers, which measure angular velocity, provide a more valid recording of rotation of a body segment in space.[164,165] Goniometers are useful for measuring rotational motion at single joints.[168]

All transducers must be mounted appropriately on a body part for tremor to be measured effectively.[154] A wearable transducer mounted on the wrist will not capture hand motion, and such a transducer provides only a partial assessment of the complex translational and rotational motion of the upper limb in three-dimensional space. A transducer on the hand will be influenced by rotation at the shoulder, elbow, and wrist, and the distribution of joint involvement may vary with time and task. Tremor in the torso can be transmitted to the head and to all four limbs. Transducers are blind to these complexities.

The potential advantages of wearable transducers are their ability to record tremor continuously for a day or more, during spontaneous daily activities. Most wearables use triaxial accelerometers, and the limitations of accelerometers have been noted. Gyroscopic transducers measure rotation in space, independent of their distance from the axis of rotation and uninfluenced by earth's gravity,[154] and such devices are available in some wearables.[158]

ET occurs during voluntary postures and movements, and all motion will be recorded to some extent by a wearable transducer. Signal analysis algorithms must then be developed to reliably distinguish tremor from other movements, which has proven to be a difficult task. Tremor is a relatively high-frequency oscillatory movement (> 3 Hz, except for myorhythmia), and most voluntary movements are less than 3 Hz, but there is some overlap. The presence or occurrence of tremor can be determined with fairly good accuracy, but determining the amplitude of tremor is far more difficult, due to concomitant voluntary movement and to the limitations of a single transducer to accurately measure complex translational and rotational motion in three-dimensional space. For example, hand tremor during finger-nose-finger testing is much less reliably measured than tremor in a posture.[158,169] Furthermore, variability in voluntary activities will add to the already large random fluctuations in tremor, resulting in reduced test-retest reliability and larger minimum detectable change. At this time, at-home testing with standardized assessment protocols appears to be a better approach than trying to record tremor during spontaneous, unspecified activities.[158,169]

A clinician or researcher must ask if any of this technology is worth the trouble. The answer to this question depends on the circumstances and reasons for considering technology. Technology currently cannot replace a skilled clinician armed with a well-validated rating scale. Standardized assessments with transducers can be performed by patients at home,[166] and technology can be used to corroborate the results of a rating scale.[167] However, one should not use technology with the expectation of detecting smaller clinical change that exceeds random fluctuations. In short, the limitations of available technology must be considered before incorporating technology into a clinical practice or therapeutic trial.

CONCLUSION

Our understanding and treatment of ET are now accelerating at a promising pace. The ET phenotype is very common and has very strong heritability, but the genetic complexity of ET remains largely undefined. The absence of Axis 2 etiologies and the likelihood of polygenic inheritance

in most patients should not deter us from proceeding with clinical trials. Animal models of tremorogenic oscillation and our understanding of tremorogenesis in the corticobulbocerebellothalamocortical loop have provided many therapeutic targets for ET, and there is thankfully a growing investment by the pharmaceutical and device industries that can be monitored on ClinicalTrials.gov.

REFERENCES

1. Louis ED, Broussolle E, Goetz CG, Krack P, Kaufmann P, Mazzoni P. Historical underpinnings of the term essential tremor in the late 19th century. *Neurology*. 2008;71:856–859. doi: 10.1212/01.wnl.0000325564.38165.d1

2. Critchley M. Observations on essential (heredofamilial) tremor. *Brain*. 1949;72:113–139. doi: 10.1093/brain/72.2.113

3. Bhatia KP, Bain P, Bajaj N, et al. Consensus Statement on the classification of tremors. From the task force on tremor of the International Parkinson and Movement Disorder Society. *Mov Disord*. 2018;33:75–87. doi: 10.1002/mds.27121

4. Whaley NR, Putzke JD, Baba Y, Wszolek ZK, Uitti RJ. Essential tremor: phenotypic expression in a clinical cohort. *Parkinsonism Relat Disord*. 2007;13:333–339. doi: 10.1016/j.parkreldis.2006.12.004

5. Louis ED, Ford B, Wendt KJ, Cameron G. Clinical characteristics of essential tremor: data from a community-based study. *Mov Disord*. 1998;13:803–808. doi: 10.1002/mds.870130508

6. Elble RJ. Do we belittle essential tremor by calling it a syndrome rather than a disease? No. *Front Neurol*. 2020;11:586606. doi: 10.3389/fneur.2020.586606

7. Deuschl G, Bain P, Brin M. Consensus statement of the Movement Disorder Society on Tremor. Ad Hoc Scientific Committee. *Mov Disord*. 1998;13 (Suppl 3):2–23. doi: 10.1002/mds.870131303

8. Louis ED, Hernandez N, Michalec M. Prevalence and correlates of rest tremor in essential tremor: cross-sectional survey of 831 patients across four distinct cohorts. *Eur J Neurol*. 2015;22:927–932. doi: 10.1111/ene.12683

9. Louis ED. "Essential tremor plus": a problematic concept: implications for clinical and epidemiological studies of essential tremor. *Neuroepidemiology*. 2020;54:180–184. doi: 10.1159/000502862

10. Fasano A, Lang AE, Espay AJ. What is "essential" about essential tremor? A diagnostic placeholder. *Mov Disord*. 2018;33:58–61. doi: 10.1002/mds.27288

11. Deuschl G, Bhatia KP, Elble R, Hallett M. Understanding the new tremor classification.

Mov Disord. 2018;33:1267–1268. doi: 10.1002/mds.27368

12. Stamelou M, Charlesworth G, Cordivari C, et al. The phenotypic spectrum of DYT24 due to ANO3 mutations. *Mov Disord.* 2014;29:928–934. doi: 10.1002/mds.25802

13. Rajalingam R, Breen DP, Lang AE, Fasano A. Essential tremor plus is more common than essential tremor: insights from the reclassification of a cohort of patients with lower limb tremor. *Parkinsonism Relat Disord.* 2018;56:109–110. doi: 10.1016/j.parkreldis.2018.06.029

14. Patel A, Deeb W, Okun MS. Deep brain stimulation management of essential tremor with dystonic features. *Tremor Other Hyperkinet Mov (N Y).* 2018;8:557. doi: 10.7916/D8P85VBQ

15. Fearon C, Espay AJ, Lang AE, et al. Soft signs in movement disorders: friends or foes? *J Neurol Neurosurg Psychiatry.* 2019;90:961–962. doi: 10.1136/jnnp-2018-318455

16. Shaikh AG, Beylergil SB, Scorr L, et al. Dystonia and tremor: a cross-sectional study of the dystonia coalition cohort. *Neurology.* 2020. doi: 10.1212/wnl.0000000000011049

17. Becktepe J, Gövert F, Balint B, et al. Exploring interrater disagreement on essential tremor using a standardized tremor elements assessment. *Mov Disord Clin Pract.* 2021. doi: 10.1002/mdc3.13150

18. Pandey S, Bhattad S. Questionable dystonia in essential tremor plus: a video-based assessment of 19 patients. *Mov Disord Clin Pract.* 2019;6:722–723. doi: 10.1002/mdc3.12838

19. Merchant SH, Kuo SH, Qiping Y, et al. Objective predictors of 'early tolerance' to ventral intermediate nucleus of thalamus deep brain stimulation in essential tremor patients. *Clin Neurophysiol.* 2018;129:1628–1633. doi: 10.1016/j.clinph.2018.05.012

20. Picillo M, Paramanandam V, Morgante F, et al. Dystonia as complication of thalamic neurosurgery. *Parkinsonism Relat Disord.* 2019;66:232–236. doi: 10.1016/j.parkreldis.2019.08.008

21. Ghosh D, Brar H, Lhamu U, Rothner AD, Erenberg G. A series of 211 children with probable essential tremor. *Mov Disord Clin Pract.* 2017;4:231–236. doi: 10.1002/mdc3.12385

22. Louis ED, Ferreira JJ. How common is the most common adult movement disorder? Update on the worldwide prevalence of essential tremor. *Mov Disord.* 2010;25:534–541. doi: 10.1002/mds.22838

23. Inzelberg R, Mazarib A, Masarwa M, Abuful A, Strugatsky R, Friedland RF. Essential tremor prevalence is low in Arabic villages in Israel: door-to-door neurological examinations. *J Neurol.* 2006;253:1557–1560. doi: 10.1007/s00415-006-0253-5

24. Aharon-Peretz J, Badarny S, Ibrahim R, Gershoni-Baruch R, Hassoun G. Essential tremor prevalence is low in the Druze population in Northern Israel. *Tremor Other Hyperkinet Mov (N Y).* 2012;2. doi: 10.7916/D8GF0S7H

25. Benito-Leon J, Bermejo-Pareja F, Morales JM, Vega S, Molina JA. Prevalence of essential tremor in three elderly populations of central Spain. *Mov Disord.* 2003;18:389–394. doi: 10.1002/mds.10376

26. Dogu O, Sevim S, Camdeviren H, et al. Prevalence of essential tremor: door-to-door neurologic exams in Mersin Province, Turkey. *Neurology.* 2003;61:1804–1806. doi: 10.1212/01.wnl.0000099075.19951.8c

27. Bergareche A, De La Puente E, Lopez De Munain A, et al. Prevalence of essential tremor: a door-to-door survey in Bidasoa, Spain. *Neuroepidemiology.* 2001;20:125–128. doi: 10.1159/000054771

28. Wenning GK, Kiechl S, Seppi K, et al. Prevalence of movement disorders in men and women aged 50–89 years (Bruneck Study cohort): a population-based study. *Lancet Neurol.* 2005;4:815–820. doi: 10.1016/S1474-4422(05)70226-X

29. Dogu O, Louis ED, Sevim S, Kaleagasi H, Aral M. Clinical characteristics of essential tremor in Mersin, Turkey—a population-based door-to-door study. *J Neurol.* 2005;252:570–574. doi: 10.1007/s00415-005-0700-8

30. Rautakorpi I, Takala J, Marttila RJ, Sievers K, Rinne UK. Essential tremor in a Finnish population. *Acta Neurol Scand.* 1982;66:58–67. doi: 10.1111/j.1600-0404.1982.tb03129.x

31. Louis ED, Barnes L, Albert SM, et al. Correlates of functional disability in essential tremor. *Mov Disord.* 2001;16:914–920. doi: 10.1002/mds.1184

32. Lorenz D, Poremba C, Papengut F, Schreiber S, Deuschl G. The psychosocial burden of essential tremor in an outpatient—and a community-based cohort. *Eur J Neurol.* 2011;18:972–979. doi: 10.1111/j.1468-1331.2010.03295.x

33. Bain PG, Findley LJ, Thompson PD, et al. A study of hereditary essential tremor. *Brain.* 1994;117(Pt 4):805–824. doi: 10.1093/brain/117.4.805

34. Lorenz D, Frederiksen H, Moises H, Kopper F, Deuschl G, Christensen K. High concordance for essential tremor in monozygotic twins of old age. *Neurology.* 2004;62:208–211. doi: 10.1212/01.wnl.0000103236.26934.41

35. Hopfner F, Ahlf A, Lorenz D, et al. Early- and late-onset essential tremor patients represent clinically distinct subgroups. *Mov Disord.* 2016;31:1560–1566. doi: 10.1002/mds.26708

36. Deuschl G, Petersen I, Lorenz D, Christensen K. Tremor in the elderly: essential and aging-related tremor. *Mov Disord.* 2015;30:1327–1334. doi: 10.1002/mds.26265

37. Deuschl G, Elble R. Essential tremor—neurodegenerative or nondegenerative disease towards a working definition of ET. *Mov Disord.* 2009;24:2033–2041. doi: 10.1002/mds.22755

38. Stark RS, Walch J, Kagi G. The phenotypic variation of a Parkin-related Parkinson's disease family and the role of heterozygosity. *Mov Disord Clin Pract*. 2019;6:700–703. doi: 10.1002/mdc3.12826

39. O'Hearn E, Holmes SE, Calvert PC, Ross CA, Margolis RL. SCA-12: tremor with cerebellar and cortical atrophy is associated with a CAG repeat expansion. *Neurology*. 2001;56:299–303. doi: 10.1212/wnl.56.3.299

40. Kay L, Jorgensen T, Lanng C. Irritable bowel syndrome: which definitions are consistent? *J Intern Med*. 1998;244:489–494.

41. Elble RJ. Essential tremor is a useful concept? No. *Mov Disord Clin Pract*. 2017;4:663–665. doi: 10.1002/mdc3.12514

42. Jankovic J. Essential tremor: a heterogenous disorder. *Mov Disord*. 2002;17:638–644. doi: 10.1002/mds.10221

43. Marsden CD, Obeso JA, Rothwell JC. Benign essential tremor is not a single entity. In: Yahr MD, ed. *Current Concepts of Parkinson's Disease and Related Disorders*. Excerpta Medica; 1983: 31–46.

44. Elble RJ. Physiologic and essential tremor. *Neurology*. 1986;36:225–231. doi: 10.1212/wnl.36.2.225

45. Louis ED, Agnew A, Gillman A, Gerbin M, Viner AS. Estimating annual rate of decline: prospective, longitudinal data on arm tremor severity in two groups of essential tremor cases. *J Neurol Neurosurg Psychiatry*. 2011;82:761–765. doi: 10.1136/jnnp.2010.229740

46. Putzke JD, Whaley NR, Baba Y, Wszolek ZK, Uitti RJ. Essential tremor: predictors of disease progression in a clinical cohort. *J Neurol Neurosurg Psychiatry*. 2006;77:1235–1237. doi: 10.1136/jnnp.2006.086579

47. Deuschl G, Raethjen J, Hellriegel H, Elble R. Treatment of patients with essential tremor. *Lancet Neurol*. 2011;10:148–161. doi: 10.1016/S1474-4422(10)70322-7

48. Benito-Leon J, Louis ED, Bermejo-Pareja F, Neurological disorders in central Spain study G. Elderly-onset essential tremor is associated with dementia. *Neurology*. 2006;66:1500–1505. doi: 10.1212/01.wnl.0000216134.88617.de

49. Becktepe JS, Govert F, Kasiske L, Yalaz M, Witt K, Deuschl G. Pupillary response to light and tasks in early and late onset essential tremor patients. *Parkinsonism Relat Disord*. 2019;66:62–67. doi: 10.1016/j.parkreldis.2019.07.004

50. Muthuraman M, Deuschl G, Anwar AR, Mideksa KG, von Helmolt F, Schneider SA. Essential and aging-related tremor: differences of central control. *Mov Disord*. 2015;30:1673–1680. doi: 10.1002/mds.26410

51. Deuschl G. Locus coeruleus dysfunction: a feature of essential or senile tremor? *Mov Disord*. 2012;27:1–2. doi: 10.1002/mds.24885

52. Papengut F, Raethjen J, Binder A, Deuschl G. Rest tremor suppression may separate essential from parkinsonian rest tremor. *Parkinsonism Relat Disord*. 2013;19:693–697. doi: 10.1016/j.parkreldis.2013.03.013

53. Jankovic J, Schwartz KS, Ondo W. Re-emergent tremor of Parkinson's disease. *J Neurol Neurosurg Psychiatry*. 1999;67:646–650. doi: 10.1136/jnnp.67.5.646

54. Agnew A, Frucht SJ, Louis ED. Supine head tremor: a clinical comparison of essential tremor and spasmodic torticollis patients. *J Neurol Neurosurg Psychiatry*. 2012;83:179–181. doi: 10.1136/jnnp-2011-300823

55. Kim CY, Louis ED. "Spooning": a subtle sign of limb dystonia. *Tremor Other Hyperkinet Mov (N Y)*. 2018;8:607. doi: 10.7916/D8B00NRV

56. Kuhlenbaumer G, Hopfner F, Deuschl G. Genetics of essential tremor: meta-analysis and review. *Neurology*. 2014;82:1000–1007. doi: 10.1212/WNL.0000000000000211

57. Diez-Fairen M, Bandres-Ciga S, Houle G, et al. Genome-wide estimates of heritability and genetic correlations in essential tremor. *Parkinsonism Relat Disord*. 2019;64:262–267. doi: 10.1016/j.parkreldis.2019.05.002

58. Wu YR, Foo JN, Tan LC, et al. Identification of a novel risk variant in the FUS gene in essential tremor. *Neurology*. 2013;81:541–544. doi: 10.1212/WNL.0b013e31829e700c

59. Hopfner F, Stevanin G, Muller SH, et al. The impact of rare variants in FUS in essential tremor. *Mov Disord*. 2015;30:721–724. doi: 10.1002/mds.26145

60. Sun QY, Xu Q, Tian Y, et al. Expansion of GGC repeat in the human-specific NOTCH2NLC gene is associated with essential tremor. *Brain*. 2020;143:222–233. doi: 10.1093/brain/awz372

61. Unal Gulsuner H, Gulsuner S, Mercan FN, et al. Mitochondrial serine protease HTRA2 p.G399S in a kindred with essential tremor and Parkinson disease. *Proc Natl Acad Sci U S A*. 2014;111:18285–18290. doi: 10.1073/pnas.1419581111

62. Muller SH, Girard SL, Hopfner F, et al. Genome-wide association study in essential tremor identifies three new loci. *Brain*. 2016;139:3163–3169. doi: 10.1093/brain/aww242

63. Hopfner F, Haubenberger D, Galpern WR, et al. Knowledge gaps and research recommendations for essential tremor. *Parkinsonism Relat Disord*. 2016;33:27–35. doi: 10.1016/j.parkreldis.2016.10.002

64. Benagiano V, Rizzi A, Lorusso L, et al. The functional anatomy of the cerebrocerebellar circuit: a review and new concepts. *J Comp Neurol*. 2018;526:769–789. doi: 10.1002/cne.24361

65. Elble RJ. Tremor disorders. *Curr Opin Neurol*. 2013;26:413–419. doi: 10.1097/WCO.0b013e3283632f46

66. Louis ED, Kerridge CA, Chatterjee D, et al. Contextualizing the pathology in the essential tremor cerebellar cortex: a patholog-omics approach. *Acta Neuropathol.* 2019;138:859–876. doi: 10.1007/s00401-019-02043-7
67. Louis ED, Faust PL, Vonsattel JP, et al. Torpedoes in Parkinson's disease, Alzheimer's disease, essential tremor, and control brains. *Mov Disord.* 2009;24:1600–1605. doi: 10.1002/mds.22567
68. Rajput AH, Robinson CA, Rajput ML, Rajput A. Cerebellar Purkinje cell loss is not pathognomonic of essential tremor. *Parkinsonism Relat Disord.* 2011;17:16–21. doi: 10.1016/j.parkreldis.2010.08.009
69. Shill HA, Adler CH, Sabbagh MN, et al. Pathologic findings in prospectively ascertained essential tremor subjects. *Neurology.* 2008;70:1452–1455. doi: 10.1212/01.wnl.0000310425.76205.02
70. Lee D, Gan SR, Faust PL, Louis ED, Kuo SH. Climbing fiber-Purkinje cell synaptic pathology across essential tremor subtypes. *Parkinsonism Relat Disord.* 2018;51:24–29. doi: 10.1016/j.parkreldis.2018.02.032
71. Jain S, Lo SE, Louis ED. Common misdiagnosis of a common neurological disorder: how are we misdiagnosing essential tremor? *Arch Neurol.* 2006;63:1100–1104. doi: 10.1001/archneur.63.8.1100
72. Schrag A, Munchau A, Bhatia KP, Quinn NP, Marsden CD. Essential tremor: an overdiagnosed condition? *J Neurol.* 2000;247:955–959. doi: 10.1007/s004150070053
73. Bajaj N, Hauser RA, Grachev ID. Clinical utility of dopamine transporter single photon emission CT (DaT-SPECT) with (123I) ioflupane in diagnosis of parkinsonian syndromes. *J Neurol Neurosurg Psychiatry.* 2013;84:1288–1295. doi: 10.1136/jnnp-2012-304436
74. Erro R, Schneider SA, Stamelou M, Quinn NP, Bhatia KP. What do patients with scans without evidence of dopaminergic deficit (SWEDD) have? New evidence and continuing controversies. *J Neurol Neurosurg Psychiatry.* 2016;87:319–323. doi: 10.1136/jnnp-2014-310256
75. Longardner K, Undurraga FV, Nahab FB, Hallett M, Haubenberger D. How do I assess tremor using novel technology? *Mov Disord Clin Pract.* 2019;6:733–734. doi: 10.1002/mdc3.12818
76. Elble RJ, Deuschl G. Tremor. In: Brown WF, Bolton CF, Aminoff M, eds. *Neuromuscular Function and Disease: Basic, Clinical and Electrodiagnostic Aspects.* W. B. Saunders Co.; 2002: 1759–1779.
77. Bourdain F, Apartis E, Trocello JM, et al. Clinical analysis in familial cortical myoclonic tremor allows differential diagnosis with essential tremor. *Mov Disord.* 2006;21:599–608. doi: 10.1002/mds.20725
78. McKeon A, Pittock SJ, Glass GA, et al. Whole-body tremulousness: isolated generalized polymyoclonus. *Arch Neurol.* 2007;64:1318–1322. doi: 10.1001/archneur.64.9.1318
79. Morgan JC, Sethi KD. Drug-induced tremors. *Lancet Neurol.* 2005;4:866–876. doi: 10.1016/S1474-4422(05)70250-7
80. Ferreira JJ, Mestre TA, Lyons KE, et al. MDS evidence-based review of treatments for essential tremor. *Mov Disord.* 2019;34:950–958. doi: 10.1002/mds.27700
81. Zesiewicz TA, Elble RJ, Louis ED, et al. Evidence-based guideline update: treatment of essential tremor: report of the Quality Standards subcommittee of the American Academy of Neurology. *Neurology.* 2011;77:1752–1755. doi: 10.1212/WNL.0b013e318236f0fd
82. O'Suilleabhain P, Dewey RB, Jr. Randomized trial comparing primidone initiation schedules for treating essential tremor. *Mov Disord.* 2002;17:382–386. doi: 10.1002/mds.10083
83. Elble R, Comella C, Fahn S, et al. Reliability of a new scale for essential tremor. *Mov Disord.* 2012;27:1567–1569. doi: 10.1002/mds.25162
84. Kamel JT, Cordivari C, Catania S. Treatment of upper limb tremor with botulinum toxin: an individualized approach. *Mov Disord Clin Pract.* 2019;6:652–655. doi: 10.1002/mdc3.12832
85. Justicz N, Hapner ER, Josephs JS, Boone BC, Jinnah HA, Johns MM, 3rd. Comparative effectiveness of propranolol and botulinum for the treatment of essential voice tremor. *Laryngoscope.* 2016;126:113–117. doi: 10.1002/lary.25485
86. Mittal SO, Lenka A, Jankovic J. Botulinum toxin for the treatment of tremor. *Parkinsonism Relat Disord.* 2019;63:31–41. doi: 10.1016/j.parkreldis.2019.01.023
87. Samotus O, Lee J, Jog M. Personalized bilateral upper limb essential tremor therapy with botulinum toxin using kinematics. *Toxins (Basel).* 2019;11:doi: 10.3390/toxins11020125
88. Samotus O, Lee J, Jog M. Personalized botulinum toxin type A therapy for cervical dystonia based on kinematic guidance. *J Neurol.* 2018;265:1269–1278. doi: 10.1007/s00415-018-8819-6
89. Elble RJ, Shih L, Cozzens JW. Surgical treatments for essential tremor. *Expert Rev Neurother.* 2018;18:303–321. doi: 10.1080/14737175.2018.1445526
90. Weintraub D, Elias WJ. The emerging role of transcranial magnetic resonance imaging-guided focused ultrasound in functional neurosurgery. *Mov Disord.* 2017;32:20–27. doi: 10.1002/mds.26599
91. Higuchi Y, Matsuda S, Serizawa T. Gamma knife radiosurgery in movement disorders: indications and limitations. *Mov Disord.* 2017;32:28–35. doi: 10.1002/mds.26625
92. Cosman ER, Nashold BS, Bedenbaugh P. Stereotactic radiofrequency lesion making. *Appl*

Neurophysiol. 1983;46:160–166. doi: 10.1159/000101256

93. Nowacki A, Debove I, Rossi F, et al. Targeting the posterior subthalamic area for essential tremor: proposal for MRI-based anatomical landmarks. *J Neurosurg.* 2018;131:820–827. doi: 10.3171/2018.4.JNS18373

94. Neudorfer C, Maarouf M. Neuroanatomical background and functional considerations for stereotactic interventions in the H fields of Forel. *Brain Struct Funct.* 2018;223:17–30. doi: 10.1007/s00429-017-1570-4

95. Schreglmann SR, Krauss JK, Chang JW, Bhatia KP, Kagi G. Functional lesional neurosurgery for tremor: a systematic review and meta-analysis. *J Neurol Neurosurg Psychiatry.* 2018;89:717–726. doi: 10.1136/jnnp-2017-316302

96. Barbe MT, Liebhart L, Runge M, et al. Deep brain stimulation of the ventral intermediate nucleus in patients with essential tremor: stimulation below intercommissural line is more efficient but equally effective as stimulation above. *Exp Neurol.* 2011;230:131–137. doi: 10.1016/j.expneurol.2011.04.005

97. Al-Fatly B, Ewert S, Kubler D, Kroneberg D, Horn A, Kuhn AA. Connectivity profile of thalamic deep brain stimulation to effectively treat essential tremor. *Brain.* 2019;142:3086–3098. doi: 10.1093/brain/awz236

98. Dembek TA, Petry-Schmelzer JN, Reker P, et al. PSA and VIM DBS efficiency in essential tremor depends on distance to the dentatorubrothalamic tract. *Neuroimage Clin.* 2020;26:102235. doi: 10.1016/j.nicl.2020.102235

99. Gallay MN, Moser D, Jeanmonod D. MR-guided focused ultrasound cerebellothalamic tractotomy for chronic therapy-resistant essential tremor: anatomical target reappraisal and clinical results. *J Neurosurg.* 2020;1–10. doi: 10.3171/2019.12.JNS192219

100. Awad A, Blomstedt P, Westling G, Eriksson J. Deep brain stimulation in the caudal zona incerta modulates the sensorimotor cerebello-cerebral circuit in essential tremor. *Neuroimage.* 2020;209:116511. doi: 10.1016/j.neuroimage.2019.116511

101. Fytagoridis A, Sandvik U, Astrom M, Bergenheim T, Blomstedt P. Long term follow-up of deep brain stimulation of the caudal zona incerta for essential tremor. *J Neurol Neurosurg Psychiatry.* 2012;83:258–262. doi: 10.1136/jnnp-2011-300765

102. Gallay MN, Jeanmonod D, Liu J, Morel A. Human pallidothalamic and cerebellothalamic tracts: anatomical basis for functional stereotactic neurosurgery. *Brain Struct Funct.* 2008;212:443–463. doi: 10.1007/s00429-007-0170-0

103. Alonso F, Latorre MA, Goransson N, Zsigmond P, Wardell K. Investigation into deep brain stimulation lead designs: a patient-specific simulation study. *Brain Sci.* 2016;6. doi: 10.3390/brainsci6030039

104. Astrom M, Diczfalusy E, Martens H, Wardell K. Relationship between neural activation and electric field distribution during deep brain stimulation. *IEEE Trans Biomed Eng.* 2015;62:664–672. doi: 10.1109/TBME.2014.2363494

105. Madler B, Coenen VA. Explaining clinical effects of deep brain stimulation through simplified target-specific modeling of the volume of activated tissue. *AJNR Am J Neuroradiol.* 2012;33:1072–1080. doi: 10.3174/ajnr.A2906

106. Blomstedt P, Sandvik U, Tisch S. Deep brain stimulation in the posterior subthalamic area in the treatment of essential tremor. *Mov Disord.* 2010;25:1350–1356. doi: 10.1002/mds.22758

107. Morishita T, Foote KD, Wu SS, et al. Brain penetration effects of microelectrodes and deep brain stimulation leads in ventral intermediate nucleus stimulation for essential tremor. *J Neurosurg.* 2010;112:491–496. doi: 10.3171/2009.7.JNS09150

108. Watson C, Lind CR, Thomas MG. The anatomy of the caudal zona incerta in rodents and primates. *J Anat.* 2014;224:95–107. doi: 10.1111/joa.12132

109. Barbe MT, Liebhart L, Runge M, et al. Deep brain stimulation in the nucleus ventralis intermedius in patients with essential tremor: habituation of tremor suppression. *J Neurol.* 2011;258:434–439. doi: 10.1007/s00415-010-5773-3

110. Barbe MT, Reker P, Hamacher S, et al. DBS of the PSA and the VIM in essential tremor: a randomized, double-blind, crossover trial. *Neurology.* 2018;91:e543–e550. doi: 10.1212/WNL.0000000000005956

111. Zrinzo L, Foltynie T, Limousin P, Hariz MI. Reducing hemorrhagic complications in functional neurosurgery: a large case series and systematic literature review. *J Neurosurg.* 2012;116:84–94. doi: 10.3171/2011.8.JNS101407

112. Binder DK, Rau GM, Starr PA. Risk factors for hemorrhage during microelectrode-guided deep brain stimulator implantation for movement disorders. *Neurosurgery.* 2005;56:722–732; discussion 722-32. doi: 10.1227/01.neu.0000156473.57196.7e

113. Kimmelman J, Duckworth K, Ramsay T, Voss T, Ravina B, Emborg ME. Risk of surgical delivery to deep nuclei: a meta-analysis. *Mov Disord.* 2011;26:1415–1421. doi: 10.1002/mds.23770

114. Schreglmann SR, Krauss JK, Chang JW, et al. Functional lesional neurosurgery for tremor: back to the future? *J Neurol Neurosurg Psychiatry.* 2018;89:727–735. doi: 10.1136/jnnp-2017-316301

115. Dallapiazza RF, Lee DJ, De Vloo P, et al. Outcomes from stereotactic surgery for essential tremor. *J Neurol Neurosurg Psychiatry.* 2019;90:474–482. doi: 10.1136/jnnp-2018-318240

116. Schuurman PR, Bosch DA, Bossuyt PM, et al. A comparison of continuous thalamic stimulation and thalamotomy for suppression of severe tremor. *N Engl J Med.* 2000;342:461–468. doi: 10.1056/NEJM200002173420703

117. Niranjan A, Raju SS, Kooshkabadi A, Monaco E, 3rd, Flickinger JC, Lunsford LD. Stereotactic radiosurgery for essential tremor: retrospective analysis of a 19-year experience. *Mov Disord.* 2017;32:769–777. doi: 10.1002/mds.26925

118. Martinez-Moreno NE, Sahgal A, De Salles A, et al. Stereotactic radiosurgery for tremor: systematic review. *J Neurosurg.* 2018;1–12. doi: 10.3171/2017.8.JNS17749

119. Harary M, Segar DJ, Hayes MT, Cosgrove GR. Unilateral thalamic deep brain stimulation versus focused ultrasound thalamotomy for essential tremor. *World Neurosurg.* 2019;126:e144–e152. doi: 10.1016/j.wneu.2019.01.281

120. Kim M, Jung NY, Park CK, Chang WS, Jung HH, Chang JW. Comparative evaluation of magnetic resonance-guided focused ultrasound surgery for essential tremor. *Stereotact Funct Neurosurg.* 2017;95:279–286. doi: 10.1159/000478866

121. Hariz MI. Surgical probings into the basal ganglia: hemorrhage and hardware-related risks, and costs of microelectrode recording. *Mov Disord.* 2011;26:1375–1377. doi: 10.1002/mds.23785

122. Pouratian N, Baltuch G, Elias WJ, Gross R. American Society for Stereotactic and Functional Neurosurgery position statement on magnetic resonance-guided focused ultrasound for the management of essential tremor. *Neurosurgery.* 2020;87:E126–E129. doi: 10.1093/neuros/nyz510

123. Sillay KA, Larson PS, Starr PA. Deep brain stimulator hardware-related infections: incidence and management in a large series. *Neurosurgery.* 2008;62:360–366; discussion 366-7. doi: 10.1227/01.neu.0000316002.03765.33

124. Niranjan A, Raju SS, Monaco EA, Flickinger JC, Lunsford LD. Is staged bilateral thalamic radiosurgery an option for otherwise surgically ineligible patients with medically refractory bilateral tremor? *J Neurosurg.* 2018;128:617–626. doi: 10.3171/2016.11.JNS162044

125. Monaco EA, III, Shin SS, Niranjan A, Lunsford LD. Radiosurgical thalamotomy. *Prog Neurol Surg.* 2018;33:135–148. doi: 10.1159/000481081

126. Prajakta G, Horisawa S, Kawamata T, Taira T. Feasibility of staged bilateral radiofrequency ventral intermediate nucleus thalamotomy for bilateral essential tremor. *World*

127. Alshaikh J, Fishman PS. Revisiting bilateral thalamotomy for tremor. *Clin Neurol Neurosurg.* 2017;158:103–107. doi: 10.1016/j.clineuro.2017.04.025

128. Huss DS, Dallapiazza RF, Shah BB, Harrison MB, Diamond J, Elias WJ. Functional assessment and quality of life in essential tremor with bilateral or unilateral DBS and focused ultrasound thalamotomy. *Mov Disord.* 2015;30:1937–1943. doi: 10.1002/mds.26455

129. Mitchell KT, Larson P, Starr PA, et al. Benefits and risks of unilateral and bilateral ventral intermediate nucleus deep brain stimulation for axial essential tremor symptoms. *Parkinsonism Relat Disord.* 2019;60:126–132. doi: 10.1016/j.parkreldis.2018.09.004

130. Hwynn N, Hass CJ, Zeilman P, et al. Steady or not following thalamic deep brain stimulation for essential tremor. *J Neurol.* 2011;258:1643–1648. doi: 10.1007/s00415-011-5986-0

131. Roemmich R, Roper JA, Eisinger RS, et al. Gait worsening and the microlesion effect following deep brain stimulation for essential tremor. *J Neurol Neurosurg Psychiatry.* 2019;90:913–919. doi: 10.1136/jnnp-2018-319723

132. Abosch A, Timmermann L, Bartley S, et al. An international survey of deep brain stimulation procedural steps. *Stereotact Funct Neurosurg.* 2013;91:1–11. doi: 10.1159/000343207

133. Kundu B, Schrock L, Davis T, House PA. Thalamic deep brain stimulation for essential tremor also reduces voice tremor. *Neuromodulation.* 2018;21:748–754. doi: 10.1111/ner.12739

134. Avecillas-Chasin JM, Poologaindran A, Morrison MD, Rammage LA, Honey CR. Unilateral thalamic deep brain stimulation for voice tremor. *Stereotact Funct Neurosurg.* 2018;96:392–399. doi: 10.1159/000495413

135. Sandstrom L, Blomstedt P, Karlsson F. Long-term effects of unilateral deep brain stimulation on voice tremor in patients with essential tremor. *Parkinsonism Relat Disord.* 2019;60:70–75. doi: 10.1016/j.parkreldis.2018.09.029

136. Barbe MT, Pochmann J, Lewis CJ, et al. Utilization of predefined stimulation groups by essential tremor patients treated with VIM-DBS. *Parkinsonism Relat Disord.* 2014;20:1415–1418. doi: 10.1016/j.parkreldis.2014.09.021

137. Seier M, Hiller A, Quinn J, Murchison C, Brodsky M, Anderson S. Alternating thalamic deep brain stimulation for essential tremor: a trial to reduce habituation. *Mov Disord Clin Pract.* 2018;5:620–626. doi: 10.1002/mdc3.12685

138. Paschen S, Forstenpointner J, Becktepe J, et al. Long-term efficacy of deep brain stimulation for essential tremor: an observer-blinded study.

Neurology. 2019;92:e1378–e1386. doi: 10.1212/WNL.0000000000007134

139. Fasano A, Helmich RC. Tremor habituation to deep brain stimulation: underlying mechanisms and solutions. *Mov Disord.* 2019;34:1761–1773. doi: 10.1002/mds.27821

140. Reich MM, Brumberg J, Pozzi NG, et al. Progressive gait ataxia following deep brain stimulation for essential tremor: adverse effect or lack of efficacy? *Brain.* 2016;139:2948–2956. doi: 10.1093/brain/aww223

141. Quinn NP, Schneider SA, Schwingenschuh P, Bhatia KP. Tremor-some controversial aspects. *Mov Disord.* 2011;26:18–23. doi: 10.1002/mds.23289

142. Kochanski RB, Bus S, Brahimaj B, et al. The impact of microelectrode recording on lead location in deep brain stimulation for the treatment of movement disorders. *World Neurosurg.* 2019;132:e487–e495. doi: 10.1016/j.wneu.2019.08.092

143. Kochanski RB, Sani S. Awake versus asleep deep brain stimulation surgery: technical considerations and critical review of the literature. *Brain Sci.* 2018;8. doi: 10.3390/brainsci8010017

144. Jacob RL, Geddes J, McCartney S, Burchiel KJ. Cost analysis of awake versus asleep deep brain stimulation: a single academic health center experience. *J Neurosurg.* 2016;124:1517–1523. doi: 10.3171/2015.5.JNS15433

145. Chen T, Mirzadeh Z, Chapple K, Lambert M, Dhall R, Ponce FA. "Asleep" deep brain stimulation for essential tremor. *J Neurosurg.* 2016;124:1842–1849. doi: 10.3171/2015.6.JNS15526

146. Ben-Haim S, Falowski SM. Evaluation of patient perspectives toward awake, frame-based deep-brain stimulation surgery. *World Neurosurg.* 2018;111:e601–e607. doi: 10.1016/j.wneu.2017.12.122

147. Rebelo P, Green AL, Aziz TZ, et al. Thalamic directional deep brain stimulation for tremor: spend less, get more. *Brain Stimul.* 2018;11:600–606. doi: 10.1016/j.brs.2017.12.015

148. Steffen JK, Reker P, Mennicken FK, et al. Bipolar directional deep brain stimulation in essential and Parkinsonian tremor. *Neuromodulation.* 2020;23:543–549. doi: 10.1111/ner.13109

149. Choe CU, Hidding U, Schaper M, et al. Thalamic short pulse stimulation diminishes adverse effects in essential tremor patients. *Neurology.* 2018;91:e704–e713. doi: 10.1212/WNL.0000000000006033

150. Kroneberg D, Ewert S, Meyer AC, Kuhn AA. Shorter pulse width reduces gait disturbances following deep brain stimulation for essential tremor. *J Neurol Neurosurg Psychiatry.* 2019;90:1046–1050. doi: 10.1136/jnnp-2018-319427

151. Groppa S, Herzog J, Falk D, Riedel C, Deuschl G, Volkmann J. Physiological and anatomical decomposition of subthalamic neurostimulation effects in essential tremor. *Brain.* 2014;137:109–121. doi: 10.1093/brain/awt304

152. Elble R, Bain P, Forjaz MJ, et al. Task force report: scales for screening and evaluating tremor: critique and recommendations. *Mov Disord.* 2013;28:1793–1800. doi: 10.1002/mds.25648

153. Haubenberger D, Abbruzzese G, Bain PG, et al. Transducer-based evaluation of tremor. *Mov Disord.* 2016;31:1327–1336. doi: 10.1002/mds.26671

154. Elble RJ, McNames J. Using portable transducers to measure tremor severity. *Tremor Other Hyperkinet Mov (N Y).* 2016;6:375. doi: 10.7916/D8DR2VCC

155. Daneault JF, Carignan B, Codere CE, Sadikot AF, Duval C. Using a smart phone as a stand-alone platform for detection and monitoring of pathological tremors. *Front Hum Neurosci.* 2012;6:357. doi: 10.3389/fnhum.2012.00357

156. Fahn S, Tolosa E, Marín C. Clinical rating scale for tremor. In: Jankovic J, Tolosa E, eds. *Parkinson's disease and movement disorders.* 2nd ed. Williams & Wilkins; 1993:225–234.

157. Elble RJ. Estimating change in tremor amplitude using clinical ratings: recommendations for clinical trials. *Tremor Other Hyperkinet Mov (N Y).* 2018;8:600. doi: 10.7916/D89C8F3C

158. Lopez-Blanco R, Velasco MA, Mendez-Guerrero A, et al. Essential tremor quantification based on the combined use of a smartphone and a smartwatch: the NetMD study. *J Neurosci Methods.* 2018;303:95–102. doi: 10.1016/j.jneumeth.2018.02.015

159. Haubenberger D, Kalowitz D, Nahab FB, et al. Validation of digital spiral analysis as outcome parameter for clinical trials in essential tremor. *Mov Disord.* 2011;26:2073–2080. doi: 10.1002/mds.23808

160. Elias WJ, Lipsman N, Ondo WG, et al. A randomized trial of focused ultrasound thalamotomy for essential tremor. *N Engl J Med.* 2016;375:730–739. doi: 10.1056/NEJMoa1600159

161. Fahn S, Tolosa E, Marin C. Clinical rating scale for tremor. In: Jankovic J, Tolosa E, eds. *Parkinson's Disease and Movement Disorders.* Urban & Schwarzenberg; 1988: 225–234.

162. Ondo W, Hashem V, LeWitt PA, et al. Comparison of the Fahn-Tolosa-Marin Clinical Rating Scale and the Essential Tremor Rating Assessment Scale. *Mov Disord Clin Pract.* 2018;5:60–65. doi: 10.1002/mdc3.12560

163. Vial F, McGurrin P, Osterholt T, Ehrlich D, Haubenberger D, Hallett M. Tremoroton, a new free online platform for tremor analysis. *Clin Neurophysiol Pract.* 2020;5:30–34. doi: 10.1016/j.cnp.2019.11.004

164. Elble RJ, Hellriegel H, Raethjen J, Deuschl G. Assessment of head tremor with accelerometers versus gyroscopic transducers. *Mov Disord Clin Pract.* 2017;4:205–211. doi: 10.1002/mdc3.12379

165. Gallego JA, Rocon E, Roa JO, Moreno JC, Pons JL. Real-time estimation of pathological tremor parameters from gyroscope data. *Sensors (Basel).* 2010;10:2129–2149. doi: 10.3390/s100302129

166. Pulliam CL, Eichenseer SR, Goetz CG, et al. Continuous in-home monitoring of essential tremor. *Parkinsonism Relat Disord.* 2014;20:37–40. doi: 10.1016/j.parkreldis.2013.09.009

167. Elble RJ, Ellenbogen A. Digitizing tablet and Fahn-Tolosa-Marin ratings of Archimedes spirals have comparable minimum detectable change in essential tremor. *Tremor Other Hyperkinet Mov (N Y).* 2017;7:481. doi: 10.7916/D89S20H7

168. Rahimi F, Debicki D, Roberts-South A, Bee C, Bapat P, Jog M. Dynamic decomposition of motion in essential and parkinsonian tremor. *Can J Neurol Sci.* 2015;42:116–124. doi: 10.1017/cjn.2015.12

169. Mostile G, Fekete R, Giuffrida JP, et al. Amplitude fluctuations in essential tremor. *Parkinsonism Relat Disord.* 2012;18:859–863. doi: 10.1016/j.parkreldis.2012.04.019

170. Elble RJ. Gravitational artifact in accelerometric measurements of tremor. *Clin Neurophysiol.* 2005;116:1638–1643. doi: 10.1016/j.clinph.2005.03.014

10

Voice Tremor

LAURA DE LIMA XAVIER AND KRISTINA SIMONYAN

INTRODUCTION

Voice tremor is characterized by involuntary oscillatory movements of muscles of the vocal tract, causing rhythmic modulations of the voice in pitch and loudness. Voice tremor may present as an isolated disorder; as a feature of other neurological disorders, including essential tremor, laryngeal dystonia, or Parkinson disease; or as a result of a physiological process.

Under various physiological conditions, a tremulous voice may manifest as a pattern of affective vocalization commonly associated with fear, sadness, wrath, or even joy. Remarkably, in its earliest referrals in the English literature, tremor was used to denote terror and was described as a shaking that happens "involuntarily as with fear or other emotion, cold, or weakness."[1] Those affected by pathological voice tremor not only suffered from difficulty speaking but were frequently mistaken to be emotional or weak. Unfortunately, these misperceptions about voice qualities tied to personality traits continue to persist to date, causing social embarrassment and anxiety for those with voice tremor, further exacerbating the condition and driving affected individuals into a vicious loop of social isolation and depression. Similarly, disorders that cause voice tremor have been misinterpreted as psychosomatic, a misconception that only increased the stigma surrounding affected individuals, while delaying investigations into the neurological underpinnings of voice tremor symptoms.

Although notable advances have been recently made in the medical and scientific understanding of voice tremor, ongoing challenges include diagnostic inconsistencies across clinical specialties and limited availability of therapeutic options. Pharmacological and neurosurgical treatments that are effective for alleviation of tremor affecting extremities often show worse results when used to treat voice tremor. The existing limitations to better treat voice tremor are due, in part, to the fact that the underlying etiopathophysiological mechanisms that generate tremor are not well understood.

This chapter aims to describe the most frequent presentations of voice tremor, their clinical features, and therapeutic options. Given the current lack of consensus between clinicians on the nomenclature or taxonomy of voice changes associated with tremor, we use "voice tremor" as an umbrella term for tremor-related terms used in the literature, including "vocal tremor,"[2] "tremulous voice," "laryngeal tremor," and "phonatory instability."[3,4] While different presentations of voice tremor can be clinically identified, recent brain imaging studies suggest that they are likely distinct manifestations of the spectrum of this disorder. Since the understanding of the voice tremor spectrum is still being developed, we also discuss the ongoing efforts and challenges in the classification of this disorder and the future diagnostic and therapeutic directions.

VOICE TREMOR AS A SYMPTOM OF ESSENTIAL TREMOR

Essential tremor (ET) is a movement disorder, whose clinical hallmark is a 4–12-Hz action tremor of the upper extremities (arms and hands). In 25–62% of patients, ET can spread to involve cranial structures, such as the larynx, soft palate, tongue, jaw, and neck, causing ET of voice (ETv) and/or head. In some, ETv may present as an isolated symptom without co-occurring tremor of extremities (Figure 10.1). The marked variability in ETv prevalence and presentations is likely due to the differences in patient cohorts studied, diagnostic methodologies applied, and the clinical expertise present across study centers.

It is worth noting that, although isolated voice tremor appears to be a focal presentation of ET based on its onset, progression, and clinical characteristics, there is still little consensus between clinicians regarding its classification.[5-7] On the one hand, the recent consensus paper of the Task Force on Tremor by the International Parkinson and Movement Disorder Society (IPMDS) excluded isolated voice and head tremors from ET classification,

- Isolated or in combination with ET of extremities
- Affects laryngeal and/or upper airway muscles
- Rhythmic tremor
- Rhythmic alterations in pitch and loudness
- No task specificity; present at passive respiration and other laryngeal/upper airway behaviors
- Common age of onset in 60s–80s
- Prevalent in females

Essential tremor of voice

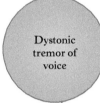

- Present only with laryngeal dystonia (~1/3 of patients)
- Affects only laryngeal muscles, together with laryngeal dystonia
- Irregular tremor
- Rhythmic alterations in pitch and loudness
- Task specific; not present at rest
- Common age of onset in 40s–50s
- Prevalent in females

Dystonic tremor of voice

FIGURE 10.1: Essential and Dystonic Voice Tremor Classification Based on Clinical Features Obtained through Medical History, Acoustic Perceptual Voice Evaluation, and Neurological and Laryngological Examinations.

restricting the latter diagnosis to at least tremor of upper extremities.[7] On the other hand, a report by the Neurolaryngology Committee of the American Academy of Otolaryngology—Head and Neck Surgery (AAO-HNS) defined isolated voice tremor as ET affecting the intrinsic muscles of the larynx and, variably, other muscles of the phonatory apparatus.[8] To reach common ground, a recent review paper strongly recommended to reconsider the inclusion of isolated voice tremor as a clinical variant of ET, highlighting that both isolated and ET-associated forms of voice tremor demonstrate the similar spread of disease through structures in the speech apparatus and share similar familial prevalence and female preponderance.[9] Supporting this recommendation, a recent brain imaging study in patients with voice tremor, both isolated and with ET affecting extremities, has identified only subtle differences in cortical thickness within parietal and temporal cortices, without any other differences in functional, white matter, or volumetric gray matter organization between the two cohorts.[10] Based on similarities of brain alterations in isolated voice tremor and ET, this study provided a pathophysiological justification for a re-classification of isolated voice tremor as a focal phenotype of ET.

Similar to ET affecting other body regions, the diagnosis of ETv, both isolated to the vocal tract and combined with tremor in the extremities, depends on a careful analysis of case history and neurological and otolaryngologic evaluations to rule out other tremor etiologies. The onset of ETv is more prevalent in females in their 60–80s,[2,6,11,12] with patients most often presenting with the intensity fluctuations associated with a perception of increased phonatory effort (Figure 10.1). Additionally, muscular discomfort and fatigue may also result from compensatory efforts to stabilize the vocal tract.

On clinical examination, voice tremor is best appreciated during phonation of prolonged vowels, such as /i/or/a/ at a normal pitch, and usually decreases at the high pitches.[13] ETv, both isolated and combined with ET affecting extremities, may become so severe that a stoppage of voice occurs, making it easily misdiagnosed as dystonic tremor of voice (DTv) present in laryngeal dystonia (LD). Differentiation between essential and dystonic tremor is reliant on the task specificity of laryngeal behavior to volitional speech tasks in DTv compared to non-volitional respiration (i.e., tidal breathing) in ETv. Therefore, voice tremor that does *not* have task specificity, occurring during both respiration and speech tasks, is characterized as ETv (Figure 10.1). This differentiation is best notable with stroboscopic examination of oscillation of the laryngeal musculature and oral articulators (e.g., pharyngeal constrictors, tongue, soft palate, jaw, and lips) during both speech tasks and passive respiration. Electromyography (EMG) may also help determine the anatomical source of tremor within the laryngeal and upper airway structures. The EMG recordings performed in experimental settings have shown that the intrinsic laryngeal muscles, specifically thyroarytenoid muscles, are the most frequently involved, with the frequency of about 5 to 7 Hz.[14] Other distinguishing factors in ETv compared to voice tremors in other neurological disorders include higher rates of a family history of tremor and alleviation of symptoms with alcohol intake, i.e., alcohol responsiveness.[2,15]

The current standard of care of voice tremor is the management of symptoms with onabotulinum toxin A injection (BoNT) into the overactive laryngeal or upper airway musculature.[16] Response to BoNT injections may vary significantly, depending on the affected structures by voice tremor. The isolated lateral variant, which involves intrinsic laryngeal (thyroarytenoid) muscles, receives greater benefits from BoNT treatment into adductor muscles compared to tremors originating from extralaryngeal sources. On average, a lower BoNT dose requirement and less pronounced effects are observed in ETv compared to DTv and LD.

Regarding the pharmaceutical treatment, there is some evidence that patients with ETv may exhibit similar improvement in voice symptomatology as those with ET of extremities.[17–21] Medications used to manage ETv typically include propranolol and primidone, although their effects are not as beneficial in voice tremor as in action tremors of extremities in ET or Parkinson disease.[22] Similarly, ETv has shown variable responsiveness to deep brain stimulation (DBS) of the ventral intermediate nucleus and caudal zona incerta of the thalamus, with better outcomes at bilateral stimulation.[23–25] Currently, DBS is reserved for ET patients with a treatment-refractory severe tremor of upper extremities who may or may not have associated ETv. Whether severe voice tremor can become itself an indication for DBS depends on future research studies to identify different tremorgenic brain networks and link these to specific anatomical end-target(s). Additionally, speech and language therapy (SLP) can equip patients with complementary strategies to improve voice loudness and speech intelligibility, although widely variable outcomes across patients should be considered.

VOICE TREMOR AS A SYMPTOM OF DYSTONIA

DTv is observed in about one-third of patients with LD. It is most commonly present in patients with adductor type of LD, where irregular contractions of the thyroarytenoid and lateral cricoarytenoid muscles produce strained and effortful voicing and voice breaks. Less commonly, it can be associated with the abductor type, where dystonic contractions of the posterior cricoarytenoid muscle lead to breathy voicing and voice breaks. DTv is characterized by irregular, isometric contractions of the affected laryngeal muscles during dystonic activity (Figure 10.1). Notably, it is characterized by task specificity, that is, DTv is present only with LD and selectively affects speech production, while being absent during respiration and other laryngeal or upper airway behaviors. Similar to LD, DTv may be responsive to sensory tricks, e.g., application of topical anesthesia.[9,26–28] Clinically, patients with DTv have similarities and differences with both LD without tremor and ETv. Patients with DTv show intermediate age and sex distributions between those with ETv and LD without tremor.[28–31] A family history of dystonia is rare in patients with and without a tremor, but higher than in the general population, with the variability from 1% to 16%.[31,32] A family history of tremor is, however, more common in LD patients with DTv compared to LD patients without tremor.[15,31] This difference is consistent with the fact that tremor conditions, both dystonic and essential, have a stronger underlying genetic predisposition, while purely dystonic disorders are more commonly sporadic than familial.

The pathophysiology of DTv is thought to broadly overlap with LD, while also sharing some similarities with ETv (Figure 10.2). Recent studies investigating alterations in brain structure and function in LD vs. DTv and ETv vs. DTv have proposed that these disorders may be characterized within the same pathophysiological spectrum, presenting both common and distinct patterns of neural alterations. Compared to healthy individuals, all patients have been shown to share the involvement of cortical brain regions controlling sensory and motor aspects of speech production. In addition, DTv and LD patients share functional and structural abnormalities in the sensorimotor cortex, basal ganglia, and thalamus, while being distinguished by greater cerebellar and middle frontal cortical changes in DTv. On the other hand, ETv and DTv show common changes in the primary sensorimotor cortex, superior and inferior parietal lobules, and inferior temporal gyrus, with distinct greater alterations of cortical vs. cerebellar changes in DTv vs. ETv.[10,33,34] It has been further determined that hyperexcitable parietal—> putaminal and right—> left interhemispheric premotor cortical information flow underlies the pathophysiological network alterations in both LD and DTv,

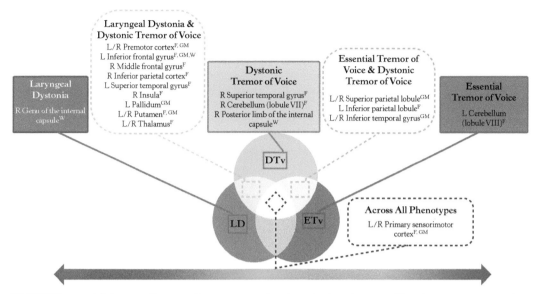

FIGURE 10.2: A Schematic Diagram Summarizing the Main Findings Retrieved from Neuroimaging Studies on Functional and Structural Abnormalities in Neurologic Disorders that Present with Voice Tremor.[10,33,34] Solid panels list abnormalities that are characteristic to laryngeal dystonia, dystonic tremor of voice, and essential tremor of voice tremor; panels with dashed lines and white background list regions where the alterations of brain function and structure are present across the spectrum of these disorders. Abbreviations: L = left; R = right; LD = laryngeal dystonia; DTv = dystonic tremor of voice; ETv = essential tremor of voice; F = functional alterations; GM = gray matter alterations; W = white matter alterations.

whereas decreased self-inhibitory influences of these brain regions contribute to differences between LD with and without DTv.[34]

Despite differences in the pathophysiology, the primary treatment of DTv is the same as for LD and ETv and consists of BoNT injections into the affected laryngeal muscles. BoNT injections yield an intermediate response in DTv, with better outcomes in LD without tremor, and worse in ETv.[15,35,36] In contrast, alcohol responsiveness is more common in ETv, followed by DTv and LD without tremor, which has been proposed to be associated with the varying degree of cerebellar involvement across these disorders.[17,37]

In alcohol-responsive patients with LD and DTv, sodium oxybate (Xyrem®) has recently shown efficacy in treating symptoms of both dystonia and tremor in an open-label study.[38,39] As a potentially novel oral therapeutic agent, sodium oxybate mimics the effects of alcohol and acts on the GABAergic neurotransmission, which is deficient in these patients. A brain imaging study in these patients has demonstrated that sodium oxybate significantly reduces hyperfunctional activity of cerebellar, thalamic, and primary/secondary sensorimotor cortical regions, with Xyrem-induced LD and DTv symptom improvement being

correlated with decreased to normal levels of cerebellar activity.[40] These studies outlined the first use of a pathophysiologically relevant, centrally acting medication; results are being confirmed in a double-blind, placebo-controlled clinical trial of LD and DTv, as well as ETv (NCT03292458). Clinical observations of the use of sodium oxybate in other forms of dystonia and ET.[6,41,42] point to a broader indication of this drug in these disorders, further tying in the pathophysiology of their different clinical phenotypes.

Other therapies available for LD with and without DTv include recurrent laryngeal nerve (RLN) section,[43] selective laryngeal adductor branch denervation and reinnervation,[44] and laryngoplasty.[45] However, these invasive and irreversible operations do not address disorder pathophysiology, offer only compensatory management of symptoms, and carry a higher risk of inconsistent outcomes.

VOICE TREMOR IN OTHER NEUROLOGICAL DISORDERS

Voice tremor can also be associated with other neurological disorders, such as Parkinson disease, multisystem atrophy, progressive supranuclear palsy, multiple sclerosis, or cerebellar diseases. As a comorbidity in these disorders, voice tremor is usually accompanied by other cranial nerve abnormalities, arises from sources other than the laryngeal musculature, cannot be managed well by BoNT injections, and often responds poorly to other treatment modalities.

In Parkinson disease (PD), voice dysfunction is one of the earliest signs of speech motor impairment. These symptoms affect as many as 89% of patients and may include hypokinetic dysarthria, stuttering, breathy or strained voice, and spastic dysarthria, along with voice tremor. It is unclear how many people with PD have clinically identified voice tremor; studies have shown a range from 13% to 68%.[46-48] Although voice tremor represents a functionally significant factor for patients with PD, little is known about the underlying anatomical sources and pathophysiological mechanisms. Voice tremor in PD can involve many structures of the voice apparatus, including the palate, but less often the vocal folds.[49] Available treatments of PD have also shown variable outcomes related to voice symptoms. For example, levodopa and DBS of the subthalamic nucleus (STN) can mildly improve or significantly impair speech production.[50-55] The effects of DBS specifically on voice tremor are even less well understood. In one study, STN-DBS ameliorated voice tremor and speech intensity but deteriorated overall speech intelligibility in most patients.[56]

Cerebellar lesions and disorders frequently affect voice and speech production and give rise to distinct articulatory and phonatory deficits, generally categorized as ataxic dysarthria.[57] Among these deficits, amplitude, and frequency of voice fluctuations during sustained vowel productions underlie voice tremor. The tremor rate in ataxic speakers is distinctively slower than in normal speakers and other voice tremor phenotypes, at a frequency of about 3 Hz.[3,58,59] As with DTv, it seems to preferentially affect volitional phonation.[60] While the cerebellum is known to be involved in speech motor control, the specific range of alterations affecting voice and speech production are less known. The cerebellum is functionally connected to various cortical and subcortical brain regions engaged in speech motor control, including movement preparation and motor execution processes.[57] Speech motor deficits have been described as predominantly bound to left-sided paravermal lesions (lobules VI and VII).[61] Why voice tremor affects only a subset of dysarthric ataxic patients and what therapies can be used to treat it warrant further research.

CONCLUSIONS

In summary, the most frequent clinical presentations of voice tremor fall within the broad pathophysiological spectrum of ET and LD. Current differential diagnosis of voice tremor is largely based on a syndromic approach, and its targeted treatment is lacking. Identification of specific clinical features and pathophysiological mechanisms underlying different clinical representations of voice tremor would not only explain its underpinning causes but also open new avenues for the objective differential diagnosis and selective treatment of affected individuals.

REFERENCES

1. Louis ED, Palmer CC. Tremble and tremor: etymology, usage patterns, and sound symbolism in the history of English. *Neurology*. 2017;88(7):706–710. doi: 10.1212/WNL.0000000000003576
2. Massey EW, Paulson GW. Essential vocal tremor: clinical characteristics and response to therapy. *South Med J*. 1985;78(3):316–317.
3. Boutsen F, Duffy JR, Dimassi H, Christman SS. Long-term phonatory instability in ataxic dysarthria. *Folia Phoniatr Logop*. 2011;63(4):216–220. doi: 10.1159/000319971
4. Gillivan-Murphy P, Miller N. Voice tremor: what we know and what we do not know. *Curr Opin Otolaryngol Head Neck Surg*. 2011;19(3):155–159. doi: 10.1097/MOO.0b013e328345970c
5. Albanese A, Del Sorbo F. Dystonia and tremor: the clinical syndromes with isolated tremor. *Tremor Other Hyperkinet Mov*. 2016;6:319. doi: 10.5334/tohm.315
6. Patel A, Frucht SJ. Isolated vocal tremor as a focal phenotype of essential tremor: a retrospective case review. *J Clin Mov Disord*. 2015;2(1):1–5. doi: 10.1186/s40734-015-0016-5
7. Bhatia KP, Bain P, Bajaj N, et al. Consensus statement on the classification of tremors. From the task force on tremor of the International Parkinson and Movement Disorder Society. *Mov Disord*. 2018;33(1):75–87. doi: 10.1002/mds.27121
8. Merati AL, Heman-Ackah YD, Abaza M, Altman KW, Sulica L, Belamowicz S. Common movement disorders affecting the larynx: a report from the neurolaryngology committee of the AAO-HNS. *Otolaryngol Head Neck Surg*. 2005;133(5):654–665. doi: 10.1016/j.otohns.2005.05.003
9. Barkmeier-Kraemer JM. Isolated voice tremor: a clinical variant of essential tremor or a distinct clinical phenotype? *Tremor Other Hyperkinet Mov*. 2020;10. doi: 10.7916/tohm.v0.738
10. de Lima Xavier L, Simonyan K. *Neural Representations of the Voice Tremor*; 2020 [in press].
11. Louis ED, Dure LS, Pullman S. Essential tremor in childhood: a series of nineteen cases.

Mov Disord. 2001;16(5):921–923. doi: 10.1002/mds.1182

12. Louis ED, Ferreira JJ. How common is the most common adult movement disorder? Update on the worldwide prevalence of essential tremor. *Mov Disord.* 2010;25(5):534–541. doi: 10.1002/mds.22838

13. Ludlow CL, Adler CH, Berke GS, et al. Research priorities in spasmodic dysphonia. *Otolaryngol Head Neck Surg.* 2008;139(4):495–505. doi: 10.1016/j.otohns.2008.05.624

14. Koda J, Ludlow CL. An evaluation of laryngeal muscle activation in patients with voice tremor. *Otolaryngol Head Neck Surg.* 1992;107(5):684–696. doi: 10.1177/019459989210700510

15. Sulica L, Louis ED. Clinical characteristics of essential voice tremor: a study of 34 cases. *Laryngoscope.* 2010;120(3):516–528. doi: 10.1002/lary.20702

16. Richards AL. Vocal tremor: where are we at? *Curr Opin Otolaryngol Head Neck Surg.* 2017;25(6):475–479. doi: 10.1097/MOO.0000000000000412

17. Guglielmino G, Moraes BT, Villanova LC, Padovani M, Biase NGD. Comparison of botulinum toxin and propranolol for essential and dystonic vocal tremors. *Clinics.* 2018;73:e87. doi: 10.6061/clinics/2018/e87

18. Justicz N, Hapner ER, Josephs JS, Boone BC, Jinnah HA, Johns MM, 3rd. Comparative effectiveness of propranolol and botulinum for the treatment of essential voice tremor. *Laryngoscope.* 2016;126(1):113–117. doi: 10.1002/lary.25485

19. Nida A, Alston J, Schweinfurth J. Primidone therapy for essential vocal tremor. *JAMA Otolaryngol Head Neck Surg.* 2016;142(2):117–121. doi: 10.1001/jamaoto.2015.2849

20. Busenbark K, Ramig L, Dromey C, Koller WC. Methazolamide for essential voice tremor. *Neurology.* 1996;47(5):1331–1332. doi: 10.1212/wnl.47.5.1331

21. Lowell SY, Kelley RT, Monahan M, Hosbach-Cannon CJ, Colton RH, Mihaila D. The effect of octanoic acid on essential voice tremor: a double-blind, placebo-controlled study. *Laryngoscope.* 2019;129(8):1882–1890. doi: 10.1002/lary.27695

22. Schneider SA, Deuschl G. The treatment of tremor. *Neurotherapeutics.* 2014;11(1):128–138. doi: 10.1007/s13311-013-0230-5

23. Ho AL, Choudhri O, Sung CK, DiRenzo EE, Halpern CH. Deep brain stimulation for essential vocal tremor: a technical report. *Cureus.* 2015;7(3):e256. doi: 10.7759/cureus.256

24. Ravikumar VK, Ho AL, Parker JJ, Erickson-DiRenzo E, Halpern CH. Vocal tremor: novel therapeutic target for deep brain stimulation. *Brain Sci.* 2016;6(4). doi: 10.3390/brainsci6040048

25. Sandström L, Blomstedt P, Karlsson F. Voice tremor response to deep brain stimulation in relation to electrode location in the posterior subthalamic area. *World Neurosurg X.* 2019;3:100024. doi: 10.1016/j.wnsx.2019.100024

26. Mor N, Simonyan K, Blitzer A. Central voice production and pathophysiology of spasmodic dysphonia. *Laryngoscope.* 2018;128(1):177–183. doi: 10.1002/lary.26655

27. Blitzer A, Brin MF, Simonyan K, Ozelius LJ, Frucht SJ. Phenomenology, genetics, and CNS network abnormalities in laryngeal dystonia: a 30-year experience. *Laryngoscope.* 2018;128 (Suppl 1):S1–S9. doi: 10.1002/lary.27003

28. Blitzer A, Brin MF, Stewart CF. Botulinum toxin management of spasmodic dysphonia (laryngeal dystonia): a 12-year experience in more than 900 patients. *Laryngoscope.* 2015;125(8):1751–1757. doi: 10.1002/lary.25273

29. Patel AB, Pollei TR, Bansberg SF, Adler CH, Lott DG, Crujido LR. The Mayo Clinic spasmodic dysphonia experience: a demographic analysis of 686 patients. *Otolaryngol Head Neck Surg.* 2014;151(1_suppl):P73–P73. doi: 10.1177/0194599814541627a138

30. Tisch SHD, Brake HM, Law M, Cole IE, Darveniza P. Spasmodic dysphonia: clinical features and effects of botulinum toxin therapy in 169 patients—an Australian experience. *J Clin Neurosci.* 2003;10(4):434–438. doi: 10.1016/s0967-5868(03)00020-1

31. Patel PN, Kabagambe EK, Starkweather JC, et al. Defining differences in patient characteristics between spasmodic dysphonia and laryngeal tremor. *Laryngoscope.* 2019;129(1):170–176. doi: 10.1002/lary.27245

32. Schweinfurth JM, Billante M, Courey MS. Risk factors and demographics in patients with spasmodic dysphonia. *Laryngoscope.* 2002;112(2):220–223. doi: 10.1097/00005537-200202000-00004

33. Kirke DN, Battistella G, Kumar V, et al. Neural correlates of dystonic tremor: a multimodal study of voice tremor in spasmodic dysphonia. *Brain Imaging Behav.* 2017;11(1):166–175. doi: 10.1007/s11682-016-9513-x

34. Battistella G, Simonyan K. Top-down alteration of functional connectivity within the sensorimotor network in focal dystonia. *Neurology.* 2019;92(16):e1843–e1851. doi: 10.1212/WNL.0000000000007317

35. Brin MF, Blitzer A, Stewart C. Laryngeal dystonia (spasmodic dysphonia): observations of 901 patients and treatment with botulinum toxin. *Adv Neurol.* 1998;78:237–252.

36. Gurey LE, Sinclair CF, Blitzer A. A new paradigm for the management of essential vocal tremor with botulinum toxin. *Laryngoscope.* 2013;123(10):2497–2501. doi: 10.1002/lary.24073

37. Kirke DN, Frucht SJ, Simonyan K. Alcohol responsiveness in laryngeal dystonia: a survey study. *J Neurol.* 2015;262(6):1548–1556. doi: 10.1007/s00415-015-7751-2

38. Rumbach AF, Blitzer A, Frucht SJ, Simonyan K. An open-label study of sodium oxybate in sSpasmodic dysphonia. *Laryngoscope.* 2017;127(6):1402–1407. doi: 10.1002/lary.26381

39. Simonyan K, Frucht SJ. Long-term effect of sodium oxybate (xyrem(r)) in spasmodic dysphonia with vocal tremor. *Tremor Other Hyperkinet Mov (N Y).* 2013;3. eCollection 2013.

40. Simonyan K, Frucht SJ, Blitzer A, Sichani AH, Rumbach AF. A novel therapeutic agent, sodium oxybate, improves dystonic symptoms via reduced network-wide activity. *Sci Rep.* 2018;8(1):16111. doi: 10.1038/s41598-018-34553-x

41. Frucht SJ, Houghton WC, Bordelon Y, Greene PE, Louis ED. A single-blind, open-label trial of sodium oxybate for myoclonus and essential tremor. *Neurology.* 2005;65(12):1967–1969.

42. Frucht SJ, Bordelon Y, Houghton WH, Reardan D. A pilot tolerability and efficacy trial of sodium oxybate in ethanol-responsive movement disorders. *Mov Disord.* 2005;20(10):1330–1337. doi: 10.1002/mds.20605

43. Dedo HH, Behlau MS. Recurrent laryngeal nerve section for spastic dysphonia: 5- to 14-year preliminary results in the first 300 patients. *Ann Otol Rhinol Laryngol.* 1991;100(4 Pt 1):274–279. doi: 10.1177/000348949110000403

44. Berke GS, Verneil A, Blackwell KE, Jackson KS, Gerratt BR, Sercarz JA. Selective laryngeal adductor denervationreinnervation: a new surgical treatment for adductor spasmodic dysphonia. *Ann Otol Rhinol Laryngol.* 1999;108(3):227–231. doi: 10.1177/000348949910800302

45. Isshiki N, Haji T, Yamamoto Y, Mahieu HF. Thyroplasty for adductor spasmodic dysphonia: further experiences. *Laryngoscope.* 2001;111(4 Pt 1):615–621. doi: 10.1097/00005537-200104000-00011

46. Perez KS, Ramig LO, Smith ME, Dromey C. The Parkinson larynx: tremor and videostroboscopic findings. *J Voice.* 1996;10(4):354–361. doi: 10.1016/s0892-1997(96)80027-0

47. Logemann JA, Fisher HB, Boshes B, Blonsky ER. Frequency and cooccurrence of vocal tract dysfunctions in the speech of a large sample of Parkinson patients. *J Speech Hear Disord.* 1978;43(1):47–57. doi: 10.1044/jshd.4301.47

48. Chenery HJ, Murdoch BE, Ingram JCL. Studies in Parkinson's disease: i. perceptual speech analyses. *Aust J Hum Commun Disord.* 1988;16(2):17–29. doi: 10.3109/asl2.1988.16.issue-2.02

49. Gillivan-Murphy P, Carding P, Miller N. Vocal tract characteristics in Parkinson's disease. *Curr Opin Otolaryngol Head Neck Surg.* 2016;24(3):175–182. doi: 10.1097/MOO.0000000000000252

50. D'Alatri L, Paludetti G, Contarino MF, Galla S, Marchese MR, Bentivoglio AR. Effects of bilateral subthalamic nucleus stimulation and medication on parkinsonian speech impairment. *J Voice.* 2008;22(3):365–372. doi: 10.1016/j.jvoice.2006.10.010

51. Tripoliti E, Zrinzo L, Martinez-Torres I, et al. Effects of subthalamic stimulation on speech of consecutive patients with Parkinson disease. *Neurology.* 2011;76(1):80–86. doi: 10.1212/WNL.0b013e318203e7d0

52. Tripoliti E, Limousin P, Foltynie T, et al. Predictive factors of speech intelligibility following subthalamic nucleus stimulation in consecutive patients with Parkinson's disease. *Mov Disord.* 2014;29(4):532–538. doi: 10.1002/mds.25816

53. Tsuboi T, Watanabe H, Tanaka Y, et al. Characteristic laryngoscopic findings in Parkinson's disease patients after subthalamic nucleus deep brain stimulation and its correlation with voice disorder. *J Neural Transm.* 2015;122(12):1663–1672. doi: 10.1007/s00702-015-1436-y

54. Sauvageau VM, Roy J-P, Cantin L, Prud'Homme M, Langlois M, Macoir J. Articulatory changes in vowel production following STN DBS and levodopa intake in Parkinson's disease. *Parkinson's Dis.* 2015;2015:1–7. doi: 10.1155/2015/382320

55. Tsuboi T, Watanabe H, Tanaka Y, et al. Early detection of speech and voice disorders in Parkinson's disease patients treated with subthalamic nucleus deep brain stimulation: a 1-year follow-up study. *J Neural Transm.* 2017;124(12):1547–1556. doi: 10.1007/s00702-017-1804-x

56. Tsuboi T, Watanabe H, Tanaka Y, et al. Distinct phenotypes of speech and voice disorders in Parkinson's disease after subthalamic nucleus deep brain stimulation. *J Neurol Neurosurg Psychiatry.* 2015;86(8):856–864. doi: 10.1136/jnnp-2014-308043

57. Ackermann H, Mathiak K, Riecker A. The contribution of the cerebellum to speech production and speech perception: clinical and functional imaging data. *Cerebellum.* 2007;6(3):202–213. doi: 10.1080/14734220701266742

58. Ackermann H, Ziegler W. Acoustic analysis of vocal instability in cerebellar dysfunctions. *Ann Otol Rhinol Laryngol.* 1994;103(2):98–104. doi: 10.1177/000348949410300203

59. Kent RD, Kent JF, Duffy JR, Thomas JE, Weismer G, Stuntebeck S. Ataxic dysarthria. *J Speech Lang Hear Res.* 2000;43(5):1275–1289. doi: 10.1044/jslhr.4305.1275

60. Ackermann H, Ziegler W. Cerebellar voice tremor: an acoustic analysis. *J Neurol Neurosurg Psychiatry.* 1991;54(1):74–76. doi: 10.1136/jnnp.54.1.74

61. Lechtenberg R, Gilman S. Speech disorders in cerebellar disease. *Ann Neurol.* 1978;3(4):285–290. doi: 10.1002/ana.410030402

11

Tremor, Dystonia, and Dystonic Tremor

H. A. JINNAH AND AASEF G. SHAIKH

INTRODUCTION

Tremor is defined as a disorder of rhythmical oscillations of a body region.[1-4] The term *rhythmical* implies a regular tempo, so *regularity* is sometimes also included in definitions for tremor. There are many different types of tremor, with the most common prototypical examples being the action-induced oscillations of both upper limbs in essential tremor (ET) or the unilateral resting hand oscillations of Parkinson disease (PD). These more common types of tremor tend to have a roughly similar speed in both directions of oscillation, so the term *sinusoidal* is frequently included in definitions of tremor as well. The term *tremor* is used to describe both a clinical sign in disorders such as PD, or a specific diagnosis such as ET.

Dystonia is defined as a disorder of involuntary sustained or intermittent muscular contractions.[5-7] Sustained contractions often cause abnormal postures, while intermittent contractions typically cause repetitive movements. Whether sustained or intermittent, the abnormal movements tend to follow a recurring pattern. Occasionally, repetitive and patterned movements are the dominant problem, without obvious abnormal posturing, and the abnormal movements of dystonia have an appearance similar to more common types of tremor. Like the term *tremor*, the term *dystonia* can be used to describe a clinical sign or a specific diagnosis.

Although tremor and dystonia are clinically defined as distinct movement disorders, there are multiple areas of overlap. Distinctions between these two movement disorders are important, because they have different etiologies to address in the workup, and different treatment strategies. However, there are no widely available laboratory tests that can lead to a definitive diagnosis of dystonia or tremor. Electromyography (EMG) can help to discriminate them in some cases, but findings are not always diagnostic and some physiological features overlap. Even genes considered

as causes for dystonia may produce a clinical syndrome that appears clinically indistinguishable from ET. The nature and causes of these many overlapping features remain to be determined.

COHORT STUDIES LINKING DYSTONIA AND TREMOR

Many cohort studies for individuals diagnosed with dystonia have described a high prevalence of tremor.[8] Depending on the cohort, the prevalence of tremor varies from 10–90% (Table 11.1).[9-27] The wide variation in these reports is likely to arise from multiple factors, such as the types of dystonia included in the cohort, whether data were collected prospectively or from review of medical records or clinical databases, how dystonia and tremor were defined and ascertained, and the interests and expertise of the investigators doing the study. For example, studies focusing predominantly on cohorts with cervical dystonia or hand dystonia typically described a much higher frequency of tremor than cohorts focusing on blepharospasm or laryngeal dystonia (Table 11.1). Most tremors are postural or kinetic, although smaller numbers of individuals with dystonia may also have a rest tremor.[28] In a large multi-center study of 2362 subjects with all types of isolated dystonia, the overall frequency of tremor was 53%.[29] This frequency varied according to several variables. These included the body regions affected by dystonia, the severity and duration of dystonia, the age of the subject, and the recruitment site (Figure 11.1). The impact of recruitment site was thought to reflect variations in diagnostic habits of individual investigators, not an effect of geographical location. Sex and race did not have a significant impact on the frequency of tremor.

By the same token, several cohort studies of patients diagnosed with ET have described a high prevalence of dystonia. Depending on the cohort, the frequency of dystonia has been reported to

TABLE 11.1: REPORTS OF TREMOR AMONG SUBJECTS DIAGNOSED WITH DYSTONIA

Study	Main types of dystonia	Total cases	Percent with tremor
Jankovic et al., 1983[9]	BL* (± OMD, CD and/or LD)	100	31.0
Chan et al., 1991[10]	CD (± SD)	266	27.9
Jankovic et al., 1991[11]	CD (± BL, OMD, LD and/or HD)	300	71.3
Dubinsky et al., 1993[12]	Mixed FD, SD, MD	296	10.8
Deuschl et al., 1997[13]	CD	55	60.0
Pal et al., 2000[14]	CD	114	68.4
Schweinfurth et al., 2002[15]	LD (±HD)	168	26.2
Tisch et al., 2003[16]	LD	169	13.1
Godeiro-Junior, 2008[17]	CD*	118	42.4
White et al., 2011[18]	LD	146	32.0
Defazio et al., 2013[19]	Mixed FD, SD, MD	429	16.7
Rudzinska et al., 2013[20]	Mixed FD, SD, MD	123	48.8
Erro et al., 2013[21]	Mixed FD, SD, MD	473	55.4
Jhunjhunwala et al., 2015[22]	HD	125	28.8
Gigante et al., 2016[23]	Mixed FD, SD, MD	173	34.0
LeDoux et al., 2016[24]	CD	1000	62.0
Williams et al., 2016[25]	Mixed FD, SD	375	16.8–23.8
Pandey et al., 2017[26]	Mixed FD	90	45.6
Hvizdosova et al., 2020[27]	CD	120	58.3

This table summarizes the prevalence of tremors for patients diagnosed with dystonia from reports published after 1980 that included at least 50 cases. The vast majority of reported cases were idiopathic adult-onset focal dystonias, sometimes with segmental or multifocal patterns. A minority of cases (noted by asterisks) included cases caused by medications, trauma, birth injury or psychogenic causes. Abbreviations: BL = blepharospasm; CD = cervical dystonia; FD = focal dystonia; HD = hand dystonia; LD = laryngeal dystonia; MD = multifocal dystonia; OMD = oromandibular dystonia; SD = segmental dystonia. The overall weighted average of 35.1% is likely to reflect an under-estimate, because some reports reported tremor only in selected body regions such as the head or hands.

vary from 0–47% (Table 11.2).[30–37] The variations among these studies reflect some of the same factors described for dystonia cohorts, and especially differences in operational definitions for ET. When the diagnostic entity of ET was first conceived, it was considered a diagnosis for individuals with tremor only. In keeping with this concept, some investigators excluded any cases with co-existing dystonia, and none of their subjects had dystonia. However, many investigators later used the diagnosis of ET more loosely to describe any tremor with clinical characteristics resembling other cases of ET, even if they had mild dystonia. As a result, the different criteria used to define ET historically led to heterogeneous cohorts, sometimes with mild dystonia, although severe dystonia was often excluded. As a result, the overall prevalence of dystonia in some cohorts diagnosed with ET is not zero, but tends to be lower than the prevalence reported in dystonia cohorts.

In summary, cohort studies reveal that tremor and dystonia co-occur far more frequently than predicted by chance. Overall, about half of all dystonia subjects have tremor, but this figure depends on the type of dystonia, as well as its severity and duration. Studies that included ET subjects with mild dystonic posturing, now sometimes referred to as ET-plus,[1] also reveal a high prevalence of dystonia in subjects with ET.

DYSTONIC TREMOR, TREMOR-DOMINANT DYSTONIA, AND TREMULOUS DYSTONIA

Dystonic movements occasionally have a tremor-like appearance because they can be oscillatory, appear rhythmic, and repetitive. These tremor-like movements were first given the term *dystonic tremor* by Fahn.[38] Two main features were thought to discriminate dystonic tremors from other more common tremors (Table 11.3). First, dystonic tremors were thought to be irregular, in contrast to the relatively regular movements of more common tremors. This irregularity could be seen in both the frequency and shape. Second, dystonic tremors had a jerky quality, in contrast to the more sinusoidal quality of more common tremors. This jerkiness resulted from a rapid movement in one direction followed by a slower movement in the opposite direction. Another feature typical of dystonic tremors was a *geste antagoniste* to suppress

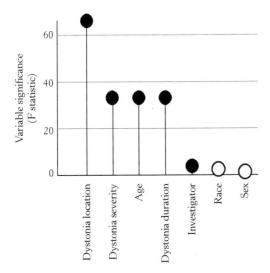

FIGURE 11.1: Factors Related to Occurrence of Tremor among Patients with Dystonia. Tremor was evaluated in 2,362 subjects with different types of isolated dystonia, and evaluated by logistic regression. Variables significantly associated with tremor (in order of impact) included location of body affected by dystonia, severity of dystonia, subject age at evaluation, duration of dystonia, and recruiting investigator. The impact of each parameter is estimated by the length of the line. Variables that had a statistically significant impact on the regression model are shown as solid circles, while those that were not significant (race and sex) are shown as open circles.

the tremor. Finally, dystonic tremors typically had a *null point* where abnormal movements abated or disappeared. Occasionally, an irregular and jerky tremor could be the dominant or even only manifestation of dystonia, so the presence of overt twisting movements or postures was not

viewed as a requirement for dystonic tremor. In the latter case, the term *tremor-dominant dystonia* was applied.[38]

The original definition for dystonic tremor had some limitations, because of the subjective nature of its criteria (Table 11.3). Oscillations that are grossly irregular and jerky are easy to observe at the bedside. However, more subtle abnormalities of regularity or jerkiness may be more difficult to ascertain clinically, and may require more objective measures. The geste antagoniste and null point were not always present, and sometimes had only partial effects that were difficult to interpret. Because of these limitations, Fahn's original definition for dystonic tremor was altered by an expert committee of the Movement Disorders Society (MDS) in 1998,[39] and further revised in 2018.[1] Both committees recognized that dystonic tremors were typically irregular and jerky, and might have a geste antagoniste and null point. However, these features were considered unreliable because of their subjective nature. Instead, dystonic tremor was redefined as any tremor that occurred in a body region that simultaneously demonstrated more obvious dystonia (Table 11.3). These committees also described a new entity, *tremor associated with dystonia* (TAD), to account for situations where dystonia might occur in one body region with tremor in another body region.

The revised definition from the MDS expert committee has not been universally adopted for several reasons. First, the co-existence of dystonic movements often is subjective.[40] Overt dystonia is easy to identify, but mild dystonia can be difficult to discriminate from normal motor behavior or compensatory behaviors to a disability. Second, the revised definition conflicts with the concept of tremor-dominant dystonia, where an irregular and

TABLE 11.2: REPORTS OF DYSTONIA AMONG SUBJECTS DIAGNOSED WITH TREMOR

Study	Type of tremor	Type of study	Total cases	Percent with dystonia
Lou & Jankovic, 1991[30]	Essential tremor	Database review	350	47.1
Koller et al.,[31]	Essential tremor	Database review	678	6.9
Jankovic et al., 1997[32]	Essential tremor	Database review	251	15.0
Shatunov et al., 2006[33]	Essential tremor	Database review	325	4.6
Hedera et al., 2010[34]	Essential tremor	Prospective	463	21.1
Rana et al., 2012[35]	Essential tremor	Chart review	274	0
Louis et al., 2013[36]	Essential tremor	Prospective	100	15.0
Lenka et al., 2015[37]	Essential tremor	Chart review	234	13.7

This table summarizes the prevalence of dystonia for patients diagnosed with tremor from reports published after 1980 that included at least 50 cases. The vast majority of reported cases were diagnosed with "essential tremor" although the operational definitions differed among the reports. The numbers are likely to reflect an under-estimate, because some studies reported only specific types of dystonia in their tremor cohorts, while others did not specify which subtypes of dystonia were evaluated.

TABLE 11.3: TWO COMMONLY USED DEFINITIONS FOR DYSTONIC TREMOR

Criterion	Fahn definition[38]	MDS task force definition[1]
Major features		
Jerkiness	yes	no
Irregularity	yes	no
Coincides with dystonia	no	yes
Supportive features		
Geste antagoniste	yes	yes
Null point	yes	yes
Weaknesses		
Too subjective to be reliable	Jerkiness and irregularity	Coincidence with mild dystonia
Eliminates tremor-dominant dystonia	no	yes
Merges overlapping tremors	no	yes

jerky tremor cannot be diagnosed as a dystonic tremor, because of the lack of overt signs of dystonia. Third, the revised definition assumes that any type of tremor in a dystonic body part should be considered a dystonic tremor. This assumption obscures the possibility of a coincidental tremor of another type, such as the tremor of PD or ET.

As a result of the uncertainty regarding the nature and definition of oscillatory movements in dystonia, some experts have continued to use the original definition described by Fahn, which emphasizes irregular and jerky qualities, even without co-existing dystonia.[4,37,41,42] Others have adopted the revised definition, which emphasizes any type of tremor that occurs co-existing with dystonia, even without irregular or jerky qualities.[42,43] Others have used alternative terminology, such as *tremulous dystonia*.[44,45] These ongoing debates have led to calls for a re-evaluation of concepts for dystonic tremor.[8,46–57]

TASK-SPECIFIC OSCILLATIONS: TREMOR, DYSTONIA, BOTH, OR NEITHER?

The oscillations of ET usually occur during various actions, for example holding sustained postures or performing various motor tasks. In some cases, oscillations emerge exclusively during the performance of one task. The most common task-specific oscillations occur with writing (primary writing tremor, PWT), although in some individuals, other tasks may trigger tremor. There has been a long debate regarding whether these task-specific oscillations should be considered a subtype of ET, a subtype of dystonia, or a distinct nosological entity.[58,59]

A summary of some of the most instructive studies of PWT is provided in Table 11.4.[60–65] Several studies have pointed out that subjects with PWT often share clinical features with ET, such as the typical regular and sinusoidal movement pattern of ET at 4–7Hz, good responses to alcohol or ET medications such as primidone or propranolol, or strong family history of ET.[60,63,66,67] For adult-onset focal dystonias, a positive family history of dystonia is uncommon (10–15%), benefits from alcohol are much less obvious,[68] and clinical responses to propranolol or primidone are not common. Other studies have described features more consistent with dystonia, such as jerky movement patterns with irregular tempo more typical of dystonia, subtle concurrent signs of dystonia such as spooning of the hand or mirror movements, dystonic co-activation of antagonistic muscles on EMG, or response to anti-dystonic medications such as anticholinergics or botulinum toxins.[62,63,67,69,70] Some investigators have favored the concept that PWT is a distinct nosological entity, because physiological or functional imaging features are different from both ET and dystonia.[65,66,71–73]

Authors of individual studies tend to favor placing PWT into a single nosological category. However, the larger studies provided hints for heterogeneity in PWT.[63,66,67] In these studies, some individuals had clinical features more typical of ET while other individuals had features of dystonia. In one study, EMG and accelerometry revealed 2 distinct types of oscillations, but some cases had both combined.[67] These observations raise concern that small studies may reach incorrect conclusions due to a sampling bias. Conclusions that task-specific tremors are a nosological entity distinct from ET or dystonia must

TABLE 11.4: REPORTS OF TASK-SPECIFIC PRIMARY WRITING TREMOR

Citation	Study description	Subjects with PWT	Findings
Kachi et al., 1985[60]	Clinical study of PWT	9	Many cases had features resembling ET including rhythmical and sinusoidal oscillations, and response to ET medications
Cohen et al., 1987[61]	Clinical study of one family	1	1 member had PWT, 2 members had ET, 2 had dystonic writer's cramp, and 1 had ET-plus writer's cramp
Rosenbaum et al., 1988[63]	Clinical study of PWT, with or without dystonia	10	Some cases had features of ET, while others had features of dystonia, a heterogeneous group with overlapping clinical features
Elble et al., 1990[67]	EMG and accelerometry study of PWT	5	Some cases had features of ET, some had features of dystonia, and some had both suggesting two distinct but overlapping disorders in some cases
Jedynak et al., 1991[69]	EMG study of PWT	5	Irregular EMG discharges were suggestive of dystonia, not ET
Bain et al., 1995[66]	Clinical, EMG, and accelerometry study of PWT	21	Some features did not resemble ET or dystonia, suggesting a distinct nosological entity
Soland et al., 1996[62]	Clinical study of PWT	9	3 cases had subtle clinical features of dystonia
Berg et al., 2000[71]	Functional MRI study of PWT vs. normal controls	3	Brain regions activated were not typical for either ET or writer's cramp
Modugno et al., 2002[72]	Physiological study of PWT vs. normal controls	7	Unlike writer's cramp, reciprocal inhibition and cortical excitability were normal
Ljubisavljevic et al., 2006[73]	Physiology of PWT vs. normal controls	6	Multiple measures from EMG and TMS were distinct from writer's cramp or ET
Papapetropoulos and Singer 2006[70]	Treatment study of PWT	5	3 of 5 subjects had mirror dystonia, and 4 responded to botulinum toxin
Meunier et al., 2011[65]	Treatment study of PWT	9	Unlike writer's cramp, transcutaneous electrical nerve stimulation worsened PWT
Hirschbickler et al., 2015[64]	Clinical study of one family	1	1 member had PWT, 1 had writer's cramp, another had dystonic tremor that was not task-specific

This table summarizes studies of PWT that included more than one case, or where an individual case was particularly instructive. Additional case reports are summarized in several reviews.[58,59]
PWT = primary writing tremor, ET = essential tremor, TMS = transcranial magnetic stimulation

also be considered in light of potential etiological heterogeneity. These conclusions are often based on physiological findings such as measures of spinal or brain inhibition which are abnormal in dystonia but not ET. It is important to note that the absolute magnitude of differences using these measures is often small, while individual variability is large. Potential etiological heterogeneity can therefore have a significant impact on group

comparisons that rely on averaging individuals together.

Family studies have also been instructive. In one family, 2 members had ET, 2 had dystonic writer's cramp, 1 had PWT, and 1 had ET with writer's cramp.[61] In another family, 1 had PWT, 1 had writer's cramp, another had a mixed postural/resting tremor of one upper limb with no task specificity.[64] These families imply an inherited predisposition

ET, PWT, writer's cramp, or dystonic tremor that is not task-specific. A woman with PWT of the dominant hand was reported to developed writer's cramp when she switched to the non-dominant hand.[74] This report also suggests two different manifestations of one underlying biological predisposition, in one individual. In a genome-wide association study for tremor, one of three candidate loci was identified in two families with ET with dystonia, but not in families with ET alone.[33]

These observations demonstrate that task-specific tremors have clinical features that overlap with ET or dystonia, making them difficult to discriminate clinically. They also point out the limitations of clinical ascertainment, particularly for individuals with subtle postural abnormalities, which may reflect mild dystonia, a normal variant, or even a behavioral compensation. Most importantly, they imply that oscillations with features of ET or dystonia may be combined, even in the same individual. Altogether, these observations imply that task-specific tremors such as isolated writer's tremor are not a homogenous group. They may sometimes reflect tremor syndromes such as ET, may other times reflect dystonia, and may occasionally reflect tremor and dystonia combined in the same individual.

ISOLATED TREMORS WITHOUT TREMOR OF THE UPPER LIMBS

Typical ET. According to the 2018 consensus group definition of different types of tremors, the diagnosis of ET requires involvement of the upper limbs.[1] In ET with involvement of the upper limbs, other regions may also be involved, most commonly the head or the voice. In earlier studies that used broader definitions of ET, the limbs were most commonly affected but rare cases considered to be ET had isolated tremors of the head or voice.[2,30,31,75–78] Under the 2018 consensus guidelines, the diagnostic nosology isolated tremors without involvement of the upper limbs has become uncertain.[49,50] Some evidence suggests these tremors should be considered among the tremor disorders, while other evidence suggests they should be considered as tremor-dominant dystonia.

Isolated head tremors (IHT). Isolated tremors affecting the head (without simultaneous upper limb involvement) have been described in the literature as *isolated head tremor, essential head tremor, essential tremor of the head,* or merely *head tremor.* The literature on IHT is difficult to interpret for several reasons. First, many studies of "prominent" head tremor or head tremor as a "presenting" feature do not describe assessment procedures for hand tremor or subtle signs of dystonia. This limitation makes it difficult to know if head tremor was truly isolated. Second, many studies included very small numbers of subjects, so a sampling bias could obscure identification of clinical heterogeneity. Finally, some investigators with firm beliefs that IHT is a type of dystonia automatically exclude them from studies of ET, producing a bias against the identification of cases.

A summary of some of the most instructive studies of IHT is shown in Table 11.5.[14,45,55,69,79–83] Some studies of IHT imply that is a subtype of ET, while others imply it is a subtype of dystonia. Evidence in favor of IHT as subtype of ET includes the regular and sinusoidal movement pattern of the head, response to anti-tremor medications, and family history of ET. It is important to emphasize that these observations apply only to some cases of IHT, and not all cases. The observation that severe tremor of the head may overshadow less prominent tremor of the upper limb[82] combined with evidence that laboratory methods are more sensitive than the clinical exam,[84] makes it feasible that some ET cases may present clinically with apparent IHT when careful evaluation to rule out mild hand tremor has not been conducted.

Evidence in favor of IHT being a subtype of dystonia includes studies that show that IHT precedes cervical dystonia in some cases,[10,11,14,19,37,69,85] sensory tricks characteristic of dystonia reduce tremor amplitude in IHT but not ET,[45] and temporal discrimination is abnormal in IHT and dystonia, but not ET.[83] For studies of sensory tricks and temporal discrimination, it is important to note that the magnitude of differences among groups is often small, with significant overlap between groups, obscuring potential subgroup heterogeneity and leading to potential over-generalizations.

Overall, it seems likely that clinically ascertained cases of IHT are a heterogeneous group. Some cases may reflect ET with severe head tremor but clinically inapparent upper limb tremor, or head tremor emerging before upper limb tremors emerge. Other cases may reflect tremor-dominant cervical dystonia, before more overt posturing movements of the head becomes obvious. Long-term studies of the evolution of a large number of cases, along with objective measures such as EMG or motion sensors are needed.

Isolated vocal tremors (IVT). Isolated tremors affecting the voice (without simultaneous upper limb involvement) have been described in the literature using several terms including *isolated voice tremor, isolated vocal tremor, primary*

TABLE 11.5: REPORTS OF ISOLATED HEAD TREMOR

Citation	Study description	Subjects with IHT	Conclusions/caveats
Rivest & Marsden 1990[79]	Clinical study of 12 subjects with severe head/trunk tremors	5	IHT may be a subtype of dystonia, because many subjects with IHT later developed more obvious dystonia
Jedynak et al., 1991[69]	EMG study of 45 subjects with idiopathic dystonia or tremor	3	Tremor and dystonia frequently overlap
Valls-Sole et al., 1997[80]	EMG study of 30 subjects with prominent head tremor	3	IHT may be a subtype of ET
Louis et al., 2000[81]	Clinical study of 115 subjects with ET	2	ET is not a homogenous population
Masuhr et al., 2000[45]	EMG/accelerometry study of 60 subjects with prominent head tremor	3	Authors defined 3 groups: tremulous CD, dystonic head tremor, and essential head tremor. Sensory trick reduces tremor in dystonia but not ET
Pal et al., 2000[14]	Clinical study of 114 subjects with CD	8	Dystonia and tremor are related
Louis & Dogu, 2009[82]	Clinical study of 583 subjects with ET	0	IHT is a rare or non-existent subtype of ET, although 2.7% had prominent head tremor with mild hand tremor
Conte et al., 2015[83]	Temporal discrimination study of 61 subjects with tremor or dystonia	8	Temporal discrimination is abnormal in dystonia and IHT, but normal in ET
Prasad & Pal, 2019[55]	Clinical study of 252 cases with ET	5	New tremor classification system makes ET rare

vocal tremor, essential voice tremor, essential vocal tremor, laryngeal essential tremor, and others.[86] Similar to IHT, some studies favor the view that IVT is a subtype of ET, a subtype of dystonia, or a distinct nosological entity.

Evidence favoring the view that IVT might be a subtype of ET includes observations that its clinical features are similar to those of ET of the upper limbs. These similarities include average age at presentation, frequent family history of ET, and clinical responses of at least some patients to alcohol, propranolol, or primidone. Other studies have shown that a portion of cases diagnosed with IVT sometimes have a subtle tremor of the hands after careful exam.[87] This observation again points out the limitations in the diagnostic certainty of tremor based only on what is clinically apparent on exam. Long-term studies have also shown that individuals with IVT may later develop tremors of the upper limbs, making a diagnosis of ET more obvious.

Evidence for the view that IVT is a subtype of dystonia or a distinct entity comes from studies showing that the vast majority of cases with ET have involvement of the upper limbs. Thus, IVT is unusual. Other studies have suggested that IVT and dystonia affecting the voice are frequently misdiagnosed.[87] In one study, a group of voice experts used audio recordings of the voice during standardized vocal tasks to provide a diagnosis for subjects who had voice tremor, laryngeal dystonia, or both problems combined.[88] When multiple experts reviewed these recordings, diagnostic agreement was poor, indicating that voice experts cannot reliably distinguish among these groups. This poor agreement could reflect many issues including inadequate diagnostic features to discriminate these problems, differences in opinion regarding how diagnostic features should be applied, disorders that cannot be discriminated because they have overlapping clinical features, or disorders that co-exist with each other.

When considering IVT, some significant differences in viewpoints also must be considered.[86] Neurologists are willing to consider IVT as a subtype of dystonia, because the concept of tremor-dominant dystonia is well accepted. However, otolaryngologists and speech-language pathologists recognize either tremor or dystonia of the voice, or their combined occurrence; they do not recognize a tremor-dominant dystonic voice disorder. On the other hand, otolaryngologists and speech pathologists recognize a diagnostic entity known as *muscle tensions dysphonia*, a concept that is rarely found in the neurological lexicon. It will be necessary for experts across all disciplines to come to agreement on such fundamental issues before the nosological position of IVT can be firmly established.

Data from studies of IVT typically involved small numbers of subjects, so any conclusions must be taken with a grain of salt. The main evidence that IVT is not a subtype of ET relates to unreliability of the diagnosis when there is not also more obvious involvement of the upper limbs. Good studies have shown that clinical features of ET and dystonia overlap so much that they cannot be reliably discriminated, even by voice experts, and many cases may reflect laryngeal dystonia. However, detailed examinations of individual cases showing hand involvement along with observations that IVT may evolve over time to include hand dystonia suggest some cases may reflect ET. Thus, IVT may not be a homogeneous group.

THE RELEVANCE OF DIAGNOSTIC ACCURACY

Misdiagnosis in the clinic. Individuals' various types of tremors are frequently misdiagnosed in the clinic.[89-91] Some cases diagnosed with ET actually have dystonic tremor or PD. Conversely, other cases diagnosed with dystonia or PD have ET. The consequence of clinical misdiagnosis means that patients may be treated for many years with inappropriate therapies, when more effective therapies may be available.

Misdiagnosis in the literature. The high frequency of misdiagnoses may reflect poor education of practicing clinicians. However, the peer-reviewed expert literature similarly contains numerous examples of misdiagnosis.[8,43,48,50,89,91-98] Unfortunately, diagnostic uncertainties have led to concerns regarding the interpretation of some studies. For example, in therapeutic clinical trials, cohorts of study subjects with incorrect diagnoses may explain the marked variations in therapeutic responses to anti-tremor medications (e.g., propranolol or primidone), anti-dystonic medications (e.g., anticholinergics or botulinum toxins), and surgical treatments (e.g., deep brain stimulation or focused ultrasound).[41,42,99-102] Some of the largest clinical studies of PD included PET scans to document dopaminergic deficits in the basal ganglia (Table 11.6).[103-108] All of these studies contained a significant portion of subjects who had scans without evidence of dopaminergic deficit (SWEDD). Although some cases later evolved to have dopaminergic deficits consistent with PD, many were thought to reflect misdiagnosed cases of ET or dystonic tremor.[92,109-111] Clearly, including up to 20% of cases with the wrong diagnosis will increase experimental variance and affect study outcomes.

In family studies aiming to map a genetic locus, misdiagnosis of a single case can have a dramatic impact on the outcome. This issue is important, because many family studies of ET have included varying proportions of members who also had dystonia.[32-34,36] One of the most detailed studies included 463 individuals in 97 families with ET.[34] Among all family members, 363 had pure tremor, and 98 also had dystonia. Among those with dystonia, 88 had tremor with dystonia and 10 had pure dystonia. In another family study of ET that involved 100 members of 28 families, re-evaluation disclosed that 10% of ET probands also has dystonia, and in 93% the dystonia was not recognized.[36] The inclusion of mixed cohorts may explain the many challenges associated with identifying genes for ET.[52,97] Imprecise diagnoses can have similar deleterious effects on other studies addressing physiology, imaging, or biomarkers.

TABLE 11.6: SCANS WITHOUT EVIDENCE OF DOPAMINERGIC DEFICIT (SWEDD) IN LARGE CLINICAL TRIALS OF PARKINSON DISEASE

Study	Target population	Goal of study	SWEDDs (%)
CALM-PD[103]	PD	Compare therapy with levodopa to pramipexole	3.6
InSPECT[104]	PD	Compare therapy with levodopa to pramipexole	13.3
European FP-CIT[105]	PD	Compare clinical features of PD with imaging result	19.6
Real-PET[106]	PD	Compare therapy with ropinirole to pramipexole	11.2
ELLDOPA[107]	PD	Compare early versus late levodopa therapy	14.7
PRECEPT[108]	PD	Evaluate potential neuroprotective therapy	11.3

(A)

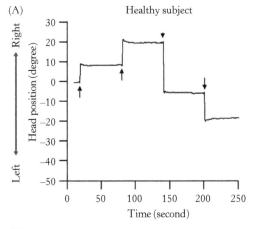

Healthy subject

(B)

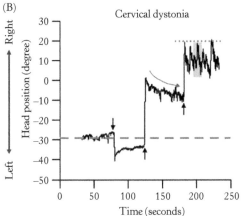

Cervical dystonia

(C)

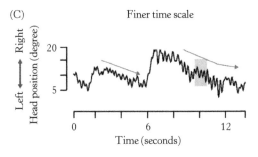

Finer time scale

(D)

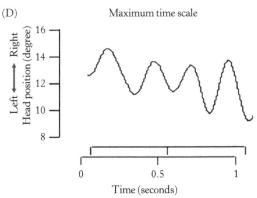

Maximum time scale

CLINICAL VS. OBJECTIVE ASCERTAINMENT OF TREMOR

Studies of oscillatory tremor-like movements in subjects with dystonia have often relied solely on clinical ascertainment, an approach with several limitations. First, the clinical exam can miss subtle or intermittent tremors. Second, the clinical exam cannot reliably discriminate phenomenologically distinct tremors, for example, relating to regularity or jerkiness. Third, determinations based only on clinical exams are subjective and vary among examiners.

Objective measures provide more sensitive and specific tools for studying tremor-like oscillations of all types.[84] Many different types of objective measures are available, each with different strengths and weaknesses. They include EMG, accelerometry, gyroscopic devices, magnetic position detectors, digital tablets, quantitative analysis of video recordings of movement, and others. These methods have provided important insights not discernible by clinical exam alone.

One of the most quantitatively precise series of studies involved measurements of tremor-like oscillations of the head in 14 subjects with cervical dystonia using a magnetic search coil to track head movements with great spatial and temporal resolution.[112–114] These studies revealed several important findings. First, tremor-like oscillations could be detected in all subjects, including those

FIGURE 11.2: Evaluation of Oscillatory Movements Resembling Tremor in Subjects with Cervical Dystonia. Panel A shows the movement traces for the head measured by a magnetic head coil when a normal subject was asked to turn the head right, then left. The head moves quickly, stays on target, and there are minimal head oscillations. Panel B shows head movement traces in cervical dystonia. Here, the subject moves the head quickly, but the head does not remain on target. In addition, oscillatory movements emerge. Evaluation of the oscillatory movements in cervical dystonia with greater temporal resolution showed two distinct types of oscillations in panels C and D. Panel C shows 2 large oscillations, with low frequency, high amplitude, and a sawtooth pattern mirroring jerky movements of the head. Panel D shows even greater temporal resolution with a higher frequency, lower amplitude, sinusoidal oscillation resembling ET that is superimposed on the larger jerky oscillation. This figure clearly shows two distinct oscillatory movements of the head in cervical dystonia.

in whom overt head tremor could not be detected on clinical exam. This finding echoes numerous other studies that found objective measures are more sensitive than the clinical exam.[84] Second, the tremor-like oscillations fell into two phenomenologically distinct subtypes. This finding also echoes other studies using EMG or motion detection devices in identifying different types of oscillations with very different characteristics.[67,115,116] Third, the two distinct subtypes were sometimes combined in the same subject. The combination of overlapping types of oscillations is not detectable with all measurement tools, but has been reported in most studies where discerning overlapping phenomenologies was feasible.[67,112–114]

Figure 11.2 depicts an example of head oscillations in a subject who had cervical dystonia and its comparison with a healthy subject. The arrow depicts the time when the subject was asked to turn the head. All healthy subjects could turn and hold the head steady at the desired orientation without any difficulty (Figure 11.2A). In contrast, those with cervical dystonia had difficulty turning the head, as well as two distinct types of head oscillations (Figure 11.2B). One type of oscillation had a high amplitude but low frequency, and it appeared as if the head was drifting slowly in one direction and then making a more rapid reversal in the other direction. These two different movements produced a jerky quality and a "sawtooth" pattern during measurement (Figure 11.2C). A second type of oscillation appeared as a smaller and more regular sinusoidal movement. These oscillations resembled those seen in ET. The combination of two types of oscillations was seen in the majority of cases studied, but their relative amounts differed. For example, the first subject shown in Figure 11.3 had a "pure" jerky movement with minimal sinusoidal oscillation. In contrast the second subject had predominantly sinusoidal oscillations with minimal jerky waveforms. A third subject had both types of oscillations. In addition to differences in their qualitative appearance, the two types of head oscillations had quantitative disparities including the mean per-cycle amplitude and frequency. The characteristics of the one type of oscillation are consistent with the definition of "dystonic tremor" according to Fahn's criteria.[38] However, sinusoidal oscillating waveforms resembling ET may co-exist. If the given subject also had overt dystonia, then either type of oscillation could be classified as "dystonic tremor" according to the 1998 and 2018 consensus definition.[1,39] This study highlights a serious limitation of the MDS consensus definition, because it conflates two different types of oscillations under a single label.

The final finding from the detailed studies of head oscillation in cervical dystonia was that the tremor-like oscillations could be predicted by a mathematical model known as the neural integrator.[117] The trajectory of the jerky oscillations had two components, one was a slow drift in head position. There was a subsequent fast phase, quickly moving the head in the opposite direction. In addition, there was also a head position dependence of the drift velocity. Velocity was minimal when the head was in the preferred "null" orientation, while it increased as the head shifted farther away from null. The direction of the drifts also reversed as the head shifted from one side of the null to the other. Such features of jerky head oscillations can be explained by a network model, whose property is to mathematically integrate the head velocity signal to maintain stable head position.[114]

The sinusoidal oscillations had several differences compared to the jerky oscillations. Their amplitude reduced but their frequency remained stable in different orientations of the head. A striking feature of the sinusoidal oscillations is that their amplitude and phase "reset" after a fast voluntary head movement, a key feature of oscillations originating from a neural integrator network.[113] Although sinusoidal and jerky oscillations both suggest abnormalities in neural integration, they are not explained by the same types of deficit. Mathematical models account for a defective neural integrator, due to suboptimal feedback, cause jerky oscillations. In contrast, an unstable neural integrator, due to excessive feedback, results in sinusoidal oscillations. Nevertheless, it is possible for two types of deficits be present in the same patient at different extents and perhaps may suggest different neural substrates.

NEUROBIOLOGICAL CONSTRUCTS TO ACCOUNT FOR OVERLAP BETWEEN DYSTONIA AND TREMOR

Evidence for overlapping biological mechanisms. The many clinical overlaps for tremor and dystonia may result from overlapping biological mechanisms. For example, some individuals may have an isolated tremor for years with a diagnosis of ET, followed later by the emergence of dystonic movements in the same or a different body region.[10,11,14,19,37,69,85] Conversely, an individual with

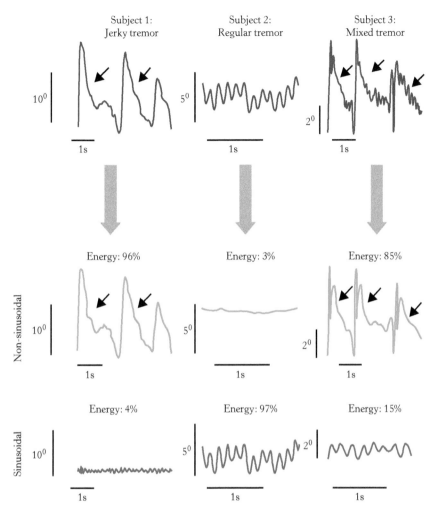

FIGURE 11.3: Kinematically Distinct Oscillatory Movements of the Head in Cervical Dystonia. This figure shows three different subjects with cervical dystonia. The first subject had large amplitude oscillatory movements that were jerky. The "energy" of the oscillations was estimated by measuring the area under the curve. This strategy revealed that the majority of oscillations (96% energy) to be non-sinusoidal. The second subject had oscillatory movements that were smaller, sinusoidal, and resembled those of ET. Here, 97% of the energy of oscillations was sinusoidal. The third subject had both types of oscillations combined, with 85% non-sinusoidal and 15% sinusoidal oscillations.

long-standing dystonia may subsequently develop tremor.[11,14,19,94] Although the development of the two disorders may be coincidental, the high frequency argues instead for evolution of overlapping biological mechanisms.

Additional evidence that tremor and dystonia share biological overlap comes from studies addressing their neuroanatomical substrates. An extensive body of evidence indicates that ET results from abnormal function of cerebellar circuits.[118,119] The cerebellum also plays an important role in the motor network that causes dystonia.[120–123] One study compared regional

brain activity in subjects with ET or dystonia using fluro-deoxyglucose PET.[124] Regions of abnormality overlapped considerably between the two disorders, although there were some differences too. Another study used fMRI to characterize regions of abnormality in subjects with ET or dystonic tremor.[125] Once again, there were extensive regions of overlap in these two populations, along with some differences. Histopathologically, patients with ET[126] or dystonia[127,128] have been reported to have similar abnormalities of the cerebellum including loss of Purkinje cells and torpedo inclusion bodies. However, the biological significance of these neuropathological findings is uncertain because they are subtle and they are not specific for tremor or dystonia.[129,130] All together, these studies imply overlapping brain regions responsible for ET and dystonia.

Further evidence for overlapping neuroanatomical substrates comes from a recent study which compared the physiological activity of single neurons of the globus pallidus among patients with cervical dystonia who had sinusoidal head oscillations resembling ET, jerky head oscillations resembling Fahn's definition of dystonic tremor, and no head oscillations.[131] Burst neurons of the internal pallidum were more common, and the number of spikes and inter-burst intervals was shorter in pure dystonia and those with jerky head oscillations compared to those with sinusoidal oscillations. The study found more pause neurons with more irregular firing in subjects with pure tremor compared to pure dystonia or jerky head oscillations. Bi-hemispheric asymmetry was present in spontaneous firing discharge in subjects who had pure dystonia and jerky head oscillations, but such a disparity was not present in subjects with sinusoidal oscillations. This study shows that the same neurons may be involved, although in different ways. In other words, the brain regions involved in ET or dystonia may overlap, but the pathophysiological changes involving the neural integrator may differ.

Further evidence for overlapping biological mechanisms comes from genetic studies. Family studies have repeatedly revealed individual family members with tremor, dystonia, or both.[31–34,36] These observations imply a shared genetic factor, with ultimate clinical expression that is influenced by other genetic or environmental factors. In fact, some potential genetic variants have been identified already. An isolated tremor syndrome resembling ET or PD tremor with no apparent dystonia has been reported for mutations in several "dystonia" genes, including *TOR1A, THAP1, ANO3,* and *SCGE.*[95,96,109,132–135] Although some such cases may represent misdiagnoses, it seems more likely that the occurrence of tremor syndromes with "dystonia" genes represents the sometimes highly varied pleiomorphic clinical phenotypes associated with some genetic mutations.

Hypothetical biological mechanisms for overlap. There are three main biological models to explain potential relationships between tremor and dystonia. The first model (phenocopy model) is that tremor and dystonia are entirely distinct disorders at the biological level, but a movement indistinguishable from pure tremor may occur

in dystonia (Figure 11.4A). In this model, the tremor of dystonia is a phenocopy of the tremor of ET. This model is inherent in the 1998 definition of dystonic tremor, which treats any tremor-like movement in dystonia to be distinct from pure tremor disorders.[39] This model also is an underlying assumption in articles implying that a syndrome of tremor with dystonia is distinct from syndromes of isolated tremor or dystonia.[43] However, this model is not consistent with the biological evidence. First, cases with dystonia may later develop tremor, or vice versa. This observation argues for evolution of a single biological process leading to different clinical phenomena. Second, imaging and pathological studies have provided plausible evidence that overlapping brain areas are affected. Third, there is frequent familial clustering of dystonia and/or tremor, and some "dystonia genes" can cause isolated tremor resembling ET. This observation demonstrates a single gene can cause either dystonia or tremor.

The second model (spectrum model) is that tremor and dystonia are pleiomorphic manifestations of the same biological disorder, falling at different ends of a continuous spectrum (Figure 11.4B). One end of the spectrum has oscillatory movements that are more regular and sinusoidal resembling ET, while the other end of the spectrum has irregular and jerky movements consistent with early definitions of dystonic tremor. This model is intuitively attractive because it explains why the two disorders may sometimes be clinically impossible to discriminate, and it can accommodate temporal evolution of dystonia and tremor in individual cases, familial clustering of dystonia and tremor, and genes causing dystonia or tremor. However, this model implies a continuous spectrum of movement abnormalities between dystonia and tremor, and such evidence is currently lacking. In fact, there is evidence from EMG and kinematic studies that argues for a dichotomous distinction (but the two tremors may co-exist) rather than a continuous spectrum between tremor in dystonia and pure tremor disorders.[67,80,113–116,136]

The third model (overlap model) postulates that tremor and dystonia are biologically different disorders, but they frequently overlap because the biological processes that cause them overlap (Figure 11.4C). For example, tremor and dystonia may involve different pathological processes, but in the same brain region. In this model a regular sinusoidal tremor resembling ET may be caused by one process, and an irregular jerky tremor resembling early definitions of dystonic tremor may be

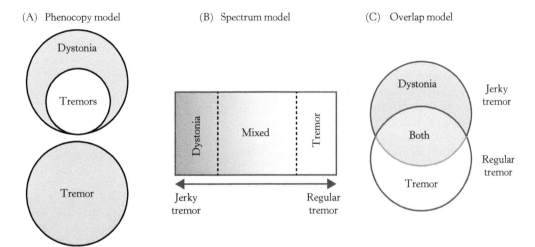

FIGURE 11.4: Biological Models to Explain Overlap between Dystonia and Tremor. For the phenocopy model (A), dystonia and tremor are biologically distinct disorders, but a movement disorder phenomenologically indistinguishable from tremor occurs also in dystonia. In this model, tremor in subjects with dystonia is biologically distinct, but a phenomenological resembles tremor. For the spectrum model (B), dystonia and tremor share the same biology, with dystonia and tremor falling on a continuum. Thus, dystonia and tremor are merely distinct clinical phenomenologies resulting from similar biological processes. In the overlap model (C), dystonia and tremor are biologically distinct but partly overlapping. In this model tremor occurring in subjects with dystonia reflect a coincidental disorder; however, the high frequency of overlap results from partly similar biological mechanisms.

caused by another process. However, these processes overlap in the same brain region, so that it is possible to find evidence for two types of tremor in the same individual. This model accommodates temporal evolution of dystonia and tremor, familial clustering, and genetic pleiomorphism. However, it does not imply a continuous spectrum of movement abnormalities between dystonia and tremor like the second model. Instead, it predicts overlap of distinct abnormalities. In fact, this is the only model that can accommodate EMG and kinematic evidence showing that some individuals may simultaneously have both a regular/sinusoidal and an irregular/jerky tremor.[67,112–114,137]

We favor the overlap model, because it best accommodates all currently available data. The main argument against this model is that the law of parsimony in medicine favors the application of a single diagnosis rather than two overlapping diagnoses. On the other hand, many examples of clinical observations are best accommodated by two separate but co-occurring conditions rather than a single unifying one. Examples include well-known associations between myocardial infarction and stroke, obesity and diabetes, and others. Similarly, it is well recognized that many individuals with PD have two distinct types of

tremor: a fine, high-frequency postural tremor and a coarse resting tremor. Further, individuals with long-standing ET may later develop PD. The overlaps between tremor and dystonia may reflect a similar situation already recognized for bilateral upper limb action tremors resembling ET in PD. Unfortunately, the search for objective biological evidence for this overlap has been hampered by current definitions that lump all types of tremors in dystonic body regions as dystonic tremors.

CONCLUSIONS

Although tremor and dystonia are distinct disorders, their clinical phenomenology and biology overlap in many areas. They are usually easy to discriminate on clinical exam alone. However, numerous studies have now shown that there are certain situations where the clinical exam alone is insufficient to establish or exclude a definitive diagnosis of tremor or dystonia. In these situations, or where a more definitive diagnosis is needed, additional physiological or motion-sensing tools may need to developed and implemented more consistently. Challenging areas where additional objective data are needed include the concepts of dystonic tremor and tremor-dominant dystonia, isolated tremors of the head or voice that do not also include the upper limbs, and task-specific tremors. Fortunately, numerous tools are now available, and we should see broader applications in the future.

Historically, clinical studies have been driven by the clinical exam and by expert opinion regarding criteria that discriminate tremor and dystonia. Biological studies have been similarly driven by the clinical exam. This clinical exam–based approach often begins with the premise that tremor and dystonia are distinct disorders (phenocopy model), and two groups are compared to find differences. This approach rarely considers the spectrum model or overlap model. It may be time to begin to design studies based on biological models, rather than traditional models based on expert clinical opinion.

ACKNOWLEDGMENTS

The review was supported in part by grants to the Dystonia Coalition, a consortium of the Rare Diseases Clinical Research Network (RDCRN) that is supported by the Office of Rare Diseases Research (ORDR) at the National Center for Advancing Clinical and Translational Studies (NCATS; U54 TR001456) in collaboration with the National Institute for Neurological Diseases and Stroke (NINDS; U54 NS065701 and U54 NS116025). Aasef Shaikh has received a Dystonia Medical Research Foundation (DMRF) Clinical Fellowship, DMRF/Dystonia Coalition Career Development Award, an American Academy of Neurology Career Development Award, the American Parkinson's Disease Association George C. Cotzias Memorial Fellowship, and philanthropic funds to the Department of Neurology at University Hospitals (Penni and Stephen Weinberg Chair and Brain Health and Allan Woll Fund).

REFERENCES

1. Bhatia KP, Bain P, Bajaj N, et al. Consensus statement on the classification of tremors. from the task force on tremor of the International Parkinson and Movement Disorder Society. *Mov Disord.* 2018;33:75–87.
2. Massey EW, Paulson GW. Essential vocal tremor: clinical characteristics and response to therapy. *South Med J.* 1985;78:316–317.
3. Louis ED. Tremor. *Continuum.* 2019;25(4): 959–975.
4. Elias WJ, Shah BB. Tremor. *JAMA.* 2014;311: 948–954.
5. Albanese A, Bhatia K, Bressman SB, et al. Phenomenology and classification of dystonia: a consensus update. *Mov Disord.* 2013;28:863–873.
6. Jinnah HA. The dystonias. *Continuum.* 2019;25:976–1000.
7. Balint B, Mencacci NE, Valente EM, et al. Dystonia. *Nat Rev Dis Primers.* 2018;4:2s5.
8. Pandey S, Sarma N. Tremor in dystonia. *Parkinsonism Relat Disord.* 2016;29:s.
9. Jankovic J, Ford J. Blepharospasm and orofacial-cervical dystonia: clinical and pharmacological findings in 100 patients. *Ann Neurol.* 1983;13:402–411.
10. Chan J, Brin MF, Fahn S. Idiopathic cervical dystonia: clinical characteristics. *Mov Disord.* 1991;6:119–126.
11. Jankovic J, Leder S, Warner D, Schwartz K. Cervical dystonia: clinical findings and associated movement disorders. *Neurology.* 1991;41:1088–1091.
12. Dubinsky RM, Gray CS, Koller WC. Essential tremor and dystonia. *Neurology.* 1993;43:2382–2384.
13. Deuschl G, Heinen F, Guschlbauer B, Schneider S, Glocker FX, Lucking CH. Hand tremor in patients with spasmodic torticollis. *Mov Disord.* 1997;12:547–552.
14. Pal PK, Samii A, Schulzer M, Mak E, Tsui JK. Head tremor in cervical dystonia. *Can J Neurol Sci.* 2000;27:137–142.
15. Schweinfurth JM, Billante M, Courey MS. Risk factors and demographics in patients with spasmodic dysphonia. *Laryngoscope.* 2002;112:220–223.
16. Tisch SHD, Brake H, Law M, Cole I, Darveniza P. Spasmodic dysphonia: clinical features and effects of botulinum toxin therapy in 169 patients—an Australian experience. *J Clin Neurosci.* 2003;10:434–438.
17. Godeiro-Junior C, Felicio AC, Aguiar PC, Borges V, Silva SM, Ferraz HB. Head tremor in patients with cervical dystonia: different outcome? *Arq Neuropsiquiatr.* 2008;66:805–808.
18. White LJ, Klein AM, Hapner ER, et al. Coprevalence of tremor with spasmodic dysphonia: a case-control study. *Laryngoscope.* 2011;121:1752–1755.
19. Defazio G, Gigante AF, Abbruzzese G, et al. Tremor in primary adult-onset dystonia: prevalence and associated clinical features. *J Neurol Neurosurg Psychiatry.* 2013;84:404–408.
20. Rudzinska M, Krawczyk M, Wojcik-Pedziwiatr M, Szczudlik A, Wasielewska A. Tremor associated with focal and segmental dystonia. *Neurol Neurochir Pol.* 2013;47:223–231.
21. Erro R, Rubio-Agusti I, Saifee TA, et al. Rest and other types of tremor in adult-onset primary dystonia. *J Neurol Neurosurg Psychiatry.* 2013;85:965–968.
22. Jhunjhunwala K, Lenka A, Pal PK. A clinical profile of 125 patients with writer's cramp. *Eur Neurol.* 2015;73:316–320.

23. Gigante AF, Berardelli A, Defazio G. Rest tremor in idiopathic adult-onset dystonia. *Eur J Neurol.* 2016;23:935–939.

24. LeDoux MS, Vemula SR, Xiao J, et al. Clinical and genetic features of cervical dystonia in a large multicenter cohort. *Neurol Genet.* 2016;2:e69.

25. Williams L, McGovern E, Kimmich O, et al. Epidemiological, clinical and genetic aspects of adult onset isolated focal dystonia in Ireland. *Eur J Neurol.* 2016;24:73–81.

26. Pandey S, Sarma N. Tremor in dystonia: a cross-sectional study from India. *Mov Disord Clin Pract.* 2017;4:858–863.

27. Hvizdosova L, Nevrly M, Otruba P, Hlustik P, Kanovsky P, Zapletalova J. The prevalence of dystonic tremor and tremor associated with dystonia in patients with cervical dystonia. *Sci Rep.* 2020;10:1436.

28. Gupta N, Pandey S. Rest tremor in dystonia: epidemiology, differential diagnosis, and pathophysiology. *Neurol Sci.* 2020;41(9):2377–2388. doi: 10.1007/s10072-020-04402-9

29. Shaikh AG, Beylergil SB, Scorr L, et al. Dystonia & tremor: a cross-sectional study of the Dystonia Coalition cohort. *Neurology.* 2021;96(4):e563–e574. doi: 10.1212/WNL.0000000000011049

30. Lou JS, Jankovic J. Essential tremor: clinical correlates in 350 patients. *Neurology.* 1991;41:234–238.

31. Koller WC, Busenbark K, Miner K. The relationship of essential tremor to other movement disorders: report on 678 patients. Essential Tremor Study Group. *Ann Neurol.* 1994;35:717–723.

32. Jankovic J, Beach J, Pandolfo M, Patel PI. Familial essential tremor in 4 kindreds. Prospects for genetic mapping. *Arch Neurol.* 1997;54:289–294.

33. Shatunov A, Sambuughin N, Jankovic J, et al. Genomewide scans in North American families reveal genetic linkage of essential tremor to a region on chromosome 6p23. *Brain.* 2006;129:2318–2331.

34. Hedera P, Phibbs FT, Fang JY, Cooper MK, Charles PD, Davis TL. Clustering of dystonia in some pedigrees with autosomal dominant essential tremor suggests the existence of a distinct subtype of essential tremor. *BMC Neurol.* 2010;10:66.

35. Rana AQ, Kabir A, Dogu O, Patel A, Khondker S. Prevalence of blepharospasm and apraxia of eyelid opening in patients with parkinsonism, cervical dystonia and essential tremor. *Eur Neurol.* 2012;68:318–321.

36. Louis ED, Hernandez N, Alcalay RN, Tirri DJ, Ottman R, Clark LN. Prevalence and features of unreported dystonia in a family study of "pure" essential tremor. *Parkinsonism Relat Disord.* 2013;19:359–362.

37. Lenka A, Bhalsing KS, Jhunjhunwala KR, Chandran V, Pal PK. Are patients with limb and head tremor a clinically distinct subtype of essential tremor? *Can J Neurol Sci.* 2015;42:181–186.

38. Fahn S. The varied clinical expressions of dystonia. *Neurol Clin.* 1984;2:541–554.

39. Deuschl G, Bain P, Brin M. Consensus statement of the movement disorder society on tremor. *Mov Disord.* 1998;13(Suppl. 3):2–23.

40. Pandey S, Bhattad S, Hallett M. The problem of questionable dystonia in the diagnosis of "essential tremor-plus." *Tremor Other Hyperkinet Mov (N Y).* 2020;10:27.

41. Puschmann A, Wszolek ZK. Diagnosis and treatment of common forms of tremor. *Semin Neurol.* 2011;31(1):65–77. doi: 10.1055/s-0031-1271312

42. Fasano A, Bove F, Lang AE. The treatment of dystonic tremor: a systematic review. *J Neurol Neurosurg Psychiatry.* 2014;85:759–769.

43. Defazio G, Conte A, Gigante AF, Fabbrini G, Berardelli A. Is tremor in dystonia a phenotypic feature of dystonia? *Neurology.* 2015;84:1053–1059.

44. Charlesworth G, Plagnol V, Holmstrom KM, et al. Mutations in ANO3 cause dominant craniocervical dystonia: ion channel implicated in pathogenesis. *Am J Hum Genet.* 2012;91:1041–1050.

45. Masuhr F, Wissel J, Muller J, Scholz U, Poewe W. Quantification of sensory trick impact on tremor amplitude and frequency in 60 patients with head tremor. *Mov Disord.* 2000;15:960–964.

46. Govert F, Deuschl G. Tremor entities and their classification: an update. *Curr Opin Neurol.* 2015;28:393–399.

47. Elble RJ. What is essential tremor? *Curr Neurol Neurosci Rep.* 2013;13:353.

48. Elble RJ. Defining dystonic tremor. *Curr Neuropharmacol.* 2013;11:48–52.

49. Quinn NP, Schneider SA, Schwingenschuh P, Bhatia KP. Tremor—some controversial aspects. *Mov Disord.* 2011;26(1):18–23.

50. Albanese A, Sorbo FD. Dystonia and tremor: the clinical syndromes with isolated tremor. *Tremor Other Hyperkinet Mov (N Y).* 2016;6:319.

51. Louis ED. The evolving definition of essential tremor: What are we dealing with? *Parkinsonism Relat Disord.* 2018;46(Suppl 1):S87–S91. doi: 10.1016/j.parkreldis.2017.07.004

52. Hopfner F, Haubenberger D, Galpern WR, et al. Knowledge gaps and research recommendations for essential tremor. *Parkinsonism Relat Disord.* 2016;33:27–35.

53. Rajalingam R, Breen DP, Lang AE, Fasano A. Essential tremor plus is more common than essential tremor: insights from the reclassification of a cohort of patients with lower limb tremor. *Parkinsonism Relat Disord.* 2018;56:109–110.

54. Louis ED. Essential tremor "plus" or "minus": perhaps now is the time to adopt the term "the essential tremors". *Parkinsonism Relat Disord.* 2018;56:111–112.

55. Prasad S, Pal PK. Reclassifying essential tremor: implications for the future of past research. *Mov Disord*. 2019;34:437.

56. Albanese A. Classifying tremor: language matters. *Mov Disord*. 2018;33:3–4.

57. Fasano A, Lang AE, Espay AJ. What is "essential" about essential tremor? a diagnostic placeholder. *Mov Disord*. 2018;33:58–61.

58. Rana AQ, Vaid HM. A review of primary writing tremor. *Int J Neurosci*. 2012;122:114–118.

59. Hai C, Yu-ping W, Hua W, Ying S. Advances in primary writing tremor. *Parkinsonism Relat Disord*. 2010;16:561–565.

60. Kachi T, Rothwell JC, Cowan JM, Marsden CD. Writing tremor: its relationship to benign essential tremor. *J Neurol Neurosurg Psychiatry*. 1985;48:545–550.

61. Cohen LG, Hallett M, Sudarsky L. A single family with writer's cramp, essential tremor, and primary writing tremor. *Mov Disord*. 1987;2:109–116.

62. Soland VL, Bhatia KP, Volonte MA, Marsden CD. Focal task-specific tremors. *Mov Disord*. 1996;11:665–670.

63. Rosenbaum F, Jankovic J. Focal task-specific tremor and dystonia: categorization of occupational movement disorders. *Neurology*. 1988;38:522–527.

64. Hirschbickler ST, Rothwell JC, Bhatia KP. Primary writing tremor is a dystonic trait: Evidence from an instructive family. *J Neurol Sci*. 2015;356:210–211.

65. Meunier S, Bleton JP, Mazevet D, et al. TENS is harmful in primary writing tremor. *Clin Neurophysiol*. 2011;122:171–175.

66. Bain PG, Findley LJ, Britton TC, et al. Primary writing tremor. *Brain*. 1995;118:1461–1472.

67. Elble RJ, Moody C, Higgins C. Primary writing tremor. A form of focal dystonia? *Mov Disord*. 1990;5(2):118–126.

68. Junker J, Brandt V, Berman BD, et al. Predictors of alcohol responsiveness in dystonia. *Neurology*. 2018;91:e2020–e2026.

69. Jedynak CP, Bonnet AM, Agid Y. Tremor and idiopathic dystonia. *Mov Disord*. 1991;6:230–236.

70. Papapetropoulos S, Singer C. Treatment of primary writing tremor with botulinum toxin type a injections: report of a case series. *Clin Neuropharmacol*. 2006;29:364–367.

71. Berg D, Preibisch C, Hofmann E, Naumann M. Cerebral activation pattern in primary writing tremor. *J Neurol Neurosurg Psychiatry*. 2000;69:780–786.

72. Modugno N, Nakamura Y, Bestmann S, Curra A, Berardelli A, Rothwell J. Neurophysiological investigations in patients with primary writing tremor. *Mov Disord*. 2002;17:1336–1340.

73. Ljubisavljevic M, Kacar A, Milanovic S, Svetel M, Kostic VS. Changes in cortical inhibition during task-specific contractions in primary writing tremor patients. *Mov Disord*. 2006;21:855–859.

74. Pita Lobo P, Quattrocchi G, Jutras MF, et al. Primary writing tremor and writer's cramp: two faces of a same coin? *Mov Disord*. 2013;28:1306–1307.

75. Hornabrook RW, Nagurney JT. Essential tremor in Papua, New Guinea. *Brain*. 1976;99:659–672.

76. Whaley NR, Putzke JD, Baba Y, Wszolek ZK, Uitti RJ. Essential tremor: phenotypic expression in a clinical cohort. *Parkinsonism Relat Disord*. 2007;13:333–339.

77. Chuang WL, Lu CS, Huang YZ, Chen RS. Clinical characteristics of essential tremor in Taiwan: an exploratory-comparative study. *Eur J Neurol*. 2012;19:135–141.

78. Chen W, Hopfner F, Szymczak S, et al. Topography of essential tremor. *Parkinsonism Relat Disord*. 2017;40:58–63.

79. Rivest J, Marsden CD. Trunk and head tremor as isolated manifestations of dystonia. *Mov Disord*. 1990;5:60–65.

80. Valls-Sole J, Tolosa ES, Nobbe F, et al. Neurophysiological investigations in patients with head tremor. *Mov Disord*. 1997;12:576–584.

81. Louis ED, Ford B, Barnes LF. Clinical subtypes of essential tremor. *Arch Neurol*. 2000;57:1194–1198.

82. Louis ED, Dogu O. Isolated head tremor: part of the clinical spectrum of essential tremor? Data from population-based and clinic-based case samples. *Mov Disord*. 2009;24:2281–2285.

83. Conte A, Ferrazzano G, Manzo N, et al. Somatosensory temporal discrimination in essential tremor and isolated head and voice tremors. *Mov Disord*. 2015;30:822–827.

84. Haubenberger D, Abbruzzese G, Bain PG, et al. Transducer-based evaluation of tremor. *Mov Disord*. 2016;31:1327–1336.

85. Rondot P, Marchand MP, Dellatorlas G. Spasmodic torticollis-review of 220 patients. *Can J Neurol Sci*. 1991;18:143–151.

86. Barkmeier-Kraemer JM. Isolated voice tremor: a clinical variant of essential tremor or a distinct clinical phenotype? *Tremor Other Hyperkinet Mov (N Y)*. 2020;10. doi: 10.7916/tohm.v0.738. PMID: 32015933; PMCID: PMC6988183.

87. Sulica L, Louis ED. Clinical characteristics of essential voice tremor: a study of 34 cases. *Laryngoscope*. 2010;120:516–528.

88. Ludlow CL, Domangue R, Sharma D, et al. Consensus-based attributes for identifying patients with spasmodic dysphonia and other voice disorders. *JAMA Otolaryngol Head Neck Surg*. 2018;144(8):657–665. doi: 10.1001/jamaoto.2018.0644. PMID: 29931028; PMCID: PMC6143004.

89. Lalli S, Albanese A. The diagnostic challenge of primary dystonia: evidence from misdiagnosis. *Mov Disord*. 2010;25:1619–1626.

90. Schrag A, Munchau A, Bhatia KP, Quinn NP, Marsden CD. Essential tremor: an overdiagnosed condition? *J Neurol.* 2000;247:955–959.

91. Jain S, Lo SE, Louis ED. Common misdiagnosis of a common neurological disorder: how are we misdiagnosing essential tremor? *Arch Neurol.* 2006;63:1100–1104.

92. Schneider SA, Edwards MJ, Mir P, et al. Patients with adult-onset dystonic tremor resembling parkinsonian tremor have scans without evidence of dopaminergic deficit (SWEDDs). *Mov Disord.* 2007;22:2210–2215.

93. Albanese A, Lalli S. Is this dystonia? *Mov Disord.* 2009;24:1725–1731.

94. Schiebler S, Schmidt A, Zittel S, et al. Arm tremor in cervical dystonia: is it a manifestation of dystonia or essential tremor? *Mov Disord.* 2011;26:1789–1792.

95. Cardoso F. Difficult diagnoses in hyperkinetic disorders—a focused review. *Front Neurol.* 2012;3:151.

96. Klepitskaya O, Neuwelt AJ, Nguyen T, Leehey M. Primary dystonia misinterpreted as Parkinson disease: video case presentation and practical clues. *Neurol Clin Pract.* 2013;3(6):469–474. doi: 10.1212/CPJ.0b013e3182a78eb5. PMID: 24353921; PMCID: PMC3863978.

97. Testa CM. Key issues in essential tremor genetics research: where are we now and how can we move forward? *Tremor Other Hyperkinet Mov (N Y).* 2013;3:tre-03-105-1843-1. doi: 10.7916/D8Q23Z0Z

98. Macerollo A, Superbo M, Gigante AF, Livrea P, Defazio G. Diagnostic delay in adult-onset dystonia: Data from an Italian movement disorder center. *J Clin Neurosci.* 2015;22:608–610.

99. Morishita T, Foote KD, Haq IU, Zeilman P, Jacobson CE, Okun MS. Should we consider Vim thalamic deep brain stimulation for select cases of severe refractory dystonic tremor. *Stereotact Funct Neurosurg.* 2010;88:98–104.

100. Pauls KA, Hammesfahr S, Moro E, et al. Deep brain stimulation in the ventrolateral thalamus/subthalamic area in dystonia with head tremor. *Mov Disord.* 2014;29:953–959.

101. Misra VP, Ehler E, Zakine B, Maisonobe P, Simonetta-Moreau M, group IIC. Factors influencing response to Botulinum toxin type A in patients with idiopathic cervical dystonia: results from an international observational study. *BMJ Open.* 2012;2(3):e000881. doi: 10.1136/bmjopen-2012-000881

102. Tsuboi T, Au KLK, Deeb W, et al. Motor outcomes and adverse effects of deep brain stimulation for dystonic tremor: a systematic review. *Parkinsonism Relat Disord.* 2020;76:32–41.

103. Parkinson Study G. Pramipexole vs levodopa as initial treatment for Parkinson disease: A randomized controlled trial. Parkinson Study Group. *JAMA.* 2000;284:1931–1938.

104. Parkinson Study G. Dopamine transporter brain imaging to assess the effects of pramipexole vs levodopa on Parkinson disease progression. *JAMA.* 2002;287:1653–1661.

105. Benamer HT, Oertel WH, Patterson J, et al. Prospective study of presynaptic dopaminergic imaging in patients with mild parkinsonism and tremor disorders: part 1. Baseline and 3-month observations. *Mov Disord.* 2003;18(9):977–984. doi: 10.1002/mds.10482

106. Whone AL, Watts RL, Stoessl AJ, et al. Slower progression of Parkinson's disease with ropinirole versus levodopa: the REAL-PET study. *Ann Neurol.* 2003;54(1).

107. Fahn S, Oakes D, Shoulson I, et al. Levodopa and the progression of Parkinson's disease. *N Engl J Med.* 2004;351:2498–2508.

108. Parkinson Study Group PI. Mixed lineage kinase inhibitor CEP-1347 fails to delay disability in early Parkinson disease. *Neurology.* 2007;69:1480–1490.

109. Erro R, Schneider SA, Stamelou M, Quinn NP, Bhatia KP. What do patients with scans without evidence of dopaminergic deficit (SWEDD) have? New evidence and continuing controversies. *J Neurol Neurosurg Psychiatry.* 2016;87:319–323.

110. Batla A, Erro R, Stamelou M, et al. Patients with scans without evidence of dopaminergic deficit: a long-term follow-up study. *Mov Disord.* 2014;29:1820–1825.

111. Marek K, Seibyl J, Eberly S, et al. Longitudinal follow-up of SWEDD subjects in the PRECEPT Study. *Neurology.* 2014;82:1791–1797.

112. Beylergil SB, Singh AP, Zee DS, Jinnah HA, Shaikh AG. Relationship between jerky and sinusoidal oscillations in cervical dystonia. *Parkinsonism Relat Disord.* 2019;66:130–137.

113. Shaikh AG, Zee DS, Jinnah HA. Oscillatory head movements in cervical dystonia: Dystonia, tremor, or both? *Mov Disord.* 2015;30:834–842.

114. Shaikh AG, Wong AL, Zee DS, Jinnah HA. Keeping your head on target. *J Neurosci.* 2013;33:11281–11295.

115. Yanagisawa N, Goto A. Dystonia musculorum deformans. Analysis with electromyography. *J Neurol Sci.* 1971;13:39–65.

116. Ansari KA, Webster DD. Quantitative measurements in spasmodic torticollis. Description of a method and results of measurement. *Dis Nerv Syst.* 1974;35:44–47.

117. Shaikh AG, Zee DS, Crawford JD, Jinnah HA. Cervical dystonia: a neural integrator disorder. *Brain.* 2017;139:2590–2599.

118. Raethjen J, Deuschl G. The oscillating central network of essential tremor. *Clin Neurophysiol.* 2012;123:61–64.

119. Louis ED. Essential tremor and the cerebellum. *Handb Clin Neurol.* 2018;155:245–258.

120. Neychev VK, Gross R, Lehericy S, Hess EJ, Jinnah HA. The functional neuroanatomy of dystonia. *Neurobiol Dis.* 2011;42:185–201.

121. Prudente CN, Hess EJ, Jinnah HA. Dystonia as a network disorder: what is the role of the cerebellum? *Neuroscience.* 2014;260:23–35.

122. Shakkottai VG, Batla A, Bhatia K, et al. Current opinions and areas of consensus on the role of the cerebellum in dystonia. *Cerebellum.* 2017;16(2):577–594.

123. Jinnah HA, Neychev V, Hess EJ. The anatomical basis for dystonia: the motor network model. *Tremor Other Hyperkinet Mov (N Y).* 2017;7:506.

124. Belenky V, Stanzhevsky A, Klicenko O, Skoromets A. Brain positron emission tomography with 2-18F-2-deoxi-D-glucose of patients with dystonia and essential tremor detects differences between these disorders. *Neuroradiol J.* 2017:1971400917719912.

125. DeSimone JC, Archer DB, Vaillancourt DE, Wagle Shukla A. Network-level connectivity is a critical feature distinguishing dystonic tremor and essential tremor. *Brain.* 2019;142:1644–1659.

126. Louis ED. Essential tremor: evolving clinicopathological concepts in an era of intensive post-mortem enquiry. *Lancet Neurol.* 2010;9:613–622.

127. Prudente CN, Pardo CA, Xiao J, et al. Neuropathology of cervical dystonia. *Exp Neurol.* 2012;241:95–104.

128. Ma K, Babij R, Cortes E, Vonsattel JP, Louis ED. Cerebellar pathology of a dual clinical diagnosis: patients with essential tremor and dystonia. *Tremor Other Hyperkinet Mov.* 2012;2:1–6.

129. Symanski C, Shill HA, Dugger B, et al. Essential tremor is not associated with cerebellar Purkinje cell loss. *Mov Disord.* 2014;29:496–500.

130. Shill HA, Adler CH, Sabbagh MN, et al. Pathologic findings in prospectively ascertained essential tremor subjects. *Neurology.* 2008;70:1452–1455.

131. Sedov A, Usova S, Semenova U, et al. Pallidal activity in cervical dystonia with and without head tremor. *Cerebellum.* 2020;19(3):409–418.

132. Cheng FB, Ozelius LJ, Wan XH, et al. THAP1/DYT6 sequence variants in non-DYT1 early-onset primary dystonia in China and their effects on RNA expression. *J Neurol.* 2012;259:342–347.

133. Stamelou M, Charlesworth G, Cordivari C, et al. The phenotypic spectrum of DYT24 due to ANO3 mutations. *Mov Disord.* 2014;29:928–934.

134. LeDoux MS, Xiao J, Rudzinska M, et al. Genotype-phenotype correlations in THAP1 dystonia: molecular foundations and description of new cases. *Parkinsonism Relat Disord.* 2012;18:414–425.

135. Cilia R, Reale C, Castagna A, et al. Novel DYT11 gene mutation in patients without dopaminergic deficit (SWEDD) screened for dystonia. *Neurology.* 2014;83:1155–1162.

136. Deuschl G, Heinen F, Kleedorfer B, Wagner M, Lucking CH, Poewe W. Clinical and polymyographic investigation of spasmodic torticollis. *J Neurol.* 1992;239:9–15.

137. Panyakaew P, Cho HJ, Lee SW, Wu T, Hallett M. The pathophysiology of dystonic tremors and comparison with essential tremor. *J Neurosci.* 2020;40:9317–9326.

Parkinson's Disease and Parkinsonian Tremor

MICHIEL F. DIRKX AND RICK C. HELMICH

DEFINITION

Parkinsonian tremor falls into the category of the combined tremor syndromes (axis 1) and is clinically defined as tremor accompanied by parkinsonism (bradykinesia and rigidity).[1] The underlying etiology (axis 2) is defined by the underlying hypokinetic-rigid syndrome (e.g., idiopathic neurodegenerative disorders such as Parkinson disease (PD) or multiple system atrophy, acquired parkinsonism, or a genetic disorder associated with parkinsonism). Classical parkinsonian tremor is characterized by a 4- to 7-Hz rest tremor of the hand ("pill-rolling" tremor), lower limb, jaw, tongue, or foot. However, other types of tremor (e.g., postural/kinetic) are also seen in patients with parkinsonism. Conversely, a rest tremor that phenomenologically resembles the classical parkinsonian tremor but is not accompanied by other symptoms of parkinsonism also occurs. In these cases, one should classify this type of tremor "isolated rest tremor," since the term parkinsonian tremor is reserved for tremor accompanied by parkinsonism (see "differential diagnosis of parkinsonian tremor," later in the chapter).

TREMOR IN PARKINSON DISEASE

Phenomenology and subtypes of tremor in Parkinson disease

Tremor is one of the cardinal motor symptoms in PD and was first described by James Parkinson in his "essay on the shaking palsy."[2] Classically, it is characterized by an involuntary, alternating agonist-antagonist contraction of the rest hand in a frequency of 4–7 Hz.[3] The presence and severity of tremor waxes and wanes spontaneously and may have a "pill-rolling"-like appearance. However, the appearance and severity of tremor in PD is highly heterogeneous. Furthermore, besides the classical rest tremor, PD harbors many different types of tremors (Table 12.1). Here, we will first describe the appearance and heterogeneity of the classical rest tremor and next elaborate on the other subtypes of tremor in PD.

Rest tremor

The classical rest tremor usually presents in one limb (typically an arm or leg) but as the disease progresses may spread to other limbs or to the tongue or jaw.[4] Remarkably, in a number of patients tremor may decrease or even completely disappear in the later stages of the disease.[5] Similar to the other cardinal motor symptoms (e.g., bradykinesia and rigidity) tremor is usually characterized by a unilateral onset and persisting asymmetry throughout the disease course. In a minority of patients, tremor may occur contralaterally to the otherwise most affected side, also called "wrong-sided tremor."[6] Its presence and amplitude are influenced by a number of factors. For example, both psychological stress and cognitive load (e.g., serial subtraction) are able to increase tremor amplitude, a phenomenon that is often used by clinicians when examining tremor.[7,8] Furthermore, tremor also increases during voluntary movements of non-tremulous limbs such as walking.[7] Conversely, rest tremor usually decreases after performing a voluntary movement with the trembling limb, such as a swift extension of the trembling hand, although after a brief period of time tremor usually re-emerges in a stable postural position. This "resetting phenomenon" (i.e., decrement of rest tremor amplitude upon posturing) is highly specific for PD and can be used in the clinic to differentiate it from other rest tremors (such as the one rarely seen in essential tremor;[9] see also Chapter 9: Essential tremor).

Rest tremor does not always respond as well to dopaminergic medication compared to bradykinesia and rigidity. One hypothesis is that tremor may sometimes require higher dosages of levodopa,[10] or that dopamine agonists are superior in treating tremor.[11] This phenomenon has also been referred to as "pseudo-dopamine-resistant" tremor.[12] However, there is also evidence that there are in fact two similar appearing rest tremor phenotypes each with presumed distinct pathophysiologies: dopamine-responsive versus dopamine-resistant tremor.[13]

Postural, kinetic, and orthostatic tremor
Besides the classical rest tremor, it is well-known that other types of tremor exist in PD: "other types of tremor may coexist in patients with parkinsonism, such as postural or kinetic tremor with the same or different frequency as rest tremor."[1] First, the most common type of postural tremor is the so-called re-emergent tremor, i.e., rest tremor that diminishes after a rapid movement of the trembling limb, only to return in a stable postural position after a variable amount of time (usually seconds but may take up to several minutes).[14] This type of postural tremor has a similar frequency, amplitude, and response to dopaminergic medication as rest tremor and is therefore considered an extension of the classical rest tremor (Figure 12.1).[15] However, it should be noted that there are slight but consistent differences between rest and re-emergent tremor. Specifically, re-emergent tremor has a slightly but statistically significant higher frequency than rest tremor (+0.4 Hz) and on average a lower response to dopaminergic medication (Figure 12.2). Since postural tremor in PD can be worse in some limb postures than in others, during clinical examination it is worth systematically evaluating tremor during different limb positions (arms outstretched or in bat winging position, hand pronated or supinated). Another subtype of parkinsonian postural tremor is pure postural

tremor, which is seen in a smaller proportion of patients and starts immediately upon change of a resting to a postural position of the hand, displays a clearly higher frequency than rest tremor (>1.5 Hz), smaller amplitude, and does not respond to dopaminergic medication (Figure 12.1). In the past, some have considered it to be an incidental co-occurring essential tremor.[16] but recent data suggest that this type of tremor is actually inherent to PD.[15] Kinetic tremor is defined as tremor of an actively moving limb (such as reaching or grasping movements or when drawing a spiral) and is frequently seen in PD, sometimes even in the absence of rest or postural tremor.[17] The frequency of kinetic tremor appears to be higher than rest tremor (+ 1 Hz), and therefore it was suggested that this type of tremor has a different pathophysiology than rest tremor.[18] This type of higher-frequency tremor appears to be insensitive to dopaminergic medication.[19]

Third, position-dependent orthostatic tremor during standing may be seen in PD, referred to as OT-plus (as it is accompanied by parkinsonism). Both classical OT (i.e., frequency range of 13–18 Hz) and slow OT (i.e., <13 Hz) have been reported. As it may sometimes respond to dopaminergic medication it has been argued to be a manifestation of PD.[20] In addition, orthostatic myoclonus (OM) may also be seen in PD or atypical parkinsonism. In fact, in up to one-third of cases OM is accompanied by parkinsonism.[21]

Epidemiology of Parkinson's tremor
Approximately 75% of patients with PD will develop classical rest tremor, of which 40–65% will be present at disease onset.[22–25] In roughly 90% of

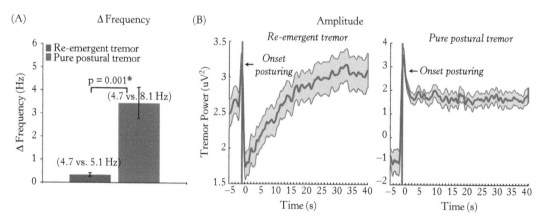

FIGURE 12.1: Comparison of Re-emergent and Pure Postural Tremor Showing that Pure Postural Tremor. (A) Has a Higher Frequency with Respect to Rest Tremor; (B) Starts Immediately upon Posturing. Adapted from [15].

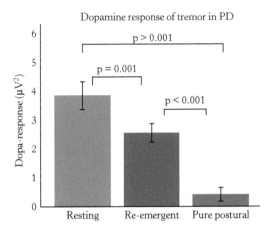

Dopamine response of tremor in PD

FIGURE 12.2: Comparison of the dopaminergic response (calculated as mean EMG power during OFF minus ON) of rest (orange), re-emergent (blue) and pure postural tremor (red) in Parkinson's disease. Abbreviation: PD = Parkinson's disease

Adapted from [15].

patients, tremor will present in the upper limbs, 6% in the lower limbs, and 5% in both lower and upper limbs.[24] As the disease progresses, tremor may spread to new sites in 39% of cases, including the (contralateral) limb, jaw, or lip.[24] The risk of developing or spreading of rest tremor during the disease course is not influenced by sex or side of motor symptom onset. However, a higher age of disease onset may predict an increased risk of rest tremor spread.[24] It should be noted that tremor expression and severity may be linked to etiology such as the specific genetic background. For example, tremor is rarer in case of PARK1 and, if present, is usually less severe.[26]

The most common type of postural tremor in PD is re-emergent tremor, which occurs in approximately two-thirds of patients.[14,15,27] Pure postural tremor is less prevalent and estimated to be present in 15% of patients with postural tremor,[15] although this may be an underestimation, as this type of tremor may become overshadowed by re-emergent tremor as the disease progresses.

Estimations of kinetic tremor in PD vary depending on the definition of kinetic tremor. In an earlier consensus statement on tremor, it was postulated that almost all PD patients exhibit at least a mild form of kinetic tremor.[28] Several studies seem to confirm this finding. For example, one large study that tested spiral drawing according to Bain and Findley.[29] in 870 PD patients showed that only 1.3% drew a completely normal spiral

and 47.1% showed a marked to very severe kinetic tremor.[17] Furthermore, another study analyzed kinetic tremor in a reach-to-grasp movement in 13 tremor-dominant PD patients, showing that 85% of patients exhibited some form of kinetic tremor.[18]

Tremor-dominant versus non-tremor PD

While some patients with PD have a prominent and disabling tremor, others never develop this motor sign. This variability is the basis for classifying patients into tremor-dominant and non-tremor subtypes.[30] In the past, several classification methods of tremor and non-tremor subtypes have been used. First, a number of subtypes based on differences in motor score have been defined. For example, a tremor-dominant (TD) phenotype has been contrasted with a postural instability and gait difficulty (PIGD) subtype. To this end, the DATATOP database has been used, which contains more than 800 early, untreated Parkinson patients who were classified into TD and PIGD based on subscores of the Unified Parkinson's Disease Rating Scale (UPDRS).[31] The PIGD subtype incorporates non-tremor motor symptoms including hypokinesia and postural instability. Furthermore, tremor-dominant PD has been contrasted with a PD subtype dominated by bradykinesia and rigidity,[32] also based on UPDRS subscores (but excluding axial items). In addition, several studies have defined a tremor-dominant phenotype based on an UPDRS rest tremor score of ≥ 2 in the OFF dopaminergic state.[33] Second, in addition to subtyping based on UPDRS motor-scores, several data-driven automated clustering methods identified not only tremor-dominant and non-tremor subtypes, but also other subtypes characterized by age of onset, speed of disease progression, and non-motor symptoms.[34-36]

A general picture that emerges is that tremor is indicative of a more benign disease course. First, several studies have confirmed that patients presenting with tremor have a slower disease progression than those with a PIGD subtype.[31,37] In addition, survival may be longer for tremor-dominant compared to the PIGD subtype,[38,39] although not all studies are able to confirm this finding.[40] Second, non-motor symptoms such as cognitive decline, depression, and apathy tend to be less prominent in patients with tremor-dominant PD.[41-43] Last, olfaction may be more impaired in the akinetic-rigid than the tremor-dominant subtype.[44] These findings have suggested that the disease course of tremor-dominant

TABLE 12.1: OVERVIEW OF THE VARIOUS TREMOR SUBTYPES THAT ARE FOUND
IN PARKINSON DISEASE

Tremor type	Prevalence	Frequency	Amplitude	Response to dopaminergic medication	Response to non-dopaminergic medication	Clinical characteristics
Rest tremor	75%	4–7 Hz	Medium - large	+[n]	+/-[m]	– Asymmetric, distal – Pill-rolling aspect – Suppressed by voluntary movement – Spontaneous waxing/waning – Increase with cognitive/motor activation
Re-emergent postural tremor	66%	4–7 Hz (±0.4 Hz higher than rest)	Medium - large	+[n]	?	– Onset seconds to minutes after posturing
Pure postural tremor	15%	7–12 Hz	Small	-	?	– Starts immediately upon posturing
Kinetic tremor	>80%	5–8 Hz (±1 Hz higher than rest)	Medium	-	?	– May resemble enhanced physiologic tremor
(Pseudo-) orthostatic tremor	Rare	4–18 Hz	Small	+/-	?	– Should be considered in patients with unsteadiness

[m] No reliable clinical trials, but beta-blockers, anticholinergics, or clozapine are sometimes effective.
[n] On average, good response to dopaminergic medication; however, large inter-subject variability.

patients is relatively benign when compared to other subtypes, although one should not underestimate the disabling potential that tremor may have on physical and psychological well-being.[45] Furthermore, it should be noted that in a number of patients, an initial tremor-dominant phenotype eventually transforms into another subtype such as PIGD,[43] which may already occur as early as 12 months after the initial diagnosis of PD.[46] Interestingly, the transition from the TD to PIGD subtype seems to be accompanied by an increased risk of cognitive decline, which is consistent with the notion that the non-tremor subtypes have an increased risk of cognitive disability.

PATHOPHYSIOLOGY OF PARKINSON DISEASE TREMOR

Tremor has a different pathophysiology than the other cardinal motor symptoms in PD (e.g., bradykinesia and rigidity). For example, tremor does not increase at the same pace as the other motor symptoms and accordingly does not correlate with the severity of bradykinesia and rigidity.[47] This suggests that tremor has a unique pathophysiological substrate that is different from other motor symptoms, which is the topic of this section.

Biochemical basis of Parkinson disease tremor

The pathological hallmark of PD is nigrostriatal dopamine depletion, but the relationship between dopamine and tremor is more complicated. Specifically, unlike bradykinesia and rigidity, tremor does not correlate with striatal dopamine depletion (referred to as the dopamine paradox)[48] and the effects of dopaminergic medication on tremor are rather unpredictable.[49] Nevertheless, levodopa therapy remains the best available treatment,[50] indicating that dopamine must at the very least be partly involved. One hypothesis for the dopamine paradox comes from the observation that tremor is correlated with pallidal rather than striatal dopamine depletion,[51] but a larger study could not confirm this.[52] Another explanation comes from recent evidence that dopaminergic medication targets tremor-related activity not only in the basal ganglia, but also in the thalamus (ventrolateral nucleus, pars ventralis (VLpv)), a region that plays an important role in the pathophysiology of PD tremor.[53] Indeed, the human thalamus is densely innervated by dopaminergic projections[54]—albeit to a lesser extent than the basal ganglia. Interestingly, postmortem studies show that the retrorubral area—which sends dopaminergic projections to the ventrolateral thalamus and the pallidum—is specifically degenerated in tremor-dominant PD patients.[55] These findings suggest that dopaminergic depletion outside the basal ganglia may play a role in the pathophysiology of tremor as well.

In addition to dopamine, several other neurotransmitters may be involved in the generation of tremor (Figure 12.3). First, several studies point toward a role of serotonin. Specifically, in a large cohort of 345 drug-naïve PD patients, raphe serotonin transporter availability was decreased in tremor-dominant patients and tremor severity was correlated with serotonin transporter depletion.[56] Moreover, the raphe/putamen binding ratio of ^{123}I-FP-CIT measured transporter binding (in other words raphe serotonin transporter availability normalized to putamen dopamine transporter availability) correlated with tremor and its response to dopaminergic medication.[52] This means that patients with a relatively dopamine-resistant tremor show relatively low raphe serotonergic transporter availability and a relatively spared putamen dopamine transporter availability. Thus, serotonin may play a larger role in the pathogenesis of patients with a relative dopamine-resistant tremor. The observation that non-dopaminergic brain areas play a larger role in patients with a clinical dopamine-resistant tremor is supported by a functional MRI study showing that the cerebellum is more active in patients with a dopamine-resistant tremor.[13]

Second, there are several pieces of evidence which link Parkinson's tremor to the noradrenergic system. For example, tremor-dominant Parkinson patients have less degeneration of the locus coeruleus (the main source of cerebral noradrenalin), and noradrenalin receptor binding in the locus coeruleus is increased in PD patients versus controls,[57] and particularly in tremor-dominant patients.[58] Furthermore, activation of the noradrenergic system via stress, cognitive load, or direct intravenous injection of adrenaline leads to tremor amplification in PD.[59-61] Accordingly, interventions aimed at attenuating noradrenergic activity (such as usage of beta-blockers or guided relaxation imagery) may ameliorate this amplification.[62,63] These findings suggest that the noradrenergic system has a modulatory (amplification) role in Parkinson's tremor.

Last, acetylcholine may also have a role in the generation of tremor, indicated by the effectiveness of anticholinergic medication over placebo in treating tremor.[64] The exact mechanisms remain largely unclear, but it has been suggested that striatal cholinergic interneurons are overactive due to a dopamine deficiency, which in turn inhibits further dopamine release,[65] but this remains speculative.

The cerebral circuit of Parkinson's tremor

Many studies have addressed the question which cerebral circuit is involved in Parkinson's tremor, using a variety of methods. The general picture that emerges is that both the basal ganglia and a cerebello-thalamo-cortical circuit play a role in tremor. Specifically, (1) magneto-encephalography (MEG) studies showed tremor-related oscillatory activity in the cerebellum and a diencephalic region that is probably the thalamus;[66] (2) PET studies show tremor-related hypermetabolism of the cerebello-thalamo-cortical circuit and putamen;[67] (3) deep brain recordings have found tremor oscillations in the ventral intermediate nucleus of the thalamus (VIM), which is a recipient of cerebellar input;[68] (4) deep brain stimulation of both the basal ganglia (GPi and STN) and cerebellar thalamus (VIM) are highly effective in reducing tremor;[69-71] and (5) several functional MRI studies have confirmed tremor-related activity is present in the cerebello-thalamo-cortical circuit and basal ganglia.[13,33,51] Thus, it is clear that both basal ganglia and a cerebello-thalamo-cortical circuit are involved, but the exact mechanisms underlying the initiation and propagation of tremor are open to interpretation. In the following part we will elaborate on several theories.

The first question that arises is whether there is a cerebral oscillator that acts as the tremor pacemaker. Several studies have argued that either the basal ganglia or thalamus may be responsible for this, mostly based on local recordings of a limited

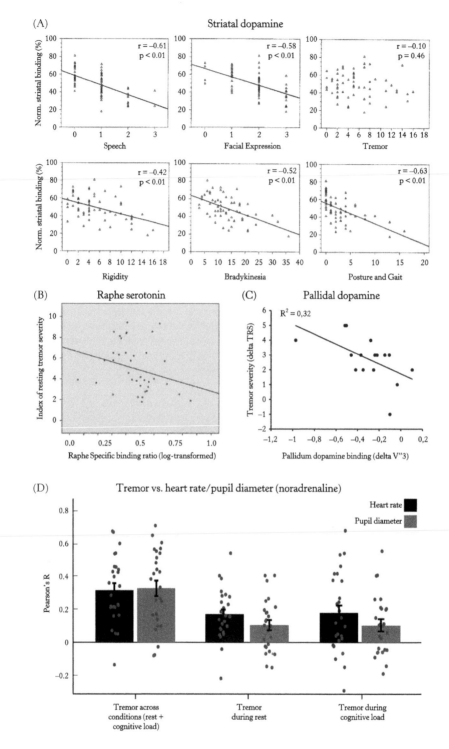

FIGURE 12.3: Neurochemical Correlates of Parkinson's Disease Tremor. (A) Correlation between age-normalized striatal ^{123}I beta-CIT binding and UPDRS motor subscores for speech, facial expression, tremor (rest and action tremor), rigidity, bradykinesia, and posture and gait (n = 59). *Adapted from* [48]. (B) Correlation between ^{123}I-FP-CIT SPECT in the raphe and index of tremor severity (β = −0.322; p<0.05; n = 37). *Adapted from* [56]; (C) Correlation showing raphe/putamen ^{123}I-FP-CIT uptake ratio of 38 patients plotted against their respective percentage rest tremor amplitude improvement. Line of best fit is shown. Patients taking levodopa only are represented by a green dot; patients taking a dopamine agonist only are represented by a blue square. The raphe/putamen ratio is associated with the percentage improvement of rest tremor amplitude (b = 0.457, P-value < 0.01). *Adapted from (Pasquini et al., 2018).* (D) Correlation between rest tremor power (measured with EMG) and proxy measures of the noradrenergic system (i.e., heart rate and pupil diameter) during periods of rest and cognitive load. *Adapted from* [59]. These data show that tremor severity is not correlated with dopamine depletion in the striatum (A), but with serotonin depletion in the raphe (B), and activity of the noradrenergic system (D), while the dopamine response of rest tremor is correlated with the ratio of striatal dopamine (DA)/raphe serotonin (SER) (C).

set of neurons (Figure 12.4). One of the first hypotheses was the thalamic pacemaker theory, which suggested that hyperpolarized cells in the thalamus might act as the tremor pacemaker.[72,73] Specifically, slightly depolarized thalamic cells oscillate at 10 Hz, whereas hyperpolarized cells oscillate at 6 Hz. However, the presence of this 6 Hz oscillatory mode has been questioned in PD patients.[74] Other studies have argued that the basal ganglia give rise to the tremor pacemaker. For example, the loss-of-segregation hypothesis[75] postulates that excessive synchronization of neurons in the dopamine depleted pallidum result in tremor.[75] However, deep brain stimulation of both the basal ganglia and thalamus are effective treatments of tremor, suggesting that both regions play a key role in the generation of tremor. One study tackled this issue by suggesting that both the basal ganglia (subthalamic nucleus (STN)) and thalamus (VIM) have pacemaker properties, as

evidenced by the ability of deep brain stimulation to entrain activity in these regions.[76] This would not, however, explain why basal ganglia oscillations are only transiently and inconsistently present with tremor,[77,78] whereas fluctuations in the VIM are highly synchronous,[79] see Figure 12.4.

One hypothesis that provides an explanatory framework for the role and interaction of both basal ganglia and cerebello-thalamo-cortical circuit is the dimmer-switch model, which hypothesizes that the basal ganglia initiate a tremor episode (analogous to a light switch) and that a cerebello-thalamo-cortical circuit subsequently produces and amplifies the tremor (analogous to a light dimmer), see Figure 12.5.[82] This model originated from combined functional MRI-EMG studies, which showed that spontaneous fluctuations in tremor amplitude correlates with activity in the cerebello-thalamo-cortical circuit, whereas changes in tremor amplitude

(A) Peri-operative VLp recordings in a tremor-dominant PD patient

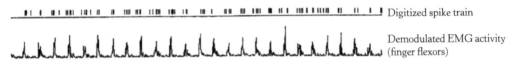

(B) Peri-operative GPi recordings in a tremor-dominant PD patient

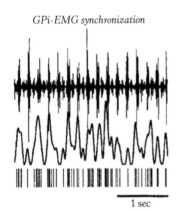
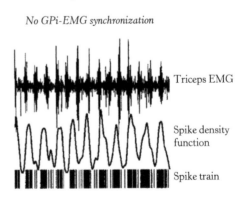

FIGURE 12.4: Neuronal Correlates of Parkinson's Disease Tremor. (A) Simultaneous recording of thalamic posterior VL (VLp) single-unit activity and peripheral EMG during tremor in a parkinsonian patient. These data show continuous synchronization between internal globus pallidus activity and peripheral EMG. *Adapted from* [80], *Copyright 1988 Society for Neuroscience.* (B) Simultaneous recording of internal globus pallidus (GPi) multi-unit activity and peripheral EMG during tremor in a patient with Parkinson's disease (PD). The two plots illustrate the raw signals of two epochs of data sampled 5 min apart. Note that in the left trace the peaks in the spike density function coincide with the EMG bursts, whereas in the right trace the oscillations in the spike density function occur at a lower frequency than the EMG. These data show that synchronization between neuronal activity in internal globus pallidus and peripheral EMG is transient in nature. *Adapted from* [81], *Copyright 1999 National Academy of Sciences.* Abbreviations: PD = Parkinson's disease; VLp = posterior ventrolateral nucleus of thalamus; GPi = internal globus pallidus; EMG = electromyography

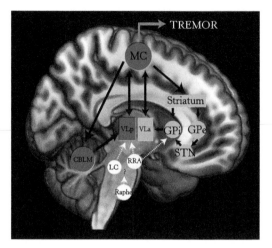

FIGURE 12.5: Illustration of the Cerebral Network Underlying Parkinson's Disease Rest Tremor Involving Both the Basal Ganglia (Blue) and Cerebello-Thalamo-Cortical Circuit (Red). According to the dimmer-switch model the basal ganglia initiate a tremor episode (analogous to a light switch) whereas the cerebello-thalamo-cortical circuit produces and modulates tremor amplitude (analogous to a light dimmer). Importantly, multiple neurotransmitter systems are involved, including the dopaminergic retrorubral area (which influences the cerebral tremor circuit through basal ganglia and VLp), noradrenergic locus coeruleus (which influences the cerebral tremor circuit through the VLp) and serotonergic raphe nuclei (unsure where this region targets the cerebral tremor circuit). Abbreviations: MC = motor cortex, GPe = globus pallidus externa, GPi = globus pallidus interna, STN = subthalamic nucleus, VLa = anterior ventrolateral nucleus of the thalamus, VLp = posterior ventrolateral nucleus of the thalamus, CBLM = cerebellum, LC = locus coeruleus, RRA = retrorubral area.

(i.e., maximal at the onset of tremor episodes) correlate with activity in the basal ganglia.[33,51] This model has been confirmed in subsequent studies where additionally computational network analyses show that tremor originates in the basal ganglia and subsequently reaches the cerebello-thalamo-cortical circuit via the motor cortex, where both circuits anatomically converge.[13,33] Furthermore, subsequent studies show that this model can also be used to explain differences in clinical phenotypes of tremor, such as (1) dopamine-resistant versus dopamine-responsive tremor, which shows that the cerebellum is more active in patients with dopamine-resistant tremor;[13] and (2) how cognitive load amplifies Parkinson's tremor through excitatory network

influences onto the thalamus, i.e., both via a bottom-up ascending arousal system and top-down cognitive-control network.[59] However, like any model, the dimmer-switch model has a number of limitations. For instance, given the limited temporal resolution of functional MRI, it cannot answer the question of whether tremor oscillations originate from one or more cerebral region(s) or perhaps from the interplay of the cerebral tremor network as a whole. The idea that tremor oscillations originate from the interplay of multiple cerebral nodes fits with studies showing that stimulation of several regions within the tremor circuitry (via intracranial electrodes or transcranial magnetic stimulation) is able to entrain tremor.[76,83,84] This indicates that tremor may be the result of several competing cerebral oscillators. Another limitation is that concurrent EMG-fMRI recordings are able to identify musculo-cerebral correlations, but it is difficult to infer causality. In other words, it is unsure whether the observed cerebral activity is afferent or efferent with respect to the tremor. Finally, although the STN is an important region regarding Parkinson's tremor (as evidenced by the ability of STN-DBS to successfully treat tremor[85]), the role of the STN within the dimmer-switch model remains unsure since no cerebral activity within this region was found, possibly due to the small volume of this region. An interesting case reports supports the role of the STN in the dimmer-switch model.[86] Using local field potentials from the STN in a single, tremor-dominant Parkinson patient, it was found that alpha/low-beta power in the STN increased transiently around tremor onset, after which persistent beta suppression and increased oscillatory activity at tremor frequency in the STN and motor cortex were associated with tremor maintenance. This suggests that the STN plays a role both in the switch and in the dimmer ("spider in the web"), given its connections to both basal ganglia and cerebello-thalamo-cortical circuit.[87] Future studies focused on these questions may elucidate the accuracy of the dimmer-switch model.

TREMOR IN ATYPICAL PARKINSONISM

Although less frequent, tremor may also be seen in atypical parkinsonism. Typically, tremor in atypical parkinsonism is more symmetrical, is more often seen in action than during rest, and may have a jerky aspect.[88] However, this depends on the specific underlying etiology. In this paragraph we will elaborate on the types of tremor seen in the most prevalent atypical parkinsonism syndromes.

In multiple system atrophy (MSA), multiple types of tremor can be observed including postural, rest, and intention tremor. Postural tremor is the most frequent type of tremor and is documented in 28–67% of cases.[89] Furthermore, postural tremor is most often observed in the parkinsonian subtype of MSA (MSA-P) compared to the cerebellar subtype (MSA-C). This type of postural tremor may have a jerkier/more irregular aspect, and it has even been suggested that these irregular and small-amplitude involuntary movements may correspond to myoclonus rather than tremor.[90,91] Indeed, neurophysiological investigations show that jerky postural movements in MSA consists of small-amplitude irregular oscillations with no predominant peak in the Fourier frequency spectrum analyses as compared to PD tremor.[92] However, in most studies no clinical differentiation between jerky postural tremor and myoclonus was made, and therefore larger studies including electrophysiological recordings are needed to specify and characterize tremulous versus myoclonic movements in MSA. For this, the clinical observation can be used that tremor is characterized by symmetrical, rhythmic movements of all fingers, whereas polyminimyoclonus is characterized by independent, jerky movements of individual fingers. Besides postural tremor, also intention tremor can be seen in MSA, which is typically part of cerebellar pathology and therefore mostly seen in MSA-C (33%) compared to MSA-P (11% of cases).[93] Intention tremor can be present at onset, but typically arises throughout the disease course. Finally, rest tremor is documented in 25–43% of cases and is more common in MSA-P compared to MSA-C.[89] Rarely, this is similar to the classical pill-rolling tremor, as seen in PD (8–11%), but if so, this can create a diagnostic dilemma.

Tremor in progressive nuclear palsy (PSP) is seen in 42% of patients and may include postural, rest, and intention tremor.[94] Although details of reported tremor are not always available, postural tremor seems to be the most prevalent type of tremor in PSP and is reported in 31% of patients with tremor, followed by rest tremor (23%) and intention tremor (8%). Tremor in PSP is usually present in the upper limbs, but may also be seen in the lower limbs or face. Furthermore, in roughly half of the cases tremor is symmetrical.[94] It should be noted that in general tremor is a relatively mild feature, especially compared to other

symptoms in PSP, and therefore often does not receive as much attention.

In corticobasal syndrome (CBS), tremor is a prominent feature occurring in 20% of cases at presentation and in 39% at some point in the disease course.[95] Again, postural tremor is the most frequent type of tremor, although rest and action tremor do occur. In general, tremor in CBS is jerkier, more irregular, and faster (6–8 Hz) than tremor in PD.[96] Stimulus-sensitive myoclonus is present in 27% of cases and may be superimposed on postural tremor.[95]

Drug-induced parkinsonism (DIP) is another frequent cause of a hypokinetic-rigid syndrome and is usually the result of usage of antipsychotic medication.[97] Classically, it is described as bilateral and symmetric parkinsonism without tremor at rest. However, asymmetrical parkinsonism with rest tremor may be present in up to 30–50% of patients, making it sometimes hard to distinguish from PD.[98] In addition, postural tremor is seen in roughly half of patients with drug-induced parkinsonism and generally accompanies rest tremor. Although tremor in DIP is poorly characterized, it may be very similar to tremor in PD, and some have even suggested that patients with DIP may have a preclinical stage of PD whose symptoms have been unmasked by the offending drug.[98] However, despite apparent clinical similarities, one electrophysiological study shows that EMG characteristics of rest tremor may be used to differentiate DIP from PD, as the former showed a slightly higher frequency (5.9 versus 4.7 Hz), longer burst duration (103 vs. 88 ms), smaller amplitude (0.16 vs. 0.41 mV), and a different muscle agonist-antagonist pattern (synchronous versus alternating).[99]

Parkinsonism with a vascular etiology (VP) is generally characterized by the absence of rest tremor, which may be used to differentiate it from Parkinson disease,[100] in addition to the main distinguishing feature—that is, predominant lower body parkinsonism in VP versus PD. However, postural tremor is frequently observed in VP (in roughly two-thirds of patients), and some studies even report a higher prevalence of postural tremor in VP than PD.[101,102]

Finally, another entity named *benign tremulous parkinsonism* has been described in patients with predominant rest tremor that resembles PD tremor, but with otherwise mild bradykinesia/rigidity, absence of gait disorder, and mild progression of parkinsonism other than tremor despite many years of disease.[103] It is unsure

TABLE 12.2: COMPARISON OF TREMOR IN VARIOUS PARKINSONISM AND DIFFERENTIAL DIAGNOSIS

Etiology	Rest tremor	Postural tremor	Kinetic tremor	Characteristics
Parkinson disease	+++	++	++	See Table 12.1
Multiple system atrophy	+	+++	++	– Jerky aspect, sometimes difficult to differentiate from myoclonus – Intention tremor (MSA-C > MSA-P) – Rest tremor usually not pill-rolling
Progressive supranuclear palsy	+	++	+/-	– Usually presents in upper limb – 50% symmetrical
Drug-induced parkinsonism	+	++	+	– Usually symmetrical postural tremor – Sometimes hard to differentiate from PD tremor
Corticobasal syndrome	+/-	+	+/-	– Jerkier, more irregular, and faster than PD tremor
Vascular parkinsonism	+/-	++	+/-	– Most frequently symmetrical postural tremor
Benign tremulous parkinsonism	+++	++	++	– Same as PD tremor, but with only mild non-tremor symptoms
Essential tremor	+/-	+++	++	– Symmetrical postural tremor of upper limbs – No resetting phenomenon – No bradykinesia/ rigidity
Dystonic tremor	+	++	++	– Position-dependent – Jerkier than parkinsonian rest tremor – No resetting phenomenon – Thumb extension rather than thumb flexion

whether this is a separate disease entity or a subtype of PD.

DIFFERENTIAL DIAGNOSIS OF PARKINSONIAN TREMOR

As stated earlier, parkinsonian tremor is defined as tremor that is accompanied by parkinsonism (bradykinesia and rigidity). Therefore, tremor in the absence of parkinsonism is by definition not parkinsonian tremor. However, some types of tremor may phenotypically resemble the classical parkinsonian tremor, which may sometimes lead to a difficult diagnostic dilemma, especially when in doubt about the presence of bradykinesia. In this paragraph we will describe the most important differential diagnosis based on phenotypical resemblance (i.e., Axis 1) of classical parkinsonian rest tremor.

Essential tremor (ET) is a symmetrical, upper-limb action tremor that is generally easily differentiated from the predominant asymmetrical rest tremor in PD. However, in some cases there is some phenotypical overlap between (subtypes of) tremor in both entities. For example, in severe cases ET may also occur at rest (up to 20% of patients). In this case, absence of a resetting phenomenon (i.e., amplitude decrement upon posturing) can be used to differentiate it from PD rest tremor.[9] Furthermore, a bilateral postural tremor frequently occurs in PD that may sometimes resemble ET, especially in the case of the "pure postural tremor" subtype. These observations, among others, have led to the question of whether there is a relationship between the occurrence of ET and PD and, more specifically, whether ET is a risk factor for developing PD.[104] That is, ET in some patients evolves into a different clinical syndrome including PD.[105] There is conflicting evidence as to whether patients with ET have an increased risk of developing PD.[106,107] Reliable longitudinal studies where patients with ET are followed over a long period of time are necessary to clarify the relationship between ET and PD, but these are lacking at the moment.[106]

In some cases, tremor associated with dystonia may be hard to differentiate from PD: dystonic symptoms often occur in patients with parkinsonism,[108] and dystonia can affect finger tapping, which could be mistaken for bradykinesia. In the past, dystonic tremor has frequently been misdiagnosed as PD, evidenced by large PD research studies showing that a significant number of patients (4–20%) enrolled did not have abnormal DAT-SPECT scans, which were labeled as SWEDD (scans without evidence of dopaminergic deficit).[109] In subsequent studies it was shown that a small number of these patients actually did have PD (with false negative scans), but most of them had a different etiology, especially dystonic tremor.[110,111] In general, position-dependent postural tremor is more prominent than rest tremor in case of dystonia. Furthermore, dystonic tremor has a jerkier character than Parkinson's tremor, the tremor movement is different (thumb extension tremor in dystonia; thumb flexion tremor in PD), dystonic tremor is more often position dependent compared to Parkinson's tremor, and there is no resetting phenomenon upon posturing in dystonic rest tremor.[27,88]

TREATMENT APPROACHES IN PARKINSONIAN TREMOR

As outlined previously, parkinsonism harbors multiple subtypes of tremor, each likely having its own pathophysiology. Therefore, the treatment of parkinsonian tremor should be tailored not only to the underlying etiology (e.g., PD), but also to the specific subtype of tremor. In this paragraph we will summarize the most important treatment strategies of parkinsonian tremor. For more extensive information we refer to Chapter 19: Treatment of tremor.

In PD, dopaminergic drugs are the first-choice therapy for treating rest and re-emergent tremor.[50] Some have suggested that dopamine agonists are superior and may even treat dopamine-resistant tremor; however, this has never been properly tested.[11] In addition to dopaminergic drugs, anticholinergic medication is an effective treatment for rest tremor as well,[64] but due to the frequent cognitive side effects (especially in elderly patients), their role is limited in daily practice. Beta-blockers may be used in PD patients with pure postural tremor or rest or re-emergent tremor that clearly increases with stress. However, strong empirical evidence regarding the effectiveness of beta-blockers in treating tremor is lacking.[112] Finally, in patients with

a multi-resistant tremor, clozapine can be tried, although the evidence for this is limited to a few case reports and there is a risk of serious side effects (agranulocytosis).[113]

In addition to these pharmacological treatments, stereotactic lesioning of both the basal ganglia (i.e., internal globus pallidus (GPi) and the subthalamic nucleus (STN)) and cerebello-thalamo-cortical circuit (i.e., ventrolateral intermediate nucleus of the thalamus (VIM)) are effective in treating tremor in PD.[69,85] Stereotactic interventions include deep brain stimulation (DBS) and focal lesioning. These effects appear similar for different subtypes of tremor including rest, postural, and action tremor, although no distinction between re-emergent and pure postural tremor was made.[114] Interestingly, DBS is an effective treatment of tremor regardless of the response to dopaminergic medication.[85] Although some of these patients may have been underdosed in terms of dopaminergic medication (i.e., pseudo-resistant), this also raises the possibility that the therapeutic effect of DBS on the specified regions is stronger than can be attained with dopaminergic medication, perhaps because multiple (non-dopaminergic) neurotransmitters are also involved. In addition to DBS, MR-guided focused ultrasound deep brain lesioning is another promising therapy. Specifically, high-intensity focused ultrasound is a noninvasive method that can induce a focal lesion in tremor-related brain areas such as the VIM, the GPi, or the STN.[115,116] Although initial results are promising,[117] large studies investigating the effectiveness and safety are still required.

In atypical parkinsonism, treatment of tremor is generally not one of the priorities, as other symptoms usually predominate the clinical spectrum. In general, a similar approach as in PD can be used, although treatment is often less effective. Specifically, levodopa can be tried to improve hypokinetic-rigid symptoms including rest tremor, but the effects are generally limited given the post- rather than pre-synaptic pathology in atypical parkinsonism.[118] Furthermore, there is some anecdotal evidence for the use of anticholinergics and beta-blockers, especially in the treatment of postural and action tremor.[119]

CONCLUSION

Besides the classical pill-rolling rest tremor, other types of tremor including postural and action tremor are frequently observed in PD and atypical parkinsonism. The pathophysiological substrate of parkinsonian tremor involves both the basal ganglia and the cerebello-thalamo-cortical circuit, as well as multiple neurotransmitter systems (dopamine, noradrenalin, serotonin). However, these mechanisms may be different on a patient-to-patient basis, and they also vary between tremor phenotypes (rest tremor, re-emergent tremor, pure postural tremor). Advances in the recognition of specific subtypes and their underlying pathophysiology may help the development of new tailor-made treatments.

REFERENCES

1. Bhatia KP, Bain P, Bajaj N, et al. Consensus statement on the classification of tremors. from the task force on tremor of the International Parkinson and Movement Disorder Society. *Mov Disord.* 2018;33(1):75–87. doi:10.1002/mds.27121

2. Parkinson J. *Essay on the Shaking Palsy.* Sherwood, Neely, and Jones. Published online 1817.

3. Deuschl G, Krack P, Lauk M, Timmer J. Clinical neurophysiology of tremor. *J Clin Neurophysiol.* 1996;13(2):110–121. http://www.ncbi.nlm.nih.gov/pubmed/8849966

4. Jankovic J. Parkinson's disease: clinical features and diagnosis. *J Neurol Neurosurg Psychiatry.* 2008;79(4):368–376. doi: 10.1136/jnnp.2007.131045

5. Toth C, Rajput M, Rajput AH. Anomalies of asymmetry of clinical signs in parkinsonism. *Mov Disord.* 2004;19(2):151–157. doi: 10.1002/mds.10685

6. Koh SB, Kwon DY, Seo WK, et al. Dissociation of cardinal motor signs in Parkinson's disease patients. *Eur Neurol.* 2010;63(5):307–310. doi: 10.1159/000314179

7. Raethjen J, Austermann K, Witt K, Zeuner KE, Papengut F, Deuschl G. Provocation of Parkinsonian tremor. *Mov Disord.* 2008;23(7):1019–1023. doi:10.1002/mds.22014

8. Zach H, Dirkx M, Bloem BRBR, Helmich RCRC. The clinical evaluation of Parkinson's tremor. *J Parkinsons Dis.* 2015;5(3):471–474. doi: 10.3233/JPD-150650

9. Papengut F, Raethjen J, Binder A, Deuschl G. Rest tremor suppression may separate essential from parkinsonian rest tremor. *Parkinsonism Relat Disord.* 2013;19(7):693–697. doi: 10.1016/j.parkreldis.2013.03.013

10. Obeso JA, Stamelou M, Goetz CG, et al. Past, present, and future of Parkinson's disease: a special essay on the 200th anniversary of the shaking palsy. *Mov Disord.* 2017;32(9):1264–1310. doi: 10.1002/mds.27115

11. Pogarell O, Gasser T, van Hilten JJ, et al. Pramipexole in patients with Parkinson's disease and marked drug resistant tremor: a randomised, double blind, placebo controlled multicentre study. *J Neurol Neurosurg Psychiatry.* 2002;72(6):713–720. http://www.ncbi.nlm.nih.gov/pubmed/12023411

12. Nonnekes J, Timmer MH, de Vries NM, Rascol O, Helmich RC, Bloem BR. Unmasking levodopa resistance in Parkinson's disease. *Mov Disord.* 2016;31(11):1602–1609. doi: 10.1002/mds.26712

13. Dirkx MFF, Zach H, Van Nuland A, Bloem BRR, Toni I, Helmich RCC. Cerebral differences between dopamine-resistant and dopamine-responsive Parkinson's tremor. *Brain.* 2019;142(10):3144–3157. doi: 10.1093/brain/awz261

14. Jankovic J, Schwartz KS, Ondo W. Re-emergent tremor of Parkinson's disease. *J Neurol Neurosurg Psychiatry.* 1999;67(5):646–650. http://www.ncbi.nlm.nih.gov/pubmed/10519872

15. Dirkx MFF, Zach H, Bloem BRR, Hallett M, Helmich RCC. The nature of postural tremor in Parkinson disease. *Neurology.* 2018;90(13):e1095–e1103. doi: 10.1212/WNL.0000000000005215

16. Louis ED, Frucht SJ. Prevalence of essential tremor in patients with Parkinson's disease vs. Parkinson-plus syndromes. *Mov Disord.* 2007;22(10):1402–1407. doi: 10.1002/mds.21383

17. Kraus PH, Lemke MR, Reichmann H. Kinetic tremor in Parkinson's disease—an underrated symptom. *J Neural Transm.* 2006;113(7):845–853. doi: 10.1007/s00702-005-0354-9

18. Wenzelburger R, Raethjen J, Löffler K, Stolze H, Illert M, Deuschl G. Kinetic tremor in a reach-to-grasp movement in Parkinson's disease. *Mov Disord.* 2000;15(6):1084–1094. doi: 10.1002/1531-8257(200011)15:6<1084::AID-MDS1005>3.0.CO;2-Y

19. Raethjen J, Pohle S, Govindan RB, Morsnowski A, Wenzelburger R, Deuschl G. Parkinsonian action tremor: interference with object manipulation and lacking levodopa response. *Exp Neurol.* 2005;194(1):151–160. doi: 10.1016/j.expneurol.2005.02.008

20. Leu-Semenescu S, Roze E, Vidailhet M, et al. Myoclonus or tremor in orthostatism: an under-recognized cause of unsteadiness in Parkinson's disease. *Mov Disord.* Published online 2007. doi: 10.1002/mds.21651

21. Hassan A, Van Gerpen JA. Orthostatic tremor and orthostatic myoclonus: weight-bearing hyperkinetic disorders: a systematic review, new insights, and unresolved questions. *Tremor Other Hyperkinet Mov.* 2016;6(0):417. doi: 10.5334/tohm.325

22. Liu K, Gu Z, Dong L, et al. Clinical profile of Parkinson's disease in the Gumei community of Minhang district, Shanghai. *Clinics.* Published online 2014. doi: 10.6061/clinics/2014(07)03

23. Uitti RJ, Baba Y, Wszolek ZK, Putzke DJ. Defining the Parkinson's disease phenotype: initial symptoms and baseline characteristics in a clinical

cohort. *Parkinsonism Relat Disord*. Published online 2005. doi: 10.1016/j.parkreldis.2004.10.007

24. Gigante AF, Pellicciari R, Iliceto G, et al. Rest tremor in Parkinson's disease: body distribution and time of appearance. *J Neurol Sci*. 2017;375:215–219. doi: 10.1016/j.jns.2016.12.057

25. Hughes AJ, Lees AJ, Daniel SE, Blankson S. A clinicopathologic study of 100 cases of Parkinson's disease. *Arch Neurol*. Published online 1993. doi: 10.1001/archneur.1993.00540020018011

26. Golbe LI, Di Iorio G, Bonavita V, Miller DC, Duvoisin RC. A large kindred with autosomal dominant Parkinson's disease. *Annals of Neurology*. Published online 1990. doi:10.1002/ana.410270309

27. Schwingenschuh P, Ruge D, Edwards MJ, et al. Distinguishing SWEDDs patients with asymmetric resting tremor from Parkinson's disease: a clinical and electrophysiological study. *Mov Disord*. 2010;25(5):560–569. doi:10.1002/mds.23019

28. Deuschl G, Bain P, Brin M. Consensus statement of the Movement Disorder Society on Tremor Ad hoc scientific committee. *Mov Disord*. 1998;13 (Suppl 3):2–23. https://www.ncbi.nlm.nih.gov/pubmed/9827589

29. Bain PG, Findley LJ, Atchison P, et al. Assessing tremor severity. *J Neurol Neurosurg Psychiatry*. Published online 1993. doi: 10.1136/jnnp.56.8.868

30. Thenganatt MA, Jankovic J. Parkinson disease subtypes. *JAMA Neurology*. 2014;71(4):499–504. doi: 10.1001/jamaneurol.2013.6233

31. Jankovic J, McDermott M, Carter J, et al. Variable expression of Parkinson's disease: a base-line analysis of the DATATOP cohort. The Parkinson Study Group. *Neurology*. 1990;40(10):1529–1534. https://www.ncbi.nlm.nih.gov/pubmed/2215943

32. Schiess MC, Zheng H, Soukup VM, Bonnen JG, Nauta HJW. Parkinson's disease subtypes: clinical classification and ventricular cerebrospinal fluid analysis. *Parkinsonism Relat Disord*. Published online 2000. doi: 10.1016/S1353-8020(99)00051-6

33. Dirkx MF, den Ouden H, Aarts E, et al. The cerebral network of Parkinson's tremor: an effective connectivity fMRI study. *J Neurosci*. 2016;36(19):5362–5372. doi: 10.1523/JNEUROSCI.3634-15.2016

34. Van Rooden SM, Heiser WJ, Kok JN, Verbaan D, Van Hilten JJ, Marinus J. The identification of Parkinson's disease subtypes using cluster analysis: a systematic review. *Mov Disord*. Published online 2010. doi: 10.1002/mds.23116

35. Lawton M, Baig F, Rolinski M, et al. Parkinson's disease subtypes in the Oxford Parkinson Disease Centre (OPDC) discovery cohort. *J Parkinson's Dis*. 2015;5(2):269–279. doi: 10.3233/jpd-140523

36. Fereshtehnejad SM, Zeighami Y, Dagher A, Postuma RB. Clinical criteria for subtyping Parkinson's disease: biomarkers and longitudinal progression. *Brain*. Published online 2017. doi: 10.1093/brain/awx118

37. Jankovic J, Kapadia AS. Functional decline in Parkinson disease. *Arch Neurol*. Published online 2001. doi: 10.1001/archneur.58.10.1611

38. Forsaa EB, Larsen JP, Wentzel-Larsen T, Alves G. What predicts mortality in Parkinson disease? *Neurology*. Published online 2010. doi: 10.1212/WNL.0B013E3181F61311

39. Lo RY, Tanner CM, Albers KB, et al. Clinical features in early Parkinson disease and survival. *Arch Neurol*. Published online 2009. doi: 10.1001/archneurol.2009.221

40. Selikhova M, Williams DR, Kempster PA, Holton JL, Revesz T, Lees AJ. A clinico-pathological study of subtypes in Parkinson's disease. *Brain*. Published online 2009. doi: 10.1093/brain/awp234

41. Burn DJ, Landau S, Hindle JV, et al. Parkinson's disease motor subtypes and mood. *Mov Disord*. Published online 2012. doi: 10.1002/mds.24041

42. Nègre-Pagès L, Grandjean H, Lapeyre-Mestre M, et al. Anxious and depressive symptoms in Parkinson's disease: the French cross-sectionnal DoPAMiP study. *Mov Disord*. 2010;25(2):157–166. doi: 10.1002/mds.22760

43. Alves G, Larsen JP, Emre M, Wentzel-Larsen T, Aarsland D. Changes in motor subtype and risk for incident dementia in Parkinson's disease. *Mov Disord*. Published online 2006. doi: 10.1002/mds.20897

44. Iijima M, Kobayakawa T, Saito S, et al. Differences in odor identification among clinical subtypes of Parkinson's disease. *Eur J Neurol*. Published online 2011. doi: 10.1111/j.1468-1331.2010.03167.x

45. Politis M, Wu K, Molloy S, Bain PG, Chaudhuri KR, Piccini P. Parkinson's disease symptoms: the patient's perspective. *Mov Disord*. 2010;25(11):1646–1651. doi: 10.1002/mds.23135

46. Simuni T, Caspell-Garcia C, Coffey C, Lasch S, Tanner C, Marek K. How stable are Parkinson's disease subtypes in de novo patients?: analysis of the PPMI cohort *Parkinsonism Relat Disord*. Published online 2016. doi: 10.1016/j.parkreldis.2016.04.027

47. Louis ED, Tang MX, Cote L, Alfaro B, Mejia H, Marder K. Progression of parkinsonian signs in Parkinson disease. *Arch Neurol*. 1999;56(3):334–337. https://www.ncbi.nlm.nih.gov/pubmed/10190824

48. Pirker W. Correlation of dopamine transporter imaging with parkinsonian motor handicap: how close is it? *Mov Disord*. 2003;18(Suppl 7):S43–S51. doi: 10.1002/mds.10579

49. Koller WC, Hubble JP. Levodopa therapy in Parkinson's disease. *Neurology*. 1990;40(10 Suppl 3):Suppl 40–7; discussion 47–9. https://www.ncbi.nlm.nih.gov/pubmed/2215973

50. Connolly BS, Lang AE. Pharmacological treatment of Parkinson disease: a review. *JAMA*. 2014;311(16):1670–1683. doi: 10.1001/jama.2014.3654

51. Helmich RC, Janssen MJ, Oyen WJ, Bloem BR, Toni I. Pallidal dysfunction drives a cerebellothalamic circuit into Parkinson tremor. *Ann Neurol*. 2011;69(2):269–281. doi: 10.1002/ana.22361

52. Pasquini J, Ceravolo R, Qamhawi Z, et al. Progression of tremor in early stages of Parkinson's disease: a clinical and neuroimaging study. *Brain*. Published online 2018. doi: 10.1093/brain/awx376

53. Dirkx MF, den Ouden HE, Aarts E, et al. Dopamine controls Parkinson's tremor by inhibiting the cerebellar thalamus. *Brain*. 2017;140(3):721–734. doi: 10.1093/brain/aww331

54. Sanchez-Gonzalez MA, Garcia-Cabezas MA, Rico B, Cavada C. The primate thalamus is a key target for brain dopamine. *J Neurosci*. 2005;25(26):6076–6083. doi: 10.1523/JNEUROSCI.0968-05.2005

55. Hirsch EC, Mouatt A, Faucheux B, et al. Dopamine, tremor, and Parkinson's disease. *Lancet*. 1992;340(8811):125–126. http://www.ncbi.nlm.nih.gov/pubmed/1352004

56. Qamhawi Z, Towey D, Shah B, et al. Clinical correlates of raphe serotonergic dysfunction in early Parkinson's disease. *Brain*. 2015;138(Pt 10):2964–2973. doi: 10.1093/brain/awv215

57. Lewis SJ, Pavese N, Rivero-Bosch M, et al. Brain monoamine systems in multiple system atrophy: a positron emission tomography study. *Neurobiol Dis*. 2012;46(1):130–136. doi: 10.1016/j.nbd.2011.12.053

58. Isaias IU, Marotta G, Pezzoli G, et al. Enhanced catecholamine transporter binding in the locus coeruleus of patients with early Parkinson disease. *BMC Neurol*. 2011;11:88. doi: 10.1186/1471-2377-11-88

59. Dirkx MF, Zach H, Nuland A van, Bloem BR, Toni I, Helmich RC. Cognitive load amplifies Parkinson's tremor through excitatory network influences onto the thalamus Journal: Published 2020. Accessed May 18, 2020. https://academic.oup.com/brain/advance-article-abstract/doi/10.1093/brain/awaa083/5827585

60. Isaias IU, Marzegan A, Pezzoli G, et al. A role for locus coeruleus in Parkinson tremor. *Front Hum Neurosci*. 2011;5:179. doi: 10.3389/fnhum.2011.00179

61. Barcroft H, Peterson E, Schwab RS. Action of adrenaline and noradrenaline on the tremor in Parkinson's disease. *Neurology*. 1952;2(2):154–160. http://www.ncbi.nlm.nih.gov/pubmed/14910821

62. Marsden CD, Owen DA. Mechanisms underlying emotional variation in parkinsonian tremor. *Neurology*. 1967;17(7):711–715. http://www.ncbi.nlm.nih.gov/pubmed/6067490

63. Schlesinger I, Benyakov O, Erikh I, Suraiya S, Schiller Y. Parkinson's disease tremor is diminished with relaxation guided imagery. *Mov Disord*. 2009;24(14):2059–2062. doi: 10.1002/mds.22671

64. Katzenschlager R, Sampaio C, Costa J, Lees A. Anticholinergics for symptomatic management of Parkinson's disease. *Cochrane Database Syst Rev*. 2003;(2):CD003735. doi: 10.1002/14651858.CD003735

65. Perez-Lloret S, Barrantes FJ. Deficits in cholinergic neurotransmission and their clinical correlates in Parkinson's disease. *NPJ Parkinsons Dis*. 2016;2(1). doi: 10.1038/npjparkd.2016.1

66. Timmermann L, Gross J, Dirks M, Volkmann J, Freund HJ, Schnitzler A. The cerebral oscillatory network of parkinsonian resting tremor. *Brain*. 2003;126(Pt 1):199–212. http://www.ncbi.nlm.nih.gov/pubmed/12477707

67. Mure H, Hirano S, Tang CC, et al. Parkinson's disease tremor-related metabolic network: characterization, progression, and treatment effects. *Neuroimage*. 2011;54(2):1244–1253. doi: 10.1016/j.neuroimage.2010.09.028

68. Lenz FA, Kwan HC, Martin RL, Tasker RR, Dostrovsky JO, Lenz YE. Single unit analysis of the human ventral thalamic nuclear group. Tremor-related activity in functionally identified cells. *Brain*. 1994;117 (Pt 3):531–543. http://www.ncbi.nlm.nih.gov/pubmed/8032863

69. Krack P, Pollak P, Limousin P, Benazzouz A, Benabid AL. Stimulation of subthalamic nucleus alleviates tremor in Parkinson's disease. *Lancet*. 1997;350(9092):1675. http://www.ncbi.nlm.nih.gov/pubmed/9400514

70. Benabid AL, Pollak P, Gervason C, et al. Long-term suppression of tremor by chronic stimulation of the ventral intermediate thalamic nucleus. *Lancet*. 1991;337(8738):403–406. http://www.ncbi.nlm.nih.gov/pubmed/1671433

71. Lozano AM, Lang AE, Galvez-Jimenez N, et al. Effect of GPi pallidotomy on motor function in Parkinson's disease. *Lancet*. 1995;346(8987):1383–1387. http://www.ncbi.nlm.nih.gov/pubmed/7475819

72. Llinas RR. The intrinsic electrophysiological properties of mammalian neurons: insights into central nervous system function. *Science (80-)*. 1988;242(4886):1654–1664. https://www.ncbi.nlm.nih.gov/pubmed/3059497

73. Jahnsen H, Llinas R. Ionic basis for the electroresponsiveness and oscillatory properties of guinea-pig thalamic neurones in vitro. *J Physiol*. 1984;349:227–247. https://www.ncbi.nlm.nih.gov/pubmed/6737293

74. Magnin M, Morel A, Jeanmonod D. Single-unit analysis of the pallidum, thalamus and

subthalamic nucleus in parkinsonian patients. *Neuroscience.* 2000;96(3):549–564. http://www.ncbi.nlm.nih.gov/pubmed/10717435

75. Bergman H, Feingold A, Nini A, et al. Physiological aspects of information processing in the basal ganglia of normal and parkinsonian primates. *Trends Neurosci.* 1998;21(1):32–38. http://www.ncbi.nlm.nih.gov/pubmed/9464684

76. Cagnan H, Little S, Foltynie T, et al. The nature of tremor circuits in parkinsonian and essential tremor. *Brain.* 2014;137(Pt 12):3223–3234. doi: 10.1093/brain/awu250

77. Raz A, Vaadia E, Bergman H. Firing patterns and correlations of spontaneous discharge of pallidal neurons in the normal and the tremulous 1-methyl-4-phenyl-1,2,3,6-tetrahydropyridine vervet model of parkinsonism. *J Neurosci.* 2000;20(22):8559–8571. http://www.ncbi.nlm.nih.gov/pubmed/11069964

78. Hurtado JM, Lachaux JP, Beckley DJ, Gray CM, Sigvardt KA. Inter- and intralimb oscillator coupling in parkinsonian tremor. *Mov Disord.* 2000;15(4):683–691. https://www.ncbi.nlm.nih.gov/pubmed/10928579

79. Pollak P, Krack P, Fraix V, et al. Intraoperative micro- and macrostimulation of the subthalamic nucleus in Parkinson's disease. *Mov Disord.* 2002;17 (Suppl 3):S155–S61. http://www.ncbi.nlm.nih.gov/pubmed/11948771

80. Lenz FA, Tasker RR, Kwam HC, et al. Single unit analysis of the human ventral thalamic nuclear group: correlation of thalamic "tremor cells" with the 3–6 Hz component of Parkinsonian tremor. *J Neurosci.* Published online 1988. doi: 10.1523/jneurosci.08-03-00754.1988

81. Hurtado JM, Gray CM, Tamas LB, Sigvardt KA. Dynamics of tremor-related oscillations in the human globus pallidus: a single case study. *Proc Natl Acad Sci U S A.* 1999;96(4):1674–1679. http://www.ncbi.nlm.nih.gov/pubmed/9990083

82. Helmich RC, Hallett M, Deuschl G, Toni I, Bloem BR. Cerebral causes and consequences of parkinsonian resting tremor: a tale of two circuits? *Brain.* 2012;135(Pt 11):3206–3226. doi: 10.1093/brain/aws023

83. Brittain JS, Probert-Smith P, Aziz TZ, Brown P. Tremor suppression by rhythmic transcranial current stimulation. *Curr Biol.* 2013;23(5):436–440. doi: 10.1016/j.cub.2013.01.068

84. Brittain JS, Cagnan H, Mehta AR, Saifee TA, Edwards MJ, Brown P. Distinguishing the central drive to tremor in Parkinson's disease and essential tremor. *J Neurosci.* 2015;35(2):795–806. doi: 10.1523/jneurosci.3768-14.2015

85. Lozano AM, Dostrovsky J, Chen R, Ashby P. Deep brain stimulation for Parkinson's disease: disrupting the disruption. *Lancet Neurol.*

2002;1(4):225–231. https://www.ncbi.nlm.nih.gov/pubmed/12849455

86. Hirschmann J, Abbasi O, Storzer L, et al. Longitudinal recordings reveal transient increase of alpha/low-beta power in the subthalamic nucleus associated with the onset of parkinsonian rest tremor. *Front Neurol.* Published online 2019. doi: 10.3389/fneur.2019.00145

87. Helmich RC. The cerebral basis of Parkinsonian tremor: a network perspective. *Mov Disord.* Published online 2017. doi:10.1002/mds.27224

88. Van De Wardt J, van der Stouwe AMM, Dirkx M, et al. Systematic clinical approach for diagnosing upper limb tremor. Published online 2020:1–9. doi: 10.1136/jnnp-2019-322676

89. Kaindlstorfer C, Granata R, Wenning GK. Tremor in multiple system atrophy—a review. *Tremor Other Hyperkinet Mov (N Y).* 2013;3:1–9. doi: 10.7916/D8NV9GZ9

90. Salazar G, Valls-Solé J, Martí MJ, Chang H, Tolosa ES. Postural and action myoclonus in patients with parkinsonian type multiple system atrophy. *Mov Disord.* Published online 2000. doi: 10.1002/1531-8257(200001)15:1<77::AID-MDS1013>3.0.CO;2-N

91. Wenning GK, Geser F, Krismer F, et al. The natural history of multiple system atrophy: a prospective European cohort study. *Lancet Neurol.* Published online 2013. doi: 10.1016/S1474-4422(12)70327-7

92. Okuma Y, Fujishima K, Miwa H, Mori H, Mizuno Y. Myoclonic tremulous movements in multiple system atrophy are a form of cortical myoclonus. *Mov Disord.* Published online 2005. doi: 10.1002/mds.20346

93. Wenning GK, Ben Shlomo Y, Magalhães M, Danie SE, Quinn NP. Clinical features and natural history of multiple system atrophy: an analysis of 100 cases. *Brain.* Published online 1994. doi: 10.1093/brain/117.4.835

94. Fujioka S, Algom AA, Murray ME, et al. Tremor in progressive supranuclear palsy. *Parkinsonism Relat Disord.* Published online 2016. doi: 10.1016/j.parkreldis.2016.03.015

95. Shimohata T, Aiba I, Nishizawa M. Criteria for the diagnosis of corticobasal degeneration. *Brain Nerve.* 2015;67(4):513–523. doi: 10.11477/mf.1416200168

96. Mahapatra RK, Edwards MJ, Schott JM, Bhatia KP. Corticobasal degeneration. *Neurology.* 2004;3(December):736–743. http://www.ncbi.nlm.nih.gov/pubmed/15556806

97. G.K. W, S. K, K. S, et al. Prevalence of movement disorders in men and women aged 50–89 years (Bruneck Study cohort): a population-based study. *Lancet Neurol.* Published online 2005.

98. Shin HW, Chung SJ. Drug-induced parkinsonism. *J Clin Neurol.* 2012;8(1):15–21. doi: 10.3988/jcn.2012.8.1.15

99. Nisticò R, Fratto A, Vescio B, et al. Tremor pattern differentiates drug-induced resting tremor from Parkinson disease. *Parkinsonism Relat Disord*. 2016;25:100–103. doi: 10.1016/j.parkreldis.2016.02.002

100. Kalra S, Grosset DG, Benamer HTS. Differentiating vascular parkinsonism from idiopathic Parkinson's disease: a systematic review. *Mov Disord*. 2010;25(2):149–156. doi: 10.1002/mds.22937

101. Rampello L, Alvano A, Battaglia G, Raffaele R, Vecchio I, Malaguarnera M. Different clinical and evolutional patterns in late idiopathic and vascular parkinsonism. *J Neurol*. 2005;252(9):1045–1049. doi: 10.1007/s00415-005-0811-2

102. Demirkiran M, Bozdemir H, Sarica Y. Vascular parkinsonism: a distinct, heterogeneous clinical entity. *Acta Neurol Scand*. 2001;104(2):63–67. doi: 10.1034/j.1600-0404.2001.104002063.x

103. Josephs KA, Matsumoto JY, Ahlskog JE. Benign tremulous parkinsonism. *Arch Neurol*. Published online 2006. doi: 10.1001/archneur.63.3.354

104. Fekete R, Jankovic J. Revisiting the relationship between essential tremor and Parkinson's disease. *Mov Disord*. Published online 2011. doi: 10.1002/mds.23512

105. Stark RS, Walch J, Kägi G. The phenotypic variation of a parkin-related parkinson's disease family and the role of heterozygosity. *Mov Disord Clin Pract*. Published online 2019. doi: 10.1002/mdc3.12826

106. Algarni M, Fasano A. The overlap between essential tremor and Parkinson disease. *Parkinsonism Relat Disord*. 2018;46(Suppl 1):S101–S104. doi: 10.1016/j.parkreldis.2017.07.006

107. Thenganatt MA, Jankovic J. The relationship between essential tremor and Parkinson's disease. *Parkinsonism Relat Disord*. 2016;22 (Suppl 1):S162–5. doi: 10.1016/j.parkreldis.2015.09.032

108. Klepitskaya O, Neuwelt A, Nguyen T, Leehey M. Primary dystonia misinterpreted as Parkinson disease. *Neurol Clin Pract*. 2013;3(6):469–474.

109. Erro R, Schneider SA, Stamelou M, Quinn NP, Bhatia KP. What do patients with scans without evidence of dopaminergic deficit (SWEDD) have? New evidence and continuing controversies. *J Neurol Neurosurg Psychiatry*. Published online 2016. doi: 10.1136/jnnp-2014-310256

110. Menéndez-González M, Tavares F, Zeidan N, Salas-Pacheco JM, Arias-Carrión O. Diagnoses behind patients with hard-to-classify tremor and normal DaT-SPECT: a clinical follow up study. *Front Aging Neurosci*. Published online 2014. doi: 10.3389/fnagi.2014.00056

111. Schneider SA, Edwards MJ, Mir P, et al. Patients with adult-onset dystonic tremor resembling Parkinsonian tremor have scans without evidence of dopaminergic deficit (SWEDDs). *Mov Disord*. Published online 2007. doi: 10.1002/mds.21685

112. Crosby NJ, Deane KH, Clarke CE. Beta-blocker therapy for tremor in Parkinson's disease. *Cochrane Database Syst Rev*. 2003;(1):CD003361. doi: 10.1002/14651858.CD003361

113. Friedman JH. Atypical antipsychotic drugs in the treatment of Parkinson's disease. *J Pharm Pract*. 2011;24(6):534–540. doi: 10.1177/0897190011426556

114. Sturman MM, Vaillancourt DE, Metman LV, Bakay RA, Corcos DM. Effects of subthalamic nucleus stimulation and medication on resting and postural tremor in Parkinson's disease. *Brain*. 2004;127(Pt 9):2131–2143. doi: 10.1093/brain/awh237

115. Kinfe TM. Stereotactic MR-guided focused ultrasound deep brain lesioning: the resurrection of posteroventral pallidotomy and thalamotomy for PD? *Acta Neurochir (Wien)*. Published online 2017. doi: 10.1007/s00701-017-3161-9

116. R. M-F, R. R-R, M. del Á, et al. Focused ultrasound subthalamotomy in patients with asymmetric Parkinson's disease: a pilot study. *Lancet Neurol*. Published online 2018. doi: 10.1016/S1474-4422(17)30403-9 LK - http://sfx.library.uu.nl/utrecht?sid=EMBASE&issn=14744465&id=doi:10.1016%2FS1474-4422%2817%2930403-9&atitle=Focused+ultrasound+subthalamotomy+in+patients+with+asymmetric+Parkinson%27s+disease%3A+a+pilot+study&stitle=Lancet+Neurol.&title=The+Lancet+Neurology&volume=17&issue=1&spage=54&epage=63&aulast=Mart%C3%ADnez-Fern%C3%A1ndez&aufirst=Raul&auinit=R.&aufull=Mart%C3%ADnez-Fern%C3%A1ndez+R.&coden=LNAEA&isbn=&pages=54-63&date=2018&auinit1=R&auinitm=

117. Magara A, Bühler R, Moser D, Kowalski M, Pourtehrani P, Jeanmonod D. First experience with MR-guided focused ultrasound in the treatment of Parkinson's disease. *J Ther Ultrasound*. Published online 2014. doi: 10.1186/2050-5736-2-11

118. Stamelou M, Bhatia KP. A typical Parkinsonism diagnosis and treatment. *Neurol Clin*. Published online 2015. doi: 10.1016/j.ncl.2014.09.012

119. Levin J, Kurz A, Arzberger T, Giese A, Höglinger GU. The differential diagnosis and treatment of atypical parkinsonism. *Dtsch Arztebl Online*. Published online 2016. doi: 10.3238/arztebl.2016.0061

Tremor and Ataxia

CHEN-YA YANG AND SHENG-HAN KUO

INTRODUCTION

Tremor is characterized by rhythmic and oscillatory movements. Specifically, tremor can occur at rest or in action. When tremor occurs at rest, the rhythmic and oscillatory movements drive specific body parts to move from the rest state. When tremor happens during action, the volitional movements are entrained into specific rhythm, leading to the deviation from intended movements. On the other hand, the core feature for ataxia is irregularity and imprecision. For example, ataxia in the gait leads to variable in stride length and directions whereas ataxia in the hands causes overshoot in finger chase or incoordination in rhythmic, repetitive movements. Despite tremor and ataxia are seemingly distinctive movement disorders phenomenology, sometimes it is difficult to separate in the clinical setting because both movement patterns are causing the disruption of normal, volitional movements. Oftentimes, intentional tremor is difficult to discern from dysmetria. To add more to the issue, the pathophysiologies of tremor and ataxia are both related to the dysfunctional cerebellum. Clinically, patients with cerebellar ataxia can have tremor, and vice versa. These two symptoms are both very challenging to treat, causing a great deal of disability in patients with ataxia and tremor (Video 13.1).

Essential tremor is the prototypical tremor disorder. People with essential tremor suffer from involuntary, rhythmic, and oscillatory movement of the hands, head, and voice,[1] which can be highly disabling to one's ability to perform daily activities, such as writing, drawing, drinking, and eating. Recent neuroimaging studies[2,3] and pathological studies[4,5] have denoted that the cerebellum is one of the brain regions involved in tremor generation. In addition, essential tremor patients often demonstrate subtle signs of ataxia, such as impaired tandem gait.[6,7] In some essential tremor patients, frank gait ataxia can occur.[8] Therefore, essential tremor maybe considered as a disorder with prominent hand tremor and some gait ataxia. To better describe ataxia symptoms in essential tremor, the Movement Disorders Society Tremor Task Force Classification suggests some patients with essential tremor may be categorized into essential tremor plus (tremor with the characteristic essential tremor and additional neurological signs of uncertain significance such as impaired tandem gait).[1] In addition, it has been proposed that essential tremor with frank ataxia be called "tremor syndrome with prominent additional signs." As there are no defined criteria to distinguish what is "ataxia of uncertain significance" and what is "frank ataxia," these classifications may only be used for research and the use of these terms has recently been questioned.[9]

On the other end of the spectrum, classical ataxia patients can also have tremor. For example, patients with gait variability and discoordination in repetitive hand movements can also have oscillatory, rhythmic hand posture tremor. These patients often have prominent ataxia, whereas tremor can be an associated feature. Some ataxic disorders, such as spinocerebellar ataxia type 2 (SCA2) and SCA12, seem to have more tremor than is seen in ataxia disorders of other etiologies.

Understanding the phenotypic overlapping and underlying pathophysiology of different cerebellar disorders will help us advance the knowledge of ataxia and certain types of tremor, such as essential tremor and orthostatic tremor, which appear to have a cerebellar network origin. In addition to the cerebellum, the broader network of cerebello-thalamo-cortical loop is also implicated in both ataxia and tremor.[10–12] In this chapter, we will first review the current understanding of anatomy, physiology, and an animal model of ataxia and tremor, highlighting the symptomatology and distinct anatomy, and we will discuss the common ataxia disorders with tremor or common tremor disorders with ataxia.

CEREBELLAR ANATOMICAL CHANGES OF ATAXIA AND TREMOR

From the above-mentioned disorders, ataxia and tremor are two often co-occurring clinical symptoms related to cerebellar dysfunction. What are the structural changes in the cerebellum that could generate these two different types of clinical symptoms? To understand this, quantitative structural analysis of postmortem human brains with ataxia and tremor was performed.[13,14] The analysis included patients with essential tremor, a prototypical tremor disorder with relatively subtle ataxia, as well as patients with spinocerebellar ataxia type 1 (SCA1) and multiple system atrophy cerebellar type (MSA-C), two prototypical degenerative cerebellar ataxic disorders with some degree of tremor.

Purkinje cell loss as well as Purkinje cell axonal torpedoes were found in both essential tremor patients and cerebellar ataxia patients,[14,15] which are indicative of a cerebellar degenerative process. A system biology approach was implemented to further investigate the pathological signatures for ataxia and tremor.[13] Investigators found that while ataxic disorders and essential tremor share Purkinje cell loss and axonopathy, patients with ataxia have much more severe Purkinje cell pathology than patients with essential tremor. Among all the pathological features analyzed, climbing fiber synaptic pathology seems to differ between ataxia and tremor.[13,14] Essential tremor patients have climbing fiber synapses extending into the outer part of the molecular layer, which should have been the parallel fiber synaptic territory. On the other hand, this study observed that SCA1 and MSA-C cases had climbing fiber synapses distributed only in the inner part of the molecular layer, demonstrating regressive changes.[13,14] This is because climbing fibers originate from the inferior olive, which is known to be an intrinsic rhythm generator. The abnormal climbing fiber synaptic organization could directly contribute to the motor discoordination in tremor and ataxia. In fact, an animal model with essential tremor–like climbing fiber synaptic pathology can recapitulate the key tremor features and pharmacological responses of essential tremor patients,[16] which strongly supports the link between this cerebellar pathology and action tremor in essential tremor. Whether the regressive pathology of climbing fibers along with Purkinje cell degeneration can cause ataxia will require further studies. Future studies of more detailed, quantitative pathological analyses in broader tremor and ataxic disorders are required to elucidate the full pictures of neuropathology of tremor and ataxia.

PURKINJE CELL PATHOPHYSIOLOGY IN ATAXIA AND TREMOR

In addition to structural changes in the cerebellum, Purkinje cell firing patterns have been linked to ataxia and tremor. In several SCA mouse models, abnormal Purkinje cell firing patterns, specifically slow and irregular firing rates, have been identified.[17] On the other hand, harmaline-induced rodent tremor has enhanced the regularity of Purkinje cell firing patterns.[18] In other words, the clinical presentations of ataxia vs. tremor could depend on the particular spatial and temporal distribution of Purkinje cell firing patterns, and as the underlying disease progresses, Purkinje cell firing patterns might change over the disease course, generating diverse yet overlapping symptoms of ataxia and tremor. Most of the knowledge of pathophysiology of ataxia and tremor comes from animal model studies. Whether and to what degree these findings could be translated to patients for clinical applications requires further determination.

LEARNINGS FROM THE ANIMAL MODEL: INTERACTION BETWEEN TREMOR AND ATAXIA IN SHAKER RATS

One of the most studied animal models to help us understand tremor and ataxia is the Shaker rat. The Shaker rat is an animal model of spontaneous genetic mutation, resulting in progressive Purkinje cell degeneration and 5Hz whole-body tremor involving extremities, head, and trunk, as well as wide-based, ataxic movements. Interestingly, the Shaker rat exhibits bimodal distribution of tremor symptoms in that the tremor intensity peaks first at around 9 weeks and gradually reduces, with another peak at 23 weeks.[19] Tremor becomes less as the Shaker rats get even older; however, the overall motor coordination becomes worse during aging, suggesting the progression of ataxia.[19] Therefore, the stereotypical progression of tremor and ataxia, modulated by aging, can help us to understand the pathological underpinning of ataxia and tremor. In pathological analysis, Shaker rats have age-dependent Purkinje cell loss in the anterior lobe,[20] suggesting that a milder form of Purkinje cell degenerative changes may be associated with tremor, whereas severe Purkinje cell loss may result in ataxia. The detailed pathological underpinning and causal relationship still requires further determination. Interestingly, deep brain stimulation (DBS) in the bilateral dorsal dentate nuclei could improve ataxia and tremor at 30Hz stimulation, whereas stimulation over 100Hz did not suppress tremor but worsened ataxia in Shaker rats.[19] These data suggest that cerebellar DBS may hold promise in normalizing brain circuitry for tremor and ataxia but fine-tuning the specific targets and frequency of stimulation could be important.

While Shaker rats are valuable tools to study tremor and ataxia, human tremor and ataxia disorders often become worse over time, rather than evolving from tremor to ataxia. In addition, the determination of specific tremor types (action vs. rest) and cerebellar physiology will be important for us to further understand the interactions of tremor and ataxia.

HOLMES TREMOR

Holmes tremor was first described by Gordon Holmes as a 3–4 Hz flexion-extension oscillatory movement, which is present at rest, aggravated by posture, and further intensified with action.[21] The Consensus Statement of the Movement Disorder Society on Tremor further defines Holmes tremor as a syndrome of rest, postural, and intention tremor that usually emerges from proximal and distal rhythmic muscle contraction at low frequency (<5 Hz).[22]

Holmes tremor is caused by lesions in the cerebellar outflow tract (i.e., the connection between the cerebellum and the thalamus) or the nigrostriatal system.[23,24] Sometimes lesions in the red nucleus, thus termed rubral tremor, can also produce similar rest, postural, and intention tremor of low frequency and may be incorporated into a broader Holmes tremor category. However, whether a discrete lesion in the red nucleus could produce tremor is still under debate, since experimental lesions in animal models fail to elicit persistent tremor.[25–27] Holmes tremor can be produced by lesions in distinct brain circuitry, demonstrating that similar tremor syndromes may have either a cerebellar or a non-cerebellar pathway.

Holmes tremor usually develops between 1 and 24 months after insults to the cerebello-thalamo-cortical or nigrostriatal circuits, which suggests the underlying plastic reorganizing process, rather than merely loss of functional connectivity.[27] Some Holmes tremor patients may have multiple lesions along these brain circuits,[28–30] whereas others may have micro-lesions not observed in neuroimaging.[31] A rare report of Holmes tremor pathology showed neuronal loss in the cerebellar cortex, dentate nucleus, and inferior olive.[32] Holmes tremor associated with cerebellar network lesions is often associated with appendicular ataxia in the same limb(s) and gait ataxia.

Pharmacologic treatment is often unsatisfactory but should be tried. Clonazepam and levodopa treatment can provide some degree of symptomatic relief.[33–36] Surgeries such as thalamotomy or DBS can be an option for drug-resistant cases. The DBS targets for Holmes tremor include the ventral intermediate nucleus of the thalamus (VIM), the subthalamic nucleus (STN), and the globus pallidus interna (GPi), yet the most optimal target for treating Holmes tremor is still under debate,[37,38] and the efficacy is variable.[39] It is possible that optimal targets for DBS may depend on the brain circuits involved. For example, VIM DBS might be useful for Holmes tremor with predominant cerebello-thalamo-cortical dysfunction, whereas STN or GPi DBS might be helpful for Holmes tremor with predominant nigrostriatal involvement.

TREMOR IN MULTIPLE SCLEROSIS

The cerebellum is a commonly affected brain region in multiple sclerosis,[40] and a subset of patients with multiple sclerosis lesions in either cerebellar white matter (i.e., myelinated Purkinje cell axons) or cerebellar outflow tracts will develop tremor. Therefore, certain type of multiple sclerosis–related tremor may be regarded as Holmes tremor.[41]

The prevalence of tremor in multiple sclerosis patients is approximately 25–60%, with severe tremor in 3–15% of the multiple sclerosis patients.[42,43] Tremor in multiple sclerosis is often observed in upper extremities and associated with truncal titubation, which has a detrimental effect on gait and balance. Tremor often confers a great impact on daily function in multiple sclerosis patients.[44] Intention tremor and postural tremor are two major components in multiple sclerosis tremor.

Multiple sclerosis tremor secondary to cerebellar pathway lesions is often refractory to pharmacological intervention. Several medications were tested mainly for either multiple sclerosis–related postural or kinetic tremor, including cannabis, propranolol, levetiracetam, ondansetron, isoniazid. However, treatment options were proven to be ineffective or yielded variable results across studies.[45-49] Some medications have unfavorable side effect profiles that are poorly tolerated.[50-52] Due to unsatisfactory results from pharmacological treatments, surgical intervention such as VIM thalamotomy and VIM DBS were studied in multiple sclerosis tremor. Most of the studies are small-scale retrospective studies with suboptimal qualitative measurement. However, immediate tremor reduction after thalamotomy can be observed in almost all patients, and approximately 70% of patients continue to benefit from thalamotomy even after a follow-up period of one year.[53] Sixty-nine percent to 100% of the patients experienced tremor reduction in three studies on VIM DBS with a follow-up period longer than one year.[54,55] Despite observations of multiple sclerosis tremor reduction after surgical intervention, the degree of functional improvement after surgeries varies.

The major obstacle to therapy development for multiple sclerosis tremor is that multiple sclerosis tremor involves heterogeneous brain circuitries and has overlapping clinical presentations. Therefore, therapies targeting a specific subgroup of multiple sclerosis tremor that shares similar pathologic brain circuitries or tremor subtypes (postural vs. action vs. intention) are likely to be the key to future clinical trials. For example, isoniazid has been shown to be effective specifically for action tremor, whereas levetiracetam has no effects on intention tremor in multiple sclerosis patients.[49,56,57] The detailed documentation and separation of different tremor subtypes and ataxia symptoms will shed light on pharmacological responses in multiple sclerosis patients.

FRAGILE X-ASSOCIATED TREMOR ATAXIA SYNDROME

Fragile X-associated tremor/ataxia syndrome (FXTAS) is a late-onset neurodegenerative disorder most frequently seen in male premutation carriers (CGG repeat expansions of 55–200 repeats) of the *FMR1* gene on the X chromosome.

Tremor is the most frequent symptom and is seen in 80% of patients; cerebellar ataxia involving mainly gait is seen in 50%, and parkinsonism in 30%.[58] Most patients have mixed tremor, with both rest and action tremor. In addition to motor features, cognitive deficits are common, especially progressive loss of executive functions and early-onset dementia.[58] Patients with FXTAS also have increased risk of anxiety and depression.[59,60] Besides cognitive and aforementioned motor symptoms, FXTAS can also be a multisystemic disorder with an increased incidence of neuropathy, sleep disorders, autonomic dysfunction, thyroid diseases, fibromyalgia, migraine, and hypertension.[61] FXTAS also has age-dependent penetrance, and patients often begin to develop symptoms in their early sixties. Magnetic resonance imaging in FXTAS patients often shows T2-hyperintensity in the bilateral middle cerebellar peduncles, which is characteristic for this disease (Figure 13.1).

The prevalence of the *FMR1* premutation is 1 in 150–300 females, and 1 in 400–850 males.[62] Approximately 40% of men and 8–16% of women carrying premutations will develop FXTAS.[63] This corresponds to an estimated prevalence of FXTAS among the general population of around 1 in 2,000 for both women and men over the age of 50.[64]

The premutation of the *FMR1* gene (55–200 CGG triplets) leads to the production of expanded messenger RNA, which initiates a mechanism that is toxic to the central nervous system. On the other hand, fragile X syndrome is caused by the full mutation of *FMR1* gene (> 200 CGG triplets), resulting in silencing the *FMR1* gene expression. Therefore, molecular therapies for FXTAS and fragile X syndrome should target different disease mechanisms.

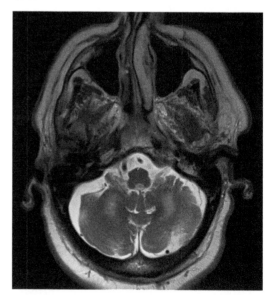

FIGURE 13.1: Neuroimaging Features of FXTAS. T2 hyperintensity in the bilateral middle cerebellar peduncles in a patient with fragile X-associated ataxia and tremor syndrome.

FMR1-associated conditions exhibit X-linked inheritance pattern. However, in male carriers, unexplained mechanisms that occur during spermatogenesis prevent further triplet repeat expansions.[65] As a result, continuing expansion of triplet repeats usually occurs in female germ cells only, and that is the reason why fragile X syndrome almost exclusively affects children of female premutation carriers. A typical family history is maternal grandfather with FXTAS and the grandson with fragile X syndrome.[66] Detailed family history is therefore crucial to the initial diagnostic workup. It is important to ask whether an individual's first- or second-degree relatives include women with early menopause, indicating premature ovarian failure; persons over the age of 50 with ataxia, tremor, and/or parkinsonism features; or children diagnosed with developmental disorders.[67]

Current treatment for FXTAS is mainly symptomatic. Various medications have been reported to be beneficial on tremor in case studies; these medications include primidone, β-blockers, and levetiracetam.[68,69] Memantine failed to demonstrate clinical efficacy on tremor in FXTAS in a randomized controlled trial.[70] Case reports show that DBS to either the ventro-oralis posterior thalamic nucleus and zona incerta or the VIM has produced mixed results in FXTAS, often improving tremor but sometimes worsening gait ataxia and speech.[71,72] Therefore, this strategy is better reserved for patients with debilitating tremor but relatively subtle ataxia.

While FXTAS may also be considered a prototypical disorder for ataxia and tremor, the widespread brain pathology associated with multifaceted symptoms, including cognitive decline, makes it difficult to determine whether ataxia and tremor originate from the same source or an overlapping pathophysiological link. In the future, determining whether both ataxia and tremor will worsen as the disease progresses in the natural history study will provide important insight. Finally, intervention studies showing that VIM DBS can improve tremor but worsen ataxia give us some clues that the cerebellum could be involved in both ataxia and tremor in FXTAS, and that perhaps a different pathophysiology of the cerebellum governs these two symptoms.

TREMOR IN SPINOCEREBELLAR ATAXIA (SCA)

SCAs are autosomal dominant neurodegenerative disorders involving the cerebellum and related brain structures.[73] While gait disturbance is the predominant feature of SCAs,[74] tremor, especially intention tremor, could be observed in the majority of SCA patients.[75] In addition to intention tremor, postural tremor, and, to a lesser degree, rest tremor can sometimes occur in SCA patients (Video 13.2).[75]

Among all SCAs, SCA2 and SCA12 are known to present with tremor in the early disease stage, and can be a predominant feature[76,77] Tremor in SCA2 is often characterized as postural intention tremor with hyporeflexia and slow saccades, whereas SCA12 patients typically have hyperreflexia and action tremor.[75,78] Rest tremor can occur in SCA2 and SCA3 patients in the setting of parkinsonism features, which can present in isolation, before ataxic features become manifest in later stages, or can co-exist with ataxia.[79] Among SCA patients with tremor, the severity of tremor increases as the ataxia progresses,[80] suggesting that an underlying pathomechanism aggravates the motor discoordination of both ataxia and tremor.

SCA42 patients have genetic mutations in *CACNA1G*, which encodes the T-type calcium channel, Cav3.1, and patients with SCA42 have ataxia and often tremor.[81,82] In addition, recent genetic studies in an essential tremor family have also identified mutations in *CACNA1G*, highlighting the role of the T-type calcium channel in ataxia and tremor.[83]

Currently, no Food and Drug Administration (FDA)-approved treatment is available for SCAs. Some studies showed encouraging promises to improve ataxia severity and perhaps also help tremor. Riluzole is considered a treatment option for SCAs and has shown some clinical benefits in gait, ataxia, dysarthria, and even intention tremor.[84,85] While these two studies included heterogeneous cerebellar disorders, a significant proportion of patients were genetically confirmed SCAs. Another small double-blind, placebo-controlled, randomized trial of 20 patients demonstrates that varenicline can help with ataxic symptoms, including intention tremor, in SCA3 patients.[86] Sometimes medications for essential tremor can be used for postural and intention tremor in SCAs, such as propranolol or primidone.[87] Rest tremor in SCAs sometimes responds to levodopa.[88,89]

DBS in the subthalamic-thalamic region or VIM has been reported to improve pharmacologically refractory tremor in a patient with SCA2.[90,91] VIM DBS was used to treat severe action tremor in 2 SCA6 patients, 1 SCA31 patient, and 2 sporadic ataxia patients with good tremor suppressing effects.[92] Another report also demonstrated the beneficial effects of VIM DBS on tremor in a SCA2 patient.[93] However, the utility of DBS in patients with SCA is currently not entirely clear because there are only a few case reports. The optimal brain targets to treat both ataxia and tremor in SCAs remain to be determined. One of the concerns is that VIM DBS could worsen ataxia, as it does in patients with essential tremor.[94] The novel directional leads of DBS and/or closed-loop design to deliver currents and voltages based on the physiological signals could hold promise in future therapies for tremor in SCAs.[95]

ATAXIA WITH VITAMIN E DEFICIENCY

Ataxia with vitamin E deficiency (AVED) is a progressive neurologic disorder affecting motor control and balance. AVED is caused by autosomal recessive mutations of the *TTPA* gene, which encodes the α-tocopherol transfer protein.[96] The α-Tocopherol transfer protein is responsible for transporting vitamin E, an antioxidant. Therefore, patients with *TTPA* gene mutations will have vitamin E deficiency and neuronal vulnerability to oxidative stress.[97] Individuals with AVED generally manifest ataxic symptoms between ages 5 and 15 years.[98] One of the key features for AVED is head tremor, which can be characteristic; therefore, it is mentioned in this chapter. Other associated features are peripheral neuropathy and retinitis pigmentosa. Treatment for AVED is oral vitamin E supplements, which will prevent or slow down ataxia progression. However, the specific effect of vitamin E in head tremor is unclear and yet to be determined.[99]

MULTIPLE SYSTEM ATROPHY (MSA)

MSA is a rare adult-onset neurodegenerative disorder characterized by progressive autonomic dysfunction, cerebellar ataxia, and parkinsonism. Depending on the predominant symptoms, MSA can be further divided into parkinsonian type (MSA-P) or cerebellar type (MSA-C). Autonomic dysfunction is a shared characteristic in both types of MSAs and can be the initial clinical presentation.[100]

Up to 80% of MSA patients have some degree of tremor; MSA-P patients are more commonly affected.[101] Postural tremor has been documented in about half of the MSA population and is frequently referred to as jerky postural tremor, with overlapping features of mini-polymyoclonus on neurophysiological examination.[101-103] In contrast to Parkinson disease, rest tremor has been reported in about one-third of MSA patients, and only 10% show typical parkinsonian "pill-rolling" rest tremor.[104,105] Some patients exhibit intention tremor associated with cerebellar dysmetria in the same limb, particularly in MSA-C patients.[102,103]

MSA has a prevalence of 1.9–4.9 cases per 100,000[106,107] and an incidence of 0.6/100,000, occurring in up to 3/100,000 in people older than 50 years.[108] Onset of MSA usually occurs during the sixth decade of life, and MSA-C patients generally have slower progression than MSA-P patients.

The pathological hallmark of MSA is the accumulation of aggregated α-synuclein in oligodendrocytes, forming glial cytoplasmic inclusions on either the striatonigral or olivopontocerebellar system, or both.[109] This complex neuropathology may explain why MSA patients can have more than one tremor type. The relative extent and degree of pathological changes in the aforementioned brain regions may explain the emergence of largely diverse clinical presentations of tremor.[110] The pathophysiological basis underlying the distinct manifestations of tremor remains to be studied in detail.

Tremor in MSA is usually not a significant target for pharmacological intervention, since akinesia-rigidity and dysautonomia pose even more debilitating impact on a patient's quality of life.[111] Amantadine has shown to improve parkinsonian symptoms in MSA, including tremor.[112]

POST-TRAUMATIC TREMOR

Tremor following traumatic brain injury is usually associated with insults to the cerebellum. The symptoms can occur within months to years after the trauma incident with variable manifestations, including rest, postural, kinetic, and intention tremor.[113] Occasionally, the tremor can exhibit a dystonic component as well. Similar to Holmes tremor or multiple sclerosis tremor, the delayed occurrence of tremor following traumatic brain injury suggests that plastic reorganization of the brain circuitry is required for tremor generation. Therefore, the secondary ataxia and tremor syndromes (Holmes tremor, multiple sclerosis tremor, and post-traumatic tremor) may have distinct pathomechanisms from primary ataxia and tremor syndromes (FXTAS, SCA and MSA).

A survey of 221 traumatic brain injury patients who were admitted with a Glasgow Coma Scale score of 8 or less showed that 19% of them developed tremor, with significant associations between generalized brain edema and the later development of kinetic tremor.[114] This study indicates that more severe brain trauma could predict the likelihood of tremor development. However, the underlying pathomechanisms and plastic reorganization of post-traumatic tremor are still not clear. Post-traumatic tremor is a unique research topic in terms of understanding tremor because there is a defined time course from insult to tremor emergence, which can be monitored by neuroimaging in patients or studied in animal models. Understanding the plastic reorganization of post-traumatic tremor will shed light on the mechanism of tremor generation.

Pharmacological treatment of post-traumatic tremors is challenging. Propranolol and primidone could be used to treat postural and intention tremor, and levodopa can be tried for rest tremor. Dystonia component of tremor can be treated with botulinum toxin. DBS for post-traumatic tremor has been proven less successful than for essential tremor or parkinsonian tremor. So far, VIM is the most well-established target, with evidence to support its efficacy.[115] However, other concomitant symptoms in post-traumatic disorder might limit the benefit of DBS, such as psychological and cognitive deficits, ataxia, dysarthria, paresis, and oculomotor deficits.[116]

UNSOLVED QUESTIONS AND FUTURE RESEARCH DIRECTION

Ataxia and tremor (mainly action tremor) are two predominant symptoms that may occur in patients with cerebellar disorders. While these two symptoms are phenomenologically distinct, both are very challenging to treat. To develop effective symptomatic treatment for ataxia and tremor, we will need to have detailed understanding of the structural changes and brain circuitry alterations of ataxia and tremor, specifically, the postmortem human studies in diverse ataxia and tremor syndromes. In addition, DBS and transcranial direct current stimulations have been shown to be helpful in ataxia and tremor patients.[117] However, it still remains unknown how to monitor cerebellar physiology in real time to fine-tune the stimulation targets and parameters, which can pose obstacles to effective neuromodulation. Studies have shown that cerebellar electroencephalogram or magnetoencephalogram can interrogate cerebellar activity.[16,118] Further studies will need to determine cerebellar physiology in patients with ataxia and patients with tremor. The combinatorial understanding of anatomical and physiological alterations in the cerebellum in ataxia and tremor will likely yield important therapeutic targets for future therapy development.

REFERENCES

1. Bhatia KP, et al. Consensus statement on the classification of tremors from the task force on tremor of the International Parkinson and Movement Disorder Society. *Mov Disord*. 2018;33(1):75–87.
2. Cerasa A, Quattrone A. Linking essential tremor to the cerebellum—neuroimaging evidence. *Cerebellum*. 2016;15(3):263–275.
3. Schnitzler A, et al. Synchronized brain network associated with essential tremor as revealed by magnetoencephalography. *Mov Disord*. 2009;24(11):1629–1635.
4. Louis ED, et al. Neuropathological changes in essential tremor: 33 cases compared with 21 controls. *Brain*. 2007;130(12): 3297–3307.
5. Lee D, et al. Climbing fiber-Purkinje cell synaptic pathology across essential tremor subtypes. *Parkinsonism Relat Disord*. 2018;51:24–29.
6. Arkadir D, Louis ED. The balance and gait disorder of essential tremor: what does this mean for patients? *Ther Adv Neurol Disord*. 2013;6(4):229–236.
7. Stolze H, et al. The gait disorder of advanced essential tremor. *Brain*. 2001;124(11):2278–2286.
8. Rao AK, Louis ED. Ataxic gait in essential tremor: a disease-associated feature? *Tremor Other Hyperkinet Mov (N Y)*. 2019;9. doi: 10.7916/d8-28jq-8t52.
9. Louis ED, et al. Essential tremor-plus: a controversial new concept. *Lancet Neurol*. 2020;19(3):266–270.
10. Hallett M. Tremor: pathophysiology. *Parkinsonism Relat Disord*. 2014;20(Suppl 1):S118–22.
11. Lenka A, et al. Role of altered cerebello-thalamo-cortical network in the neurobiology of essential tremor. *Neuroradiology*. 2017;59(2):157–168.
12. Muthuraman M, et al. Essential and aging-related tremor: differences of central control. *Mov Disord*. 2015;30(12):1673–1680.
13. Louis ED, et al. Contextualizing the pathology in the essential tremor cerebellar cortex: a patholog-omics approach. *Acta Neuropathol*. 2019;138(5):859–876.
14. Kuo SH, et al. Climbing fiber-Purkinje cell synaptic pathology in tremor and cerebellar degenerative diseases. *Acta Neuropathol*. 2017;133(1):121–138.
15. Louis ED, et al. Neuropathological changes in essential tremor: 33 cases compared with 21 controls. *Brain*. 2007;130(Pt 12):3297–307.

16. Pan MK, et al. Cerebellar oscillations driven by synaptic pruning deficits of cerebellar climbing fibers contribute to tremor pathophysiology. *Sci Transl Med.* 2020;12(526).

17. Jayabal S, et al. 4-aminopyridine reverses ataxia and cerebellar firing deficiency in a mouse model of spinocerebellar ataxia type 6. *Sci Rep.* 2016;6:29489.

18. Llinas R, Muhlethaler M. Electrophysiology of guinea-pig cerebellar nuclear cells in the in vitro brain stem-cerebellar preparation. *J Physiol.* 1988;404:241–258.

19. Anderson CJ, et al. Deep cerebellar stimulation reduces ataxic motor symptoms in the shaker rat. *Ann Neurol.* 2019;85(5):681–690.

20. Clark BR, LaRegina M, Tolbert DL. X-linked transmission of the shaker mutation in rats with hereditary Purkinje cell degeneration and ataxia. *Brain Res.* 2000;858(2):264–273.

21. Holmes G. On certain tremors in organic cerebral lesions. *Brain.* 1904;27(3):327–375.

22. Bhatia KP, et al. Consensus Statement on the classification of tremors. from the task force on tremor of the International Parkinson and Movement Disorder Society. *Mov Disord.* 2018;33(1):75–87.

23. Kim M, et al. Vim thalamotomy for Holmes' tremor secondary to midbrain tumour. *J Neurol, Neurosurg Psychiatry.* 2002;73(4):453–455.

24. Krack P, et al. Delayed onset of "rubral tremor" 23 years after brainstem trauma. *Mov Disord.* 1994;9(2):240–242.

25. Remy P, et al. Peduncular rubral tremor and dopaminergic denervation: a PET study. *Neurology.* 1995;45(3):472–477.

26. Rieder CR, Rebouças RG, Ferreira MP. Holmes tremor in association with bilateral hypertrophic olivary degeneration and palatal tremor: chronological considerations. Case report. *Arq Neuropsiquiatr.* 2003;61(2B):473–477.

27. Samie MR, Selhorst JB, Koller WC. *Post-traumatic midbrain tremors. Neurology.* 1990;40(1):62–66.

28. Shepherd GM, et al. Midbrain tremor and hypertrophic olivary degeneration after pontine hemorrhage. *Mov Disord.* 1997;12(3):432–437.

29. Defer G-L, et al. Rest tremor and extrapyramidal symptoms after midbrain haemorrhage: clinical and 18F-dopa PET evaluation. *J Neurol Neurosurg Psychiatry.* 1994;57(8):987–989.

30. Vidailhet M, et al. Pathology of symptomatic tremors. *Mov Disord.* 1998;13(S3):49–54.

31. Gajos A, et al. The clinical and neuroimaging studies in Holmes tremor. *Acta Neurol Scand.* 2010;122(5):360–366.

32. Rydz D, et al. Pathological findings of anti-Yo cerebellar degeneration with Holmes tremor. *J Neurol Neurosurg Psychiatry.* 2015;86(1):121–122.

33. Fujieda T, et al. Effect of levodopa on tremor in Benedikt's syndrome. *Br Med J.* 1974;1(5905):456.

34. Findley L, Gresty M. Suppression of "rubral" tremor with levodopa. *Br Med J.* 1980;281(6247):1043.

35. Woo JH, et al. Holmes tremor after brainstem hemorrhage, treated with levodopa. *Ann Rehab Med.* 2013;37(4):591.

36. Boelmans K, Gerloff C, Munchau A. Long-lasting effect of levodopa on holmes' tremor. *Mov Disord.* 2012;27(9):1097–1098.

37. Kudo M, et al. Bilateral thalamic stimulation for Holmes' tremor caused by unilateral brainstem lesion. *Mov Disord.* 2001;16(1):170–174.

38. Romanelli P, et al. Possible necessity for deep brain stimulation of both the ventralis intermedius and subthalamic nuclei to resolve Holmes tremor: case report. *J Neurosurg.* 2003;99(3):566–571.

39. Ramirez-Zamora A, Okun MS. Deep brain stimulation for the treatment of uncommon tremor syndromes. *Expert Rev Neurother.* 2016;16(8):983–997.

40. Wilkins A. Cerebellar dysfunction in multiple sclerosis. *Front Neurol.* 2017;8:312.

41. Boonstra F, et al. Tremor in multiple sclerosis is associated with cerebello-thalamic pathology. *J Neural Transm (Vienna).* 2017;124(12):1509–1514.

42. Pittock SJ, et al. Prevalence of tremor in multiple sclerosis and associated disability in the Olmsted County population. *Mov Disord.* 2004;19(12):1482–1485.

43. Alusi SH, et al. A study of tremor in multiple sclerosis. *Brain.* 2001;124(4):720–730.

44. Weinshenker BG, et al. The natural history of multiple sclerosis: a geographically based study: 3. multivariate analysis of predictive factors and models of outcome. *Brain.* 1991;114(2):1045–1056.

45. Zajicek J, et al. Cannabinoids for treatment of spasticity and other symptoms related to multiple sclerosis (CAMS study): multicentre randomised placebo-controlled trial. *Lancet.* 2003;362(9395):1517–1526.

46. Fox P, et al. The effect of cannabis on tremor in patients with multiple sclerosis. *Neurology.* 2004;62(7):1105–1109.

47. Koller WC. Pharmacologic trials in the treatment of cerebellar tremor. *Arch Neurol.* 1984;41(3):280–281.

48. Striano P, et al. Levetiracetam for cerebellar tremor in multiple sclerosis: an open-label pilot tolerability and efficacy study. *J Neurol.* 2006;253(6):762–766.

49. Feys P, et al. The effect of levetiracetam on tremor severity and functionality in patients with multiple sclerosis. *Mult Scler.* 2009;15(3):371–378.

50. Duquette P, Pleines J, du Souich P. Isoniazid for tremor in multiple sclerosis: a controlled trial. *Neurology.* 1985;35(12):1772–1775.

51. Hallett M, et al. Controlled trial of isoniazid therapy for severe postural cerebellar tremor in multiple sclerosis. *Neurology.* 1985;35(9):1374–1377.

52. Hallett M. Isoniazid and action tremor in multiple sclerosis. *J Neurol Neurosurg Psychiatry.* 1985;48(9):957.

53. Riechert T. Stereotaktische operationen zur behandlung des tremors der multiplen sklerose. 1972.

54. Geny C, et al. Improvement of severe postural cerebellar tremor in multiple sclerosis by chronic thalamic stimulation. *Mov Disord.* 1996;11(5):489–494.

55. Schulder M, Sernas TJ, Karimi R. Thalamic stimulation in patients with multiple sclerosis: long-term follow-up. *Stereotact Funct Neurosurgery.* 2003;80(1–4):48–55.

56. Sabra AF, et al. Treatment of action tremor in multiple sclerosis with isoniazid. *Neurology.* 1982;32(8):912–913.

57. Twomey J, Espir M. Paroxysmal symptoms as the first manifestations of multiple sclerosis. *J Neurol Neurosurg Psychiatry.* 1980;43(4):296–304.

58. Robertson EE, et al. Fragile X-associated tremor/ataxia syndrome: phenotypic comparisons with other movement disorders. *Clin Neuropsychol.* 2016;30(6):849–900.

59. Bourgeois JA, et al. Lifetime prevalence of mood and anxiety disorders in fragile X premutation carriers. *J Clin Psychiatry.* 2011;72(2):175–182.

60. Seritan AL, et al. Psychiatric disorders associated with FXTAS. *Curr Psychiatry Rev.* 2013;9(1):59–64.

61. Hagerman RJ, et al. Neuropathy as a presenting feature in fragile X-associated tremor/ataxia syndrome. *Am J Med Genet A.* 2007;143(19):2256–2260.

62. Hagerman RJ, Hagerman P. Fragile X-associated tremor/ataxia syndrome—features, mechanisms and management. *Nat Rev Neurol.* 2016;12(7):403–412.

63. Tassone F, Hagerman R. The fragile X-associated tremor ataxia syndrome. Results Probl *Cell Differ.* 2012;54:337–357.

64. Grigsby J. The fragile X mental retardation 1 gene (FMR1): historical perspective, phenotypes, mechanism, pathology, and epidemiology. *Clin Neuropsychol.* 2016;30(6):815–833.

65. Reyniers E, et al. The full mutation in the FMR-1 gene of male fragile X patients is absent in their sperm. *Nat Genet.* 1993;4(2):143–146.

66. Berry-Kravis E, et al. Fragile X-associated tremor/ataxia syndrome: clinical features, genetics, and testing guidelines. *Mov Disord.* 2007;22(14):2018–2030.

67. Chonchaiya W, Schneider A, Hagerman RJ. Fragile X: a family of disorders. *Adv Pediatr.* 2009;56:165–186.

68. Hall DA, et al. Symptomatic treatment in the fragile X-associated tremor/ataxia syndrome. *Mov Disord.* 2006;21(10):1741–1744.

69. Hagerman RJ, et al. Treatment of fragile X-associated tremor ataxia syndrome (FXTAS) and related neurological problems. *Clin Interv Aging.* 2008;3(2):251–262.

70. Seritan AL, et al. Memantine for fragile X-associated tremor/ataxia syndrome: a randomized, double-blind, placebo-controlled trial. *J Clin Psychiatry.* 2014;75(3):264–271.

71. dos Santos Ghilardi MG, et al. Long-term improvement of tremor and ataxia after bilateral DBS of VoP/zona incerta in FXTAS. *Neurology.* 2015;84(18):1904–1906.

72. Xie T, et al. Treatment of fragile X-associated tremor/ataxia syndrome with unilateral deep brain stimulation. *Mov Disord.* 2012;27(6):799–800.

73. Fratkin JD, Vig P. Neuropathology of degenerative ataxias. *Handb Clin Neurol.* 2012;103:111–125.

74. Luo L, et al. The initial symptom and motor progression in spinocerebellar ataxias. *Cerebellum.* 2017;16(3):615–622.

75. Gan SR, et al. Postural tremor and ataxia progression in spinocerebellar ataxias. *Tremor Other Hyperkinet Mov (N Y).* 2017;7:492.

76. Bonnet C, et al. Tremor-spectrum in spinocerebellar ataxia type 3. *J Neurol.* 2012;259(11): 2460–2470.

77. Schöls L, et al. Extrapyramidal motor signs in degenerative ataxias. *Arch Neurol.* 2000;57(10): 1495–1500.

78. O'Hearn E, et al. SCA-12: tremor with cerebellar and cortical atrophy is associated with a CAG repeat expansion. *Neurology.* 2001;56(3):299–303.

79. van Gaalen J, Giunti P, van de Warrenburg BP. Movement disorders in spinocerebellar ataxias. *Mov Disord,* 2011;26(5):792–800.

80. Lai RY, et al. Tremor in the degenerative cerebellum: towards the understanding of brain circuitry for tremor. *Cerebellum.* 2019;18(3):519–526.

81. Hara N, et al. Zonisamide can ameliorate the voltage-dependence alteration of the T-type calcium channel Ca(V)3.1 caused by a mutation responsible for spinocerebellar ataxia. *Mol Brain.* 2020;13(1):163.

82. Kimura M, et al. SCA42 mutation analysis in a case series of Japanese patients with spinocerebellar ataxia. *J Hum Genet.* 2017;62(9):857–859.

83. Odgerel Z, et al. Whole genome sequencing and rare variant analysis in essential tremor families. *PLoS One.* 2019;14(8):e0220512.

84. Romano S, et al. Riluzole in patients with hereditary cerebellar ataxia: a randomised, double-blind, placebo-controlled trial. *Lancet Neurol.* 2015;14(10):985–991.

85. Ristori G, et al. Riluzole in cerebellar ataxia: a randomized, double-blind, placebo-controlled pilot trial. *Neurology.* 2010;74(10):839–845.

86. Zesiewicz TA, et al. A randomized trial of varenicline (Chantix) for the treatment of spinocerebellar ataxia type 3. *Neurology.* 2012;78(8):545–550.

87. Zesiewicz TA, Kuo SH. Essential tremor. *BMJ Clin Evid*. 2015;2015.

88. Nandagopal R, Moorthy SG. Dramatic levodopa responsiveness of dystonia in a sporadic case of spinocerebellar ataxia type 3. *Postgrad Med J*. 2004;80(944):363–365.

89. Wilkins A, Brown JM, Barker RA. SCA2 presenting as levodopa-responsive parkinsonism in a young patient from the United Kingdom: a case report. *Mov Disord*. 2004;19(5):593–595.

90. Freund HJ, et al. Subthalamic-thalamic DBS in a case with spinocerebellar ataxia type 2 and severe tremor-A unusual clinical benefit. *Mov Disord*. 2007;22(5):732–735.

91. Isobe T, et al. Long-term suppression of disabling tremor by thalamic stimulation in a patient with spinocerebellar ataxia type 2. *Stereotact Funct Neurosurg*. 2019;97(4):241–243.

92. Hashimoto T, et al. Neuronal activity and outcomes from thalamic surgery for spinocerebellar ataxia. *Ann Clin Transl Neurol*. 2018;5(1):52–63.

93. Oyama G, et al. Deep brain stimulation for tremor associated with underlying ataxia syndromes: a case series and discussion of issues. *Tremor Other Hyperkinet Mov (N Y)*. 2014;4:228.

94. Reich MM, et al. Progressive gait ataxia following deep brain stimulation for essential tremor: adverse effect or lack of efficacy? *Brain*. 2016;139(11):2948–2956.

95. Ramirez-Zamora A, Okun MS. Deep brain stimulation for the treatment of uncommon tremor syndromes. *Expert Rev Neurother*. 2016;16(8):983–997.

96. Di Donato I, Bianchi S, Federico A. Ataxia with vitamin E deficiency: update of molecular diagnosis. *Neurol Sci*. 2010;31(4):511–515.

97. Copp RP, et al. Localization of α-tocopherol transfer protein in the brains of patients with ataxia with vitamin E deficiency and other oxidative stress related neurodegenerative disorders. *Brain Res*. 1999;822(1–2):80–87.

98. Schuelke M. *Ataxia with Vitamin E Deficiency*. In: *GeneReviews®[Internet]*. University of Washington, Seattle; 2016.

99. Gabsi S, et al. Effect of vitamin E supplementation in patients with ataxia with vitamin E deficiency. *Eur J Neurol*. 2001;8(5):477–481.

100. McKay JH, Cheshire WP. First symptoms in multiple system atrophy. *Clin Auton Res*. 2018;28(2):215–221.

101. Kaindlstorfer C, Granata R, Wenning GK. Tremor in multiple system atrophy—a review. *Tremor Other Hyperkinet Mov (N Y)*. 2013;3.

102. Salazar G, et al. Postural and action myoclonus in patients with parkinsonian type multiple system atrophy. *Mov Disord*. 2000;15(1):77–83.

103. Wenning GK, et al. The natural history of multiple system atrophy: a prospective European cohort study. *Lancet Neurol*. 2013;12(3):264–274.

104. Wenning GK, et al. Clinical features and natural history of multiple system atrophy. An analysis of 100 cases. *Brain*. 1994;117(Pt 4):835–845.

105. Tison F, et al. Parkinsonism in multiple system atrophy: natural history, severity (UPDRS-III), and disability assessment compared with Parkinson's disease. *Mov Disord*. 2002;17(4):701–709.

106. Schra A, Ben-Shlomo Y, Quinn N. Prevalence of progressive supranuclear palsy and multiple system atrophy: a cross-sectional study. *Lancet*. 1999;354(9192):1771–1775.

107. Wenning GK, et al. Multiple system atrophy. *Lancet Neurol*. 2004;3(2):93–103.

108. Bower JH, et al. Incidence of progressive supranuclear palsy and multiple system atrophy in Olmsted County, Minnesota, 1976 to 1990. *Neurology*. 1997;49(5):1284–1288.

109. Brettschneider J, et al. Converging patterns of alpha-synuclein pathology in multiple system atrophy. *J Neuropathol Exp Neurol*. 2018;77(11):1005–1016.

110. Terao Y, et al. Is multiple system atrophy with cerebellar ataxia (MSA-C) like spinocerebellar ataxia and multiple system atrophy with parkinsonism (MSA-P) like Parkinson's disease?—a saccade study on pathophysiology. *Clin Neurophysiol*. 2016;127(2):1491–1502.

111. Kaindlstorfer C, Granata R, Wenning GK. Tremor in multiple system atrophy—a review. *Tremor Other Hyperkinet Mov*. 2013;3.

112. Rajrut AH, et al. *Amantadine effectiveness in multiple system atrophy and progressive supranuclear palsy. Parkinsonism Relat Disord*. 1997;3(4):211–214.

113. Issar NM, et al. Treating post-traumatic tremor with deep brain stimulation: report of five cases. *Parkinsonism Relat Disord*. 2013;19(12):1100–1105.

114. Foote KD, et al. Dual electrode thalamic deep brain stimulation for the treatment of posttraumatic and multiple sclerosis tremor. *Oper Neurosurg*. 2006;58(suppl_4):ONS-280-ONS-286.

115. Issar NM, et al. Treating post-traumatic tremor with deep brain stimulation: report of five cases. *Parkinsonism Relat Disord*. 2013;19(12):1100–1105.

116. Ellison PH. Propranolol for severe post-head injury action tremor. *Neurology*. 1978;28(2):197–199.

117. Maas R, Helmich RCG, van de Warrenburg BPC. The role of the cerebellum in degenerative ataxias and essential tremor: insights from non-invasive modulation of cerebellar activity. *Mov Disord*, 2020;35(2):215–227.

118. Marty B, et al. Neuromagnetic cerebellar activity entrains to the kinematics of executed finger movements. *Cerebellum*. 2018;17(5):531–539.

14

Myoclonus

SHABBIR MERCHANT AND MARK HALLETT

The term "myoclonus" is used to define the clinical category of hyperkinetic movement disorders characterized by sudden, brief "jerk-like" movements.[1-3] Several movement disorders such as tics, chorea, dystonia, ballism, and functional movements have associated "jerk-like" movements, and, as such, there are several limitations to the current clinically defined category of myoclonus.[4,5] Another movement disorder that has frequent overlap in terms of clinical characteristics with the category of myoclonus is tremor. Tremors are defined as rhythmic oscillatory movements around a particular joint.[6-8] When "jerk-like" movements or myoclonus occur repetitively, even though they are neither rhythmic or oscillatory around a joint, they can clinically look like tremor. By contrast, the neurophysiologic characteristics of different types of myoclonus are distinct, and are used to refine the characterization of myoclonus into cortical, brainstem and spinal/propriospinal subcategories.[4] Objective physiologic characterization of myoclonus into distinct categories serves to localize its origin along the neuroaxis and provides useful pathophysiologic insights that have therapeutic implications.[2,4,5,9] In this chapter we discuss two clinical syndromes, namely "cortical tremor" and "palatal tremor," which share physiologic and pathophysiologic characteristics of cortical and brainstem myoclonus, respectively. Cortical tremor can be clinically described as repetitive, irregular, jerky movements mainly involving the hand and fingers. Palatal tremor can be clinically described as repetitive jerky movements of the palatal muscles, not involving any oscillations around a joint. However, by virtue of their clinical characteristics of semi-rhythmicity, both these disorders have been categorized as tremors.[7,8]

CORTICAL TREMOR

Cortical tremor was first reported by Ikeda et al. in 1990, described as "fine shivering-like finger twitching provoked by action and posture" in two Japanese patients. Though the tremor syndrome shared notable similarities with essential tremor (ET), the additional astute clinical observations

of distal predominance, superimposed irregular, arrhythmic, and "jerk-like" movements with action were atypical.[7] The co-existence of "tremor" and "myoclonus" phenomenology in these patients led to further detailed physiologic assessments, leading in turn to the description of this distinct nosological entity as "cortical tremor" (CT), physiologically categorized as a variant of cortical reflex myoclonus, and which may be seen with many etiologies. Subsequently, over a hundred pedigrees have been identified with this clinical syndrome in different countries, and these have proven to be clinically and genetically heterogeneous.[10] The evolution of this clinical syndrome is indeed reflective of the importance of astute clinical examination combined with objective clinical neurophysiology in the diagnosis of movement disorders. There have been several different nomenclatures used previously to describe this syndrome, which has now come to be recognized as Familial Cortical Myoclonic Tremor with Epilepsy (FCMTE).[11,12]

Clinical characteristics

Phenomenology of this movement disorder can be described as a combination of tremor and myoclonus. The tremor phenomenology is characterized as distal predominant (mainly involving the digits and forearm muscles), rapid, and semi-rhythmic with fluctuating amplitude mainly provoked by action and posture. Given the semi-rhythmic rather than rhythmic quality, these movements are better characterized as "tremulous" or "tremor-like," rather than tremor. Tremulous movements are predominant in the hands with action/posture; however, they can also be noted at rest. Tremulous movements can also involve the legs, head, and trunk. Tremor is the most commonly reported presenting symptom.[6,12-18] Other clinical characteristics noted to differentiate CT from ET include worsening with fatigue, sleep deprivation, caffeine use, glucose deprivation, and vibratory as well as visual and/or auditory stimulation.[6] It is interesting to note that these same clinical characteristics used to differentiate CT from ET make CT clinically and even electrophysiologically more similar to enhanced physiologic tremor from various etiologies.[19–22]

The myoclonus phenomenology is most consistent with those noted for cortical myoclonus, characterized as spontaneous or action-induced jerks predominantly involving the distal upper limbs, sensitive to tactile and somatosensory stimuli.[1,9,23,24]

Patients with FCMTE usually have a family history with an autosomal dominant inheritance pattern. Another cardinal clinical feature of this syndrome is the presence of epilepsy. Epilepsy may be the presenting symptom in about 16% of patients.[10,25] Tremulous movements usually predate seizures, at times by several decades, or they may present simultaneously. Epilepsy is commonly the symptom that makes patients seek medical attention, as was the case with the first two patients reported.[7] FCMTE usually presents in the second or third decade, with jerky, tremulous movements in the distal upper limbs (range 3–70 years), with seizures more commonly starting in the third or fourth decades and a higher prevalence with advancing age. The semiology of the seizures is generalized tonic-clonic, but complex partial seizures, also referred to as focal seizures with impaired awareness, are also reported (International League Against Epilepsy [ILAE] 2017 classification).[26] The Japanese cohorts in general have a relatively benign course compared to European cohorts, which present with earlier onset of epilepsy and have associated neurocognitive impairments.[10,14–16,25,27–31]

Other clinical findings in FCMTE reported include presence of ataxia, gait instability (especially in patients with leg/truncal tremulousness), dysarthria, and eye movement abnormalities implicating cerebellar involvement.[13,32,33] However, it is important to note that ataxia is not one of the core clinical features of this syndrome. A wide variety of neurocognitive and psychiatric issues have also been reported. The neurocognitive impairment spectrum varies from frank mental retardation, to dementia, to only mild cognitive impairment. More profound early neurocognitive issues notable in the European cohorts. Psychiatric comorbidities noted include anxiety, personality disturbances, and even schizophrenia reported in some patients of Italian FCMTE pedigrees.[10,12,17,29,34]

Neurophysiologic characteristics

Electrophysiology is paramount in making the diagnosis of CT. All movements of CT, clinically described as tremor, tremulous movement, or myoclonus, are physiologically characterized as a variant of cortical reflex myoclonus. The physiologic studies for characterizing and making a diagnosis include those used for tremor analysis and cortical myoclonus.[2,4,35]

Electrophysiological analysis involves using surface EMG on a pair of antagonist muscles with additional use of accelerometers for better frequency resolution.[35] Continuous recordings show arrhythmic/semi-rhythmic, repetitive, short-duration (<50ms), high-frequency (usually >10 Hz) myoclonic bursts. The burst can be synchronous between antagonist muscles, which is characteristic of cortical myoclonus and importantly distinct from the neurophysiological manifestation of action tremor syndromes such as ET, which is characterized some of the time by rhythmic alternating bursts of longer duration (> 100ms).[4,35] Cortical spikes can be detected on EEG preceding the EMG bursts on jerk-locked averaging (Figure 14.1). Other features consistent with cortical reflex myoclonus include presence of giant median nerve sensory evoked potentials (SEPs) with enhanced (P25/N33) components and presence of enhanced long-latency reflex responses (LLR).[2,7,10,12,36]

Pathophysiology

The clinical and electrophysiologic characteristics of CT provide some useful pathophysiologic insights. The physiologic findings are suggestive of cortical hyperexcitability, which is the main pathophysiologic hallmark of this syndrome. There are two aspects of the involuntary movements needed to explain the pathophysiology of CT: 1) cortical myoclonus and associated disinhibited long loop reflexes (LLRs); and 2) repetitive nature of cortical myoclonic jerks presenting clinically as arrhythmic tremulous movements.

The characteristics of the jerky movements are most consistent with cortical myoclonus, implicating disinhibited sensorimotor cortex. Myoclonic jerks are mainly limited to the fingers and distal upper limbs, which have the largest cortical homuncular representation. The enhanced LLRs, presence of cortical spikes correlating with myoclonic jerks, and giant SEPs are all consistent with disinhibited sensorimotor cortex. Another cardinal feature is the presence of epilepsy with generalized spikes and waves, and photoparoxysmal and photo-myogenic response.[10,12,29,37]

One of the proposed mechanisms to explain the repetitive jerks resulting in tremulous

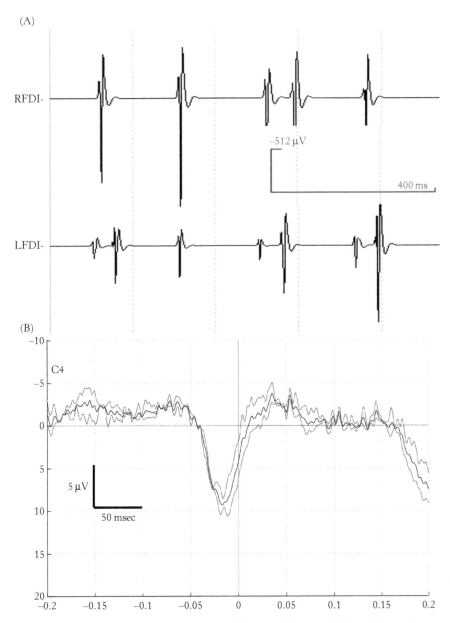

(A)

RFDI-

−512 μV

400 ms

LFDI-

(B)

C4

5 μV

50 msec

FIGURE 14.1: Physiological Findings in a Patient with Cortical Tremor. (A) Short-duration (<30 μsec bursts) arrhythmic EMG bursts recorded from bilateral FDI muscles at a frequency of ~10Hz. (B) Back-averaged cortical spike recorded from the contralateral sensorimotor cortex.

movements is to consider the degree of cortical disinhibition along a spectrum. The presence of enhanced LLRs and isolated, spontaneous, or action-induced myoclonic jerks is on the milder end of the spectrum. More severe cortical dis-inhibition resulting in repetitive myoclonic jerks manifesting clinically as tremulousness and episodes of tonic-clonic seizures, as noted in FCMTE. Malignant seizure disorders and

myoclonic epilepsies represent the most severe end of the clinical spectrum.[10,12,25]

The role of cerebellum has been implicated to explain cortical disinhibition and generation of arrhythmic myoclonic discharges originating in the sensorimotor cortex. Evidence for cerebellar involvement in FCMTE varies based on the pedi-gree being evaluated. Abnormalities in the cere-bellum were reported in certain Dutch pedigrees, including pathologic changes in Purkinje cells and changes on magnetic resonance spectroscopy (MRS).[10,12,13,30,33,38] The cerebellum has been independently implicated in the pathophysiology of several tremor, myoclonus, and epilepsy syndromes, likely through reduced GABA-mediated cortical inhibition via the cerebello-thalamo-cortical pathways.[24,38–42] The degree of cerebello-cortical disinhibition is perhaps also along a spectrum, with lower degrees of disinhibition resulting in isolated reflex, action-induced, or spontaneous jerks due to pathologic enhancement of reflex gains. Greater degrees of cerebellar disinhibition result in more repetitive myoclonic jerks and epilepsy syndromes.[25,39]

The discharges of cortical neurons resulting in arrhythmic tremor could be driven by subcortical generators or by rhythmic generators within the cortex.[43] The rhythmic oscillatory neurons in the inferior olivary nucleus and the thalamic relay nuclei have been implicated to explain the arrhythmic, tremor-like movements. Both these nuclei have relays in the cerebellum via the climbing fibers and cerebello-thalamo-cortical loops, respectively.[44] The loss of Purkinje cells in the cerebellum with subsequent downstream deficient inhibition of dentate nucleus, resulting in cortical disinhibition via cerebello-thalamo-cortical pathways, could explain the cortical myoclonus and epilepsy.[30,38,39] The cerebellar dysfunction could also explain the transformation of the normally rhythmic discharges originating in the subcortical structures into arrhythmic tremor-like movements.[13,38] Considering that several of the clinical and physiologic characteristics of CT are similar to an enhanced physiologic tremor, as well as the presence of inherent rhythmicity of the neocortex at similar frequencies, CT could perhaps best be categorized as an "enhanced" enhanced physiologic tremor.[6,7,19,22,29] The cortical disinhibition results in increased synchronization of the neocortical generated rhythms with the enhanced mechanical reflex tremors via gain in the long loop reflexes.[43,45,46] The cerebellar modulation of the reflex gain is therefore a combination of cerebello-cortical and peripheral (via modulation of stretch reflex) mechanisms.[6,47–50]

Etiology

CT can arise in any syndrome of cortical myoclonus. FCMTE is a clinically and genetically heterogenous syndrome with predominant autosomal dominant inheritance with varying degrees of severity.[10,12,25] The possible causative mutations

implicated include trinucleotide repeat expansions, missense mutations, and some candidate genes, suggesting that FCMTEs may be channelopathies.[51] Several candidate genes have been identified in different pedigrees using linkage analysis.[10,14] Table 14.1 summarizes the findings in FCMTE 1–4, with possible candidate genes and associated clinical characteristics.[51–54]

A gain of function mutation in the *ADRA2B* gene resulting in reduced GABA neurotransmission has been reported in the FCMTE2 Italian pedigrees.[55] Mutations in the aminocarboxymuconate semialdehyde decarboxylase (*ACMSD*) gene, resulting in accumulation of waste products in the kynurenine pathways and excitotoxicity via involvement of the serotonergic pathways, has been implicated in the Spanish FCMTE2 pedigree.[56] A possible role of CAG repeat expansion in the calcium channel (*CACNA1A*) gene has been implicated, considering the notable clinical (ataxia/downbeat nystagmus) and pathologic (Purkinje cell changes) similarities between Dutch cohorts with FCMTE and spinocerebellar ataxia (SCA) type 6.[32,39]

Treatment

Treatment of CT syndromes is guided toward symptomatic treatment of repetitive cortical myoclonus, which clinically manifests as tremulousness. The drugs used to treat myoclonus generally possess anticonvulsant properties,[57–62] usually by enhancing GABA inhibitory activity. Unlike most epilepsy syndromes, where it is preferred to manage patients using monotherapy, there are good reasons for considering a polypharmacy approach targeting the various pathophysiologic mechanisms implicated in the generation of varying degrees of cortical disinhibition in FCMTE syndromes. Based on neurophysiological evidence, antimyoclonic drugs may exert different actions on the sequence of events responsible for myoclonus, at least for those concerned with cortical myoclonus. Some drugs that decrease cortical myoclonus increase the size of the giant sensory-evoked potential, while others have the opposite effect. Myoclonus thus often responds best to a combination of drugs.[24,30,60,63]

Cortical myoclonus in FCMTE responds best to drugs such as sodium valproate and clonazepam, often used in combination in maximum tolerated anticonvulsant doses. The initial choice of agents can be based on the underlying etiology, consideration of potential medication-related side effects, and whether myoclonic jerks are the

TABLE 14.1: SUMMARY OF FCMTE 1–4 PEDIGREES AND DESCRIBED CLINICAL SYNDROMES

FCMTE linkage	Pedigrees	Gene region	Candidate genes	Clinical syndrome
FCMTE 1[1,52,53]	Japanese, Chinese	8q	Unknown	Benign syndrome presenting with arrhythmic distal myoclonus with late-onset epilepsy (after 3rd decade).
FCMTE 2[34,54,55]	European countries; Italian, Spanish	2p	*ACMSD* (Spanish) *ADRA2B* (Italian)	Severe myoclonus with significant disability with age. More severe and earlier-onset epilepsy. Spanish pedigree: Parkinsonism and ataxia. Italian pedigree: Psychiatric and cognitive comorbidity.
FCMTE 3[32,33]	Chinese, French, Dutch	5p	*CTNND2* (Dutch)	Chinese pedigree: Benign syndrome with late onset (4th decade). French pedigree: More profound cognitive changes, gait instability, and frontal lobe syndrome. Dutch: Mild neurocognitive impairment with aging.
FCMTE 4[54]	Thai	3q	Unknown	Myoclonus onset in second decade, and seizures in 3rd decade with no cognitive decline.

ACMSD=Aminocarboxymuconate Semialdehyde Decarboxylase; ADRA2B=alpha 2 adrenergic receptor subtype B; CTTND2=Catenin Delta 2.

primary disabling issue or a comorbidity with refractory epilepsy. It was conventional to start with sodium valproate in patients with severe myoclonus, then to add clonazepam. If symptoms remained refractory, previously piracetam was added; now levetiracetam has largely replaced it.[61,64] However, considering the better side effect profile of levetiracetam, it is now not uncommon to use it as the first agent. Primidone, a medication used to treat action tremors primarily in ET, also may be of value as an additional drug in severely affected patients, as may clobazam and acetazolamide. There is recent interest in perampanel, but not much experience yet.[65] Phenytoin, carbamazepine, lamotrigine, vigabatrin, and gabapentin may, paradoxically, worsen some types of CT and should best be avoided.[66]

PALATAL TREMOR

Abnormal rhythmic movements of the pharynx and larynx likened to nystagmus were described by Spencer in 1886.[67] The earliest pathologic descriptions related to this pathology and implicating the involvement of the inferior olivary nucleus, described as hypertrophy, were noted in the late nineteenth century.[68,69] Schenck performed the first large review describing the clinical and physiologic characteristics of this entity, establishing it as a distinctive nosological entity.[70] Deuschl et al. formally characterized and classified the two

distinctive subtypes of rhythmic palatal movements described as "symptomatic" and "essential" rhythmic palatal myoclonus.[71] This entity was renamed and came to be formally recognized as "palatal tremor" at the First International Congress of Movement Disorders in 1990 (based on an oral vote) to recognize the continuous and rhythmic nature of the palatal movements.

The two main subtypes of palatal tremor are symptomatic palatal tremor (SPT) and essential palatal tremor (EPT).[8,71,72] In the past, the term "isolated palatal tremor" (IPT) was proposed for EPT alone, with further subclassification as primary IPT where no other neurological or imaging abnormalities were identified; and secondary IPT, which is voluntary, acquired as a special skill, or functional (psychogenic).[73] It has been reported that a large majority of EPT cases have functional etiology, and as such, the term EPT has been largely replaced by the term "psychogenic palatal tremor" and, more recently, by "functional palatal tremor."[74]

Clinical characteristics

SPT is characterized most commonly by semirhythmic involuntary movements of the soft palate and pharynx. The contractions involve the levator veli palatini muscle, causing superior and posterior displacement of the soft palate and uvula. The frequency of the palatal movements is slow and fairly consistent per individual, with a range from 1.5–3 Hz.[8,72,75] Unilateral contraction may result in pulling of the palate and uvula ipsilaterally; however, even with unilateral involvement the palatal movements seem bilateral, as the levator veli palatini muscle is inserted into the medial aponeurosis.[72] Patients with SPT rarely complain of ear clicks, and the palatal movements are usually asymptomatic.[8,76] SPT persists during sleep.[8,72]

SPT rarely occurs as an isolated tremor syndrome and usually occurs as part of a larger syndrome. Most SPT patients seek medical attention for issues with other muscles twitching, most frequently involving the muscles belonging to the gill arches in the face, as well as the tongue, pharynx, larynx, muscles on the floor of the mouth, and, rarely the diaphragm.[77]

A significant proportion (about 30%) of patients with SPT develop ocular nystagmus that are most commonly vertical and pendular and less commonly can also have horizontal and torsional components. The ocular nystagmus, when present, is coherent with the palatal tremor, and the syndrome is defined as oculopalatal tremor (OPT).[8,78,79] Patients with OPT report distressing oscillopsia, impaired fixation, and associated impairments in visual acuity.[79,80] Another important clinical characteristic of SPT syndromes such as progressive ataxia and palatal tremor (discussed later in the chapter) is the presence of cerebellar signs such as unilateral or bilateral limb ataxia or axial ataxia, impairing gait and balance.[8,76,78,79,81]

EPT is characterized by the presence of palatal movements and ear clicks.[8,71] The ear clicks are often the only complaint and are variously described as ticking, crackling, or popping, or at times are likened to the ticking movements of a watch.[73,82] The palatal movements involve contraction of the tensor veli palatini muscle, which mainly involves the anterior part of the soft palate. The tensor veli palatini muscle originates along the medial pterygoid plate and membranous wall of the eustachian tube and inserts into the palatine aponeurosis in the anterior part of the soft palate after going around the pterygoid hamulus. Contraction of this muscle results in palatal movements in EPT that are almost always bilateral. The associated opening of the lateral wall of the eustachian tube results in ear clicks.[72,82] The frequency of the palatal tremor is variable between and even within individuals and can be entrained to voluntary movements. In all patients the tremor extinguishes during sleep.[8,71,73,74,76] The majority of these patients satisfy the diagnostic criteria for functional movement disorders.[73,74,83–85] Additionally, patients may have other associated functional movement disorders and other somatizations. Gait ataxia and other clinical signs to implicate organic cerebellar or brainstem involvement are usually absent in EPT.[8,71,73,74,81]

Neurophysiologic and imaging characteristics

The frequency of SPT ranges from 1.5–3 Hz, with burst duration ranging from 40–120 msec.[8] The frequency of the palatal tremor recorded from the levator veli palatini muscle is stable and time locked with twitching of the other facial muscles and the frequency of pendular nystagmus (when present).[8] The tremor frequency remains stable and persistent during sleep.[8,71,72] SPT patients have physiologic abnormalities in brainstem monosynaptic, oligosynaptic, and polysynaptic reflexes.[8] Physiologic abnormalities implicating cerebellar involvement are also described in SPT, such as impairments in classical blink conditioning and impairments in adaptation learning for limb movements.[81] Impairments in motor adaptation learning are also noted for eye movements in patients with OPT.[78] In contrast, frequency of EPT is highly variable among subjects, with frequencies ranging from <1Hz–7Hz.[8] The frequencies are also variable within subjects with additional distractibility and demonstrable entrainment.[73,74,83,84] Physiologic studies demonstrating a Bereitschaftspotential (BP) (rising negative potential in the premotor and supplementary motor areas) preceding the palatal movements, as notable in voluntary and functional movements, have also been shown in EPT.[35,83,86]

The imaging findings implicating pathology within the triangle of Guillain-Mollaret are typically noted in T2/FLAIR MRI sequences in SPT.[8,79,87,88] The classical abnormality involves the inferior olives and is typically described as hypertrophic olivary degeneration (HOD). The typical temporal evolution of the findings noted includes presence of an initial T2 hyper-signal in the inferior olives that progresses to hypertrophy over 6 months with gradual resolution of the swelling/hypertrophy and subsequent atrophy of the inferior olives over 3–4 years.[89] In rare cases the MRI signal may normalize over time. The abnormalities can be unilateral/bilateral in SPT/OPT.[8,90] Other imaging findings less commonly reported include lesions in the contralateral cerebellum or ipsilateral central tegmental tract, which can sometimes precede the onset of HOD.[88,91–95] MRI is typically normal in patients with EPT.[8,73,74]

Pathophysiology

Pathophysiologic models to explain the low-frequency arrhythmic tremor in SPT/OPT involve a preponderant role of a disinhibited inferior olivary nucleus.[88] In the normal state, the inferior olivary neurons generate a 1–2 Hz rhythmic activity that is conducted to the Purkinje cells in the cerebellar cortex via the climbing fibers through the inferior cerebellar peduncles.[96] The prevailing model suggests that pathology involving the triangle of Guillain-Mollaret along the dentato-olivary pathway would lead to downstream denervation and disinhibition of the inferior olivary neurons, resulting in electrotonic coupling among them.[97–99] As a result, the cerebellar cortex now receives a more synchronized input from electrotonically coupled, disinhibited inferior olivary neurons, which now project to a larger field of cerebellar cortical Purkinje cells.[98,99] A further refinement and learning of this arrhythmic bursting pattern is provided via projections through the vestibular nucleus, which is a displaced deep cerebellar nucleus. The vestibular nucleus receives direct inputs from cerebellar Purkinje cells and indirectly projects back to them via a mossy fiber/granule-cells parallel fiber. The repeated inferior olivary bursts reverberating through this circuit are amplified and smoothed as the Purkinje cells receive both climbing and mossy fiber projections at about the same time.[8,77,78,100,101]

Although this proposed model explains the preponderant 1–2 Hz tremor noted especially in OPT, it is unclear whether both the inferior olive and cerebellum are necessary to explain the persistence of palatal tremor. The inferior olivary hypertrophy and associated hypermetabolism resolves over time, and as such, the tremor should improve with atrophy and loss of electrotonically coupled inferior olivary cells.[96,99,102,103] Additionally, there is discordant reduction in the inferior olivary and cerebellar activity associated with treatment with clonazepam. There is persistence of inferior olivary hyperactivity despite reduction in cerebellar activity and palatal tremor improvements with clonazepam.[104] It is plausible that the repeated near-simultaneous projections to the Purkinje cells via climbing fibers and mossy fiber/granule-cell parallel fibers facilitate learning and persistence of this abnormal rhythm in this circuit via mechanisms involving establishment of Hebbian-like plasticity.[105,106] Over time, the

larger fields of electrotonically coupled Purkinje cells can perhaps result in synchronized bursting with limited climbing fiber input.[107,108]

Another pathophysiologic model that has gone out of favor is the suggestion that SPT could be the result of recurrence of an archaic phenomenon. The muscles involved in SPT/OPT belong to the embryological first to fifth branchial arches, which are part of the primitive accessory respiratory reflex in gill-breathing vertebrates. These muscles are innervated by the nucleus ambiguous and denervation of this nucleus via lesions along the central tegmental tract, proposed to be the mechanism of generation of SPT.[109] Though an interesting proposition, it does not explain the 1–2 Hz tremor as explained by the aforementioned model.[78] Additionally, the muscles involved in SPT/OPT seem more likely to involve the facial nerve nucleus rather than the nucleus ambiguous as previously thought.[8]

The majority of patients with EPT have a likely functional etiology.[74] Patients are often able to voluntarily elicit the palatal movements. EPT may reflect enhancement of a specialized motor skill, similar to those developed by musicians playing wind instruments and scuba divers who can exquisitely control middle ear air pressure by opening/closing their eustachian tubes, which is the premise of the ear clicks noted in EPT.[73,110] The idea of EPT having a central tremor generator has fallen out of favor; however, in some cases a possible generator in the vicinity of the trigeminal nerve nucleus has been proposed.[73]

Etiology

Lesions from varied etiologies along the dentato-olivary pathways in the brainstem and cerebellum involving the triangle of Guillain-Mollaret are reported to be causative of SPT/OPT. The most common lesions are secondary to monophasic disorders that result in destructive pathology within this region. Vascular etiologies, more commonly hemorrhagic than ischemic, are most common. The common causes for brainstem hemorrhages are cavernoma bleeds and hypertension. Multiple sclerosis (MS) is another common etiology and is especially more commonly noted for patients with OPT. Several patients with MS present with pendular nystagmus without the presence of palatal tremor, and as such, are misclassified as SPT/OPT. Other etiologies include brainstem tumors, brain trauma, and iatrogenic lesions secondary to surgical or gamma knife surgeries targeting the brainstem. SPT usually develops from about 1 month after the initial lesion, reaching its peak in the ensuing 5 to 24 months. Rare cases of palatal tremor have been reported to occur up to 8 years after the presumed initial lesion. The majority of patients with EPT have been deemed to have a functional etiology based on voluntary entrainment and the presence of BPs noted before palatal movements characteristic of functional movements as well as voluntary movements.[73,74,83,84]

Another distinctive syndrome that deserves a separate etiologic classification is the syndrome of Progressive Ataxia and Palatal Tremor (PAPT).[111,112] This syndrome, characterized by progressively worsening cerebellar ataxia and associated palatal tremor with notable progressive cerebellar degeneration, has been further subclassified into sporadic and familial forms.[113] Most patients with sporadic PAPT present with MRI findings of HOD and progressive cerebellar degeneration. Several cases are secondary to mitochondrial disorders, specifically polymerase gamma (POLG) mutation.[114-116] Several cases of sporadic PAPT associated with neurodegenerative tauopathies have also been reported.[113,117-119] Familial PAPT has a more complex phenotype and involves more extensive degenerative changes in the brainstem and cervical cord in addition to the olivary degeneration. Besides progressively worsening ataxia and palatal tremor, there are long tract signs implicating corticospinal involvement. Three main etiological categories of familial PAPT are Alexander disease, mitochondrial DNA POLG mutations, and spinocerebellar ataxia type 20 (SCA 20).[79,113]

Alexander disease is a leukodystrophy, most commonly resulting from de novo mutations in the gene encoding glial fibrillary acidic protein on chromosome 17q21.[120,121] It presents with progressively worsening spastic tetraparesis, cerebellar dysfunction with associated palatal tremor, and ocular motor abnormalities with a classical MRI sign characterized by medullary and upper cervical cord atrophy (tadpole sign).[113,118,121-124] POLG mutations can present with a wide spectrum of neurological syndromes in addition to PAPT, including progressive external ophthalmoplegia, ophthalmoparesis, dysarthria, sensory neuronopathy, sensory ataxia, and cranial, axial, and limb muscle weakness.[116,125-127] SCA 20 is an autosomal dominantly inherited syndrome characterized by gradually progressive ataxia and dysarthria with characteristic dentate calcifications, with a large majority of patients developing a palatal tremor.[128,129]

Treatment

Most patients with isolated SPT are asymptomatic for the palatal movements and thus do not warrant any treatment. Presence of distressing pendular nystagmus in OPT (especially in MS) warrants symptomatic treatment. Gabapentin and memantine have been most systematically studied and noted to have benefit in OPT via reduction in amplitude and irregularity of nystagmus. Trihexyphenidyl has been noted to have some beneficial effect for eye and symptomatic palatal movements (reduction in audible ear clicks). Botulinum toxin injections targeting the pendular nystagmus in OPT and ear clicks noted in cases with SPT and EPT has been noted to have some benefit. Deep brain stimulation targeting the red nucleus for palliation of OPT was noted to be ineffective.[130] Treatment of patients with EPT with functional etiology involves a multidisciplinary approach combining medical therapy with physical and psychological rehabilitation approaches best suited to the individual.[131]

Conclusion

"Cortical tremor," frequently due to FCMTE, is clinically described as tremulous movements mainly involving the distal upper limbs. Physiologically, it is characterized as repetitive myoclonus of cortical origin. FCMTE is a clinically and genetically heterogenous syndrome with an autosomal dominant inheritance, with more than 100 different pedigrees reported. Pathophysiologic models implicate disinhibited sensorimotor cortex with enhancement of long loop reflexes. Treatment is targeted toward repetitive cortical myoclonus using anti-seizure medications enhancing GABAergic inhibition.

"Palatal tremor," clinically characterized by repetitive jerky movements of the palatal muscles, can be subclassified into SPT and EPT. SPT is characterized by repetitive jerky movements of the levator veli palatini muscles and physiologically classified as repetitive brainstem myoclonus. SPT is caused by lesions from various etiologies involving the dentato-olivary pathways in the brainstem and cerebellum involving the Guillain-Mollaret triangle. PAPT is a clinical syndrome of progressive cerebellar ataxia with palatal tremor, and has sporadic and familial forms. Pathophysiologic models for SPT implicate a disinhibited inferior olivary nucleus with downstream cerebellar disinhibition. Treatment is directed toward symptomatic control of distressing pendular nystagmus and audible ear clicks (when present) using medications such as gabapentin or memantine, or targeted botulinum toxin injections to the involved muscles. EPT is characterized by palatal movements involving the tensor veli palatini muscles with associated ear clicks. Palatal movements are of variable frequency, distractible, and entrainable. Most cases of EPT are deemed to be of functional origin, with treatments involving a multidisciplinary approach.

REFERENCES

1. Shibasaki H. Neurophysiological classification of myoclonus. *Neurophysiol Clin.* 2006;36(5–6): 267–269.
2. Shibasaki H, Hallett M. Electrophysiological studies of myoclonus. *Muscle Nerve.* 2005;31(2): 157–174.
3. Caviness JN. Parkinsonism & related disorders: myoclonus. *Parkinsonism Relat Disord.* 2007;13(Suppl 3):S375–384.
4. Merchant SHI, et al. Myoclonus: an electrophysiological diagnosis. *Mov Disord Clin Pract.* 2020;7(5):489–499.
5. Merchant SH, et al. A novel exaggerated "spinobulbo-spinal like" reflex of lower brainstem origin. *Parkinsonism Relat Disord.* 2018.
6. Bourdain F, et al. Clinical analysis in familial cortical myoclonic tremor allows differential diagnosis with essential tremor. *Mov Disord.* 2006;21(5):599–608.
7. Ikeda A, et al. Cortical tremor: a variant of cortical reflex myoclonus. *Neurology.* 1990;40(10):1561–1565.
8. Deuschl G, et al. Symptomatic and essential palatal tremor. 1. Clinical, physiological and MRI analysis. *Brain.* 1994;117(Pt 4):775–788.
9. Shibasaki H. Electrophysiological studies of myoclonus. *Muscle Nerve.* 2000;23(3):321–335.
10. van den Ende T, et al. Familial cortical myoclonic tremor and epilepsy, an enigmatic disorder: from phenotypes to pathophysiology and genetics. A systematic review. *Tremor Other Hyperkinet Mov (N Y).* 2018;8:503.
11. Eyre TA, et al. The HUGO gene nomenclature database, 2006 updates. *Nucleic Acids Res.* 2006;34(Database issue):D319–321.
12. van Rootselaar AF, et al. Familial cortical myoclonic tremor with epilepsy: a single syndromic classification for a group of pedigrees bearing common features. *Mov Disord.* 2005;20(6):665–673.
13. Sharifi S, et al. Familial cortical myoclonic tremor with epilepsy and cerebellar changes: description of a new pathology case and review of the literature. *Tremor Other Hyperkinet Mov (N Y).* 2012;2.
14. Cen Z, et al. Clinical and neurophysiological features of familial cortical myoclonic tremor with epilepsy. *Mov Disord.* 2016;31(11):1704–1710.
15. Delva A, et al. Clinical and electrophysiological features of "cortical tremor." *Rev Neurol (Paris).* 2003;159(5 Pt 1):518–527.
16. Elia M, et al. Familial cortical tremor, epilepsy, and mental retardation: a distinct clinical entity? *Arch Neurol.* 1998;55(12):1569–1573.
17. Magnin E, et al. Familial cortical myoclonic tremor with epilepsy (FCMTE): clinical characteristics and exclusion of linkages to 8q and 2p in a large French family. *Rev Neurol (Paris).* 2009;165(10):812–820.
18. Striano P, et al. Familial cortical tremor and epilepsy: a well-defined syndrome with genetic heterogeneity waiting for nosological placement in the ILAE classification. *Epilepsy Behav.* 2010;19(4):669.
19. Elble RJ. *Characteristics of physiologic tremor in young and elderly adults. Clin Neurophysiol.* 2003;114(4):624–635.
20. Fargen KM, Turner RD, Spiotta AM. Factors that affect physiologic tremor and dexterity during surgery: a primer for neurosurgeons. *World Neurosurg.* 2016;86:384–389.
21. Pickles H, et al. Propranolol and sotalol as antagonists of isoproterenol-enhanced physiologic tremor. *Clin Pharmacol Ther.* 1981;30(3):303–310.
22. Elble RJ. Physiologic and essential tremor. *Neurology.* 1986;36(2):225–231.
23. Hallett M, Chadwick D, Marsden CD. Cortical reflex myoclonus. *Neurology.* 1979;29(8):1107–1125.
24. Shibasaki H, Thompson PD. Milestones in myoclonus. *Mov Disord.* 2011;26(6):1142–1148.
25. Latorre A, et al. Unravelling the enigma of cortical tremor and other forms of cortical myoclonus. *Brain.* 2020.
26. Scheffer IE, et al. ILAE classification of the epilepsies: position paper of the ILAE Commission for Classification and Terminology. *Epilepsia.* 2017;58(4):512–521.
27. Aydin Ozemi Z, et al. Autosomal dominant cortical tremor, myoclonus, and epilepsy syndrome mimicking juvenile myoclonic epilepsy. *Noro Psikiyatr Ars.* 2016;53(3):272–275.
28. Depienne C, et al. Familial cortical myoclonic tremor with epilepsy: the third locus (FCMTE3) maps to 5p. *Neurology.* 2010;74(24):2000–2003.
29. Suppa A, et al. Clinical, neuropsychological, neurophysiologic, and genetic features of a new Italian pedigree with familial cortical myoclonic tremor with epilepsy. *Epilepsia.* 2009;50(5):1284–1288.
30. Coppola A, et al. Natural history and long-term evolution in families with autosomal dominant cortical tremor, myoclonus, and epilepsy. *Epilepsia.* 2011;52(7):1245–1250.
31. Sharma CM, et al. Autosomal dominant cortical tremor, myoclonus, and epilepsy (ADCME): probable first family from India. *Ann Indian Acad Neurol.* 2014;17(4):433–436.

32. van Rootselaar AF, et al. Familial cortical tremor with epilepsy and cerebellar pathological findings. *Mov Disord.* 2004;19(2):213–217.

33. van Rootselaar AF, et al. delta-Catenin (CTNND2) missense mutation in familial cortical myoclonic tremor and epilepsy. *Neurology.* 2017;89(23):2341–2350.

34. Licchetta L, et al. A novel pedigree with familial cortical myoclonic tremor and epilepsy (FCMTE): clinical characterization, refinement of the FCMTE2 locus, and confirmation of a founder haplotype. *Epilepsia.* 2013;54(7):1298–1306.

35. Vial F, et al. How to do an electrophysiological study of tremor. *Clin Neurophysiol Pract.* 2019;4:134–142.

36. Terada K, et al. Familial cortical myoclonic tremor as a unique form of cortical reflex myoclonus. *Mov Disord.* 1997;12(3):370–377.

37. Nakatani-Enomoto S, et al. Somatosensory-evoked potential modulation by quadri-pulse transcranial magnetic stimulation in patients with benign myoclonus epilepsy. *Clin Neurophysiol.* 2016;127(2):1560–1567.

38. Striano P, Louis ED, Manto M. Autosomal dominant cortical tremor, myoclonus, and epilepsy: is the origin in the cerebellum? Editorial. *Cerebellum.* 2013;12(2):145–146.

39. Ganos C, et al. The role of the cerebellum in the pathogenesis of cortical myoclonus. *Mov Disord.* 2014;29(4):437–443.

40. Hossen A, et al. Discrimination of Parkinsonian tremor from essential tremor using statistical signal characterization of the spectrum of accelerometer signal. *Biomed Mater Eng.* 2013;23(6):513–531.

41. Muthuraman M, et al. The central oscillatory network of essential tremor. *Conf Proc IEEE Eng Med Biol Soc.* 2010;2010:154–157.

42. Schnitzler A, et al. Synchronized brain network associated with essential tremor as revealed by magnetoencephalography. *Mov Disord.* 2009;24(11):1629–1635.

43. Connors BW, Amitai Y. Making waves in the neocortex. *Neuron.* 1997;18(3):347–349.

44. Rothwell JC. Physiology and anatomy of possible oscillators in the central nervous system. *Mov Disord.* 1998;13 (Suppl 3):24–28.

45. Noth J. Long loop reflexes: concepts and consequences. *Appl Neurophysiol.* 1986;49(5):262–268.

46. Noth J, Podoll K, Friedemann HH. Long-loop reflexes in small hand muscles studied in normal subjects and in patients with Huntington's disease. *Brain.* 1985;108 (Pt 1):65–80.

47. Diener HC, et al. Characteristic alterations of long-loop "reflexes" in patients with Friedreich's disease and late atrophy of the cerebellar anterior lobe. *J Neurol Neurosurg Psychiatry.* 1984;47(7):679–685.

48. Gemba H, Sasaki K. Tonic vibration reflex and cerebellar disorders. *Exp Neurol.* 1978;60(2):213–220.

49. Rowe MJ, Ishikawa K, Kawaguchi S. Influence of muscle vibration on cerebellar Purkinje cells. *Pflugers Arch.* 1972;332(Suppl 332):R85.

50. Hagbarth KE, Eklund G. Motor effects of muscle vibration in spasticity, rigidity and cerebellar disorders. *Electroencephalogr Clin Neurophysiol.* 1968;25(4):407.

51. Cen ZD, et al. Rational search for genes in familial cortical myoclonic tremor with epilepsy, clues from recent advances. *Seizure.* 2016;34:83–89.

52. Mikami M, et al. Localization of a gene for benign adult familial myoclonic epilepsy to chromosome 8q23.3-q24.1. *Am J Hum Genet.* 1999;65(3):745–751.

53. Plaster NM, et al. Genetic localization of the familial adult myoclonic epilepsy (FAME) gene to chromosome 8q24. *Neurology.* 1999;53(6):1180–1183.

54. Yeetong P, et al. A newly identified locus for benign adult familial myoclonic epilepsy on chromosome 3q26.32-3q28. *Eur J Hum Genet.* 2013;21(2):225–228.

55. De Fusco M, et al. The alpha2B-adrenergic receptor is mutant in cortical myoclonus and epilepsy. *Ann Neurol.* 2014;75(1):77–87.

56. Marti-Masso JF, et al. The ACMSD gene, involved in tryptophan metabolism, is mutated in a family with cortical myoclonus, epilepsy, and parkinsonism. *J Mol Med (Berl).* 2013;91(12):1399–406.

57. Bhatia KP, et al. Progressive myoclonic ataxia associated with coeliac disease. The myoclonus is of cortical origin, but the pathology is in the cerebellum. *Brain.* 1995;118 (Pt 5):1087–1093.

58. Agarwal P, Frucht SJ. Myoclonus. *Curr Opin Neurol.* 2003;16(4):515–521.

59. Papero PH, et al. Neurobehavioral and psychosocial functioning of children with opsoclonus-myoclonus syndrome. *Dev Med Child Neurol.* 1995;37(10):915–932.

60. Caviness N. Treatment of myoclonus. *Neurotherapeutics.* 2014;11(1):188–200.

61. Caviness JN, Truong DD. Myoclonus. *Handb Clin Neurol.* 2011;100:399–420.

62. Chang VC, Frucht SJ. Myoclonus. *Curr Treat Options Neurol.* 2008;10(3):222–229.

63. Caviness JN. Pathophysiology and treatment of myoclonus. *Neurol Clin.* 2009;27(3):757–777, vii.

64. Espay AJ, Chen R. Myoclonus. *Continuum (Minneap Minn).* 2013;19(5 Movement Disorders):1264–1286.

65. Oi Y, et al. [Low-dose perampanel improved cortical myoclonus and basophobia in a patient with Unverricht-Lundborg disease: a case report]. *Rinsho Shinkeigaku.* 2018;58(10):622–625.

66. Asconape J, Diedrich A, DellaBadia J. Myoclonus associated with the use of gabapentin. *Epilepsia.* 2000;41(4):479–481.

67. Lapresle J. Palatal myoclonus. *Adv Neurol.* 1986;43:265–273.

68. Pearce J. Palatal myoclonus. *Proc R Soc Med.* 1969;62(3):267.

69. Pearce JM. Palatal Myoclonus (syn. Palatal Tremor). *Eur Neurol.* 2008;60(6):312–315.

70. Schenck E. Brain-nerve-myorhythmia, its pathogenesis and place in the myoclonic syndrome. Clinico-neurophysiologic study. *Monogr Gesamtgeb Neurol Psychiatr.* 1965;109:1–75.

71. Deuschl G, et al. Symptomatic and essential rhythmic palatal myoclonus. *Brain.* 1990;113(Pt 6):1645–1672.

72. Deuschl G, Toro C, Hallett M. Symptomatic and essential palatal tremor. 2. Differences of palatal movements. *Mov Disord.* 1994;9(6):676–678.

73. Zadikoff C, Lang AE, Klein C. The "essentials" of essential palatal tremor: a reappraisal of the nosology. *Brain.* 2006;129(Pt 4):832–840.

74. Stamelou M, et al. Psychogenic palatal tremor may be underrecognized: reappraisal of a large series of cases. *Mov Disord.* 2012;27(9):1164–1168.

75. Deuschl G, Wilms H. Palatal tremor: the clinical spectrum and physiology of a rhythmic movement disorder. *Adv Neurol.* 2002;89:115–130.

76. Deuschl G, Wilms H. Clinical spectrum and physiology of palatal tremor. *Mov Disord.* 2002;17(Suppl 2):S63–S66.

77. Borruat FX. Oculopalatal tremor: current concepts and new observations. *Curr Opin Neurol.* 2013;26(1):67–73.

78. Shaikh AG, et al. Oculopalatal tremor explained by a model of inferior olivary hypertrophy and cerebellar plasticity. *Brain.* 2010;133(Pt 3):923–940.

79. Tilikete C, Desestret, V. Hypertrophic olivary degeneration and palatal or oculopalatal tremor. *Front Neurol.* 2017;8:302.

80. Tilikete C, et al. Acquired pendular nystagmus in multiple sclerosis and oculopalatal tremor. *Neurology.* 2011;76(19):1650–1657.

81. Deuschl G, et al. Symptomatic and essential palatal tremor. 3. Abnormal motor learning. *J Neurol Neurosurg Psychiatry.* 1996;60(5):520–525.

82. Gotze A. Objective ear murmurs of myoclonus origin. *Orv Hetil.* 1957;98(44):1215–1218.

83. Pirio Richardson S, et al. Psychogenic palatal tremor. *Mov Disord.* 2006;21(2):274–276.

84. Williams DR. Psychogenic palatal tremor. *Mov Disord.* 2004;19(3):333–335.

85. Fahn S, Williams DT. Psychogenic dystonia. *Adv Neurol.* 1988;50:431–455.

86. Hallett M. Physiology of psychogenic movement disorders. *J Clin Neurosci.* 2010;17(8):959–965.

87. Yokota T, et al. MRI findings of inferior olives in palatal myoclonus. *J Neurol.* 1989;236(2):115–116.

88. Pierot L, et al. Palatal myoclonus and inferior olivary lesions: MRI-pathologic correlation. *J Comput Assist Tomogr.* 1992;16(1):160–163.

89. Medina LS. MR imaging of hypertrophic olivary degeneration: is there a role for metaanalysis? *AJNR Am J Neuroradiol.* 2000;21(6):998–999.

90. Jang L, Borruat FX. Oculopalatal tremor: variations on a theme by Guillain and Mollaret. *Eur Neurol.* 2014;72(3–4):144–149.

91. Yoshii F, Tomori Y, Mori T. Diffusion tensor imaging in a case of pontine bleeding showing hypertrophic olivary degeneration and cerebellar ataxia. *Case Rep Neurol.* 2018;10(3):297–301.

92. Auffray-Calvier E, et al. Hypertrophic olivary degeneration. MR imaging findings and temporal evolution. *J Neuroradiol.* 2005;32(1):67–72.

93. Gautier JC, Blackwood W. Enlargement of the inferior olivary nucleus in association with lesions of the central tegmental tract or dentate nucleus. *Brain.* 1961;84:341–361.

94. Blanco Ulla M, Lopez Carballeira A, Pumar Cebreiro JM. Magnetic resonance imaging of hypertrophic olivary degeneration. *Radiologia.* 2015;57(6):505–511.

95. Smets G, et al. The dentato-rubro-olivary pathway revisited: new MR imaging observations regarding hypertrophic olivary degeneration. *Clin Anat.* 2017;30(4):543–549.

96. De Zeeuw CI, et al. Microcircuitry and function of the inferior olive. *Trends Neurosci.* 1998;21(9):391–400.

97. Manor Y, et al. Low-amplitude oscillations in the inferior olive: a model based on electrical coupling of neurons with heterogeneous channel densities. *J Neurophysiol.* 1997;77(5):2736–2752.

98. Ruigrok TJ, de Zeeuw CI, Voogd J. Hypertrophy of inferior olivary neurons: a degenerative, regenerative or plasticity phenomenon. *Eur J Morphol.* 1990;28(2–4):224–239.

99. Sotelo C, Llinas R, Baker R. Structural study of inferior olivary nucleus of the cat: morphological correlates of electrotonic coupling. *J Neurophysiol.* 1974;37(3):541–559.

100. Lia K, et al. Impulsive head rotation resets oculopalatal tremor: examination of a model. *Prog Brain Res.* 2008;171:227–234.

101. Hong S, et al. Inferior olive hypertrophy and cerebellar learning are both needed to explain ocular oscillations in oculopalatal tremor. *Prog Brain Res.* 2008;171:219–226.

102. Dubinsky RM, et al. Increased glucose metabolism in the medulla of patients with palatal myoclonus. *Neurology.* 1991;41(4):557–562.

103. Dubinsky RM, Hallett M. Palatal myoclonus and facial involvement in other types of myoclonus. *Adv Neurol.* 1988;49:263–278.

104. Yakushiji Y, et al. Glucose utilization in the inferior cerebellar vermis and ocular myoclonus. *Neurology.* 2006;67(1):131–133.

105. Andersen N, Krauth N, Nabavi S. Hebbian plasticity in vivo: relevance and induction. *Curr Opin Neurobiol.* 2017;45:188–192.

106. Caporale N, Dan Y. Spike timing-dependent plasticity: a Hebbian learning rule. *Annu Rev Neurosci.* 2008;31:25–46.

107. Sgritta M, et al. Hebbian spike-timing dependent plasticity at the cerebellar input stage. *J Neurosci.* 2017;37(11):2809–2823.

108. Piochon C, et al. Non-Hebbian spike-timing-dependent plasticity in cerebellar circuits. *Front Neural Circuits.* 2012;6:124.

109. Stern MM. Rhythmic palatopharyngeal myoclonus, review, case report and significance. *J Nerv Ment Dis.* 1949;109(1):48–53.

110. Kadakia S, McAbee G. Volitional control of palatal myoclonus. *Mov Disord.* 1990;5(2):182–183.

111. Sperling MR, Herrmann Jr. C. Syndrome of palatal myoclonus and progressive ataxia: two cases with magnetic resonance imaging. *Neurology.* 1985;35(8):1212–1214.

112. Leger JM, Duyckaerts C, Brunet P. Syndrome of palatal myoclonus and progressive ataxia: report of a case. *Neurology.* 1986;36(10):1409–1410.

113. Samuel M, et al. Progressive ataxia and palatal tremor (PAPT): clinical and MRI assessment with review of palatal tremors. *Brain.* 2004;127(Pt 6):1252–1268.

114. Kinghorn KJ, et al. Hypertrophic olivary degeneration on magnetic resonance imaging in mitochondrial syndromes associated with POLG and SURF1 mutations. *J Neurol.* 2013;260(1):3–9.

115. Mongin M, et al. Progressive ataxia and palatal tremor: think about POLG mutations. *Tremor Other Hyperkinet Mov (N Y).* 2016;6:382.

116. Nicastro N, et al. Pure progressive ataxia and palatal tremor (PAPT) associated with a new polymerase gamma (POLG) mutation. *Cerebellum.* 2016;15(6):829–831.

117. Berlo R, Kojovic M. Palatal tremor in progressive supranuclear palsy: a case report. *Parkinsonism Relat Disord.* 2015;21(3):335–336.

118. Kulkarni PK, et al. Palatal tremor, progressive multiple cranial nerve palsies, and cerebellar ataxia: a case report and review of literature of palatal tremors in neurodegenerative disease. *Mov Disord.* 1999;14(4):689–693.

119. Suyama N, et al. Progressive supranuclear palsy with palatal myoclonus. *Acta Neuropathol.* 1997;94(3):290–293.

120. Howard KL, et al. Adult-onset Alexander disease with progressive ataxia and palatal tremor. *Mov Disord.* 2008;23(1):118–122.

121. Li R, et al. Glial fibrillary acidic protein mutations in infantile, juvenile, and adult forms of Alexander disease. *Ann Neurol.* 2005;57(3):310–326.

122. Gass JM, et al. Novel GFAP variant in adult-onset Alexander disease with progressive ataxia and palatal tremor. *Neurologist.* 2017;22(6):247–248.

123. Mari Z, et al. Clinico-pathological correlation in progressive ataxia and palatal tremor: a novel tauopathy. *Mov Disord Clin Pract.* 2014;1(1):50–56.

124. Probst EN, et al. Atypical focal MRI lesions in a case of juvenile Alexander's disease. *Ann Neurol.* 2003;53(1):118–120.

125. Tchikviladze M, et al. A diagnostic flow chart for POLG-related diseases based on signs sensitivity and specificity. *J Neurol Neurosurg Psychiatry.* 2015;86(6):646–654.

126. Bostan A, et al. Novel mutation in spacer region of POLG associated with ataxia neuropathy spectrum and gastroparesis. *Auton Neurosci.* 2012;170(1–2):70–72.

127. Ng YS, et al. Novel POLG variants associated with late-onset de novo status epilepticus and progressive ataxia. *Neurol Genet.* 2017;3(5):e181.

128. Storey E, Gardner RJM. *Spinocerebellar Ataxia Type 20.* In: Adam MP, et al., eds. *GeneReviews((R)).* University of Washington, Seattle; 1993.

129. Storey E, et al. Spinocerebellar ataxia type 20. *Cerebellum.* 2005;4(1):55–57.

130. Wang D, et al. Failed DBS for palliation of visual problems in a case of oculopalatal tremor. *Parkinsonism Relat Disord.* 2009;15(1):71–73.

131. Espay AJ, et al. Current concepts in diagnosis and treatment of functional neurological disorders. *JAMA Neurol.* 2018;75(9):1132–1141.

15

Myorhythmia

FELIPE VIAL AND MARK HALLETT

INTRODUCTION

Myorhythmia is included in the 2018 MDS tremor classification and is defined as a "very rare rhythmic movement disorder of cranial or limb muscles at rest or during action . . . the frequency is 1 to 4 Hz. It is usually associated with localizing brainstem signs and a diagnosable etiology,"[1] and is classified under the category of tremor with prominent additional signs. However, historical and pathophysiological reasons explain why this particular type of tremor has a specific name.

PHENOMENOLOGY

The term myorhythmia was first used by Herz in 1931 to describe the slow rhythmic movement seen in dystonia (movements that today would be labeled as dystonic tremor).[2] After Herz's work in 1931, the literature became confusing because several different terms have since been used to label similar phenomenologies, such as facial myoclonus/myorhythmia, skeletal myoclonus/myorhythmia, palatal myoclonus/tremor, segmental myoclonus, oculo-masticatory myorhythmia, and oculo-facio-skeletal myorhythmia. Although there are differences in the definitions of each of these terms, there is much overlap.

All these concepts are similar in describing a slow rhythmic or pseudo-rhythmic involuntary movement: branchial myoclonus/myorhythmia would involve only branchial muscles; skeletal myoclonus/myorhythmia affects skeletal (mainly limb) muscles; palatal tremor/myoclonus would involve palate muscles and sometimes limb; oculo-masticatory myorhythmia (OMM) involves masticatory muscles together with pendular vergence oscillation of the eyes (synchronous with the activity of the masticatory muscles); oculo-facio-skeletal myorhythmia (OFSM) is similar to OMM but includes other facial, neck, or limb muscles.[3] Holmes tremor may also affect cranial as well as limb muscles. For a summary, see Figure 15.1.

In their review about myorhythmia, Baizabal-Carvallo et al. (2015)[4] define myorhythmia as a repetitive, rhythmic, often jerky movement of slow (1–4 Hz) frequency, affecting mainly cranial and limb muscles. These movements usually occur at rest but may be observed in posture or action.

Ure et al. (2016),[3] on the other hand, describe it as semi-rhythmic rapid muscle contractions (but typically more sustained than in pure myoclonus), which are very mildly and variably modulated by actions. Importantly, this definition was done after reviewing 44 videos of cases reported as myorhythmia describing a particular movement consistently seen in the cases secondary to Whipple disease. The authors gave much importance to the irregular features of myorhythmia in order to differentiate it from a tremor.

Bally et al. (2018)[5] reviewed movement disorders in Whipple disease and defined myorhythmia as a form of rhythmic or semi-rhythmic segmental myoclonus, affecting either branchial or spinal muscles or both.

On the other hand, other authors have proposed that myorhythmia is just a form of segmental myoclonus,[6] a slow rest tremor,[7] or a Holmes tremor.[8]

Only a few studies are available regarding electrophysiological characterization, describing a slow oscillatory activity with bursts lasting 200ms with normal morphology showing sometimes synchronic or asynchronous activity between antagonist muscles. Sometimes there is also synchronous activation of muscles of different parts of the body.[4,9,10]

PATHOLOGY

The most extensive pathological description of cases with myorhythmia comes from the Masucci et al. (1984) series, in which 6 of the 24 patients were pathologically studied. They described myorhythmia as a slow, relatively rhythmic rest tremor that may involve single limbs, several limbs, or a combination of limbs plus face, palate, head, jaw, neck, tongue, eyes, or trunk. Many of the

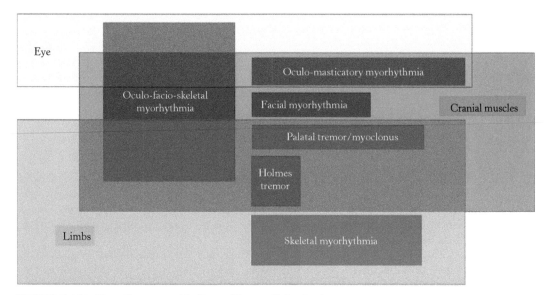

FIGURE 15.1: Venn Diagram of Different Types of Myorhythmia.

described cases also had cerebellar signs. The etiology was attributed to either brainstem vascular disease or cerebellar degeneration secondary to chronic alcoholism-nutritional deficit.[9] The most common structure affected was the substantia nigra (5/6 cases), and there was one case in which this was the only affected structure. The dentate nucleus, superior cerebellar peduncle, cerebellar hemispheres, brachium pontis, and inferior olive were affected in at least 2 of the 6 cases. The subthalamus was involved in one case, but in that case, it was the only affected structure. There were no cases with the central tegmental tract involvement. The pathological changes include atrophy, hypertrophy degenerative changes, and demyelination. Regarding the clinic pathological correlation, the authors observed that both the palatal and limb involvement were related to lesions in either the ipsilateral dentate nucleus or the superior cerebellar peduncle or to contralateral inferior olive involvement.

Considering the involvement of the brainstem and cerebellar regions described in the Masucci study, the question is whether the Guillain-Mollaret triangle is part of the pathophysiology in some cases of myorhythmia, and whether this pathophysiology is similar to that observed in cases of symptomatic palatal tremor/myoclonus, which occurs at a frequency in the same range as observed in myorhythmia. The Guillain-Mollaret triangle is classically described as a pathway between the dentate nucleus, red nucleus, and inferior olive. However, there is evidence now that

the most important connection is an inhibitory GABAergic pathway between the dentate nucleus and contralateral inferior olivary nucleus that goes through the red nucleus.[11] Many of the neurons in the inferior olivary nucleus have dendro-dendritic gap junctions, and they discharge rhythmically. So, disinhibition produced by a lesion in the GABAergic pathway coming from the contralateral dentate nucleus will transform the inferior olivary nucleus into an oscillator that will produce the rhythmic movements observed in symptomatic palatal tremor/myoclonus. This phenomenological entity is associated with inferior olivary hypertrophy. In the Masucci et al. series, 2 of the 6 cases were found to have inferior olivary involvement, and one of those had atrophy instead of hypertrophy, a finding previously described in a case of myorhythmia with no palate involvement.[12]

However, the myorhythmia as described in Whipple disease—and most of the literature about myorhythmia concerns Whipple disease—rarely has palate involvement.[5] Additionally, a finding of inferior olivary nucleus hypertrophy in imaging studies is most unusual.[4]

ETIOLOGIES

Myorhythmia in Whipple

Whipple disease is a rare infectious disease caused by *Tropheryma whipplei*, with an incidence of 0.4 –1 per 1,000,000 a year.[13] Usually, the clinical picture is dominated by gastrointestinal symptoms. The central nervous system is involved in about 50% of cases.[14] The first time myorhythmia was mentioned concerning Whipple disease was in 1963, by van Bogaert et al.[15] In 1986 Schwartz introduced the term OMM to describe slow (1–2 Hz) regular masticatory movements together with pendular vergence oscillation of the eyes.[16] Sometimes there is associated vertical nystagmus, rhythmic contraction of the eyelids, tongue protrusion, or bruxism.[4,17] The term OFSM was added later to describe a similar movement that extends to the facial, neck, or limb muscles.

In a review about movement disorders in Whipple disease that includes 146 cases, Bally et al. describe the presence of myorhythmia in 40% of the cases, with 60% of those classified as either OMM or OFSM.[5] As the authors note, the use of the terminology for the description of the phenomenology was not very consistent across different articles; however, there seems to be an agreement in that the OMM and OFSM forms of myorhythmia are almost pathognomonic of Whipple disease. Apart from myorhythmia, patients with Whipple may exhibit cognitive impairment, supranuclear ophthalmoplegia, and an altered level of consciousness.[18]

Regarding the imaging abnormalities in Whipple disease with neurological manifestations, most reports describe T2 hyperintensities in the mesial temporal lobe, midbrain, hypothalamus, and thalamus.[19] Nevertheless, these reports and their imaging abnormalities include patients with and without myorhythmia.

Cerebrovascular disease

There are many reports of involuntary movements labeled as myorhythmia secondary to cerebrovascular lesions. Again, the use of the term myorhythmia is not very consistent. Concerning the localization, most of the reports described thalamic and brainstem lesions.[20]

Thalamic lesions

There is a report of 7 cases with a posterio-lateral lesion of the thalamus and movements labeled as myorhythmia. The slow, rhythmic movements affecting limbs occurred in the context of dystonia and appeared with or were exacerbated by posture and action. The movements started between 17 days and two years after the lesion.[21] Considering that description, it is possible to argue that those movements correspond to dystonic tremor more than myorhythmia.

Brainstem lesions

In Masucci et al.'s classic series, there are 6 cases with ischemic brainstem lesions. The definition of myorhythmia in that series was described earlier in this chapter.[9]

Wu et al. (2000)[22] described two cases of slow (2.5–3.5 Hz) tremor presenting in the proximal upper limbs predominantly when at rest, aggravated by outstretched arms and by active hand movements, and secondary to brainstem stroke. In both cases, the movements started several months after the ischemic attack and were associated with inferior olivary hypertrophy.

Vancaester et al. (2013)[23] described a case of extensive midbrain hemorrhage, after which the patient developed rhythmic movements (0.9–1 Hz) of the right arm, co-occurring with the masticatory muscles.

Inflammatory-autoimmune

Myorhythmic movements have been described in anti-NMDA encephalitis in a series of 9 children, 2 of which are described as having these movements. In one of the cases, the movement is described as 1- to 2-Hz repetitive contractions of the procerus, corrugator, orbicularis oculi, and oromandibular muscles with tongue protrusion, along with slow leg tremor.[24] There are also descriptions in celiac disease[25] and steroid-responsive encephalitis.[26]

TREATMENT

In cases secondary to Whipple disease, the idea is to treat the cause (antibiotic therapy). Regarding symptomatic treatment, several drugs have been tried with poor results (baclofen, carbamazepine, clonazepam, diazepam, lorazepam, trihexyphenidyl, haloperidol, fluoxetine, tetrabenazine).[4] There are some reports of improvement with tetrabenazine in myorhythmia secondary to anti-NMDA receptor encephalitis.[24]

CONCLUSION

Myorhythmia is not a very well-defined syndrome, and the term has been used to label different phenomena. The core symptom in all the reports is a slow periodic (rhythmic or semi-rhythmic) involuntary muscle activation of some part of the body, and the pathology is usually localized in the brainstem. Many of the reported cases in the literature could well be labeled as dystonic tremor, segmental myoclonus, palatal tremor/myoclonus, or Holmes tremor. Because the term myorhythmia has been used in so many different ways, the association with the only pathological study[9] is not straightforward.

The literature is limited about myorhythmia, and it is likely that the reason this concept has survived through the years is its commonly described association with Whipple disease. In fact, the OMM and OFSM forms are phenotypically more consistently defined, including their pathognomonic association with Whipple disease.

An agreement between experts regarding the definition of myorhythmia is critical to keep using this concept. We propose to define myorhythmia as a slow periodic rhythmic or semi-rhythmic involuntary movement of some part of the body. This term would encompass OMM, OFSM, facial myorhythmia, and skeletal myorhythmia, as well as Holmes tremor and palatal tremor/myoclonus. As the movement is not always rhythmic and/or oscillatory (it does not necessarily involve a repetitive variation around a central point), it is debatable whether it should be called a tremor.

REFERENCES

1. Bhatia KP, Bain P, Bajaj N, et al. Consensus statement on the classification of tremors. from the task force on tremor of the International Parkinson and Movement Disorder Society. *Mov Disord.* 2018;33(1):75–87. doi: 10.1002/mds.27121

2. Herz K. Die amyostatischen Unruheerscheinungen: Klinisch kinematographische Analyse ihrer Kennzeichen und Begleiterscheinungen. *J Psychol Neurol.* 1931;43:146–163.

3. Ure RJ, Dhanju S, Lang AE, Fasano A. Unusual tremor syndromes: know in order to recognise. *J Neurol Neurosurg Psychiatry.* 2016;87(11):1191–1203. doi: 10.1136/jnnp-2015-311693

4. Baizabal-Carvallo JF, Cardoso F, Jankovic J. Myorhythmia: phenomenology, etiology, and treatment. *Mov Disord.* 2015;30(2):171–179. doi: 10.1002/mds.26093

5. Bally JF, Méneret A, Roze E, Anderson M, Grabli D, Lang AE. Systematic review of movement disorders and oculomotor abnormalities in Whipple's disease. *Mov Disord.* 2018;33(11):1700–1711. doi: 10.1002/mds.27419

6. Jankovic J, Pardo R. Segmental myoclonus: clinical and pharmacologic study. *Arch Neurol.* 1986;43(10):1025–1031. doi: 10.1001/archneur.1986.00520100039012

7. Donaldson IM, Marsden CD, Schneider SA, Bhatia KP. *Marsden's Book of Movement Disorders* (Chapter 19). Oxford University Press; 2012: 715.

8. Deuschl G, Bain P, Brin M. Consensus statement of the Movement Disorder Society on Tremor. *Mov Disord.* 2008;13(S3):2–23. doi: 10.1002/mds.870131303

9. Masucci EF, Kurtzke JF, Saini N. Myorhythmia: a widespread movement disorder: Clinicopathological correlations. *Brain.* 1984;107(1):53–79. doi: 10.1093/brain/107.1.53

10. Dimberg EL, Crowe SE, Trugman JM, et al. Fatal encephalitis in a patient with refractory celiac disease presenting with myorhythmia and carpal spasm. *Mov Disord.* 2007;22(3):407–411. doi: 10.1002/mds.21324

11. Shaikh AG, Hong S, Liao K, et al. Oculopalatal tremor explained by a model of inferior olivary hypertrophy and cerebellar plasticity. *Brain.* 2010;133(3):923–940. doi: 10.1093/brain/awp323

12. Garcin R, Lapresle J, Fardeau M. Myoclonies squelettiques rythmees sans nystagmus du voile. Etude anatomo-clinique avec presentation d'un film cinematographique. *Rev Neurol (Paris).* 1963;109:105–114.

13. Uryu Dr K, Sakai T, Yamamoto T, et al. Central nervous system relapse of Whipple's disease. *Intern Med.* 2012;51(15):2045–2050. doi: 10.2169/internalmedicine.51.7304

14. Verhagen WIM, Huygen PLM, Dalman JE. Central nervous system Whipple's disease [2]. *Ann Neurol.* 1997;41(4):560–561. doi: 10.1002/ana.410410424

15. van Bogaert L, Lafoh R, Pages P, Labauge R. Sur une encephalite subaigue non classable, principalement caracterisee par des myorhythmies oculo-facio-cervicales. *Rev Neurol.* 1963;109(4):443–453.

16. Schwartz MA, Selhorst JB, Ochs AL, et al. Oculomasticatory myorhythrma: a unique movement disorder occurring in Whipple's disease. *Ann Neurol.* 1986;20(6):677–683. doi: 10.1002/ana.410200605

17. Tison F, Louvet-Giendaj C, Henry P, Lagueny A, Gaujard E. Permanent bruxism as a manifestation of the oculo-facial syndrome related to systemic whipple's disease. *Mov Disord.* 1992;7(1):82–85. doi: 10.1002/mds.870070117

18. Fenollar F, Puéchal X, Raoult D. Whipple's disease. *N Engl J Med.* 2007;356(1):55–66. doi: 10.1056/NEJMra062477

19. Black DF, Aksamit AJ, Morris JM. MR imaging of central nervous system Whipple disease: a 15-year review. *Am J Neuroradiol.* 2010;31(8):1493–1497. doi: 10.3174/ajnr.A2089

20. Mehanna R, Jankovic J. Movement disorders in cerebrovascular disease. *Lancet Neurol.* 2013;12(6):597–608. doi: 10.1016/S1474-4422(13)70057-7

21. Lera G, Scipioni O, Garcia S, Cammarota A, Fischbein G, Gershanik O. A combined pattern of movement disorders resulting from posterolateral thalamic lesions of a vascular nature: a syndrome with clinico-radiologic correlation. *Mov Disord.* 2000;15(1):120–126. doi: 10.1002/1531-8257(200001)15:1<120::aid-mds1018>3.0.co;2-v

22. Wu JC, Lu CS, Ng SH. Limb myorhythmia in association with hypertrophy of the inferior olive: report of two cases. *Chang Gung Med J.* 2000;23(10):630–635. Accessed December 30, 2019. http://www.ncbi.nlm.nih.gov/pubmed/11126156.

23. Vancaester E, Hemelsoet D, De Letter M, Santens P. Masticatory myorhythmia following pontine hemorrhage. *Acta Neurol Belg.* 2013;113(3):327–329. doi: 10.1007/s13760-013-0206-6

24. Baizabal-Carvallo JF, Stocco A, Muscal E, Jankovic J. The spectrum of movement disorders in children with anti-NMDA receptor encephalitis. *Mov Disord.* 2013;28(4):543–547. doi: 10.1002/mds.25354

25. Dimberg EL, Crowe SE, Trugman JM, et al. Fatal encephalitis in a patient with refractory celiac disease presenting with myorhythmia and carpal spasm. *Mov Disord.* 2007;22(3):407–411. doi: 10.1002/mds.21324

26. Erickson JC, Carrasco H, Grimes JB, Jabbari B, Cannard KR. Palatal tremor and myorhythmia in Hashimoto's encephalopathy. *Neurology.* 2002;58(3):504–505. doi: 10.1212/WNL.58.3.504

16

Functional Tremor

PETRA SCHWINGENSCHUH

INTRODUCTION

Functional tremor (FT) and other types of functional movement disorders (FMDs) are part of the spectrum of functional neurological disorders (FND), previously known as "hysteria," "dissociative," "conversion," "somatoform," "non-organic" and "psychogenic" disorders. FNDs are defined as symptoms of altered voluntary motor or sensory function that cause clinically significant distress or impairment, and the presence of clinical findings supporting incompatibility between symptoms and neurological or medical conditions.[1] FNDs are common and account for approximately 6% of neurology outpatient contacts.[2] Despite the high frequency of this disorder and the negative impact on quality of life and working life, these patients have historically been poorly diagnosed and managed.[2] The last decade has seen remarkable progress and a clear shift in the clinical approach to these disorders.

In the fifth edition of the *Diagnostic and Statistical Manual of Mental Disorders* (DSM-5) the Somatic Symptom and Related Disorders category was created and terminology as well as diagnostic criteria for "functional neurological symptom disorder" were changed. The former term "psychogenic," which implied a psychological causation, was replaced with "functional," and the criterion of psychological stress as a prerequisite for FND was removed. Furthermore, emphasis was placed on the use of positive clinical symptoms and signs rather than the absence of a medical explanation for somatic symptoms.[1] "Conversion disorder" was kept as an alternative name for FND, although it has never been widely accepted by either nonpsychiatrists or patients.[3,4]

A negative consequence of DSM-5 was, however, that the diagnosis of somatization disorder that, according to DSM-IV-SD, encompassed individuals with functional neurological symptoms and prominent other bodily symptoms including pain, was eliminated, and somatization disorder, somatoform pain disorder, and undifferentiated somatoform disorder were collapsed into the somatic symptom disorder diagnosis.[5]

The shift in terminology from "psychogenic" to "functional"[6] underlines the conceptual evolution from brain–mind dualism to a biopsychosocial illness model, including alterations in sensorimotor and limbic brain circuits.[7,8,9,10,11]

FNDs are characterized by the unintentional production of neurological symptoms and are therefore distinct from malingering and factitious disorder. In factitious disorder, patients deliberately produce, feign, or exaggerate physical or psychological symptoms without benefits except optaining a patien's role. When behavior is motivated by external incentives such as avoiding military duty or work, or obtaining financial compensation, the appropriate term is malingering. Factitious disorder is regarded as a mental illness, while malingering is a non-medical condition encountered in medico-legal cases.[12] Although there are no tests capable of demonstrating whether symptoms are deliberately produced and there may not be a clear categorical difference between voluntary and involuntary symptoms, intentionally produced symptoms are considered relatively rare in clinical practice.[4,13] Since objective evidence of malingering or factitious disorder is rare and difficult to obtain, the requirement to exclude feigning was eliminated from the DSM-5.[1]

It is important to take into account that patients may have a combination of an "organic" disease with functional overlay.[13,14] In recent years, the term "organic" has itself become controversial.[15] The functional-organic distinction aims to distinguish symptoms, signs, and syndromes that can be explained by diagnosable biological changes from those that cannot.[16] However, all symptoms must have a biological basis, thus "recognized pathophysiological disease" might be a preferable wording.[17] FMD refers to involuntary abnormal movements that are inconsistent and incongruent with the phenotypic range of other recognized movement disorders.[18]

FMDs are estimated to represent between 2 and 25% of patients seen in movement disorder clinics.[19] FT is regarded as the most common

FMD, accounting for more than 50% of patients in published cohorts.[20,21,22] In a recent multicenter, observational study including 410 consecutive patients with functional motor disorders, the most common phenotypes were weakness (44%) and tremor (41%), followed by dystonia (29%).[23]

While FT can affect children and the elderly, it usually starts during young and middle adulthood (Schwingenschuh, Pont-Sunyer, Surtees, Edwards, & Bhatia, 2008) (Batla et al., 2013). The mean age at onset of FT in large series was 32.0 ± 24.5 (Schwingenschuh et al., 2016), 36.1 ± 13.8 (Kim et al., 1999), and 43.0 ± 14.0 years, respectively (Jankovic & Thomas, 2005). FT can affect both men and women, but a female predominance (female to male ratio 1.9–2.5:1) was shown in several studies.[24,25] In a study analyzing 196 consecutive patients with FMD, males had an older age at onset (40.5 vs. 34.1 years) and an older age at evaluation (43.8 vs. 38.1 years) compared to females.[26]

The importance of a phenotype-specific positive diagnosis rather than one of exclusion has been repeatedly emphasized.[27,28,29,30,31,32] However, high levels of diagnostic uncertainty remain, and a recent survey-based study found that nearly half the responding neurologists considered FMD an exclusionary diagnosis and almost two-thirds indicated that they were "more or very concerned" about missing another diagnosis compared to patients with other disorders.[33]

The general concern to miss an "organic" disorder stands in contrast to studies indicating that the number of misdiagnoses in functional disorders is actually low and not unlike that of other neurological disorders. A systematic review found that the rate of erroneously diagnosed functional disorders had been 4% since 1970.[34] Among 1144 new neurology outpatients in a Scottish cohort, the proportion of patients with other diagnoses who were misdiagnosed with a functional disorder was 0.4% only.[35] One of the reasons for this concern might be a wrong perception among neurologists that neurological diseases are always more serious than functional disorders.[17] This fear of missing another neurologic disorder often leads to unnecessary and expensive laboratory and imaging tests, which cause a substantial diagnostic delay, while early diagnosis is regarded as an important prognostic factor for good outcome in FMD patients.[36] Misdiagnosis can harm patients in either direction, especially as evidence-based treatment for FNDs has become available.[17]

To complicate matters further, it is relatively frequent for other movement disorders to coincide with a functional disorder, and distinguishing pure FT from another tremor disorder with functional overlay is often a diagnostic dilemma.[18]

The following sections will discuss the principles of an inclusionary diagnostic approach of FT, followed by a review of the current literature on potential overlap of FT and other movement disorders and, finally, a summary on evidence-based treatment of FT.

PATHOPHYSIOLOGY

The key clinical feature that separates patients with FT from those with other tremor disorders is that the movements have features that one would usually associate with voluntary movement, but patients report them as being involuntary and not under their control. This feature may mean either that movements are deliberately feigned or that there are brain mechanisms that allow voluntary movement to occur, but to be experienced subjectively as involuntary.[29] During the last decade, neuroscience has provided strong evidence for a neurobiological basis of FND:

Several studies found distinct patterns between feigners and FMD that support different mechanisms for both entities and confirm the involuntary nature of functional symptoms.[37,12]

Functional imaging recorded in patients during an episode of FT compared to episodes where patients were voluntarily mimicking their tremor showed hypoactivation of the temporoparietal junction during FT.[38] This area is thought to be an important comparator region: comparing actual with predicted sensory feedback and its dysfunction might producing a feeling of involuntariness associated with movement.[38] In concordance with this assumption, another study found an abnormal sense of intention that is associated with voluntary movement in patients with FT.[39] A recent fMRI study using a virtual-reality movement paradigm found impaired hemodynamic responsiveness to changes in the sense of agency in critical areas of the network in patients with FMD.[40]

FT is associated with abnormalities in activation and functional connectivity in networks involved in emotion processing and theory of mind.[9] FT patients showed increased activation in the anterior cingulate/paracingulate cortex, and tremor improvement after cognitive behavioral therapy was associated with normalized activation patterns.[41] Altered emotional processing may represent a key link between psychosocial risk factors and core features of FMD.[11] Dysfunctional emotion processing appears to play a major role in the perpetuation of symptoms for some patients.[42]

Furthermore, patients with FMD have been shown to exhibit structural gray matter abnormalities in critical components of the limbic and sensorimotor circuitry. These abnormalities may represent a premorbid trait rendering patients more susceptible to disease, to the disease itself, or to a compensatory response to disease.[43]

DIAGNOSTIC APPROACH BASED ON "RULE-IN-SIGNS"

There are several positive signs on history, physical examination, and electrophysiological testing that help make the diagnosis of a FT (also see Box 16.1).[22] Almost none are 100% diagnostic, so it is important to appreciate the whole picture.[18] However, this is not that different from many other movement disorders, in which neurologists

---

BOX 16.1
KEY POSITIVE FEATURES
INDICATIVE OF
FUNCTIONAL TREMOR

History
- Acute onset
- Rapid progression to maximum severity
- Fluctuating course with remissions or static course
- Variability of affected body part
- Somatization in the past history
- Atypical response to medication

Examination
- Unusual clinical combinations of rest, postural and kinetic tremors
- Variability in amplitude, frequency, distribution
- Increased attention toward the affected limb
- Distractibility
- Entrainability, coherence
- Variability of tremor phenomenology
- Co-contraction
- Suggestibility / Placebo responsiveness
- "Whack-a-mole" sign
- Excessive exhaustion during examination or "La belle indifférence"
- Appearance of additional and unrelated neurologic signs

---

have to deal with a certain level of diagnostic uncertainty, especially in early stages of the disease. Similar to other disorders, diagnoses may change over time, which does not necessarily mean the doctor got it wrong the first time.[35,13]

History

The time course of the disorder is very important. With the exception of some symptomatic tremors (e.g., those secondary to intoxication, vascular events, or trauma), organic tremors usually start gradually. In contrast to this, FT appears suddenly in the majority of patients, sometimes even within seconds to minutes, and maximal disability is often reached immediately.[24] Many patients with FT remember the exact moment and the circumstances when the disorder began. Patients may describe this moment as random, or as having occurred during or after a period of stress. The most common precipitating events are (minor) physical injuries.[24,44] Other precipitating physical events are surgery, infections, drug reactions, or other illnesses.[45] FT may also occur after successful treatment of an organic tremor with deep brain stimulation.[46]

Focal or segmental onset is more common than generalized onset. However, tremor often spreads to other body parts or even becomes generalized (Kim et al., 1999). Also, tremor phenomenology and tremor severity may change over time. The clinical course after maximal disability can be fluctuating, progressively worsening, or static. Patients may experience spontaneous and often transient remissions.[27,24,29] Rarely, FT presents as a paroxysmal movement disorder.[47]

Patients with FT may overestimate their daily tremor duration.[48] However, a recent study found that patients with FT had a similar association between subjective and objective tremor symptoms as compared to patients with organic tremors.[49]

A history of unresponsiveness to medications, response to placebos, and remission with psychotherapy may be present.

FND including FT usually brings other symptoms with it, and sometimes the tremor is not the worst problem these patients have.[50,51] Careful history often reveals non-motor symptoms, especially chronic pain, anxiety, and fatigue.[52] Many patients have other associated FNDs such as sensory symptoms, non-epileptic seizures, and visual symptoms.[20,23,52] Overall, there is a clear overlap between FND and other comorbid functional somatic symptoms, especially through the previous entity of "somatization disorder."[5] In one study, 8 out of 36 patients (12.5%) with FMD met criteria for "comorbid somatization disorder."[42]

Clinical examination

FT often presents with a complex clinical presentation and marked variability may be observed within one consultation (see Video 16.1). Variability can present as change in frequency, amplitude, direction (e.g., changing from pronation/supination to flexion/extension pattern), and as fluctuation of anatomic tremor distribution.[20]

Tremor of the upper limbs is most common and often presents with similar amplitudes during rest, posture, and action. Finger tremor is typically absent.[22] Other body parts frequently affected are head, legs, and the trunk.[27,29] Lower limb tremor with whole body distribution of tremor at onset is another possible clue to the diagnosis of FT.[53] Tremor of more than one body part typically has a synchronous pattern (synchronicity). Targeted clinical examination revealed positive functional signs in the majority of patients diagnosed with essential palatal tremor, for which the term "isolated palatal tremor" has also been used.[54] Combined electroencephalography and electromyography with time-locked video recordings was suggested as useful tool to support the functional origin of presumed essential palatal tremor.[55]

Simple observation of patients with FT revealed excessive attention to their affected limbs and to movements of these limbs during examination.[56] In concordance with this clinical observation, functional imaging studies in FND reported increased activity in areas associated with "self-monitoring."[57,58] Visual attention to the limb may be a marker of explicit control of movement, usually seen during the performance of novel tasks.[59] Distraction of attention away from the affected limb forms the basis of the majority of clinical tests used to distinguish FT.[60] In FT, shift of attention to other tasks often causes a decrease or suspension of tremor (see Video 16.1), in contrast to many other tremors (e.g., rest tremor in Parkinson disease) which tend to increase.

Cognitive distraction maneuvers, also referred to as cognitive load or dual tasks, include mental arithmetics (e.g., subtracting serial sevens from 100) or other cognitive tasks, such as listing the months of the year in reverse order. Motor tasks need to be adapted based on the tremor distribution. The sequential finger tapping method is commonly used in patients with upper limb tremors, where the patient is instructed to tap with the thumb and fingers II, III, IV, and V in subsequent order. At the same time, the tremor of the other hand is observed in order to detect if tremor decreases or resolves during the task (i.e., distractibility). If needed, the difficulty level can be raised by changing the tempo or the sequence order. Sudden ballistic movements or finger-to nose tests with a moving target performed with the contralateral hand may be helpful to reveal distractibility of tremor.[22]

Finger tapping or similar voluntary movements (foot tapping, rapid alternating movements) at a given frequency are also used to demonstrate entrainability, which represents another clinical hallmark of FT. Entrainment occurs if the tremor overtakes the frequency of the contralateral tapping movements.[22]

Before labeling a tremor as "not distractable," the level of difficulty and the type of the distraction task need to be adapted. Appropriate maneuvers for the lower limbs include alternating toe–heel tapping or drawing on the floor with the contralateral foot. For a head tremor, a task using repetitive eye or tongue movements may be helpful.[22] However, in some patients with FT distractibility cannot be demonstrated, at least on clinical grounds.[27]

An unexplained poor performance of the distraction task while maintaining the FT may add to the overall clinical impression that guides the differentiation of functional from other tremors (see Video 16.1).[22]

It is important to recognize that tremor variability does not necessarily indicate FT. Other tremors can also have a variable amplitude influenced by the level of anxiety and exhaustion, may be position dependent, or may appear irregular in rhythm or change direction (e.g., in the case of a dystonic tremor).[61]

FT may show a "coactivation sign," i.e., some underlying antagonistic muscle activation (cocontraction), whenever the tremor is present. If the increased muscle tone disappears, the tremor disappears too. This is demonstrated during slow, arrhythmic, passive movements—as rigidity is commonly tested.[27,22]

Sometimes FT is suggestible and varies in response to certain stimuli, such as the examiner touching a certain trigger point or applying a vibrating tuning fork to the affected body part and suggesting that this may reduce the symptoms.[28,61] Care must be taken when using suggestion as an exam maneuver, however, as this may affect the physician–patient relationship.

The "whack-a-mole" sign, which is defined as spread of tremor to another body part if the tremor is restrained by the examiner's hand, is regarded as another positive physical sign and diagnostic maneuver in patients with FT.[62]

In FMD, voluntary movements may appear to be slow when testing for bradykinesia, but without fatiguing and decrement or the typical arrests seen in Parkinson disease.[63] Some patients with FT seem to struggle and put more effort than needed into performing the tasks. During examination they may demonstrate exhaustion and excessive fatigue and may use their whole body in order to do a minor movement (see Video 16.1). Other patients with FT appear to disregard their symptoms despite showing a severe tremor on examination ("La belle indifference").[20,61]

In addition to exam findings typical of FT, patients may have other non-physiologic neurologic signs that support the diagnosis of aFMD, such as giveaway weakness with a brief burst of strength followed by a quick drop-off of strength against resistance, often out of proportion to strength displayed in voluntary movements, non-anatomical sensory loss, or convergence spasm and other dysconjugate oculomotor abnormalities.[61] Some patients with FT also have a functional gait disorder and sometimes respond with large, effortful movements on postural stability testing and tandem walking, or they may successfully complete these tasks despite self-generated large limb and trunk movement that increases the difficulty of the task.

FT may be part of a mixed FMD or a mixed functional neurologic disorder. In a recent study of 320 patients with hyperkinetic FMD, 24% had more than one phenotype.[52] Another study on functional motor disorders reported that some symptoms (weakness, tremor, dystonia, and gait disorders) occurred far more frequently in combination than in isolation.[64] It is important to remember that the presence of other functional signs does not confirm that the tremor itself is functional.[22]

Electrophysiology: tremor recordings

The electrophysiological characterization of hand tremors is regarded as a useful method to complement the history and physical exam of tremor patients and provides objective, reproducible, and diagnostic information about tremors.[65] A recent survey-based study found that 60% of practitioners performed electrophysiological testing on a regular basis for diagnostic confirmation of FT, with considerable differences between countries in practice patterns and access to testing.[33]

Clinical assessment remains the key aspect when evaluating patients with FT. However, in some patients the diagnosis remains challenging and appropriate treatment may therefore be delayed; this delay is thought to be a negative modifying factor regarding the long-term outcome. In order to support an early more sensitive and specific positive diagnosis of FT, the development of laboratory supported criteria has been suggested.[28,31,32,66]

The recommended equipment includes two accelerometers, a four-channel surface electromyography (EMG), a metronome, and a 500-gram weight.[32,65] A variety of electrophysiologic techniques have been proposed as useful in distinguishing FT from organic tremors.[67,22] These are mainly used to demonstrate the electrophysiological correlates of the clinical examination, namely entrainability, distractibility, co-contraction, and synchronicity.

FT may entrain at the frequency at which the patient is tapping with the other hand.[31,32] In some patients, mirror movements may be mistaken for tremor entrainment. Using low amplitude movements for tremor entrainment testing may help to reduce the likelihood of motor overflow confounding assessment of entrainment. Additionally, EMG coherence should be used for evaluation of tremor entrainment, since the accelerometers may erroneously report volume conduction.[65,68] More common than true entrainment is a significant absolute change and marked intraindividual variability in tremor frequency with opposite limb tapping.[69,31] Less accurate tapping performance at requested frequencies is also considered a sign of functionality.[69,31,32]

FT might influence contralateral motor performance. Contralateral voluntary tasks are strongly affected when FT is present, but are preserved when the tremor has stopped. Conversely, voluntary motor tasks are not affected by the presence of other recognized tremors on the opposite side.[70,71] This again might be explained by the shift of attention to FT if present.

Variability can be shown in tremor amplitude as well as frequency. In terms of distractibility, EMG can be used to demonstrate that ballistic movements of the contralateral hand might transiently stop FT that does not occur in other tremors.[31,70] An increase in the amplitude of the oscillation with the use of loads (500 g–1 kg) to maintain the generating mechanism of antagonistic muscle coactivation is another characteristic of FT.[69,72,31]

In some patients with FT, EMG can be used to record coactivation of agonist and antagonist muscles approximately 300 ms before the onset of tremor bursts as an electrophysiologic equivalent of the clinical "coactivation sign."[27,31]

Approximately half of the patients with FT show significant coherence between tremors of two extremities. In contrast to this, with the exception of orthostatic tremor, most patients with bilateral organic tremors have independent tremor rhythms in different limbs.[31,73] Wavelet coherence analysis enables to detect variations in coherence and phase difference between two signals over time. The percentage of time with significant coherence and the number of periods without significant coherence may be useful parameters to distinguish FT from other neurologic tremors.[74]

A simple test battery[31] consisting of tremor recordings at rest, posture (with and without loading), action, while performing tapping tasks (at 1, 3, and 5 Hz), and while performing ballistic movements with the less-affected hand was able to distinguish functional and other neurologic tremors with good sensitivity (89.5%) and specificity (95.9%) in a prospective study including 40 patients with FT and 72 patients with other tremor disorders.[32] Tonic muscular coactivation, intermanual coherence of tremor frequency, response to contralateral ballistic movement (pause of tremor), loading (increased tremor amplitude), and incorrect tapping performance to a given frequency were regarded as positive functional signs. This test battery may allow an earlier "confident" diagnosis of FT in the setting of clinical diagnostic uncertainty. In patients in whom the clinical diagnosis of FT is more obvious, the test battery can still provide objective evidence and help convey the diagnosis to a patient.[32] The same applies for other movement disorders, where electrophysiology often is useful to strengthen the diagnosis (e.g., in differentiation of myoclonus versus tremor).

Most electrophysiological studies have included only patients with pure FT; thus, we do not know if they are useful in patients with potential overlap of functional and other neurologic tremors.[32] Importantly, electrophysiology has recently been shown to be helpful to identify a central tremor of unclear origin that was masked by a FT.[68]

COEXISTENCE OF FT WITH OTHER NEUROLOGIC TREMORS AND MOVEMENT DISORDERS

One study suggested that 12% of patients with neurological disease also display functional symptoms without clear differences among broad categories of neurological disorders.[14] Patients who have a tremor disorder, such as essential tremor, dystonic tremor, or parkinsonian tremor may have "functional overlay," where they experience enhanced symptoms or additional symptoms that are unrelated to their primary problem, which are of functional origin. However, literature on the comorbidity of FT and other tremor disorders is scarce, highlighting an important knowledge gap.[33] Interestingly, a recent survey among members of the International Parkinson and Movement Disorder Society with experience in treatment of FMD showed that 41% of respondents identified comorbid "functional" and "organic" neurological disorders "sometimes" or "frequently."[33]

In a large study assessing features of FT in 70 patients, coexisting organic movement disorders were documented in 12 patients (17%). An overlay with essential tremor was found in seven patients, with dystonia in two patients, and with tardive dyskinesia, parkinsonism, and benign fasciculations in one patient each.[24]

Out of 410 consecutive patients with functional motor disorders, 17.1% had other comorbid neurological conditions, such as migraine and parkinsonism. This indicates that functional motor disorders often occur over the course of other neurological diseases. FT and functional weakness represented the most common phenotypes in this cohort.[23]

This common overlap has previously mainly been reported with Parkinson disease[75] and epilepsy.[76] In a large study of 488 patients with Parkinson disease, 7.5% had a somatoform disorder. Common functional motor symptoms in that study were paresis, abnormal postures, globus pharynges, functional parkinsonism including FT, and catatonic signs and functional sensory symptoms were anesthesia and multilocalized pain with gastrointestinal symptoms, often accompanied by body deformation delusions.[77,78] In a small series of 11 patients who developed a FMD before the diagnosis of PD or during the course of the disease, FT was reported as most common, followed by functional gait disorder and fixed dystonia.[79] Recently, the clinical features of 106 matched non-demented patients with Parkinson disease with and without comorbid functional symptoms were compared in a retrospective case–control study. FT (40%) and functional gait or balance impairment (40%) were most frequent, followed by incongruent ballistic dyskinesia (25%). Functional symptoms nearly always manifest on the more affected PD side.[75] Interestingly, while patients with coexistence of epileptic and functional seizures usually develop functional seizures after epilepsy,[76,80] functional features precede or co-occur in a substantial proportion of patients with PD.[75,78] A recent meta-analysis of somatization in Parkinson disease found nine relevant studies with a prevalence of somatization ranging from 7.0% to 66.7%.[81] Patients with somatization were more likely to suffer from cognitive decline. In a large cohort study, the prevalence of somatoform disorders was higher in patients with dementia with Lewy bodies (18%) compared to PD (7.5%).[78]

Dopamine transporter imaging can quantify with high sensitivity presynaptic striatal dopaminergic deficit, which is not present in pure FT or pure functional parkinsonism.[82] A review on functional symptoms in PD included 12 studies with a total of 121 patients. Authors of all studies proposed dopamine transporter imaging (DAT-SPECT) to support the diagnosis of underlying PD. A DAT-SPECT or a fluoro-dopa PET was performed for 81.8% of the patients and was abnormal in all of them.[83] Another study showed that the use of DAT-SPECT was significantly more frequent in patients with Parkinson disease with comorbid functional symptoms compared to those with pure organic disease (58.5% versus 30%).[75] DAT-SPECT is regarded as a useful diagnostic tool that can serve to help distinguish pure functional parkinsonism from neurodegenerative PD with functional overlay and thus guide clinical management.[82] However, a negative scan does not clinch an FT diagnosis. False negative scans and other diagnoses, primarily dystonic tremor, were observed in studies of SWEDDs(scans without evidence of dopaminergic deficit in Parkinson disease patients) (Erro, Schneider, Stamelou, Quinn, & Bhatia, 2016) (Menéndez-González, Tavares, Zeidan, Salas-Pacheco, & Arias-Carrión, 2014; Schneider et al., 2007).

On one hand, the identification of comorbid Parkinson disease in patients with FT is crucial, because accurate dopaminergic treatment might significantly improve symptoms. On the other hand, accurate diagnosis of functional symptoms in Parkinson disease is of particular importance, as functional symptoms may lead to significant disability, escalation of antiparkinsonian treatment ineffective for the driving symptom, requests for alternative therapy such as deep brain stimulation, and poorer quality of life.[75,83] It is not clear why patients with Parkinson disease are prone to functional symptoms, but neurologists need to be alert to their presence.[84] So far, the question of whether the incidence of functional symptoms

differs between patients with Parkinson disease compared to patients with other tremor disorders has not been explored.

As the cooccurrence of FT with other neurologic disorder is not rare, additional baseline diagnostic investigation may be justified if doubt remains. However, a careful approach to diagnosis that includes the consideration of functional overlay over an "organic" movement disorder should prevent diagnostic paralysis where more and more tests are requested to rule out increasingly unlikely causes.

MANAGEMENT
Optimal management of FT consists of early diagnosis, providing the patient with a credible explanation of the diagnosis, curtailing investigations, and a multidisciplinary approach to aid in the development of a patient-centered treatment plan.[85] Although this applies to any medical condition, there are reasons to suspect that the therapeutic benefit of effective communication is particularly high in patients with functional disorders. This includes taking the patient seriously, giving the problem a diagnostic label, explaining the rationale for the diagnosis, discussing how the symptoms arise, emphasizing the potential for reversibility, and referral for other treatments where appropriate.[86] The opportunity to "save face" is important for patients and the patient–doctor relationship. A clear, coherent message is also something patients can use to explain their experience to family members, friends, and colleagues.

Explanation as therapeutic tool
Sharing positive clinical signs such as entrainment or distractibility of tremor with patients illustrates how the diagnosis is made and is regarded as a powerful way of persuading them about the nature of their illness.[87] In addition, visualized electrophysiological data can be used as an objective demonstration tool.[32] If present, the "whack-a-mole" sign can be described to patients as evidence in support of a "software" problem involving broader networks, as opposed to a "hardware" problem affecting a particular anatomical location.[62]

Although explanation can sometimes be therapeutic on its own, its role is probably more important as a facilitator to other therapy.[86] There is widespread agreement that active psychiatric symptoms (e.g., depression and anxiety) and ongoing psychosocial stressors should be adequately addressed.[88] There is increasing evidence that patients with FMDs benefit from physical, occupational, and psychotherapeutic interventions, and treatment needs to be tailored to individual motor and non-motor symptoms and comorbidities.[85]

Most treatment studies included patients with various FNDs or various FMDs. The few studies that focused on treatment of FT or at least documented the number of FT patients included in their cohorts will be discussed here.

Medical treatment

Antidepressant treatment outcomes were assessed in a prospective uncontrolled cohort study in 23 patients with chronic FMDs, including 16 patients with FT.[89] Fifteen patients agreed to be treated with antidepressants. Patients received citalopram or paroxetine, and those who did not respond after 4 weeks of taking an optimal dose were switched to venlafaxine. Among treated patients, depression significantly improved, with a better outcome observed in those diagnosed with primary conversion disorder. Further well-designed studies are required to confirm these findings.

Physiotherapy

There is growing evidence that physiotherapy is an effective treatment in FMD including FT. A prospective uncontrolled cohort study in 47 patients with functional motor symptoms (including 9 patients with FT) provided evidence to support the use of specialist physiotherapy treatment in these patients.[90] Subsequently, a randomized feasibility study of a 5-day specialist physiotherapy-led intervention versus a treatment-as-usual control was conducted in patients with a clinically established diagnosis of functional motor symptoms. 5 of 29 patients in the active group and 4 of 28 patients in the control group had FT. Acceptability of the intervention was high, there were no adverse events, and clinical outcomes were promising. At 6 months, 72% of the intervention group rated their symptoms as improved, compared to 18% in the control group.[91] A future trial should consider a standardized control condition.

In a recent retrospective cohort study, the authors investigated the relationship between treatment adherence and clinical outcome in a hospital-based outpatient physical therapy program. Medical records of 50 consecutive patients with functional motor disorders, including 12 patients with FT, were reviewed. The physical

therapy intervention included a 1-hour initial assessment and the development of individualized treatment plans guided by published consensus recommendations. Treatment adherence to outpatient physical therapy program was associated with clinical improvement. Prospective observational and randomized controlled trials are needed to further optimize physical therapy for patients with functional motor symptoms in the outpatient setting.[92]

Physiotherapy in FMDs should address illness beliefs, self-directed attention, and abnormal habitual movement patterns through a process of education, movement retraining with diverted attention, and self-management strategies within a positive and non-judgmental context.[93] A major drawback is that the availability of specialists to implement this motor reprogramming protocol is limited.

Tremor retrainment

The "tremor retrainment" method has been proposed as treatment option for FT. The improvement or change of tremor when performing a rhythmic movement with an unaffected limb as biofeedback is utilized. With the help of sensory and visual feedback, affected people practice to modulate the frequency and severity of their tremor. Retrainment as therapeutic strategy has been investigated in ten patients with FT in an uncontrolled clinical trial. Retrainment was facilitated by tactile and auditory external cueing and real-time visual feedback on a computer screen and resulted in significant tremor improvement for up to 6 months in 60%.[94] The therapeutic use of retrainment strategies as adjunctive to psychotherapy or specialized physical therapy should be tested in larger studies.

Psychological therapies

Among psychotherapeutic methods, cognitive behavioral therapy (CBT) is the one that is best studied in functional disorders. CBT is a structured, time-limited therapy that helps patients identify how thinking affects emotional states or specific behaviors with an aim of inducing change in cognitions and behaviors around movements and interpersonal functioning.[41] In a recent prospective uncontrolled trial, 15 consecutive patients with FT were evaluated before and after 12 weeks of CBT. The main clinical endpoint was the tremor score adapted from the Rating Scale for Psychogenic Movement Disorders assessed by a blinded clinician. CBT significantly reduced tremor severity, with remission or near remission in 73.3% of the cohort.[41]

CBT-based guided self-help (GSH) was studied in 127 patients with functional symptoms, including 19 patients with FT. Patients were randomized to receive either usual care or usual care and GSH, which comprised a self-help manual and 4 half-hour guidance sessions. Participants allocated to GSH reported greater improvement on a clinical global improvement scale at 3 months.[95]

Besides CBT, the use of hypnosis, and other heterosuggestive interventions, the active use of placebo effects and psychodynamic interventions have been described as effective.[85] A randomized controlled trial investigated the additional effect of hypnosis in a comprehensive 8-week inpatient treatment program in 45 patients with motor conversion disorder, including 7 patients with FT. Significant improvements were found for the total sample, but the use of hypnosis had no additional effect on treatment outcome. The authors concluded that a comprehensive treatment program, either with or without hypnosis, can be worthwhile for patients with long-standing functional motor disorders.[96]

Psychodynamic psychotherapy aims to explore underlying psychopathology that may be giving rise to the functional neurological symptoms, and the emphasis is on resolving an underlying psychological conflict. In a single blinded prospective trial on 10 patients with FMDs (8 had a FT), weekly psychodynamic psychotherapy for 12 weeks with adjunctive psychiatric medication significantly improved Psychogenic Movement Disorders Rating Scale scores.[97] However, another study did not show a significant difference between psychodynamic psychotherapy versus neurological observation. Fifteen patients with FMDs, including 6 patients with FT, were included in a randomized, crossover design trial comparing the effects of 3 months of psychodynamic psychotherapy followed by observation by the neurologist versus observation by the neurologist, followed by psychiatric intervention. In this setting, movements, depression, and anxiety improved over time, but there was no specific benefit from psychodynamic psychotherapy either early or late as opposed to neurological observation and support.[98] Another retrospective, open-label design study including 30 patients with FMD who underwent treatment with psychodynamic psychotherapy found improvement in 60% of the patients (33% had good outcome and 27%

had modest improvement), while 33% had poor response. The authors suggested that patients with good insight and who are receptive of diagnosis should be encouraged to undergo psychodynamic psychotherapy, as they have the greatest likelihood for response.[99]

Botulinum toxin

In 48 patients with chronic jerky and tremulous FMD the effect of botulinum neurotoxin (BoNT) was assessed in a double-blind, randomized placebo-controlled trial with an open-label extension phase. Patients were assigned to two subsequent treatments with BoNT or placebo every 3 months. Subsequently all patients were treated with BoNT in a ten-month open-label phase. The authors reported no evidence of improved outcomes in patients treated with BoNT compared with placebo. The response to placebo, however, was very large. Despite symptom improvement, there was no change in quality of life and disability.[100] A favorable motor outcome was recently reported in the majority of this study population after a follow-up duration between three and seven years.[101]

Transcranial magnetic stimulation

A prospective randomized placebo-controlled crossover design study used low-frequency repetitive transcranial magnetic stimulation (rTMS) over the cortex contralateral to the symptoms in patients with FMD (13/33 with FT).[102] Magnetic stimulation sessions led to significant improvement in 22 patients without a significant difference between real TMS and root stimulation. The authors concluded that the therapeutic benefit of TMS in patients with FMDs is due more to a cognitive-behavioral effect than to cortical neuromodulation.

Recently, 18 patients with FT were included in a study that investigated the effects of a sham versus a real coil in a randomized, double-blind, controlled study using validated rTMS parameters that are known to induce long-lasting inhibitory changes in motor cortex excitability.[103] In a second open-label phase, patients underwent 3 weekly sessions of hypnosis combined with single sessions of real rTMS. Significant improvement of FT was found in the active rTMS group at months one, six and 12. The control group had non-significant improvement after one month and tremor scores returned to baseline by month two. The stronger and longer benefit observed in the real versus sham groups may be preliminary evidence of rTMS-induced neuromodulation of the motor cortex, although addition of hypnosis in an open-label phase of the study may have been a confounding factor.[103] Further research in this area is of interest to test pathways involved in symptom genesis and identify new treatment targets.[85]

In summary, classic symptomatic anti-tremor medications such as primidone, propranolol, or dopaminergic agents, as well as botulinum toxin, have no role in FT. Instead, there is good evidence to support the use of physiotherapy, non-medication psychotherapeutic methods, and potentially antidepressants. The development of standardized outcome measures is a crucial step in developing future randomized controlled studies designed to compare different treatment modalities and measure long-term treatment outcomes for patients (Pick et al., 2020) (LaFaver, 2020).

CONCLUSION

The last decade has seen remarkable progress in our understanding of FMDs and in the management of these patients. New evidence suggests a neurobiological basis in FND. Practitioners can use positive exam features, potentially supplemented with electrophysiology, to confidently make sensitive and specific FT diagnoses. There is a well-constructed and increasingly studied specific treatment pathway to help these patients. Regular follow-up visits by the neurologist are important.

REFERENCES

1. American Psychiatric Association. *Diagnostic and Statistical Manual of Mental Disorders (DSM-5)*. American Psychiatric Association; 2013.
2. Carson A, Lehn A. Epidemiology. *Handb Clin Neurol*. 2016;139:47–60.
3. Nicholson TR, et al. Life events and escape in conversion disorder. *Psychol Med*. 2016;46(12): 2617–2626.
4. Espay AJ, et al. Current concepts in diagnosis and treatment of functional neurological disorders. *JAMA Neurol*. 2018;75(9):1132–1141.
5. Maggio J, et al. Briquet syndrome revisited: implications for functional neurological disorder. *Brain Commun*. 2020;2(2):fcaa156.
6. Edwards MJ, Stone J, Lang AE. From psychogenic movement disorder to functional movement disorder: it's time to change the name. *Mov Disord*. 2014;29(7):849–852.
7. Roelofs JJ, Teodoro T, Edwards MJ. Neuroimaging in functional movement disorders. *Curr Neurol Neurosci Rep*. 2019;19(3):12.
8. Maurer CW, et al. Impaired self-agency in functional movement disorders: a resting-state fMRI study. *Neurology*. 2016;87(6):564–5570.
9. Espay AJ, et al. Impaired emotion processing in functional (psychogenic) tremor: a functional magnetic resonance imaging study. *Neuroimage Clin*. 2018;17:179–187.
10. Begue I, et al. Structural alterations in functional neurological disorder and related conditions: a software and hardware problem? *Neuroimage Clin*. 2019;22:101798.
11. Pick S, et al. Emotional processing in functional neurological disorder: a review, biopsychosocial model and research agenda. *J Neurol Neurosurg Psychiatry*. 2019;90(6):704–711.
12. Galli S, et al. Conversion, factitious disorder and malingering: a distinct pattern or a continuum? *Front Neurol Neurosci*. 2018;42:72–80.
13. Stone J, Reuber M, Carson A. Functional symptoms in neurology: mimics and chameleons. *Pract Neurol*. 2013;13(2):104–113.
14. Stone J, et al. Which neurological diseases are most likely to be associated with "symptoms unexplained by organic disease? *J Neurol*. 2012;259(1):33–38.
15. Stone J, Carson A. "Organic" and "non-organic": a tale of two turnips. *Pract Neurol*. 2017;17(5):417–418.
16. Bell V, et al. What is the functional/organic distinction actually doing in psychiatry and neurology? *Wellcome Open Res*. 2020;5:138.
17. Walzl D, Carson AJ, Stone J. The misdiagnosis of functional disorders as other neurological conditions. *J Neurol*. 2019;266(8):2018–2026.
18. Hallett M. Functional (psychogenic) movement disorders—clinical presentations. *Parkinsonism Relat Disord*. 2016;22 (Suppl 1):S149–S152.
19. Miyasaki JM, et al. Psychogenic movement disorders. *Can J Neurol Sci*. 2003;30(Suppl 1):S94–S100.
20. Bhatia KP, Schneider SA. Psychogenic tremor and related disorders. *J Neurol*. 2007;254(5):569–574.
21. Redondo L, Morgado Y, Duran E. Psychogenic tremor: a positive diagnosis. *Neurologia*. 2010;25(1):51–57.
22. Schwingenschuh P, Deuschl G. Functional tremor. *Handb Clin Neurol*. 2016;139:229–233.
23. Tinazzi M, et al. Clinical correlates of functional motor disorders: an Italian multicentre study. *Mov Disord Clin Pract*. 2020;7(8):920–929.
24. Kim YJ, Pakiam AS, Lang AE. Historical and clinical features of psychogenic tremor: a review of 70 cases. *Can J Neurol Sci*. 1999;26(3):190–195.
25. Jankovic J, Thomas M. *Psychogenic tremor and shaking*. In: Hallett M, et al., eds. *Psychogenic Movement Disorders*. Lippincott, Williams and Wilkins; 2005: 42–47.
26. Baizabal-Carvallo JF, Jankovic J. Gender differences in functional movement disorders. *Mov Disord Clin Pract*. 2020;7(2):182–187.

27. Deuschl G, et al. Diagnostic and pathophysiological aspects of psychogenic tremors. *Mov Disord.* 1998;13(2):294–302.

28. Gupta A, Lang AE. Psychogenic movement disorders. *Curr Opin Neurol.* 2009;22(4):430–436.

29. Edwards MJ, Bhatia KP. Functional (psychogenic) movement disorders: merging mind and brain. *Lancet Neurol.* 2012;11(3):250–260.

30. Espay AJ, Lang AE. Phenotype-specific diagnosis of functional (psychogenic) movement disorders. *Curr Neurol Neurosci Rep.* 2015;15(6):32.

31. Schwingenschuh P, et al. Moving toward "laboratory-supported" criteria for psychogenic tremor. *Mov Disord.* 2011;26(14):2509–2515.

32. Schwingenschuh P, et al. Validation of "laboratory-supported" criteria for functional (psychogenic) tremor. *Mov Disord.* 2016;31(4):555–562.

33. LaFaver K, et al. Opinions and clinical practices related to diagnosing and managing functional (psychogenic) movement disorders: changes in the last decade. *Eur J Neurol.* 2020;27(6):975–984.

34. Stone J, et al. Systematic review of misdiagnosis of conversion symptoms and "hysteria". *BMJ.* 2005;331(7523):989.

35. Stone J, et al. Symptoms "unexplained by organic disease" in 1144 new neurology out-patients: how often does the diagnosis change at follow-up? *Brain.* 2009;132(Pt 10):2878–2888.

36. Gelauff J, et al. The prognosis of functional (psychogenic) motor symptoms: a systematic review. *J Neurol Neurosurg Psychiatry.* 2014;85(2):220–226.

37. Hassa T, et al. Functional networks of motor inhibition in conversion disorder patients and feigning subjects. *Neuroimage Clin.* 2016;11:719–727.

38. Voon V, et al. The involuntary nature of conversion disorder. *Neurology.* 2010;74(3):223–228.

39. Edwards MJ, et al. Abnormal sense of intention preceding voluntary movement in patients with psychogenic tremor. *Neuropsychologia.* 2011;49(9):2791–2793.

40. Nahab FB, et al. Impaired sense of agency in functional movement disorders: an fMRI study. *PLoS ONE.* 2017;12(4):e0172502.

41. Espay AJ, et al. Clinical and neural responses to cognitive behavioral therapy for functional tremor. *Neurology.* 2019;93(19):e1787–e1798.

42. Epstein SA, et al. Insights into chronic functional movement disorders: the value of qualitative psychiatric interviews. *Psychosomatics.* 2016;57(6):566–575.

43. Maurer CW, et al. Gray matter differences in patients with functional movement disorders. *Neurology.* 2018;91(20):e1870–e1879.

44. Stone J, et al. The role of physical injury in motor and sensory conversion symptoms: a systematic and narrative review. *J Psychosom Res.* 2009;66(5):383–390.

45. Parees I, et al. Physical precipitating factors in functional movement disorders. *J Neurol Sci.* 2014;338(1–2):174–177.

46. McKeon A, Ahlskog JE, Matsumoto JY. Psychogenic tremor occurring after deep brain stimulation surgery for essential tremor. *Neurology.* 2008;70(16 Pt 2):1498–1499.

47. Ganos C, et al. Psychogenic paroxysmal movement disorders--clinical features and diagnostic clues. *Parkinsonism Relat Disord.* 2014;20(1):41–46.

48. Parees I, et al. "Jumping to conclusions" bias in functional movement disorders. *J Neurol Neurosurg Psychiatry.* 2012;83(4):460–463.

49. Kramer G, et al. Similar association between objective and subjective symptoms in functional and organic tremor. *Parkinsonism Relat Disord.* 2019;64:2–7.

50. Vechetova G, et al. The impact of non-motor symptoms on the health-related quality of life in patients with functional movement disorders. *J Psychosom Res.* 2018;115:32–37.

51. Stone J. Functional neurological disorder 2.0? *Brain Commun.* 2020;2:fcaa217.

52. Lagrand T, et al. Functional, or not functional; that is the question Can we predict the diagnosis functional movement disorder based on associated features? *Eur J Neurol.* 2021;28(1):33–39.

53. Rajalingam R, et al. The clinical significance of lower limb tremors. *Parkinsonism Relat Disord.* 2019;65:165–171.

54. Stamelou M, et al. Psychogenic palatal tremor may be underrecognized: reappraisal of a large series of cases. *Mov Disord.* 2012;27(9):1164–1168.

55. Vial F, et al. Electrophysiological evidence for functional (psychogenic) essential palatal tremor. *Tremor Other Hyperkinet Mov (N Y).* 2020;10:10.

56. van Poppelen D, et al. Attention to self in psychogenic tremor. *Mov Disord.* 2011;26(14):2575–2576.

57. Bell V, et al. Dissociation in hysteria and hypnosis: evidence from cognitive neuroscience. *J Neurol Neurosurg Psychiatry.* 2011;82(3):332–339.

58. de Lange FP, Roelofs K, Toni I. Increased self-monitoring during imagined movements in conversion paralysis. *Neuropsychologia.* 2007;45(9):2051–2058.

59. Willingham DB. A neuropsychological theory of motor skill learning. *Psychol Rev.* 1998;105(3):558–584.

60. Edwards MJ, Schrag A. Hyperkinetic psychogenic movement disorders. *Handb Clin Neurol.* 2011;100:719–729.

61. Thenganatt MA, Jankovic J. Psychogenic tremor: a video guide to its distinguishing features. *Tremor Other Hyperkinet Mov (N Y).* 2014;4:253.

62. Park JE, Maurer CW, Hallett M. The "Whack-a-Mole" Sign in Functional Movement Disorders. *Mov Disord Clin Pract.* 2015;2(3):286–288.

63. Lang AE, Koller WC, Fahn S. Psychogenic parkinsonism. *Arch Neurol.* 1995;52(8):802–810.

64. Baik JS, Lang AE. Gait abnormalities in psychogenic movement disorders. *Mov Disord.* 2007;22(3):395–399.

65. Vial F, et al. How to do an electrophysiological study of tremor. *Clin Neurophysiol Pract.* 2019;4:134–142.

66. Gironell A. Routine neurophysiology testing and functional tremor: toward the establishment of diagnostic criteria. *Mov Disord.* 2016;31(11):1763–1764.

67. Hallett M. Physiology of psychogenic movement disorders. *J Clin Neurosci.* 2010;17(8):959–965.

68. Merchant SH, Haubenberger D, Hallett M. Mirror movements or functional tremor masking organic tremor. *Clin Neurophysiol Pract.* 2018;3:107–113.

69. Zeuner KE, et al. Accelerometry to distinguish psychogenic from essential or parkinsonian tremor. *Neurology.* 2003;61(4):548–550.

70. Kumru H, et al. Transient arrest of psychogenic tremor induced by contralateral ballistic movements. *Neurosci Lett.* 2004;370(2–3):135–139.

71. Apartis E. Clinical neurophysiology of psychogenic movement disorders: how to diagnose psychogenic tremor and myoclonus. *Neurophysiol Clin.* 2014;44(4):417–424.

72. O'Suilleabhain PE, Matsumoto JY. Time-frequency analysis of tremors. *Brain.* 1998;121 (Pt 11):2127–2134.

73. McAuley J, Rothwell J. Identification of psychogenic, dystonic, and other organic tremors by a coherence entrainment test. *Mov Disord.* 2004;19(3):253–267.

74. Kramer G, et al. Wavelet coherence analysis: a new approach to distinguish organic and functional tremor types. *Clin Neurophysiol.* 2018;129(1):13–20.

75. Wissel BD, et al. Functional neurological disorders in Parkinson disease. *J Neurol Neurosurg Psychiatry.* 2018;89(6):566–571.

76. Wissel BD, et al. Which patients with epilepsy are at risk for psychogenic nonepileptic seizures (PNES)? A multicenter case-control study. *Epilepsy Behav.* 2016;61:180–184.

77. Onofrj M, et al. Cohort study on somatoform disorders in Parkinson disease and dementia with Lewy bodies. *Neurology.* 2010;74(20):1598–606.

78. Onofrj M, et al. Updates on somatoform disorders (SFMD) in Parkinson's disease and dementia with Lewy bodies and discussion of phenomenology. *J Neurol Sci.* 2011;310(1–2):166–171.

79. Parees I, et al. Functional (psychogenic) symptoms in Parkinson's disease. *Mov Disord.* 2013;28(12):1622–1627.

80. Devinsky O, et al. Clinical profile of patients with epileptic and nonepileptic seizures. *Neurology.* 1996;46(6):1530–1533.

81. Carrozzino D, et al. Somatization in Parkinson's disease: a systematic review. *Prog Neuropsychopharmacol Biol Psychiatry.* 2017;78:18–26.

82. Umeh CC, et al. Dopamine transporter imaging in psychogenic parkinsonism and neurodegenerative parkinsonism with psychogenic overlay: a report of three cases. *Tremor Other Hyperkinet Mov (N Y).* 2013;3:tre-03-188-4324-2.

83. Ambar Akkaoui M, et al. Functional motor symptoms in Parkinson's disease and functional parkinsonism: a systematic review. *J Neuropsychiatry Clin Neurosci.* 2020;32(1):4–13.

84. Hallett M. Patients with Parkinson disease are prone to functional neurological disorders. *J Neurol Neurosurg Psychiatry.* 2018;89(6):557.

85. LaFaver K. Treatment of functional movement disorders. *Neurol Clin.* 2020;38(2):469–480.

86. Stone J, Carson A, Hallett M. Explanation as treatment for functional neurologic disorders. *Handb Clin Neurol.* 2016;139:543–553.

87. Stone J, Edwards M. Trick or treat? Showing patients with functional (psychogenic) motor symptoms their physical signs. *Neurology.* 2012;79(3):282–284.

88. Perez DL, et al. A review and expert opinion on the neuropsychiatric assessment of motor functional neurological disorders. *J Neuropsychiatry Clin Neurosci.* 2021;33(1):14–26.

89. Voon V, Lang AE. Antidepressant treatment outcomes of psychogenic movement disorder. *J Clin Psychiatry.* 2005;66(12):1529–1534.

90. Nielsen G, et al. Outcomes of a 5-day physiotherapy programme for functional (psychogenic) motor disorders. *J Neurol.* 2015;262(3):674–681.

91. Nielsen G, et al. Randomised feasibility study of physiotherapy for patients with functional motor symptoms. *J Neurol Neurosurg Psychiatry.* 2017;88(6):484–490.

92. Maggio JB, et al. Outpatient physical therapy for functional neurological disorder: a preliminary feasibility and naturalistic outcome study in a U.S. cohort. *J Neuropsychiatry Clin Neurosci.* 2020;32(1):85–89.

93. Nielsen G, et al. Physiotherapy for functional motor disorders: a consensus recommendation. *J Neurol Neurosurg Psychiatry.* 2015;86(10):1113–1119.

94. Espay AJ, et al. Tremor retraining as therapeutic strategy in psychogenic (functional) tremor. *Parkinsonism Relat Disord.* 2014;20(6):647–650.

95. Sharpe M, et al. Guided self-help for functional (psychogenic) symptoms: a randomized controlled efficacy trial. *Neurology.* 2011;77(6):564–572.

96. Moene FC, et al. A randomized controlled clinical trial on the additional effect of hypnosis in a comprehensive treatment programme for inpatients with conversion disorder of the motor type. *Psychother Psychosom.* 2002;71(2):66–76.

97. Hinson VK, et al. Single-blind clinical trial of psychotherapy for treatment of psychogenic movement disorders. *Parkinsonism Relat Disord.* 2006;12(3):177–180.

98. Kompoliti K, et al. Immediate vs. delayed treatment of psychogenic movement disorders with short term psychodynamic psychotherapy: randomized clinical trial. *Parkinsonism Relat Disord.* 2014;20(1):60–63.

99. Sharma VD, Jones R, Factor SA. Psychodynamic Psychotherapy for Functional (Psychogenic) Movement Disorders. *J Mov Disord.* 2017;10(1):40–44.

100. Dreissen YEM, et al. Botulinum neurotoxin treatment in jerky and tremulous functional movement disorders: a double-blind, randomised placebo-controlled trial with an open-label extension. *J Neurol Neurosurg Psychiatry.* 2019;90(11):1244–1250.

101. Dreissen YE, et al. Botulinum neurotoxin (BoNT) treatment in functional movement disorders: long-term follow-up. *J Neurol Neurosurg Psychiatry.* 2020;91(10):1120–1121.

102. Garcin B, et al. Impact of transcranial magnetic stimulation on functional movement disorders: cortical modulation or a behavioral effect? *Front Neurol.* 2017;8:338.

103. Taib S, et al. Repetitive transcranial magnetic stimulation for functional tremor: a randomized, double-blind, controlled study. *Mov Disord.* 2019;34(8):1210–1219.

SECTION 3

Tremor in the Clinic

How to recognize, diagnose, and treat tremor is an area of exponential growth. This reflects the growth in basic research and nosology/classification work, plus the broadening of tremor clinical care and research into new territories.

This section covers traditional areas of tremor assessment and treatment. Chapters also explore the wider context of tremor clinical care. Formal consideration of inclusivity in clinical care and research is relatively new, yet important for advancing understanding of tremor etiologies as well as ensuring treatment access for all. Addressing symptom areas beyond tremor itself can play a key role in treatment. Investigating a wide range of options, from non-medication therapies to surgeries, is becoming standard in active clinical care and new therapeutic development.

After early successes, tremor treatment options remained stable for years. In contrast, this section details the new wave of work in tremor therapeutics, from treatment access and diagnostic processes, to more holistic treatment frameworks, to novel therapeutic mechanisms.

Diversity and Inclusivity in Parkinson Disease and Essential Tremor

THERESA A. ZESIEWICZ, NICOLAS DOHSE, CLIFTON L. GOOCH,
YAREMA B. BEZCHLIBNYK, AND SHAILA GHANEKAR

INTRODUCTION

Tremor is one of the most common movement disorders globally and is a cardinal symptom of various neurological disorders such as Parkinson disease (PD) and essential tremor (ET). While much research has been performed on tremor syndromes, information regarding tremor patients' ethnicity and racial diversity is limited. This information is vital to better understand potential contributions of race and ethnicity, genetics, and environment to the pathoetiology of tremor syndromes and their response to treatment, and to determine whether patients of diverse racial groups are receiving adequate healthcare. Racial and ethnic minorities currently account for 28% of the United States (US) population[1] and are predicted to account for half the population by 2040.[1] Unequal access to health care education and resources affecting different racial and economic groups is a clear contributor to poor health outcomes.[2] While healthcare disparities have been studied for many common disorders, including heart disease, diabetes, and cancer, these are less apparent in tremor syndromes, despite millions of people being affected worldwide.

We reviewed the published literature for studies analyzing racial and ethnic differences in pathoetiology and treatment response, potential bias in healthcare access and utilization, and the ways in which diversity and inclusivity impact care for patients with tremor. This review indicated that although tremor is an exceedingly common symptom, there is little information on diversity, equity, and inclusion (DEI) in movement disorders in general, apart from the limited studies on PD and ET discussed as follows. (When reporting the results of prior studies in this chapter, the term "Blacks" was used in place of the term "African American").

EPIDEMIOLOGY

Essential tremor

Essential tremor (ET) is one of the most common movement disorders in adults, affecting millions worldwide. It is characterized by bilateral postural and action tremor—by definition, affecting both hands, and often affecting the head and vocal cords[3]—and is frequently accompanied by non-motor symptoms such as depression, anxiety, and cognitive issues.[4] ET usually worsens over time and can lead to significant disability, principally because of impairment in manual activities, with approximately 15 to 25% of patients forced into an early retirement.[5]

While the prevalence and incidence of ET increases with age, there appears to be a bimodal distribution of age of onset, usually in the second and sixth decades of life,[6-8] and children can be affected.[9-11] Published estimates of prevalence and incidence vary greatly, due to the high rate of undiagnosed individuals with mild tremor, the lack of a sensitive and specific test or biological marker, and variability in diagnostic criteria.[12-15] However, the prevalence estimates for ET from published community-based studies range from 4 to 39 cases per 1000, while for people age 60 and older, the estimates are closer to 13 to 50 per 1000.[12,16] At least 5% of people 65 years of age and older are believed to suffer from ET,[13] although the prevalence may be less in some populations.[17-19] One review of the worldwide prevalence of ET from population-based epidemiological studies showed a pooled prevalence of 0.9% using a meta-analysis.[13] The incidence of ET has been estimated to be 23.7 per 100,000.[20]

Regional and ethnic differences

There is little published information regarding regional and ethnic differences in ET in the US, and only a few studies have focused on potential ethnic differences in ET presentation. One large community-based health survey of elderly persons age 65 years and older in northern Manhattan[21] assessed study participants for ET based on handwriting samples reviewed by tremor experts. The prevalence of ET was observed to be higher in Blacks and Hispanics than White patients in this cohort (5.9% versus 7.3% versus 3.1%). Logistic regression analysis found that the odds of ET (dependent variable) were positively associated with age [odds ratio (OR) = 1.14, 95% CI = 1.03–1.26, p = 0.01] and with Hispanic ethnicity versus White ethnicity (OR = 2.19, 95% CI = 1.03–4.64, p = 0.04).[21]

Conversely, an early study in Copiah County, Mississippi, which in the 1980s consisted of roughly equal percentages of Black and White people,[22,23] found a trend for ET to be more common in Whites than Blacks. However, only a screening questionnaire was utilized, allowing for possible bias of results due to varying education levels—the results could have been biased to exhibit lower ET prevalence in less-educated individuals due to a lack of understanding of the screening questionnaire.[21,24] Furthermore, only people over age 40 were included in the study, which may not account for discrepancies in age of onset between different races or ethnicities, and the personnel who performed the screening did not have expertise in medical care, and so may have missed or misdiagnosed patients.

Another large community-based study in Washington Heights, NY (N = 2117), studied a multiethnic cohort of subjects with confirmed ET.[25] All patients underwent an interview, tremor examination, and a quantitative computerized tremor analysis. They were given a total tremor score (range, 0–36, with 0 indicating no tremor and 36 indicating maximum tremor) based on 2 neurologists' ratings of the tremor examination. Sixty-two ET patients were included in this study (16 = White, 18 =Black, 28 = Hispanic) and ethnic differences were noted in the total tremor score (F = 3.68, p = .03).[25] Utilizing a regression model adjusted for age, White ET patients had a mean total tremor score 5.3 points lower than that of the other ethnicities (p = .008).[25]

Although no definitive conclusions can currently be drawn regarding regional and ethnic differences in ET based upon this highly limited data, there are several potential explanations for these studies' findings. The studies based upon the most objective assessments of individuals living in a restricted, relatively economically homogeneous geographic area (Washington Heights/Northern Manhattan) suggest substantial differences between the studied ethnic groups, with lower severity of tremor in Whites vs. non-Whites (Hispanics and Blacks). Some ethnic groups are less likely to access care for medical reasons, and patient access bias may affect epidemiologic studies. Recent data has also emerged on the effect of environmental stressors on adverse gene expression and chronic inflammation in non-White ethnic groups—often due to economic underprivilege, systemic racism, and other factors—and it is conceivable that such factors might also modulate the severity of other disorders.[26] Also, future research assessing the severity of ET and other diseases must be carefully designed to differentiate between the cultural construct of different races (e.g., Black, White, Hispanic, Asian, Latin, etc., groups that are often quite genetically heterogeneous within themselves), and truly genetically uniform cohorts (which may or may not correspond to current constructs of race and ethnicity).[27]

Bias and healthcare access

There is a great discrepancy between the high prevalence of ET and the number of patients who consult a healthcare provider for diagnosis and treatment.[28] While ET is one of the most common movement disorders worldwide, the proportion of patients who seek medical treatment is estimated to be as low as 20% in several Western countries;[29,30] this is in contrast to PD patients, for example. Without a diagnosis, these ET patients often go untreated.[28] One study reported that only 27% of ET patients discussed their tremor with physicians,[31] while a Finnish study reported that only 11% of ET patients reported their tremor to a healthcare provider.[30] A Turkish population study found that over 90% of ET patients were unaware that they had ET, while in another study, only 7% of ET patients received a diagnosis and treatment.[32] It is estimated that more than 90% of patients who do seek medical care do so because of disability due to ET.[33]

One study evaluated the prevalence of physician-diagnosed ET in elderly communities in the US to determine potential differences between Whites and Blacks.[34] Using the Cardiovascular Health Study, a sample of Medicare beneficiaries 65 years of age or older from several US communities answered a 12-question screen about ET.[34] More White respondents than Blacks indicated that they had a diagnosis of ET (1.7% vs. 0.4%; odds ratio = 4.9; 95% CI, 1.2–20.2; P = 0.028).[34]

Using logistic regression analysis, physician-diagnosed ET was significantly associated with White ethnicity (P = 0.038) rather than with other factors including age, sex, educational level, income, smoking, and alcohol consumption. Compared to Black subjects, White subjects were five times as likely to have received an ET diagnosis from a physician. A variety of factors may be responsible for under-recognition of ET by both patients and their primary care providers, including the mild severity of some tremors, the belief that the tremor is a "familial" trait, or that it is merely a sign of normal aging.[28] Furthermore, it is important to consider that many individuals in minority and underserved communities may not have sought out medical attention for ET, possibly due to economic or other factors.[34] Finally, a diagnostic bias paired with decreased access to quality health care in minority communities are potential factors.[34] Considering the aforementioned significant differences in ET diagnosis and treatment when comparing White and US minority populations, it is essential that further research be conducted to better identify and address health disparities that could be dramatically impacting ET patients.

Parkinson Disease

PD is a common neurodegenerative disease, second to Alzheimer's disease (AD). It is caused by a loss of dopaminergic neurons in the substantia nigra due to deposition of Lewy bodies containing alpha-synuclein.[35] The exact cause of PD is unknown in most cases, but genetic and environmental factors may play roles. It is estimated that almost 1 million people are affected by PD in the US.[36] The median age-standardized annual incidence rate of PD is approximately 160 per 100 000 people 65 years of age or older.[37] PD's lifetime risk is estimated to be 2% for men and 1.3% for women for people 40 years of age and older.[37] The prevalence of PD is expected to triple in the next 30 years.[1]

Regional and ethnic differences

The prevalence of PD in different races and ethnicities in the US is unclear, although several epidemiological studies have suggested that Blacks have a lower prevalence of PD than Whites.[38–41] Kessler et al. enlisted a panel of neurologists in Baltimore, Maryland, in the late 1960s to obtain community-based samples of patients with and without PD,[39] and found a lower frequency of PD among Blacks compared to Whites.[39] Another study estimated

the incidence of PD by age, gender, and ethnicity in a large prepaid health maintenance organization (HMO) in Northern California.[42] Age- and gender-adjusted PD rate per 100,000 people was highest among Hispanics, followed by non-Hispanic Whites, Asians, and Blacks, suggesting that race/ethnicity have an influence on the incidence of PD. A study of Pennsylvania State Medicaid claims from 1999–2003 found that Blacks were half as likely to be diagnosed with PD as Whites.[43] The 4-year cumulative incidence of PD was 54 per 100,000 in Whites, 23 per 100,000 in Blacks, and 40 per 100,000 in Latinos (P < 0.0001).[43] The 4-year cumulative risk of PD was 0.21% for Whites, 0.15% for Latinos, and 0.08% for Blacks, even after adjustment of age, gender, healthcare use, and location of care (RR 0.45, P < 0.0001).[43]

The previously mentioned study performed in Copiah County, Mississippi, in the 1980s[22] additionally screened elderly patients to determine whether a neurologist should further examine them for symptoms of PD.[22,23] While the study found that the rates of PD were similar in Blacks and Whites, many Blacks with PD had been previously undiagnosed.[22] As noted previously, the staff who performed the screening had no prior medical training[23] and may have been unable to determine which people needed further examination by a neurologist.[23]

In terms of phenotypic characteristics, limited information indicates Black PD patients appear to have a slightly higher risk of mortality than White PD patients,[44–48] are at a greater risk to develop dementia than other ethnic groups,[44,49] and possess a greater vascular burden than Whites in the US.[44,50,51] Thus, they may be at a greater risk of vascular dementia which may overwhelm the other PD symptoms, resulting in a lack of PD diagnosis.

Bias and healthcare access

Although the population of PD patients has practically doubled in the past 25 years, there is little information regarding biased healthcare access among different racial groups. Several studies have reported that minority groups have reduced access to outpatient care, less chance of being treated with PD medications, and greater disability with PD symptoms before treatment is sought. A review of the 2006 to 2013 Medical Expenditure Panel Survey (MEPS) for neurological care found that Black participants were almost 30% less likely to be examined by an outpatient neurologist compared to White patients (OR .72,

CI= .64-.81), while Hispanic patients were 40% less likely to be examined (OR.61, CI= .54-.69).[1] Blacks with known neurological conditions were more likely to be cared for in emergency rooms and have longer hospital stays than Whites. In the study of Pennsylvania State Medicaid claims from 1999–2003,[52] Black PD patients were less likely to receive medication or physical therapy than White patients (12 vs. 38%),[52] and were half as likely to be diagnosed with PD as White patients after adjusting for variables such as age, gender, location, and Medicaid eligibility reason.[43] One study at the Philadelphia Veterans Affairs Medical Center reported that Blacks presented for care at a later stage than White patients (median Hoehn and Yahr 2.5 vs. 2.0 for White patients, p = 0.02).[53] Another study assessed racial and socioeconomic disparities in patients with parkinsonism at a movement disorders center[54] and found that Blacks were less likely to be prescribed dopaminergic medications, particularly newer agents (Blacks: 20.6% vs. Whites: 41.1%; P=.001).[54]

Socioeconomic and racial bias may even occur on death certificates.[55] A national population-based survey was linked to death certificate data obtained from the National Death Index (NDI) to determine the concordance of PD indicated on death certificates in those who reported having this condition while living. For those patients who reported PD during life, almost 55% of them had "PD" recorded on their death certificates. However, almost 70% of people in higher income brackets had PD recorded on their death certificates compared to about 35% for those who earned $10,000 or less. Education and income were two factors associated with significant biases when reporting PD on death certificates for those who had PD during life.[55] This potential bias is important, as incidence and prevalence studies often rely on this type of data source.

Clinical trials

There is a disproportionate lack of minority representation in PD clinical trials.[56] One study evaluated minority participation in PD trials that focused on neuropsychiatric symptoms by reviewing published articles from 2000–2019.[57] Sixty-three randomized clinical trials (RCTs) with 7,973 patients were reviewed, and 17.5% reported race or ethnicity. In this data set, only 5 Blacks (0.2%), 16 Hispanics (0.64%), and 539 Asians (21.44%) were enrolled in the RCTs. The pooled prevalence for being White in these trials was 98% (CI 0.97–0.98, p < 0.001).[57] Another study published in 2004 reviewed PubMed for PD clinical trials conducted in the US over the previous 20 years and found that only 17% of them reported racial/ethnic participation;[56] in these trials, only 8% of subjects were non-White.[56] More accurate reporting of RCT's racial and ethnic composition is vital to determine the true participation of minority groups in PD clinical research.

Deep brain stimulation

Deep Brain Stimulation (DBS) is a safe and effective method to treat medically refractory tremors in patients with ET, and medically intractable tremor, stiffness, and slowness, as well as motor fluctuations and dyskinesia in PD. However, DBS may be underused in certain patient populations. One study examined the Nationwide Inpatient Sample, neurologist and neurosurgeon density data, and disease codes (ICD-9 332.0) to identify patient discharges in nonfederal hospitals (all-payer) in the US who were diagnosed with PD, and also from those who received a DBS implantation.[58] From 2002 to 2009, the review uncovered 2,408,302 PD discharges, and 18,312 of these discharges were specifically for DBS. While 4.7% of PD discharges were from Black patients, only 0.1% of DBS for PD discharges were this group. Using hierarchical multivariate analysis, male patients and increasing income quartile of patient zip code were factors that favorably predicted DBS, while predictors of non-use were Blacks (P < .001), Medicaid, (P < .001), and a higher comorbidity score (P < .001). Blacks with PD who were discharged in this study were almost 8 times less likely to undergo DBS than White patients.[58] In a large study of 665,765 Medicare beneficiaries with PD derived from outpatient, carrier, and Beneficiary Annual Summary files from 2007 to 2009, approximately 1% had undergone DBS, of which almost 95% were White.[58] Indeed, while no differences were observed between Hispanic and White PD patients, Black and Asian patients were significantly less likely to have undergone DBS compared to White patients even when accounting for the effects of comorbidities, socioeconomic status, and neurologist availability (ORs = 0.20, 95% CI 0.16–0.25 and 0.55, 95% CI 0.44–0.70, respectively). Moreover, patients in minority-serving practices were less likely to receive DBS regardless of race (OR = 0.79, 95% CI 0.66–0.87). Socioeconomic status was also found to be an important predictor of receiving

DBS, with patients living in neighborhoods with higher socioeconomic status being more likely to undergo this surgery (AOR = 1.42, 95% CI 1.33–1.53).[58]

CONCLUSIONS

Our review of the available data regarding the influence of race and ethnicity on the diagnosis and management (as well as rates of participation in clinical trials) for patients with ET and PD supports potential differences in the prevalence of these disorders among different racial groups. However, more importantly, these studies reinforce broad trends described for many years across the medical literature—primarily, that economically disadvantaged racial and ethnic minorities access the medical system at far lower rates than Whites and other economically privileged groups, and that they also participate at far lower rates in clinical trials. The reasons for this disproportion in healthcare access are many but appear to be primarily economic and related to rates of medical insurance, as well as access to transportation and employment settings, which enables time away for medical appointments.[59] Poverty also impacts access to medical therapy and to high-level surgical therapies and devices, such as those required for DBS. Poverty also impacts education quality and level, and low levels of education may influence awareness of disease symptoms, when to seek care, and the potential availability of treatments. Generational poverty and low-quality community education are two aspects of a cluster of problems affecting underprivileged minorities that, due to their structural integration into American and other societies over many years, have come to be known as manifestations of systemic racism.[60] Other potential contributors, such as inherent bias and overt racism, have not been definitively studied in regard to their impact on care for ET and PD. These data continue to demonstrate the deleterious consequences to national health—not to mention the associated cost to society, ultimately, of untreated chronic disease[61]—and support the need for a national paradigm to provide medical care to all citizens, including those who are impoverished and otherwise unable to access medical care on their own. We encourage the ongoing US national conversation around this critical issue and would urge a timely solution for our patients. In addition, there continues to be a pressing need for further research regarding the impact of race, ethnicity, and economic status on patient health, well-being, morbidity, and mortality in ET, PD, and other neurological diseases, both in the US and in other national populations.

REFERENCES

1. Saadi A, Himmelstein DU, Woolhandler S, Mejia NI. Racial disparities in neurologic health care access and utilization in the United States. *Neurology.* 2017;88(24):2268–2275. doi: 10.1212/WNL.0000000000004025
2. Riley WJ. Health disparities: gaps in access, quality and affordability of medical care. *Trans Am Clin Climatol Assoc.* 2012;123:167–174. Accessed July 11, 2020. https://www.ncbi.nlm.nih.gov/pmc/articles/PMC3540621/
3. Deuschl G, Bain P, Brin M. Consensus statement of the movement disorder society on tremor. *Mov Disord.* 1998;13(S3):2–23. doi: 10.1002/mds.870131303
4. Agarwal S, Biagioni MC. Essential tremor. In: *StatPearls.* StatPearls Publishing; 2020. Accessed July 11, 2020. http://www.ncbi.nlm.nih.gov/books/NBK499986/
5. Louis ED, Okun MS. It is time to remove the "benign" from the essential tremor label. *Parkinsonism Relat Disord.* 2011;17(7):516–520. doi: 10.1016/j.parkreldis.2011.03.012
6. Bain PG, Findley LJ, Thompson PD, et al. A study of hereditary essential tremor. *Brain J Neurol.* 1994;117(Pt 4):805–824. doi: 10.1093/brain/117.4.805
7. Lenka A, Bhalsing KS, Jhunjhunwala KR, Chandran V, Pal PK. Are patients with limb and head tremor a clinically distinct subtype of essential tremor? *Can J Neurol Sci.* 2015;42(3):181–186. doi: 10.1017/cjn.2015.23
8. Louis ED, Dogu O. Does age of onset in essential tremor have a bimodal distribution? Data from a tertiary referral setting and a population-based study. *Neuroepidemiology.* 2008;29(3–4):208–212. doi: 10.1159/000111584
9. Paulson GW. Benign essential tremor in childhood: symptoms, pathogenesis, treatment. *Clin Pediatr (Phila).* 1976;15(1):67–70. doi: 10.1177/000992287601500112
10. Louis ED, Ford B, Frucht S, Barnes LF, X-Tang M, Ottman R. Risk of tremor and impairment from tremor in relatives of patients with essential tremor: a community-based family study. *Ann Neurol.* 2001;49(6):761–769. doi: 10.1002/ana.1022
11. Tan EK, Lum SY, Prakash KM. Clinical features of childhood onset essential tremor. *Eur J Neurol.* 2006;13(12):1302–1305. doi: 10.1111/j.1468-1331.2006.01471.x
12. Findley LJ. Epidemiology and genetics of essential tremor. *Neurology.* 2000;54(11 Suppl 4):S8–S13.
13. Louis ED, Ferreira JJ. How common is the most common adult movement disorder? Update on the worldwide prevalence of essential tremor.

Mov Disord. 2010;25(5):534–541. doi: 10.1002/mds.22838

14. Dogu O, Louis ED, Sevim S, Kaleagasi H, Aral M. Clinical characteristics of essential tremorin Mersin, Turkey. *J Neurol.* 2005;252(5):570–574. doi: 10.1007/s00415-005-0700-8

15. Lorenz D, Poremba C, Papengut F, Schreiber S, Deuschl G. The psychosocial burden of essential tremor in an outpatient- and a community-based cohort. *Eur J Neurol.* 2011;18(7):972–979. doi: 10.1111/j.1468-1331.2010.03295.x

16. Louis ED, Ottman R, Hauser WA. How common is the most common adult movement disorder? Estimates of the prevalence of essential tremor throughout the world. *Mov Disord.* 1998;13(1):5–10. doi: 10.1002/mds.870130105

17. Inzelberg R, Mazarib A, Masarwa M, Abuful A, Strugatsky R, Friedland RF. Essential tremor prevalence is low in Arabic villages in Israel: door-to-door neurological examinations. *J Neurol.* 2006;253(12):1557–1560. doi: 10.1007/s00415-006-0253-5

18. Aharon-peretz J, Badarny S, Ibrahim R, Gershoni-baruch R, Hassoun G. Essential tremor prevalence is low in the Druze population in Northern Israel. *Tremor Other Hyperkinet Mov (N Y).* 2012;2. Accessed March 1, 2021. https://www.ncbi.nlm.nih.gov/pmc/articles/PMC3570042/

19. Özel L, Demir R, Özdemir G, et al. Investigation of the prevalence of essential tremor in individuals aged 18–60 in Erzurum. *Acta Neurol Belg.* 2013;113:127–131. doi: 10.1007/s13760-012-0147-5

20. Zesiewicz TA, Chari A, Jahan I, Miller AM, Sullivan KL. Overview of essential tremor. *Neuropsychiatr Dis Treat.* 2010;6:401–408. Accessed March 2, 2021. https://www.ncbi.nlm.nih.gov/pmc/articles/PMC2938289/

21. Louis ED, Thawani SP, Andrews HF. Prevalence of essential tremor in a multiethnic, community-based study in northern Manhattan, New York, N.Y. *Neuroepidemiology.* 2009;32(3):208–214. doi: 10.1159/000195691

22. Schoenberg BS, Anderson DW, Haerer AF. Prevalence of Parkinson's disease in the biracial population of Copiah County, Mississippi. *Neurology.* 1985;35(6):841–845. doi: 10.1212/wnl.35.6.841

23. Bailey M, Anderson S, Hall DA. Parkinson's disease in African Americans: a review of the current literature. *J Park Dis.* 2020;10(3):831–841. doi: 10.3233/JPD-191823

24. Haerer AF, Anderson DW, Schoenberg BS. Prevalence of essential tremor. Results from the Copiah County study. *Arch Neurol.* 1982;39(12):750–751. doi: 10.1001/archneur.1982.00510240012003

25. Louis ED, Barnes LF, Ford B, Pullman SL, Yu Q. Ethnic differences in essential tremor. *Arch Neurol.* 2000;57(5):723–727. doi: 10.1001/archneur.57.5.723

26. Thames A, Irwin M, Breen E, Cole S. Experienced discrimination and racial differences in leukocyte gene expression. *Psychoneuroendocrinology.* 2019;106:277–283. doi: 10.1016/j.psyneuen.2019.04.016

27. Bamshad M. Genetic influences on health: does race matter? *JAMA.* 2005;294(8):937–946. doi: 10.1001/jama.294.8.937

28. Rajput AH, Rajput A. Medical treatment of essential tremor. *J Cent Nerv Syst Dis.* 2014;6:29–39. doi: 10.4137/JCNSD.S13570

29. Louis ED, Rohl B, Rice C. Defining the treatment gap: what essential tremor patients want that they are not getting. *Tremor Other Hyperkinet Mov (N Y).* 2015;5. doi: 10.7916/D87080M9

30. Rautakorpi I, Takala J, Marttila RJ, Sievers K, Rinne UK. Essential tremor in a Finnish population. *Acta Neurol Scand.* 1982;66(1):58–67. doi: 10.1111/j.1600-0404.1982.tb03129.x

31. Deuschl G, Raethjen J, Hellriegel H, Elble R. Treatment of patients with essential tremor. *Lancet Neurol.* 2011;10(2):148–161. doi: 10.1016/S1474-4422(10)70322-7

32. Sur H, Ilhan S, Erdoğan H, Oztürk E, Taşdemir M, Börü UT. Prevalence of essential tremor: a door-to-door survey in Sile, Istanbul, Turkey. *Parkinsonism Relat Disord.* 2009;15(2):101–104. doi: 10.1016/j.parkreldis.2008.03.009

33. Benito-León J, Louis ED. Essential tremor: emerging views of a common disorder. *Nat Clin Pract Neurol.* 2006;2(12):666–678. doi: 10.1038/ncpneuro0347

34. Louis ED, Fried LP, Fitzpatrick AL, Longstreth Jr. WT, Newman AB. Regional and racial differences in the prevalence of physician-diagnosed essential tremor in the United States. *Mov Disord.* 2003;18(9):1035–1040. doi: 10.1002/mds.10492

35. Kouli A, Torsney KM, Kuan W-L. Parkinson's disease: etiology, neuropathology, and pathogenesis. In: Stoker TB, Greenland JC, eds. *Parkinson's Disease: Pathogenesis and Clinical Aspects.* Codon Publications; 2018. Accessed July 1, 2020. http://www.ncbi.nlm.nih.gov/books/NBK536722/

36. Marras C, Beck JC, Bower JH, et al. Prevalence of Parkinson's disease across North America. *NPJ Park Dis.* 2018;4. doi: 10.1038/s41531-018-0058-0

37. Ascherio A, Schwarzschild MA. The epidemiology of Parkinson's disease: risk factors and prevention. *Lancet Neurol.* 2016;15(12):1257–1272. doi: 10.1016/S1474-4422(16)30230-7

38. Kessler II. Epidemiologic studies of Parkinson's disease. 3. A community-based survey. *Am J Epidemiol.* 1972;96(4):242–254. doi: 10.1093/oxfordjournals.aje.a121455

39. Kessler II. Epidemiologic studies of Parkinson's disease. II. A hospital-based survey. *Am J Epidemiol.* 1972;95(4):308–318. doi: 10.1093/oxfordjournals.aje.a121399

40. Paddison RM, Griffith RP. Occurrence of Parkinson's disease in black patients at Charity Hospital in New Orleans. *Neurology.* 1974;24(7):688–690. doi: 10.1212/wnl.24.7.688

41. Wright Willis A, Evanoff BA, Lian M, Criswell SR, Racette BA. Geographic and ethnic variation in parkinson disease: a population-based study of US Medicare beneficiaries. *Neuroepidemiology.* 2010;34(3):143–151. doi: 10.1159/000275491

42. Van Den Eeden SK, Tanner CM, Bernstein AL, et al. Incidence of Parkinson's disease: variation by age, gender, and race/ethnicity. *Am J Epidemiol.* 2003;157(11):1015–1022. doi: 10.1093/aje/kwg068

43. Dahodwala N, Siderowf A, Xie M, Noll E, Stern M, Mandell DS. Racial differences in the diagnosis of Parkinson's disease. *Mov Disord.* 2009;24(8):1200–1205. doi: 10.1002/mds.22557

44. Ben-Joseph A, Marshall CR, Lees AJ, Noyce AJ. Ethnic variation in the manifestation of Parkinson's disease: a narrative review. *J Park Dis.* 10(1):31–45. doi: 10.3233/JPD-191763

45. Fernandes GC, Socal MP, Schuh AFS, Rieder CRM. Clinical and epidemiological factors associated with mortality in Parkinson's disease in a Brazilian cohort. *Park Dis.* 2015;2015. doi: 10.1155/2015/959304

46. Mayeux R, Marder K, Cote LJ, et al. The frequency of idiopathic Parkinson's disease by age, ethnic group, and sex in northern Manhattan, 1988–1993. *Am J Epidemiol.* 1995;142(8):820–827. doi:10.1093/oxfordjournals.aje.a117721

47. Djaldetti R, Hassin-Baer S, Farrer MJ, et al. Clinical characteristics of Parkinson's disease among Jewish Ethnic groups in Israel. *J Neural Transm Vienna Austria 1996.* 2008;115(9):1279–1284. doi: 10.1007/s00702-008-0074-z

48. Willis AW, Schootman M, Kung N, Evanoff BA, Perlmutter Joel S, Racette BA. Predictors of survival in Parkinson disease. *Arch Neurol.* 2012;69(5):601–607. doi: 10.1001/archneurol.2011.2370

49. Chaudhuri KR, Hu MT, Brooks DJ. Atypical parkinsonism in Afro-Caribbean and Indian origin immigrants to the UK. *Mov Disord Off J Mov Disord Soc.* 2000;15(1):18–23. doi: 10.1002/1531-8257(200001)15:1<18::aid-mds1005>3.0.co;2-z

50. Gottesman RF, Fornage M, Knopman DS, Mosley TH. Brain aging in African-Americans: the Atherosclerosis Risk in Communities (ARIC) experience. *Curr Alzheimer Res.* 2015;12(7):607–613. Accessed February 28, 2021. https://www.ncbi.nlm.nih.gov/pmc/articles/PMC4739532/

51. Mollenhauer B, Zimmermann J, Sixel-Döring F, et al. Baseline predictors for progression 4 years after Parkinson's disease diagnosis in the De Novo Parkinson Cohort (DeNoPa). *Mov Disord.* 2019;34(1):67–77. doi: 10.1002/mds.27492

52. Dahodwala N, Xie M, Noll E, Siderowf A, Mandell DS. Treatment disparities in Parkinson's disease. *Ann Neurol.* 2009;66(2):142–145. doi: 10.1002/ana.21774

53. Dahodwala N, Karlawish J, Siderowf A, Duda JE, Mandell DS. Delayed Parkinson's disease diagnosis among African-Americans: the role of reporting of disability. *Neuroepidemiology.* 2011;36(3):150–154. doi: 10.1159/000324935

54. Hemming JP, Gruber-Baldini AL, Anderson KE, et al. Racial and socioeconomic disparities in parkinsonism. *Arch Neurol.* 2011;68(4):498–503. doi: 10.1001/archneurol.2010.326

55. Pressley JC, Tang M-X, Marder K, Cote LJ, Mayeux R. Disparities in the recording of Parkinson's disease on death certificates. *Mov Disord.* 2005;20(3):315–321. doi: 10.1002/mds.20339

56. Schneider MG, Swearingen CJ, Shulman LM, Ye J, Baumgarten M, Tilley BC. Minority enrollment in Parkinson's disease clinical trials. *Parkinsonism Relat Disord.* 2009;15(4):258–262. doi: 10.1016/j.parkreldis.2008.06.005

57. Di Luca DG, Sambursky JA, Margolesky J, et al. Minority enrollment in Parkinson's disease clinical trials: meta-analysis and systematic review of studies evaluating treatment of neuropsychiatric symptoms. *J Parkinsons Dis.* 2020;10(4):1709–1716. doi: 10.3233/JPD-202045

58. Chan AK, McGovern RA, Brown LT, et al. Disparities in access to deep brain stimulation surgery for Parkinson disease: interaction between African American race and Medicaid use. *JAMA Neurol.* 2014;71(3):291–299. doi: 10.1001/jamaneurol.2013.5798

59. Egede LE. Race ethnicity, culture, and disparities in health care. *J Gen Intern Med.* 2006;21(6):667–669. doi: 10.1111/j.1525-1497.2006.0512.x

60. Evans MK, Rosenbaum L, Malina D, Morrissey S, Rubin EJ. Diagnosing and treating systemic racism. *N Engl J Med.* 2020;383(3):274–276. doi: 10.1056/NEJMe2021693

61. Gooch CL, Pracht E, Borenstein AR. The burden of neurological disease in the United States: a summary report and call to action. *Ann Neurol.* 2017;81(4):479–484. doi: 10.1002/ana.24897

18

Assessing Tremor

Diagnostic Pearls, Rating Scales, and Waveform Recording

PETER A. LEWITT, ALFONSO FASANO, AND ALBERTO J. ESPAY

INTRODUCTION

It is necessary that the peculiar nature of this tremulous motion be ascertained, as well as for the sake of giving it to its proper designation, as for assisting in forming probable conjectures, as to the nature of the malady, which it helps to characterize. Tremors were distinguished by Juncker into Active, those proceeding from sudden affectation of the minds, as terror, anger, &c. and Passive, dependant on debilitating causes, such as advanced age, palsy, &c. But a much more satisfactory and useful distinction is made by Sylvius de Boë into those tremors which are produced by attempts at voluntary motion, and those which occur whilst the body is at rest.[1]

As recognized by James Parkinson more than two centuries ago, the clinical approach to tremor calls for its differentiation into categories that reflect the diversity of its origins and disease mechanisms. An adequate understanding of the patient with tremor requires attention to the somatic distribution of the involuntary movement, its pattern (frequency, amplitude, regularity, and circumstances surrounding its initiation or suppression), and accompanying clinical features. Tremor is a common experience in adults and occasionally in the pediatric population.[2] Unlike other movement disorders, tremor has a "normal" version, physiological tremor, as well as pathological manifestations originating from the central nervous system (CNS). That physiological tremor might be a *forme fruste* of the most common tremor disorder, essential tremor (ET), has been proposed.[3] However, more recent considerations of ET have highlighted its complex identity,[4] differentiating it from physiological tremors recognized in the healthy person. Nevertheless, the notion of a continuum between normal aging-related changes and pathological tremor is

important to consider, since an upper extremity action tremor suggestive of ET can be found in as many as 5% of persons older than 65 years.[2]

Although it seems intuitive that rhythmic, sinusoidal movements should necessarily be of neurological origin, low-amplitude tremorous movements of peripheral origin are derived from the 1–1.5 Hz heartbeats and arterial pulsations (cardio-ballistic tremor) that resonate in the limbs.[5] In addition, neurological peripheral mechanical-resonant tremor (rather than CNS-derived tremor) is the major contributor to physiological tremor in both young and elderly adults.[6] Physiological tremor is expressed in the range of 8–12 Hz and is brought out by stressors such as anxiety, hypoglycemia, pain, or other hyperadrenergic states. Sometimes enhanced physiological tremor (EPT) can be intrusive and disabling.[7] Like ET, EPT usually emerges during action and with posture maintenance. It also can be brought out in resting position or during the execution of precision-demanding tasks with the hands. EPT can be brought on by vigorous exercise leading to muscular fatigue. Localized (and temporary) occurrence of EPT has also been described following a localized arm injury.[8]

The distinction between physiological and pathological tremor types has implications for the busy clinician, for whom establishing a definitive distinction between the various types of tremor might not seem the highest priority. Generally, symptoms of mild tremor of any etiology do not call for augmenting clinical testing with neuroimaging or an electromyography (EMG) study. However, even tremors of minimal amplitude should not be ignored since they may herald an underlying disorder that is potentially reversible or carries other health consequences. Examples include adverse effects from several classes of tremor-inducing medications,[9] hyperthyroidism, and other hyperadrenergic states (for example, during myocardial infarction). Mild tremulousness can be mistakenly attributed to ET instead of generalized polymyoclonus, which can be the initial manifestation of a serious underlying illness involving paraneoplastic or autoimmunity manifestation.[10] For patients who are puzzled, worried, or functionally impaired (for example, surgeons or artists) by even a mild hand tremor, their request for a definitive diagnosis may be a search for assuring their health, a wish to eliminate a cosmetically undesirable appearance, or a necessary way to maintain professional skills.

A first step for making a tremor diagnosis is to adopt a uniform definition that is sensible to both clinicians and patients. From the patient's point of view, symptoms may be described as "shaking," "twitching," "vibrating," or "jerking" rather than "tremor." In the mid-nineteenth century, as reports of individual and familial cases of tremor entered the medical literature,[11] the terminology of this disorder became more established and recognized as a specific disease state, whether inherent or acquired. The modern era has yielded a few consensus statements on a tremor definition.[12,13] A useful starting point was provided by Elble and Koller in their 1990 monograph, describing tremor as "any involuntary, *approximately* rhythmic, and *roughly* sinusoidal movement."[14] With italicized modifiers in mind, there may be an easier way to encompass the diversity that tremors can present. For example, the 2018 consensus statement from the International Parkinson and Movement Disorder Society (MDS) Task Force on Tremor defined tremor as " *. . . an involuntary, rhythmic, oscillatory movement of a body part . . .usually visible and persistent*" and recognized the co-existence of physiological tremor in unsupported limbs and head.[13] Those with access to tremor recording equipment (including an electrocardiogram, into which a Parkinson disease [PD] patient's resting tremor can intrude) can also use this information for distinguishing tremor from other hyperkinetic movement disorders. As discussed later in this chapter, smartphone apps are capable of recording limb tremor.

In contrast to most other hyperkinetic movement disorders, regularity is a hallmark of tremor. There are other hyperkinetic movement disorders with repetitiveness that resembles tremor, such as clonus,[15] which can be generated in both static and movement circumstances.[16] Another movement disorder also possessing regularity is generalized polymyoclonus.[10] Since jerky movements that resemble voluntarily produced tremor (albeit involuntary) constitutes the most common

pattern of functional (psychogenic) movement disorder, this needs to be considered in evaluating puzzling tremor-like movements. However, on examination of functional tremor, regularity is often not maintained when the examiner uses various entrainment strategies (if there is a volition component to the tremorous movements).[17] Other physiological aids can also help in diagnosing functional tremors.[18] Other irregular movements that can appear very regular to observers in a clinic setting are often classified with tremors, for example dystonic tremor and Holmes tremor.

The discussion that follows is a commentary on how the history and physical examination can guide tremor diagnostics. Tremor rating scales and the use of tremor recording apparatus are also covered.

KEY ELEMENTS OF A TREMOR-BASED HISTORY AND PHYSICAL EXAMINATION

As summarized in the 1998 MDS consensus statement, the varieties of tremor can be differentiated by their frequency and activation patterns.[12] However, since the various tremor syndromes have considerable overlap, accurate diagnosis needs a plan to sort out the phenotypic alternatives. Differentiation requires integrating neurological history (including available family information), observation of tremor, provocative testing and, if necessary, neuroimaging and electrophysiological testing. Sometimes, the best that can be accomplished is a probabilistic diagnosis. For example, ET is generally determined with the exclusion of alternative explanations for action tremor. A diagnostic impression is susceptible to revision by the arrival of new details, such as an unexpected response to a medication (like an anticholinergic drug) or the new evolution of a characteristic neurological sign (like dystonic posturing). The following strategies can help to enhance recognition and differentiation of tremors.

Tremor-based history

A patient with the complaint of tremor has a thorough story to tell. The objective features—its amplitude, body parts affected, situations in which it arises or remits, and associated neurological features—should be easy to describe. Once details of the history are recorded, the examination should be confirmatory. A checklist of objective features describing tremor is found in Box 18.1. Discussion points with a patient may focus on

---

BOX 18.1
CHECKLIST FOR INFORMATION TO BE COLLECTED IN
A TREMOR HISTORY

- When did the tremor begin and what were its first manifestations?
- How has the tremor changed over time?
- What parts of the body are affected?
- Does tremor occur during specific actions, at rest, or with holding a posture?
- Describe the amplitude of the tremor, how regular it is, and what makes it worse
- Is it felt internally without being visible
- What makes the tremor better or worse?
- Is coordination, balance, or walking affected by tremor?

---

typical situations during which tremor occurs. For example, even though tremor interfering with feeding may be suspected to be an action tremor, PD patients often complain about their rest tremor in this situation; presumably, the rested or postured hand holding a shaking utensil can be as bothersome as the tremorous hand delivering a morsel to the mouth. The clinician can inquire about activation of tremor from the patient's own history. This can be especially informative if the tremor is task specific (such as during use of a musical instrument) or arises after strenuous exercise (as does EPT). Tremors associated with dropping items or obvious clumsiness can steer the discussion to possible neurological problems such as negative myoclonus or cerebellar system dysfunction. The role of mental concentration in bringing out tremor (particularly resting tremor of PD) is a topic not well understood as to its CNS origins. A patient's history of long periods between any manifestation of tremor is an important clue for a potentially functional tremor.

The subjective side of tremor can be valuable to explore in arriving at a diagnosis. The perception of internal tremor is a relatively common experience in PD. Sometimes the PD patient experiences tremor in the upper chest or legs, where movements are difficult to observe outwardly even if muscle fibers in these regions are exhibiting tremorous firing patterns. Patients with an internal sense of parkinsonian tremor can simultaneously have observed tremor in another limb, and the hidden tremor can respond to anti-parkinsonian medication.

Tremor has other subjective elements that sometimes emerge from careful questioning.

Patients may start their description of a tremors disorder by indicating how slow they are in accomplishing tasks (because of the need to be guarded or precise in movements), how illegible their handwriting has become, or how weak their hands are in fine motor tasks ("weakness" being their description of their disability). Sometimes uncertainty as to whether tremor is present may be best answered by a short medication trial. The absence of response to ethanol or drugs for ET or PD might not be the definitive answer to excluding these disorders, but this information might open the way for searching for secondary causes of tremor such as demyelinating disease or a past history of alcoholism.

Tremor-based physical examination

Tremorous movements can be best assessed with control of the observational setting. Tremor present in specific body regions or during specific activations will usually need specific examination maneuvers. Nearly all tremor-based exam points can be covered without more than pen and paper. With lower extremity tremor, a stethoscope or surface EMG can be useful for detecting orthostatic tremor.

Jaw tremor provides a special challenge; to assess if the tremor is occurring at rest, the patient will need to be in a supine position to eliminate the effect of gravity, which would change the category to "postural" rather than "resting." The ideal position for ascertaining upper extremity rest tremor is with the hands held dangling off the seated knees or while the patient is standing, with arms held by the sides. Testing for action tremors should investigate several situations, such as excursions of the hand from a target to the face and in specific tasks such as pouring water or handwriting. Sometimes rotating the hands from horizontal to vertical positioning can bring out tremor. Drawing spirals or jagged lines can provide enduring evidence of tremor and its relative amplitude. In contrast to handwriting, this activity can be easily conducted with the non-dominant hand. A patient holding a writing instrument 1–2 cm above a dot can provide a visual measure of tremor amplitude. For the assessment of tremor while maintaining a forward posture of the arms, the observer should note whether tremor emerges immediately (as usually in ET) or becomes evident following a few seconds of delay (as is typical of parkinsonian postural tremor).[19] For postural tremor examination, a maneuver that brings out proximal components is the "wing beating" position (the arms extended forward, the forearms horizontal by flexing the elbows). Properly adopting this position is important for detection of wing-beating tremor, common in (but not specific for) Wilson disease.[20] The patient with EPT after exercise may demonstrate this phenomenon by holding the arms extended in front to bring out a fatigued (and tremorous) state. The observation of the hand moving to a target should determine the extent of regularity to observed action tremor. Alternatively, what may initially be regarded as tremor might be recognized as a more chaotic pattern of movement, with over- and under-shooting more indicative of ataxia due to cerebellar system dysfunction. Some tremor types are entirely observational, such as the hereditary disorder of chin tremor (hereditary geniospasm, occurring entirely within the territory of the mentalis muscle) or the rhythmic glottal sound production in pure voice tremor. The latter disorder can closely mimic varieties of impaired phonation in spasmodic dysphonia; visualization of vocal cords with stroboscopic light may be a necessary diagnostic tool to differentiate tremor from dystonic symptoms. Voice tremor may result from ET; some diagnostic systems consider voice tremor sufficient for ET diagnosis.[21] Using the MDS diagnostic criteria for ET adopted in 2018,[13] however, both upper limbs need to manifest tremor for establishing this diagnosis.

Like upper extremity tremors, involvement of the legs can occur during action or at rest. The latter entity is best evaluated with a patient sitting or in a supine position. The entity of orthostatic tremor, defined as leg shaking in standing, is discussed below. A person with action tremor in the lower extremities may be unaware of an action or posture maintenance component until formally examined. Leg tremor in ET is relatively uncommon. In a 1994 survey of 350 subjects with a familial pattern of action tremor (selected from 20 kindreds thought to be affected by ET), 244 had upper extremity action tremor, while only 48 had postural or action tremor affecting the legs.[22] In PD, the patient's experience of lower extremity resting tremor can be much less than that occurring in the hands since the mass and configuration of leg muscles dampens the outward appearance of tremors.

Specific "pearls" for recognizing rare tremors

Unusual forms of tremor are increasingly recognized.[23] Some of these are familiar tremor patterns originating from novel causes.[24–27] For example, a newly described addition to the spectrum of tremorous movements is an entity termed "isolated upper limb jerky tremor."[28] Though the jerky movements are elicited during action and therefore resemble ET, this movement disorder is currently classified as an "indeterminate tremor."[13] It lacks myoclonic or dystonic features, though it resembles the latter category based on evaluations of somatosensory temporal discrimination thresholds (measuring the shortest timing interval with which the subject can perceive separation of two paired electrical stimuli to a finger).[28] These methods exemplify the need for careful study to gain insight into tremor mechanisms and, ultimately, ways these movement disorders can be treated.

The topic of orthostatic tremor (OT) is covered in detail in chapter 8. Sometimes referred to a "shaky leg syndrome," it is a relative newcomer in the spectrum of tremor disorders. First reported in 1984,[29] OT is unique in both its frequency range and in the disabilities it imposes. Recognizing OT is sometimes delayed, with a circuit of evaluations for imbalance, gait disorders, and even psychological assessment before the neurological problem is recognized.[30] What puzzles the patient and physician alike is loss of ability to stand comfortably and securely, since walking is affected only in severe versions of OT.

The examination of the patient with OT is congruent with the patient's complaint of instability while standing. Flexion-extension activation of distal leg musculature can create a bouncing appearance in standing. Though not leading to collapsing weakness, it sometimes seems as if the OT patient's legs lack strength and are giving way. Walking, especially with a widened base, generally improves the shaking and the perceived instability of an upright position. Leg tremors are abolished when the sufferer is seated with the legs planted on the floor. If two examiners lift an upright patient off the floor, the tremor also disappears, as it does with the patient in a supine position (even with pressure applied to the soles) (personal observation). While the nomenclature focuses on legs, EMG manifestations of OT can also be detected in lumbar paraspinal muscles.

Palpation of muscles during standing can detect OT, as can stethoscope auscultation of upper and lower leg muscles.[31]

Though a patient's history and bedside exam are generally characteristic, it is surface EMG recording that clinches the diagnosis of this relatively rare disorder: bilateral coherence (in-phase cycles of motor activation) of tremors in both legs and an EMG frequency between 13–18 Hz are the hallmarks of OT.[32] Use of EMG in evaluation of tremor and the specifics of EMG terminology are discussed later in the Tremor Measurement section. Another finding in some cases of OT is EMG evidence for high-frequency burst patterns recorded in upper extremity muscles and synchronous with those in the legs.[33]

The 2018 MDS Task Force on Tremor designated the entity of *primary OT* as demonstrating tremor in the frequency range 13–18 Hz,[34] greater than the 4–11 Hz range of physiological tremor and ET. Primary OT is distinguished from *pseudo-OT* syndromes, which have similar symptomatology but exhibit EMG frequency of <13Hz.[35] The story may be even more complex; typical OT may possess a broader phenotype than originally recognized. For example, in about half of patients with otherwise typical OT, arms hanging at the sides during stance exhibit detectable >13 Hz tremor.[30,35] Although OT was initially considered an isolated tremor disorder, many examples have appeared in the medical literature expanding its phenotype. For example, OT with 14–15 Hz EMG findings has been encountered in some cases of cerebellar ataxia.[36] In one series, up to a quarter of cases strongly suggestive of OT had additional neurological deficits.[37] These circumstances can make the clinician's diagnostic task more challenging.

OT has some lookalikes that are even less common, including Holmes tremor, which occurs in either resting or action and originates in proximal muscles when it affects the legs. Holmes tremor is readily distinguished its frequency is 4 Hz or less. Other examples of slow-frequency tremor OT (or, as described above, *pseudo-OT*) include

patients with lesions in the pons[38] or cerebellum, or autoimmune or paraneoplastic syndromes.[39] Tremorous lower extremity movements during standing and distinctive EMG findings have been termed *orthostatic myoclonus* rather than OT.[40,41] Patients with sustained clonus at the ankles may also be subject to leg tremors especially while leaning forward (and thereby stretching the Achilles tendon). Tremorous movements of the lower leg can also be the consequence of a disorder termed *paradoxical clonus* in which repetitive 5–6 Hz muscles contractions impart lower extremity tremor while standing. In this disorder, the regular tremorous movements arise from triggering a physiological response (Westphal's shortening reaction) in ankle extensors.[42]

CLINICAL RATING SCALES FOR TREMOR

Perhaps the earliest example of tremor rating, albeit hypothetical, might be an ET sufferer's observations that there was progressively less spilling of an alcoholic beverage after ingesting increasing amounts. In fact, measuring spillage figures into two of the published tremor rating scales.[43,44] In the modern era, a range of clinical methods for quantifying tremor has evolved in parallel with the development of effective therapeutics. Of these methods, tremor recording devices (discussed later in this chapter) present a special appeal for providing the most accurate means for measurement. However, clinical observations and patients' subjective responses predominate in academic tremor research and for testing anti-tremor medications and devices. The clinical tools currently available for tremor screening and severity determination rating scales were summarized in a 2013 review.[45] Of the 12 that were reviewed, most of them characterized tremor severity by measurement of its amplitude in various body parts. Several of the published rating scales pair a clinician's observations of tremor with the patient's descriptions of specific functional disabilities and the overall impact of tremor on daily life.

While rating tremor might seem a lesser task than the challenges posed by assessing across multiple motor symptoms or assessing complex motor tasks, several aspects of tremor confound judging the impact of living with this movement disorder. Unique quirks of tremor include its situational variability and controlling for those factors that momentarily exacerbate it (such as mental concentration or conducting fine movements). With analogy to the Heisenberg uncertainty principle in nuclear physics, the rater's intervention at assessing tremor (by drawing attention to it) may result in temporary tremor enhancement. Furthermore, in assessment of pathological tremor, the rating methodology needs to contend with the possibility that some component of the observed tremor might be an underlying physiological tremor. Considerable clinimetric expertise is needed for effectively translating the phenomena of tremor into credible rating descriptions and a validated rating scale. A recent example highlighting details of this process is the development and validation of the Orthostatic Tremor Severity and Disability Scale (OT-10).[46] Ultimately, the challenge for a clinically useful rating is how well it provides correlation to patient experience of living with tremor. For testing new therapies, there is a need for assessment instruments to be readily amenable for effective standardization of rating methodology [47] Ease of use by researchers is widely recognized as critical for successful outcomes of clinical trials. Tremor assessment schemes have to be effective for teaching, validation, and translation into multiple languages. Beyond acceptance by the clinician and tremor research community, rating scales for tremor also face the challenge of acceptance by regulatory authorities in their review of proposed marketing for anti-tremor therapies.

Unlike using recording devices for tremor quantification, rating scales employ words and numbers as their means of translating observations and experiences into data. The choice of descriptors—*anchors* in clinimetrics terminology—calls for careful nomenclature. For example, distinguishing between the terms "minimal" and "mild" presents a linguistic challenge even for a native English speaker; this distinction can be even more vexing for others with less English language fluency. Most of the rating instruments have adopted a 5-element scale convention (that is, 0 to 4). More choices in the elements of a rating item might lead to more difficulty for an examiner's description of tremor severity. The incremental change between no tremor (0) and "1" might seem to be the same as from "1" to "2"; however, the tremor quantification and data analysis is not that simple. Estimating change in tremor amplitude (either displacement or angular rotation) using clinical ratings needs to recognize that simple percent computation of change from baseline will not be correct.[48]

Another dimension of understanding the threshold for discriminating differences of phenomena with small incremental differences comes from the Weber-Fechner equations for psychophysics. Using these formulations, the incremental changes between sequential rating scale points are best represented logarithmically rather than linearly. With the use of a 0–4 rating scale, a 1-point reduction in tremor ratings is roughly a 68% reduction in tremor amplitude regardless of the baseline tremor rating, as shown by correlations of ratings to objectively quantified tremor amplitude measures using recording devices.[49] Similarly, a 2-point reduction in rated tremor is approximately a 90% reduction in tremor amplitude. These observations have great relevance for tremor ratings analysis, for which treatment of percent change with conventional parametric statistical approaches may yield misleading results.

A milestone in screening and evaluating tremor was a 2013 MDS Tremor Task Force publication, in which a group of 14 experts provides critique and recommendations among 7 tremor rating scales, 6 activities of living and disability scales, 4 quality of life scales, and 5 screening instruments for tremor.[45] For most of these scales, the focus was measuring kinetic tremor (regardless of origin). The MDS Task Force report surveyed each of the published tremor assessments with the goal of critical evaluation of their use in clinical research and within specific tremor populations. Factors assessed included scale availability (i.e., accessibility in the public domain), subsequent use of the scale beyond its initial publication, overall acceptability by tremor experts and the movement disorder community, the quality of clinimetric testing, scale validity, and sensitivity to change (for example, responsiveness to interventions such as medications). Strengths and weakness were highlighted. This expert review concluded that 4 of the scales met criteria for recommendation and that no new tremor scales needed to be developed; however, existing scales needed further improvement by validation (including in pediatric populations) and expansion to languages besides English. The scales chosen for recommendation were the Fahn-Tolosa-Marín Tremor Rating Scale (FTM-TRS),[50] the Bain-Findley Clinical Tremor Rating Scale (BF-CTRS),[51] the Washington Heights-Inwood Genetic Study of Essential Tremor—Tremor Rating Scale (version 2) (WHIGET-TRS),[52,53] and the Tremor Research Group Essential Tremor Rating Scale (TETRAS).[54] No new rating scales have appeared since that time except for the OT-10 (discussed earlier).[46]

Existing tremor assessment scales

To date, the most widely used scales that focus on tremor have been those created for rating PD and ET (in particular, the FTM-TRS[50] and TETRAS[54]). The 1993 version of the FTM-TRS was revised from an initial 1988 publication. It is a combination of three sections: Part A discusses observational assessment of tremor in different body regions and whether there are resting, postural, or action components. Part B involves examination of pouring a liquid, handwriting, and spiral drawing. Activities of daily living and a global assessment of tremor severity by both examiner and patient are included in Part C. The 1993 FTM-TRS version added a review of tremor's impact on social activities and assessment of tremor while standing. In addition, it changed the definition of "severe" extremity tremor to be greater than 4 cm in amplitude rather than >2 cm.[50] In its 2013 review, the MDS Task Force commented that the FTM-TRS needed thorough training and efforts at standardization for use of the scale, especially since the verbal anchors have linguistically ambiguous definitions ("e.g., "slight," "mild," "moderate," "marked," and "severe").[45] The MDS Task Force also cited the potential problem of a ceiling effect in rating high-amplitude upper extremity tremor. This concern was borne out in a study that compared the FTM-TRS with TETRAS, which has >20cm amplitude as its top rating anchor.[47] Nonetheless, the FTM-TRS has had wide use in clinical research. Assessment of inter- and intra-rater reliability average Spearman correlation in one study was 0.87, indicating very good consistency between two videotaped tremor recordings.[55] In general, the rated observations of tremors with the FTM-TRS were better than evaluations of handwriting and spiral drawing tasks.

TETRAS is the latest of the action tremor ratings to be developed.[54] It was developed in response to recognized limitations of prior tremor rating scales. In TETRAS, there are 12 items for gauging impact of tremor on activities of daily living (ADL), capturing some of the ADL items found in other tremor ratings. The performance portion of TETRAS has 9 items for quantifying tremor of the head, face, voice, upper and lower extremities, and trunk. Another intended feature in its development, besides ease of use, was a mandate to use objective metric anchors for each of the rating categories so that experiential rating bias and uncertainty could be reduced. Specifically, descriptions of the 0–4 ratings include examiners estimates of peak-to-peak tremor amplitudes. TETRAS has undergone critical assessment leading to validation of its verbal anchors as well as other clinimetric features (such as good intra- and inter-rater reliability and sensitivity to change).[47] Unlike the FTM-TRS, it also includes assessment of tremor tested in the wing beating position. Comparison of TETRAS with FTM-TRS has shown strong correlations. However, TETRAS ratings of upper limb tremor tended to be lower than FTM-TRS ratings (attributable to the lower amplitude ranges and ceiling effects for the latter scale).[56] Although the items in TETRAS are rated "0" to "4," this rating scale permits the use of 0.5-point increments for in-between ratings. In the latest iteration, TETRAS 2.0, the heel-to-shin exam for lower extremity tremor has been dropped. In addition to achieving widespread use in ET clinical trials, it has undergone validation (for its clinical observation section) by comparison of its upper extremity and activity of daily living findings to the output of recording devices.[57,58] Although published in a peer-reviewed journal, the use of TETRAS by a commercial entity is restricted by licensing of its copyright owner, the Tremor Research Group (www.tremorresearchgroup.org).

The BF-CTRS[51] also achieved recommendation in the 2013 report. The report noted that it had been used widely by others and can be carried out easily. Only upper limb postural tremor and head tremor achieved acceptable reliability, however, and both definition and interpretation of kinetic versus intention tremor were cited as difficulties.

Observational (clinical examination) and ADL assessments for parkinsonian tremor are found in several clinical instruments, including the Unified PD Rating Scale (UPDRS)[59] and the UPDRS revision by the MDS (the MDS-UPDRS).[60] Both forms of UPDRS rate observation of resting, postural, and action tremor in the PD patient using 5-element assessments. A 5-element question on tremor impact on ADL over the previous week is also in both versions. The sensitivity of capturing the reduction of tremor by levodopa and other treatments in PD patients was studied using the FTM-TRS in comparison to the MDS-UPDRS.[61] The authors concluded that the FTM-TRS Part C (ADL section) proved to be more sensitive at capturing the effects of levodopa treatment; Part A (the clinician's examination of the tremor) showed the most effect size.

There are a few clinical instruments that focus solely on the impact of tremor on quality of life. The Quality of Life in Essential Tremor questionnaire (QUEST) comprises 30 items pertaining to activities in everyday life.[62] The 2013 MDS Task Force report recommended its use based on its clinimetric performance. However, in some investigations, QUEST was not sensitive to treatments effects and patients using this self-administered scale often did not fully respond to all of its questions.[61,62] QUEST demonstrated adequate test-retest reliability, with an ICC of 0.77 in its summary index. Furthermore, a separate scale has been developed and validated for self-assessed rating of embarrassment related to tremor.[63]

APPARATUS MEASURES OF TREMOR

The differential diagnosis of tremor syndromes is often difficult even for tremor experts deploying strategies discussed above, and misdiagnosis can affect management.[64] Moreover, there can be significant inter-observer variability in clinical assessments, especially with "soft signs."[65] Several clinical criteria have been suggested but their diagnostic accuracy is limited by a priori assumptions, underscoring the need for objective diagnostic methods.[66]

Objective evaluations of tremor have been used for more than a century, e.g., simply measuring patients' handwriting or Archimedes spirals, or using a tambour and smoked drum to record physiologic and pathologic tremors[67] (Figure 18.1). Accelerometers were introduced in the 1960s to measure tremor and understand its mechanisms.[68] Over the years, smaller, cheaper, and more sensitive motion transducers have been developed. Inertial measurement units (IMUs) host the variable combination of a triaxial accelerometer, triaxial gyroscope, triaxial magnetometer and even an altimeter; these systems are integrated with an electronic circuit for digital storage and wireless output, usually via Bluetooth protocol. In parallel, force transducers have been applied to force plates for posturography (useful to quantify stance duration in OT[69]) and digital graphics tablets have been developed to quantify tremor during writing and drawing.[70]

IMU sensors can detect motion of a body part in three-dimensional space, namely in the antero-posterior (roll), lateral (pitch), and vertical (yaw) axes. Accelerometers—the most frequently used transducers in tremor analysis—record linear inertial acceleration according to Newton's second law. Gyroscopic transducers record angular velocity and are free of gravitational artifact, in contrast with accelerometers. Many commercially available motion sensors have a triaxial accelerometer and triaxial gyroscope housed in a single IMU along with built-in analog-to-digital converters; examples include Kinesia One (Great Lakes NeuroTechnologies Inc., Cleveland, OH, USA), Opal (ERT, Philadelphia, USA) and GT9X (ActiGraph, Pensacola, FL, USA).

While accelerometry can directly measure tremor frequency and indirectly tremor amplitude, EMG cannot measure the latter. Instead, EMG allows the accurate assessment of tremor frequency and the location of affected muscles, thus revealing whether antagonist muscles (such as flexors and extensors of the wrist) are bursting at the same time or alternately to produce tremor. EMG activity may be recorded using needle, wire electrodes, or more typically in tremor surface electrodes overlying active muscles. EMG is also useful in differentiating tremor from a pseudo-rhythmic myoclonus, as the latter features very short bursts (around 100 msec or less) and can also be coupled with a back-averaged electroencephalogram to identify the cortical origin of these involuntary movements, as in so-called cortical tremor.[23]

Tremor analysis

A standard tremor study of the upper extremities requires an amplifier, bipolar surface EMG recordings with silver–silver-chloride electrodes of forearm extensors and flexors plus wrist accelerometry on both limbs (total of 6 channels). EMG electrodes are usually fixed close to the motor points of the ulnar or radial part of the hand extensor and flexor muscles of the forearm. Accelerometers are usually fixed on the third metacarpal bone bilaterally. Recordings are performed during different positions: resting on chair armrest, posture with hands outstretched, posture plus a weight loading ranging from 300 to 1000 g, and a kinetic task *slowly* performed, usually a finger-to-nose maneuver. Loading the arm with a weight is useful in extracting the different tremor components: mechanical, mechanical-reflex, and central[71] (Figure 18.2). Pathological tremors typically show constant frequencies under a weight load as the central rhythmic drive is largely independent of the peripheral mechanics.

Each recording's epoch typically lasts about 30 seconds, but longer periods are needed in certain situations, e.g., in patients with

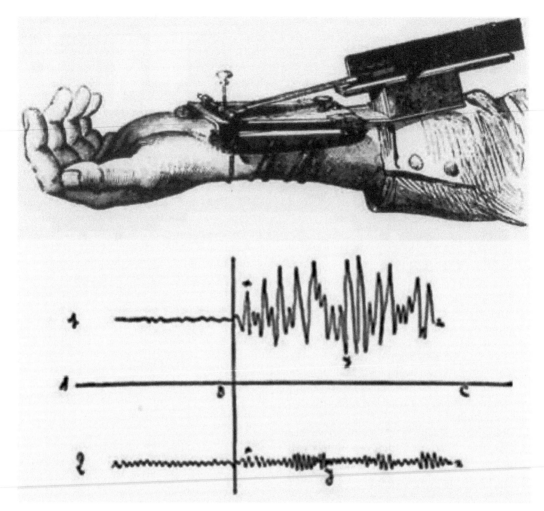

FIGURE 18.1: Nineteenth-Century French Neurologist Jean-Marie Charcot's Graphical Recording Method for Tremor ("Myographic Curves") Relied on Various Pneumatic Tambour-Like Mechanisms. The top tracing represents an intention tremor in a patient with multiple sclerosis. Segment AB indicates "at rest," and BC indicates increasing oscillations during voluntary movement. The lower tracing represents a parkinsonian tremor, with segment AB indicating a tremor at rest persisting in segment BC during voluntary movement. Modified from [67].

re-emergent rest tremor. In addition, very mild rest tremor is typically intermittent, so a 60-second recording with an augmenting task may be necessary.[72] Continuous long-term recordings have been used,[73] although longer recordings during prescribed activities such as holding a fixed posture may become impractical due to subject fatigue.

Recorded data can be analyzed with commercially available tremor analysis software,[74] some of which are also accessible online (Figure 18.2).[75] It is recommended that each lab establish its own normative data; it is estimated that at least 25 normal subjects have to be recorded to obtain normal values.[76] The tremor analysis returns several parameters (see below) useful to narrow down the differential diagnosis of tremor.[77]

Amplitude and frequency

Accelerometers allow amplitude detection expressed as root mean squared plotted versus time. This is appropriate when the tremor is stable (statistically stationary) over time.

While the experienced eye can distinguish the three main frequency ranges as high (>7 Hz), medium (4–7 Hz) and low (<4 Hz), the exact frequency measurement requires a signal analysis of accelerometric or EMG recordings. Tremor is a

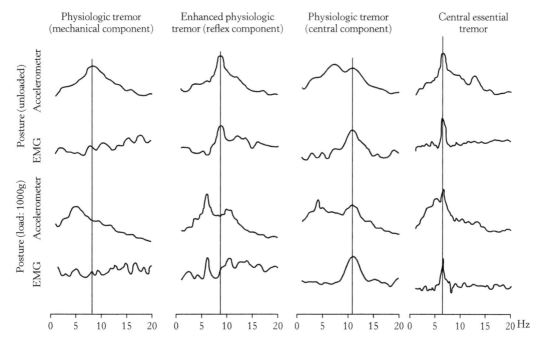

FIGURE 18.2: Accelerometer and EMG Recordings of Upper Limb Postural Tremor (With and Without Loading).

roughly sinusoidal oscillatory movement, and it can be mathematically interpreted as a periodic signal. The fast Fourier transform (FFT) is a discrete Fourier transform that is computed with a mathematical algorithm minimizing the number of computations. FFT is used to obtain the magnitudes of oscillation at any given frequency, thus generating an amplitude-frequency plot (Figure 18.2). This plot is used to determine the main peak frequency (i.e., frequency of maximum power), main peak power, number of harmonic frequencies, and also the relative power contribution to the first harmonic.[78,79]

The frequency content of voluntary movement is generally concentrated at frequencies below 2 Hz. This is particularly relevant during the recording of kinetic tremor (i.e., differentiating tremor from the movement caused by a finger-to-nose maneuver) and in cases of prolonged tremor recording, as filtering the signals can dissect tremor from other movements. However, some tremors—particularly Holmes tremor, cerebellar tremor, and myorhythmia—can occur at relatively low frequencies (3–4 Hz).[23] In addition, some voluntary actions can be interpreted as tremor (e.g., teeth brushing in the case of wearable-based prolonged recordings), and other involuntary movements, such as myoclonus, contain high-frequency content that may extend into the frequency range of tremor.[66]

Most biological tremors fall in a frequency lower than 25 Hz; thus, the sampling rate of the recording device must be at least 50 Hz (and preferably several times that) for better signal processing. Low-pass filtering and other techniques can be used to further improve the frequency window of interest.

The central rhythmic drive seen in pathological tremor causes any body part to tremble through muscles activation. Thus, another characteristic of pathological central tremors is an EMG burst activity at the same frequency of the rhythmic movements detected by the accelerometer (Figure 18.2).

FTT analysis is the most used method for analyzing time series amplitude and frequency data. However, time-domain analyses and other frequency-domain analyses are also available, e.g., wavelet analysis or Hilbert-Huang Transform. Long-term recordings of intermittent tremor are more appropriately characterized with a time-frequency analysis that shows how the signal power and frequency change over time. The most common type of time-frequency analysis produces images called spectrograms (Figure 18.3). Rhythmicity can also be quantified in terms of the variability in the period of successive tremor cycles, which is particularly relevant for more irregular tremors such as dystonic tremor[18] or tremors with inconsistent frequencies such as functional tremor.

Coherence

The 95% confidence limits and confidence intervals for the coherence (i.e., the fixed relationship) between two different signal sources can also be calculated.[80] Multiple oscillators can be determined for tremors deriving from a central mechanism in patients with multifocal or generalized tremor. Some studies, however, have found high coherence between limbs (despite amplitude asymmetry) for brief periods of time. For example, PD tremor is coupled within but less between limbs; in addition, a mental task increases the coherence between muscles of the same limb, whereas a finger-to-nose test decreases it.

Coherence values higher than 0.6 are usually considered high. Within-limb coherence tends to be high also thanks to mechanical properties, while between-limb assessment is useful in differentiating some tremor disorders. In this respect, values between 0.9 and 1 are typically reached in three conditions: 1) orthostatic tremor (where a single oscillator causes the same bilateral leg tremor); 2) the "volitional mechanism" of functional tremor (see discussion later in chapter); and 3) in the case of the rare combination of congenital mirror movements and tremor.[81]

Smart devices for tremor analysis

Non-health commercial devices—such as smartphones, smartwatches, and tablets—are versatile, ubiquitous, and easily accessible to consumers at a relatively low cost (Figure 18.4). Studies using smart devices to quantify tremor are increasingly being published.[82–85] Smartphones and smartwatches have highly accurate accelerometers and have been used to develop metrics like the tremor stability index[86] and the relative power contribution to the first harmonic.[78,79] Although none of these tools combine multiple quantitative methods (i.e., no EMG is possible), their value is mainly twofold: they can be easily used to quantify tremor in the clinical setting, such as for OT (Figure 18.4A);[87] and they can be worn by the patient for days, thus allowing a continuous monitoring of the tremor during daily activities.[88]

Data tablets are now portable and very affordable, and have been used to identify pathologic tremor in genetic studies and to assess treatment effect in interventional studies, generally by means of a computerized analysis of spiral drawing (Figure 18.4B).[89] The x- and y-axis displacement data are analyzed to produce velocity and acceleration data that can be analyzed in a variety of ways, including FFT. For example, it has been proposed that a single spiral axis is typical of ET

while no or multiple axes are seen in dystonic tremor, and that the spiral density is greater in PD than ET due to the combination of tremor and bradykinesia.

Neuroglyphics is a free tablet software for Archimedes spiral acquisition and analysis, available at: http://www.neuroglyphics.org.

Applications of apparatus-based tremor assessment

Tremor analysis can be very useful in differentiating tremor conditions, particularly functional tremor. It is fundamental for the diagnosis of OT and is increasingly used in clinical trials.

Physiological and enhanced physiological tremor vs. pathological tremors

Normal physiological tremor is usually not visible, and it can only be measured with accelerometers. An increase of the amplitude leads to EPT. Three different physiological tremor mechanisms have been established: mechanical, mechanical-reflex, and central-neurogenic. Any movable limb can be regarded as a pendulum with the capability to swing rhythmically, that is, to oscillate (mechanical mechanism). These oscillations will automatically assume the resonant frequency of the body part depending on its mechanical properties: the greater its weight, the lower its resonant frequency; the greater the joint stiffness, the higher this frequency. Consequently, normal elbow tremor has a frequency of 3–5 Hz, wrist tremor of 7–10 Hz, and metacarpophalangeal joint tremor of 17–30 Hz.[6] Any mechanical perturbation, such as those produced by irregularities in motor-unit firing and by the force of blood ejection during cardiac systole, can activate such an oscillation.[90–92] In these conditions, muscles show normal non-rhythmic isometric activity, i.e., FFT of the EMG signal lacks tremor activity. In addition, a clear reduction of the accelerometric tremor frequency by at least 1–1.5 Hz is expected under a weight load (Figure 18.2).

However, as this low-amplitude oscillation leads to rhythmic activation of muscle receptors, it activates segmental (spinal) or long (e.g., transcortical) reflex loops which can greatly enhance the oscillation itself (mechanical-reflex mechanism). The third—less frequent—mechanism (central-neurogenic) in physiological tremor is a transmission of oscillatory activity within the CNS to the peripheral muscles. It is invariably associated with modulation of motor-unit activity, not simply a passive response to sensory feedback. The rhythmic

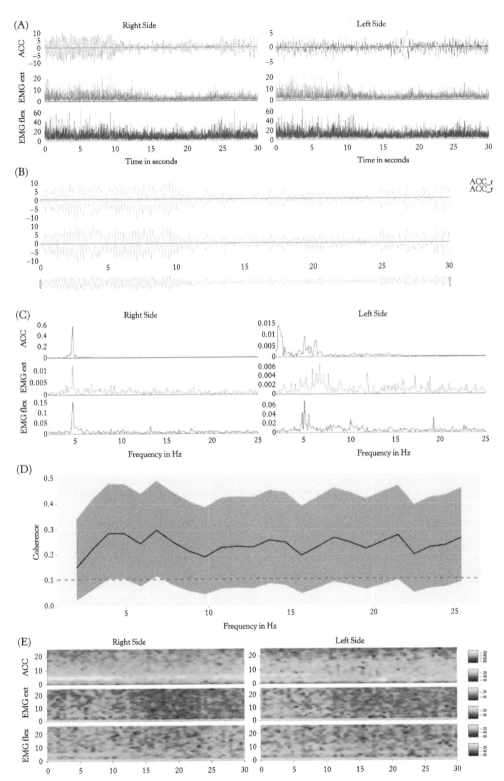

FIGURE 18.3: Tremor Recordings Made Using Wearable Devices. EMG polygraphy was performed using a setup including 4-channel surface EMG and 2-channel accelerometry (sampling rate: 1000Hz). (A) General view of the 6 channels raw signal. (B) Time domain (useful to assess amplitude variability). (C) Amplitude-frequency plot using the fast Fourier transform. (D) Coherence analysis between right and left accelerometric signals (no significant coherence is detected). (E) Tremor spectrogram. Abbreviation: ACC = Accelerometry.

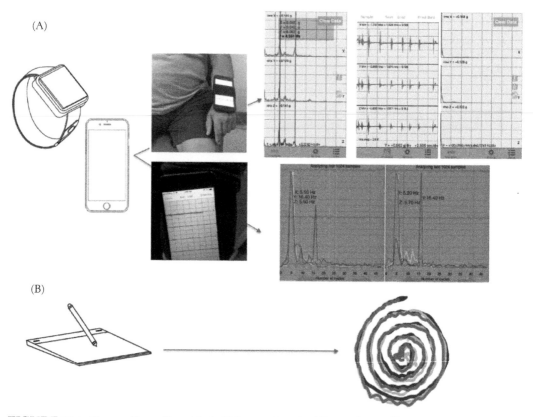

FIGURE 18.4: Tremor Recordings Made Using an Attached Smartphone (A) or a Writing Tablet (B). Tremor can be recorded using the accelerometer embedded in smart devices. Hand tremor (top panel) can be measured using a smartphone attached to the wrist with a strap-containing case. The first patient (recording on left) has a 4.5Hz rest tremor caused by Parkinson's disease, the second patient (panel on right) exhibits a myoclonic jerk for which the fast Fourier transform does not detect any peaks. Measurement of leg tremor (bottom panel) illustrates the particularly useful that the rapid oscillations of OT can be detected.

B. Archimedes spirals can be recorded and analyzed using a computerized tablet. This recording was performed with Neuroglyphics, a free software available at http://www.neuroglyphics.org.

activity of the participating motor-units then leads to 8–12 Hz tremor, i.e., FFT of the EMG signal shows tremor activity (Figure 18.2). In contrast with the mechanical-reflex oscillations, central oscillations occur at the centrally determined frequency and are independent of the limbs' mechanics.[93] An enhancement of this component is another basis for EPT and pathological centrally generated tremors.[94]

In summary, EPT has the same peripheral and central components as physiological tremor, but there is greater participation of the stretch reflex and of the 8–12 Hz central oscillator. When EPT becomes clinically symptomatic without provoking factors, it becomes phenomenologically like essential tremor (ET); therefore, it may be difficult to separate early ET from EPT. Accordingly, ET can be readily reset by external perturbations,

unlike PD tremor, thus suggesting that oscillations within spinal reflex loops also play a major role in the generation of ET.[95]

EMG is also useful in diagnosing tremor at rest, which is characterized by an EMG burst in the middle of background silence. A silent EMG in a trembling body part at rest means that the tremor is transmitted mechanically from another site. Breakthrough of action tremor in a body part at rest is instead characterized by an EMG burst in the middle of background activity, as seen in some ET patients.

Finally, although diagnostically less accurate, poly-EMG profile (i.e., simultaneous multichannel EMG) of PD rest tremor typically shows alternating (less commonly synchronous) contraction of agonist and antagonist muscles, whereas the muscle contraction patterns of the

ET, EPT, and dystonic tremor are mainly synchronous contraction.

Central tremor differential diagnosis with apparatus measures

The paragraphs above detail some major features of ET, EPT, and PD tremor. Several studies have explored the value and accuracy of instrumental differential diagnosis between ET and PD. Measuring latency of tremor occurrence when moving from rest to postural position (i.e., re-emergent tremor) and changes in tremor amplitude after mental concentration might distinguish parkinsonian tremor from tremor in ET, although these features can be easily identified on physical examination. Recently, more sophisticated metrics such as the "tremor stability index"[86] and the mean harmonic power[96,97] have been proposed.

The differential between dystonic tremor, tremor associated with dystonia, and ET is particularly challenging. EMG has been used to document the effect of sensory tricks and quantify motor overflow and mirroring, characteristic features of dystonia. In addition, either EMG or accelerometry can be used to document the effect of position, which should not affect tremor in ET, but should influence dystonic tremor.[98,99] A characteristic of dystonic tremor is indeed the "null point," a position in which the tremor almost fully abates.[100] A tremor variability greater than 50% has been proposed in the differential

between tremor in ET and tremor associated with dystonia.[101] More experimental tools, such as the triphasic EMG pattern of ballistic movements[102] or temporal discrimination,[103] have also been published.

The differential between tremor and cerebellar dysmetria is also challenging. Higher tremor frequencies are in keeping with the former. Additional tools, such as analysis of ballistic movements or object grasping, can be useful, although they are not widely available. Measuring fast, reverse-at-target, goal-directed movements has been found to reliably quantify dysmetria independently of tremor.[104]

Finally, OT is the only tremor with a pathognomonic frequency of 14–16 Hz recorded during standing. Such fast oscillation is difficult to assess clinically, thus accelerometry and/or EMG is needed in such cases. These tools are also useful in the differential diagnosis with orthostatic myoclonus, slow orthostatic tremors, and pseudo-OT,[23] as discussed in detail earlier in the chapter.

Functional tremor

A battery consisting of EMG and accelerometer recordings of upper limbs in a relaxed condition, outstretched with and without weight loading, during tapping tasks and while performing ballistic movements has been validated for a "laboratory-supported" diagnosis of functional tremor.[105] This battery has been found to have high sensitivity (90%) and specificity (96%) in

---

BOX 18.2
CHARACTERISTIC FEATURES OF FUNCTIONAL TREMOR*

- Changes in frequency during distraction (sensitivity: 42–92%, specificity of 94%).
- Changes in frequency during entrainment (sensitivity: 39–91%, specificity: 91–100%).
- Higher amplitude during loading (sensitivity: 33–69%, specificity: 75–95%).
- Higher number of periods without significant coherence.
- Large variation of tremor amplitude and frequency.
- Less accuracy in tapping performances (sensitivity: 46%, specificity: 84%).
- Reduction of amplitude or cessation when performing ballistic movement with the opposite hand (sensitivity: 67–100%, specificity: 84–100%).
- Significant coherence between the two hands in bilateral tremor (sensitivity: 56%, specificity: 96%).
- Tonic discharge of antagonist muscles approximately 300 msec before the onset of tremor bursts (sensitivity: 46–100%, specificity: 96–100%).

* Modified from[106]

differentiating functional tremor, with a positive predictive value of 92%. One unanswered question is the proportion of people with tremor for whom such tests would be necessary. Clinical examination is often sufficient to diagnose functional tremor, and it is likely that these tests will only be necessary for a small number of patients. The battery could be useful in specific contexts, such as clinical trials, in cases with suspected functional overlay, and when invasive neurosurgical treatments are being considered. Box 18.2 summarizes the published tremor analysis features of functional tremor. High coherence between different trembling body parts or during entrainment tasks (e.g., contralateral finger tapping) is a very distinct feature of these patients.[106] However, independent oscillations (i.e., low coherence) are found in some cases. The latter might be

---

BOX 18.3
CHALLENGES FOR RESEARCH INTO ASSESSMENT OF TREMOR USING TREMOR ANALYSIS BY DEVICES

- The current gold standard of clinical diagnosis of tremor is based on phenotype-based nosology dictated by clinicians;
- Several types of tremor (including functional ones) can be diagnosed on clinical grounds and with high-level confidence in most patients:
- The cost-effectiveness of augmented tremor analysis hasn't been proven;
- The value in characterizing tremors with a functional overlay is not known;
- The optimal tremor analysis protocol has not been determined—selection of motor tasks, duration of sampling, and methods of spectral analysis may vary among users;
- No standardized position for recording tremor at rest has been validated;
- Protocols may need to vary with the type of tremor being studied;
- Most studies and protocols have focused just on upper limb tremor;
- Small body parts (e.g., the finger) require minute recording devices;
- Tremor amplitude depends on the distance of the accelerometer from rotation axis, thus introducing:
- Within-subject variability (especially if transducers are removed and re-attached during measurements);
- Between-subject variability (if transducers are not attached at the same location in all subjects, a limitation that cannot be avoided because oscillation axes vary between subjects).
- Sensors worn on the wrist (similar to a watch) function poorly at capturing tremor from rotation of the wrist and finger joints.
- Between-subject variability relies on other factors, such as:
- Hand and limb sizes vary considerably person to person, thus resulting in different physiological tremor frequencies;[66]
- The greater the wrist stiffness, the larger the frequency of hand tremor;
- Writing tablets possess two major limitations:
- The motion of the pen is not detected unless the pen tip is within 1 cm of the tablet surface (and so, patients with very severe tremor frequently cannot keep the pen close to the surface of the tablet);
- Tremor is recorded only in two dimensions and movement perpendicular to the tablet will not be detected (though some tablets have pressure sensors but these sensors record in a nonlinear fashion and so must be calibrated).
- Applications using smartphones or smartwatches utilize device-specific software and so may have subtle differences across applications and between device models.

explained by a coexisting non-functional tremor or other non-volitional mechanism, namely clonus or EPT.[107]

Surgical planning

Tremor analysis before thalamic surgery (either deep brain stimulation or thalamotomy) is often needed when a functional etiology (or overlay) is suspected in a surgical candidate (personal observation). In addition, accelerometric recordings of frequency and rhythmicity may help distinguish patients with predominant tremor from those with tremor and ataxia, e.g., in multiple sclerosis.[108]

Clinical trials

Accelerometers, gyroscopes, tablets, and even posturography have been used as endpoints in clinical trials exploring a variety of tremor treatments.[69,109] Although these objective measures have good convergent validity and correlate with patient disability,[110] the correlation between a transducer measure of tremor and a relevant rating scale is logarithmic, not linear, stemming from the fact that clinical ratings are nonlinear measures, i.e., the Weber-Fechner law of psychophysics discussed above.[48] These sensitive tools are therefore able to capture significant differences even in trials with negative results on clinical scale based primary endpoints.[109]

CONCLUSIONS

Although tremor can be envisioned as a very distinctive movement disorder, as well as a physiological characteristic sometimes difficult to distinguish from its pathological counterpart, expertise in the clinical approach to tremor requires an education that is open to new findings and technologies. This chapter describes the evolution of new concepts and clinical observations since James Parkinson's comments in 1817, and over a 4-decade span during which the field of movement disorders research has refined what we know of tremor. In the current era, there has been increased insight into mechanisms of tremor, which, ultimately, might lead to better therapeutics beyond the limited medication and surgical approaches to tremor control. Rating methods for tremor have advanced greatly but still have gaps for translating observations of the movement disorder into clinically meaningful anchors and disability correlates.

Tremor recording has been an especially productive direction of research. As noted earlier,

the use of motion transducers, particularly those embedded in wearable devices, is still an active topic of research and development. Many other ways to capture tremor have been developed, such as laser transduction of velocity, force transducers to measure joint movement with two degrees of freedom, electromagnetic tracking of motion with six degrees of freedom (translational and rotational),[111] acoustic analysis for voice tremor, video image processing,[112] and even ultrasound M-Mode for tremor frequency determination.[113] Novel systems to gather large population-based data are being investigated as well, such as the analysis of keystroke dynamics during typing on smartphone touchscreens and keyboards[114] or computer mouse cursor movement of the users of a web search engine.[115] All of these advances in technology of electrophysiologic analysis of tremor must be interpreted in the context of the patient's history and neurologic exam. More research is certainly needed, particularly to address the barriers of wearables and other issues listed in Box 18.3.[71]

REFERENCES

1. Parkinson J. *An Essay on the Shaking Palsy.* Sherwood, Neely, and Jones; 1817.
2. Louis ED, Ottman R, Hauser WA. How common is the most common adult movement disorder? estimates of the prevalence of essential tremor throughout the world. *Mov Disord.* 1998;13(1):5–10.
3. Elble RJ. Physiologic and essential tremor. *Neurology.* 1986;36(2):225–231.
4. Espay AJ, Lang AE, Erro R, et al. Essential pitfalls in "essential" tremor. *Mov Disord.* 2017;32(3):325–331.
5. Brumlik J, Yap C-B. *Normal Tremor: A Comparative Study.* Charles C Thomas Company; 1970.
6. Elble RJ. Characteristics of physiologic tremor in young and elderly adults. *Clin Neurophysiol.* 2003;114(4):624–635.
7. Trenado C, Amtage F, Huethe F, et al. Suppression of enhanced physiological tremor via stochastic noise: initial observations. *PLoS One.* 2014;9(11):e112782.
8. Yoo SW, Lee M, Kim JS, Lee KS. Focal localized enhanced physiological tremor after physical insult. *Neurol Sci.* 2019;40(12):2641–2643.
9. LeWitt PA. Drug-induced tremors. In: Friedman JH, ed. *Medication-Induced Movement Disorders.* Cambridge Press; 2015: 104–109.
10. McKeon A, Pittock SJ, Glass GA, et al. Whole-body tremulousness: isolated generalized polymyoclonus. *Arch Neurol.* 2007;64(9):1318–1322.
11. Louis ED, Broussolle E, Goetz CG, Krack P, Kaufmann P, Mazzoni P. Historical underpinnings of the term essential tremor in the late 19th century. *Neurology.* 2008;71(11):856–859.

12. Deuschl G, Bain P, Brin M, Committee AHS. Consensus statement of the Movement Disorder Society on Tremor. *Mov Disord*. 1998;13(Suppl 3):2–23.
13. Bhatia KP, Bain P, Bajaj N, et al. Consensus Statement on the classification of tremors. from the task force on tremor of the International Parkinson and Movement Disorder Society. *Mov Disord*. 2018;33(1):75–87.
14. Elble RJ, Koller WG. *Tremor*. Baltimore (MD): The Johns Hopkins Press; 1991.
15. LeWitt PA, Mihaila D. Clonus. In: Aminoff M, Daroff RB, eds. *Encyclopedia of the Neurological Science*. New York: Academic Press; 2003:728–729.
16. Fraix V, Delalande I, Parrache M, Derambure P, Cassim F. Action-induced clonus mimicking tremor. *Mov Disord*. 2008;23(2):285–288.
17. Bhatia KP, Schneider SA. Psychogenic tremor and related disorders. *J Neurol*. 2007;254(5):569–574.
18. Muthuraman M, Raethjen J, Koirala N, et al. Cerebello-cortical network fingerprints differ between essential, Parkinson's and mimicked tremors. *Brain*. 2018;141(6):1770–1781.
19. Belvisi D, Conte A, Bologna M, et al. Re-emergent tremor in Parkinson's disease. *Parkinsonism Relat Disord*. 2017;36:41–46.
20. Manoj S, Hari Kumar KVS. Wing beating tremor and double panda sign. *Mov Disord Clin Pract*. 2015;2(1):47–48.
21. Silverdale MA, Schneider SA, Bhatia KP, Lang AE. The spectrum of orolingual tremor—a proposed classification system. *Mov Disord*. 2008;23(2):159–167.
22. Bain PG, Findley LJ, Thompson PD, et al. A study of hereditary essential tremor. *Brain*. 1994;117(Pt 4):805–824.
23. Ure RJ, Dhanju S, Lang AE, Fasano A. Unusual tremor syndromes: know in order to recognise. *J Neurol Neurosurg Psychiatry*. 2016;87(11):1191–1203.
24. Aggarwal A, Schneider SA, Houlden H, et al. Indian-subcontinent NBIA: unusual phenotypes, novel PANK2 mutations, and undetermined genetic forms. *Mov Disord*. 2010;25(10):1424–1431.
25. Saldarriaga-Gil W, Rodriguez-Guerrero T, Fandino-Losada A, Ramirez-Cheyne J. Tremor-ataxia syndrome and primary ovarian insufficiency in an FMR1 premutation carrier. *Colomb Med (Cali)*. 2017;48(3):148–151.
26. Termsarasab P, Thammongkolchai T, Frucht SJ. Spinal-generated movement disorders: a clinical review. *J Clin Mov Disord*. 2015;2:18.
27. Valentino P, Labate A, Pirritano D, Crescibene L, Cascini G, Quattrone A. Orolingual tremor as unusual presentation of anti-Hu paraneoplastic syndrome. *Mov Disord*. 2008;23(12):1791–1792.
28. Govert F, Becktepe J, Balint B, et al. Temporal discrimination is altered in patients with isolated asymmetric and jerky upper limb tremor. *Mov Disord*. 2020;35(2):306–315.
29. Heilman KM. Orthostatic tremor. *Arch Neurol*. 1984;41(8):880–881.
30. Gerschlager W, Munchau A, Katzenschlager R, et al. Natural history and syndromic associations of orthostatic tremor: a review of 41 patients. *Mov Disord*. 2004;19(7):788–795.
31. Brown P. New clinical sign for orthostatic tremor. *Lancet*. 1995;346(8970):306–307.
32. Hassan A, Ahlskog JE, Matsumoto JY, Milber JM, Bower JH, Wilkinson JR. Orthostatic tremor: clinical, electrophysiologic, and treatment findings in 184 patients. *Neurology*. 2016;86(5):458–464.
33. Sander HW, Masdeu JC, Tavoulareas G, Walters A, Zimmerman T, Chokroverty S. Orthostatic tremor: an electrophysiological analysis. *Mov Disord*. 1998;13(4):735–738.
34. Erro R, Bhatia KP, Cordivari C. Shaking on standing: a critical review. *Mov Disord Clin Pract*. 2014;1(3):173–179.
35. Rigby HB, Rigby MH, Caviness JN. Orthostatic tremor: a spectrum of fast and slow frequencies or distinct entities? *Tremor Other Hyperkinet Mov (N Y)*. 2015;5:324.
36. Setta F, Jacquy J, Hildebrand J, Manto MU. Orthostatic tremor associated with cerebellar ataxia. *J Neurol*. 1998;245(5):299–302.
37. Coffeng SM, Hoff JI, Tromp SC. A slow orthostatic tremor of primary origin. *Tremor Other Hyperkinet Mov (N Y)*. 2013;3.
38. Benito-Leon J, Rodriguez J, Orti-Pareja M, Ayuso-Peralta L, Jimenez-Jimenez FJ, Molina JA. Symptomatic orthostatic tremor in pontine lesions. *Neurology*. 1997;49(5):1439–1441.
39. Gilhuis HJ, van Ommen HJ, Pannekoek BJ, Sillevis Smitt PA. Paraneoplastic orthostatic tremor associated with small cell lung cancer. *Eur Neurol*. 2005;54(4):225–226.
40. Hassan A, van Gerpen JA. Orthostatic tremor and orthostatic myoclonus: weight-bearing hyperkinetic disorders: a systematic review, new insights, and unresolved questions. *Tremor Other Hyperkinet Mov (N Y)*. 2016;6:417.
41. Hassan A, Caviness J. Slow orthostatic tremor: review of the current evidence. *Tremor Other Hyperkinet Mov (N Y)*. 2019;9. doi: 10.7916/tohm.v0.721. PMID: 31832265; PMCID: PMC6886496.
42. LeWitt PA. Orthostatic tremor: the phenomenon of "paradoxical clonus." *Arch Neurol*. 1990;47(5):501–502.
43. Bain PG, Mally J, Gresty M, Findley LJ. Assessing the impact of essential tremor on upper limb function. *J Neurol*. 1993;241(1):54–61.
44. Gironell A, Martinez-Corral M, Pagonabarraga J, Kulisevsky J. The Glass scale: a simple tool to determine severity in essential tremor. *Parkinsonism Relat Disord*. 2010;16(6):412–414.

45. Elble R, Bain P, Forjaz MJ, et al. Task force report: scales for screening and evaluating tremor: critique and recommendations. *Mov Disord.* 2013;28(13):1793–1800.

46. Merola A, Torres-Russotto DR, Stebbins GT, et al. Development and validation of the Orthostatic Tremor Severity and Disability Scale (OT-10). *Mov Disord.* 2020;35(10):1796–1801.

47. Ondo WG, Pascual B, Tremor Research G. Tremor Research Group Essential Tremor Rating Scale (TETRAS): assessing impact of different item instructions and procedures. *Tremor Other Hyperkinet Mov (N Y).* 2020;10:36.

48. Elble RJ, Pullman SL, Matsumoto JY, et al. Tremor amplitude is logarithmically related to 4- and 5-point tremor rating scales. *Brain.* 2006;129(Pt 10):2660–2666.

49. Elble RJ. Estimating change in tremor amplitude using clinical ratings: recommendations for clinical trials. *Tremor Other Hyperkinet Mov (N Y).* 2018;8:600.

50. Fahn S, Tolosa E, Marin C. Clinical rating scale for tremor. In: Jankovic J, Tolosa E, eds. *Parkinson's Disease and Movement Disorders.* 2nd ed. Williams & Wilkins; 1993: 271–280.

51. Bain PG, Findley LJ, Atchison P, et al. Assessing tremor severity. *J Neurol Neurosurg Psychiatry.* 1993;56(8):868–873.

52. Louis ED, Ford B, Bismuth B. Reliability between two observers using a protocol for diagnosing essential tremor. *Mov Disord.* 1998;13(2):287–293.

53. Louis ED, Ottman R, Ford B, et al. The Washington Heights-Inwood genetic study of essential tremor: methodologic issues in essential-tremor research. *Neuroepidemiology.* 1997;16(3):124–133.

54. Elble R, Comella C, Fahn S, et al. Reliability of a new scale for essential tremor. *Mov Disord.* 2012;27(12):1567–1569.

55. Stacy MA, Elble RJ, Ondo WG, Wu SC, Hulihan J. Assessment of interrater and intrarater reliability of the Fahn-Tolosa-Marin Tremor Rating Scale in essential tremor. *Mov Disord.* 2007;22(6):833–838.

56. Ondo W, Hashem V, LeWitt PA, et al. Comparison of the Fahn-Tolosa-Marin Clinical Rating Scale and the Essential Tremor Rating Assessment Scale. *Mov Disord Clin Pract.* 2018;5(1):60–65.

57. Mostile G, Giuffrida JP, Adam OR, Davidson A, Jankovic J. Correlation between Kinesia system assessments and clinical tremor scores in patients with essential tremor. *Mov Disord.* 2010;25(12):1938–1943.

58. Mostile G, Fekete R, Giuffrida JP, et al. Amplitude fluctuations in essential tremor. *Parkinsonism Relat Disord.* 2012;18(7):859–863.

59. Fahn S, Elton RL, UPDRS program members. Unified Parkinson's Disease Rating Scale. In: Fahn S, Marsden CD, Goldstein M, Calne DB, eds. *Recent Developments in Parkinson's Disease.* Vol 2. Macmillan Healthcare Information; 1987: 153–163.

60. Goetz CG, Tilley BC, Shaftman SR, et al. Movement Disorder Society-sponsored revision of the Unified Parkinson's Disease Rating Scale (MDS-UPDRS): scale presentation and clinimetric testing results. *Mov Disord.* 2008;23(15):2129–2170.

61. Pinter D, Forjaz MJ, Martinez-Martin P, et al. Which scale best detects treatment response of tremor in parkinsonism? *J Parkinsons Dis.* 2020;10(1):275–282.

62. Troster AI, Pahwa R, Fields JA, Tanner CM, Lyons KE. Quality of life in Essential Tremor Questionnaire (QUEST): development and initial validation. *Parkinsonism Relat Disord.* 2005;11(6):367–373.

63. Traub RE, Gerbin M, Mullaney MM, Louis ED. Development of an essential tremor embarrassment assessment. *Parkinsonism Relat Disord.* 2010;16(10):661–665.

64. Sepulveda Soto MC, Fasano A. Tremor: so common, so difficult. *J Neurol Neurosurg Psychiatry.* 2020;91(8):809–810.

65. Fearon C, Espay AJ, Lang AE, et al. Soft signs in movement disorders: friends or foes? *J Neurol Neurosurg Psychiatry.* 2019;90(8):961–962.

66. Elble RJ, McNames J. Using portable transducers to measure tremor severity. *Tremor Other Hyperkinet Mov (N Y).* 2016;6:375.

67. Charcot J-M. De la paralysie agitante. In: *Oeuvres Complètes (tome 1) Leçons sur les maladies du système nerveux.* Paris: Bureaux du Progrès Médical; 1873: s.

68. Randall JE, Stiles RN. Power spectral analysis of finger acceleration tremor. *J Appl Physiol.* 1964;19:357–360.

69. Hellriegel H, Raethjen J, Deuschl G, Volkmann J. Levetiracetam in primary orthostatic tremor: a double-blind placebo-controlled crossover study. *Mov Disord.* 2011;26(13):2431–2434.

70. Elble RJ, Sinha R, Higgins C. Quantification of tremor with a digitizing tablet. *J Neurosci Methods.* 1990;32(3):193–198.

71. Fasano A, Mancini M. Wearable-based mobility monitoring: the long road ahead. *Lancet Neurol.* 2020;19(5):378–379.

72. Cleeves L, Findley LJ, Gresty M. Assessment of rest tremor in Parkinson's disease. *Adv Neurol.* 1987;45:349–352.

73. Van Someren EJ, Pticek MD, Speelman JD, Schuurman PR, Esselink R, Swaab DF. New actigraph for long-term tremor recording. *Mov Disord.* 2006;21(8):1136–1143.

74. Lauk M, Timmer J, Lucking CH, Honerkamp J, Deuschl G. A software for recording and analysis of human tremor. *Comput Methods Programs Biomed.* 1999;60(1):65–77.

75. Vial F, McGurrin P, Osterholt T, Ehrlich D, Haubenberger D, Hallett M. Tremoroton, a new free online platform for tremor analysis. *Clin Neurophysiol Pract.* 2020;5:30–34.

76. Raethjen J, Lauk M, Koster B, et al. Tremor analysis in two normal cohorts. *Clin Neurophysiol.* 2004;115(9):2151–2156.

77. Vial F, Kassavetis P, Merchant S, Haubenberger D, Hallett M. How to do an electrophysiological study of tremor. *Clin Neurophysiol Pract.* 2019;4:134–142.

78. Daneault JF, Carignan B, Codere CE, Sadikot AF, Duval C. Using a smart phone as a standalone platform for detection and monitoring of pathological tremors. *Front Hum Neurosci.* 2012;6:357.

79. Barrantes S, Sanchez Egea AJ, Gonzalez Rojas HA, et al. Differential diagnosis between Parkinson's disease and essential tremor using the smartphone's accelerometer. *PLoS One.* 2017;12(8):e0183843.

80. Halliday DM, Rosenberg JR, Amjad AM, Breeze P, Conway BA, Farmer SF. A framework for the analysis of mixed time series/point process data—theory and application to the study of physiological tremor, single motor unit discharges and electromyograms. *Prog Biophys Mol Biol.* 1995;64(2–3):237–278.

81. Isayama R, Chen R, Lang AE, Deuschl G, Fasano A. Tremor with congenital mirror movements: evidence of involvement of the primary motor cortex in tremor. *Eur J Neurol.* 2019;26(6):e66–e67.

82. Senova S, Querlioz D, Thiriez, Jedynak P, Jarraya B, Palfi S. Using the accelerometers integrated in smartphones to evaluate essential tremor. *Stereotact Funct Neurosurg.* 2015;93(2):94–101.

83. Kubben PL, Kuijf ML, Ackermans LP, Leentjens AF, Temel Y. TREMOR12: an open-source mobile app for tremor quantification. *Stereotact Funct Neurosurg.* 2016;94(3):182–186.

84. Zheng X, Vieira Campos A, Ordieres-Mere J, Balseiro J, Labrador Marcos S, Aladro Y. Continuous monitoring of essential tremor using a portable system based on smartwatch. *Front Neurol.* 2017;8:96.

85. Lopez-Blanco R, Velasco MA, Mendez-Guerrero A, et al. Essential tremor quantification based on the combined use of a smartphone and a smartwatch: the NetMD study. *J Neurosci Methods.* 2018;303:9s02.

86. di Biase L, Brittain JS, Shah SA, et al. Tremor stability index: a new tool for differential diagnosis in tremor syndromes. *Brain.* 2017;140(7):1977–1986.

87. Balachandar A, Fasano A. Characterizing orthostatic tremor using a smartphone application. *Tremor Other Hyperkinet Mov (N Y).* 2017;7:488.

88. Lopez-Blanco R, Velasco MA, Mendez-Guerrero A, et al. Smartwatch for the analysis of rest tremor in patients with Parkinson's disease. *J Neurol Sci.* 2019;401:37–42.

89. Picillo M, Moro E, Edwards M, Di Lazzaro V, Lozano AM, Fasano A. Subdural continuous theta burst stimulation of the motor cortex in essential tremor. *Brain Stimul.* 2015;8(4):840–842.

90. Elble RJ, Randall JE. Mechanistic components of normal hand tremor. *Electroencephalogr Clin Neurophysiol.* 1978;44(1):72–82.

91. Homberg V, Hefter H, Reiners K, Freund HJ. Differential effects of changes in mechanical limb properties on physiological and pathological tremor. *J Neurol Neurosurg Psychiatry.* 1987;50(5):568–579.

92. Timmer J, Lauk M, Pfleger W, Deuschl G. Cross-spectral analysis of physiological tremor and muscle activity. I. Theory and application to unsynchronized electromyogram. *Biol Cybern.* 1998;78(5):349–357.

93. Elble RJ. Central mechanisms of tremor. *J Clin Neurophysiol.* 1996;13(2):133–144.

94. Raethjen J, Lemke MR, Lindemann M, Wenzelburger R, Krack P, Deuschl G. Amitriptyline enhances the central component of physiological tremor. *J Neurol Neurosurg Psychiatry.* 2001;70(1):78–82.

95. Lee RG, Stein RB. Resetting of tremor by mechanical perturbations: a comparison of essential tremor and parkinsonian tremor. *Ann Neurol.* 1981;10(6):523–531.

96. Muthuraman M, Hossen A, Heute U, Deuschl G, Raethjen J. A new diagnostic test to distinguish tremulous Parkinson's disease from advanced essential tremor. *Mov Disord.* 2011;26(8):1548–1552.

97. Wile DJ, Ranawaya R, Kiss ZH. Smart watch accelerometry for analysis and diagnosis of tremor. *J Neurosci Methods.* 2014;230:1–4.

98. Sanes JN, Hallett M. Limb positioning and magnitude of essential tremor and other pathological tremors. *Mov Disord.* 1990;5(4): 304–309.

99. Shaikh AG, Wong AL, Zee DS, Jinnah HA. Keeping your head on target. *J Neurosci.* 2013;33(27):11281–11295.

100. Gironell A, Kulisevsky J. Diagnosis and management of essential tremor and dystonic tremor. *Ther Adv Neurol Disord.* 2009;2(4):215–222.

101. Shaikh AG, Jinnah HA, Tripp RM, et al. Irregularity distinguishes limb tremor in cervical dystonia from essential tremor. *J Neurol Neurosurg Psychiatry.* 2008;79(2):187–189.

102. Munchau A, Schrag A, Chuang C, et al. Arm tremor in cervical dystonia differs from essential tremor and can be classified by onset age and spread of symptoms. *Brain.* 2001;124(Pt 9):1765–1776.

103. Tinazzi M, Fasano A, Di Matteo A, et al. Temporal discrimination in patients with dystonia and tremor and patients with essential tremor. *Neurology.* 2013;80(1):76–84.

104. Casamento-Moran A, Yacoubi B, Wilkes BJ, et al. Quantitative separation of tremor and ataxia in essential tremor. *Ann Neurol.* 2020;88(2):375–387.

105. Schwingenschuh P, Saifee TA, Katschnig-Winter P, et al. Validation of "laboratory-supported" criteria for functional (psychogenic) tremor. *Mov Disord.* 2016;31(4):555–562.

106. Thomsen BLC, Teodoro T, Edwards MJ. Biomarkers in functional movement disorders: a systematic review. *J Neurol Neurosurg Psychiatry.* 2020;91(12):1261–1269.

107. Raethjen J, Kopper F, Govindan RB, Volkmann J, Deuschl G. Two different pathogenetic mechanisms in psychogenic tremor. *Neurology.* 2004;63(5):812–815.

108. Alusi SH, Aziz TZ, Glickman S, Jahanshahi M, Stein JF, Bain PG. Stereotactic lesional surgery for the treatment of tremor in multiple sclerosis: a prospective case-controlled study. *Brain.* 2001;124(Pt 8):1576–1589.

109. Zesiewicz TA, Ward CL, Hauser RA, Sanchez-Ramos J, Staffetti JF, Sullivan KL. A double-blind placebo-controlled trial of zonisamide (zonegran) in the treatment of essential tremor. *Mov Disord.* 2007;22(2):279–282.

110. Louis ED. More time with tremor: the experience of essential tremor versus Parkinson's disease patients. *Mov Disord Clin Pract.* 2016;3(1):36–42.

111. O'Suilleabhain PE, Dewey Jr. RB. Validation for tremor quantification of an electromagnetic tracking device. *Mov Disord.* 2001;16(2):265–271.

112. Swider M. The application of video image processing to quantitative analysis of extremity tremor in humans. *J Neurosci Methods.* 1998;84(1–2):167–172.

113. Richter D, Woitalla D, Muhlack S, Gold R, Tonges L, Krogias C. Coronal transcranial sonography and m-mode tremor frequency determination in Parkinson's disease and essential tremor. *J Neuroimaging.* 2017;27(5):524–530.

114. Arroyo-Gallego T, Ledesma-Carbayo MJ, Butterworth I, et al. Detecting motor impairment in early Parkinson's disease via natural typing interaction with keyboards: validation of the neuroQWERTY approach in an uncontrolled at-home setting. *J Med Internet Res.* 2018;20(3):e89.

115. White RW, Horvitz E. Population-scale hand tremor analysis via anonymized mouse cursor signals. *NPJ Digit Med.* 2019;2:93.

19

Treatment of Tremor

DEEPA DASH AND TIAGO A. MESTRE

INTRODUCTION

Tremor is an involuntary, rhythmic, oscillatory movement of a body part.[1] Tremor is a common phenomenology in movement disorders. Essential tremor (ET) is the paradigmatic tremor syndrome with an estimated prevalence of 0.4–0.9% worldwide across all age groups.[2] Tremor can frequently lead to significant functional disability and a reduction in quality of life.[3,4] People with tremors may experience a premature end of professional life,[5] social phobia with associated mental health problems.[6]

As a general principle, the treatment of tremor aims not only to reduce the severity of the tremor but chiefly to mitigate its detrimental functional impact. Treatment is tailored to the degree of disability, the risk associated with the treatment, and the patient's preference. Treatment options for tremor are broadly divided into pharmacological intervention, chemo-denervation or botulinum toxin, lesional surgery, and deep brain stimulation (DBS). The most robust evidence exists for ET, and there is a significant gap in knowledge to guide treatment for other tremor syndromes. In this chapter, we will review available treatment options and the supporting evidence for pharmacotherapy, surgical interventions, and non-pharmacological non-surgical interventions, with an emphasis on ET and a selection of other tremor syndromes.

PHARMACOTHERAPY

Essential tremor

The first line of treatment for ET is oral pharmacological interventions. Propranolol, primidone, and, more recently, topiramate are the medications with the more robust evidence for efficacy in ET.[7] Propranolol and primidone were evaluated in studies conducted in the 1970s and 80s. Many of these trials were randomized and placebo-controlled but were small (frequently < 20–30 patients) and had a short follow-up. Topiramate was evaluated more recently in clinical trials with a more robust design and a larger number of patients.[7] A critical gap is the lack of evidence to guide the long-term pharmacotherapy for ET. The decision for one of the first-line options is based on the supporting evidence, individual patient characteristics and preference, and consideration of additional therapeutic benefits. In clinical practice, propranolol followed by primidone are more commonly prescribed by general neurologists and movement disorders specialists, but the rate of discontinuation is approximately 50%.[8] The current evidence for ET treatment has been tabulated in Table 19.1 and Table 19.2).

TABLE 19.1: SUMMARY OF CLINICAL UTILITY OF VARIOUS TREATMENT OPTIONS FOR TREATMENT OF ET*

Clinically useful	Propranolol, primidone, topiramate (>200mg)
Possibly useful	Alprazolam, botulinum toxin type A, unilateral VIM-DBS, unilateral radiofrequency thalamotomy, unilateral MRI-focused ultrasound thalamotomy
Investigational use	Carisbamate, gabapentin, zonisamide, propranolol long-acting, nadolol, metoprolol, atenolol, sotalol, phenobarbital/phenobarbitone, T2000 (1,3-dimethoxymethyl-5,5-dephenyl-barbituric acid), flunarizine, nimodipine, methazolamide, mirtazapine, olanzapine, theophylline, bilateral VIM-DBS, unilateral gamma knife thalamotomy
Unlikely useful	Trazodone, isoniazid, acetazolamide, progabide
Not useful	Levetiracetam, pregabalin

---

* Based on the International Parkinson and Movement Disorder Society Evidence-Based Review 2018[7]

TABLE 19.2: RECOMMENDATION FOR TREATMENT OF
ESSENTIAL TREMOR (ET)*

Recommendations regarding use	Treatment
Should be offered to patients who desire treatment for limb tremor in ET, depending on concurrent medical conditions and potential side effects	Primidone, propranolol, propranolol LA
Probably effective and should be considered to reduce limb tremor in ET	Alprazolam, atenolol, gabapentin (monotherapy) Sotalol, topiramate
Probably effective and should be considered to reduce head tremor in ET or isolated head tremor	Propranolol
Possibly effective and may be considered to reduce limb tremor associated with ET	Botulinum toxin A injection of forearm muscles
Recommendations against use	Clonazepam, nadolol, nimodipine 3,4diaminopyridine, acetazolamide, isoniazid, levetiracetam, pindolol, trazodone, flunarizine, methazolamide, mirtazapine, nifedipine, verapamil, amantadine, clonidine, clozapine, glutethimide, L-tryptophan, pyridoxine, metoprolol, nicardipine, olanzapine, oxcarbazepine, phenobarbital, pregabalin, quetiapine, sodium oxybate, theophylline, tiagabine, zonisamide

* Evidence-Based Guideline Update for Treatment of ET: American Academy of Neurology, 2011[250]

Propranolol: Propranolol is a non-selective β-adrenergic receptor antagonist and the first pharmacological agent found to be effective for tremor control as early as 1965.[9] Propranolol is the most studied pharmacological intervention for the symptomatic treatment of ET. There is option of using immediate-release and long-acting formulation, both of which have comparable efficacy and safety.[10,11]

The most robust evidence for propranolol's clinical efficacy comes from 13 randomized controlled trials (RCTs) comparing immediate-release propranolol with placebo and various other active agents.[11-21] In these studies, propranolol was tested in doses up to 240–360 mg/d for a treatment duration ranging from 1.5 to 8 weeks and focused primarily on improvement of upper limb tremor. There were positive outcomes in tremor severity, task performance testing, activities of daily living (ADLs), patient-reported clinical improvement, and data collected from accelerometric devices.[7] However, functional improvement is less commonly reported.[7] The overall responder rates for limb tremor in these studies ranged from 50 to 70%.[7] Overall, propranolol was well tolerated and withdrawals due to side effects were less than 10%. The most common and dose-limiting adverse effects were bradycardia, syncope, fatigue, and erectile dysfunction.[7]

The long-term use of long-acting propranolol (80–160 mg/d) has been evaluated in an open-label study comparison with primidone (50–250 mg/d), showing sustained improvement in about 40% of patients after one year and a waning of effect in 12% of the cases. Chronic side effects occurred in 17% of the cases.[22]

As a non-selective β-blocker, propranolol is contraindicated in patients with active bronchial asthma, allergic rhinitis, or chronic obstructive pulmonary disease. Caution should be used while prescribing propranolol in people with diabetes mellitus due to the masking effect of propranolol on hypoglycemia.[23]

Other β-adrenergic antagonists have been evaluated for ET, including the non-selective β-blocker nadolol and the selective β1 receptor blockers metoprolol and atenolol. Evidence is less robust for these agents,[7] but selective β1 receptor blocking agents may be tried in patients with ET with comorbidities like bronchial asthma and allergic rhinitis.[24] Non-responders to propranolol are unlikely to respond to an alternative β-blocker.[25]

While most of the drugs in this class ameliorate tremors, there are few like pindolol with partial β-agonist activity which can worsen tremors.[26,27]

Primidone: Primidone is the other "classical" first-line pharmacological intervention used in ET. Primidone is metabolized to phenylethylmalonamide and phenobarbital. Primidone has been evaluated in eight RCTs using as comparator placebo or other active agents.[28-34] Most studies were crossover in design.[7] Primidone was evaluated in doses ranging from 150 to 750 mg/d during 3 to 52 weeks.[7] The clinical benefit of primidone was captured in clinical rating scales, task performance testing, ADLs, and accelerometric device data.[7]

Primidone may cause an acute sensation of dizziness, vertigo, or imbalance ("acute toxic reaction") coincident with the start of a treatment trial in up to 22.7% of patients,[30] which can lead to an early discontinuation. However, these symptoms usually subside after 1 to 4 days.[22,30] Overall, discontinuation rate due to side effects ranged from 7.5% to 42%.[7] Evidence does not support a particular titration algorithm[33] to mitigate acute tolerance problems. In clinical practice, the starting dose varies but is usually started at a low dose (starting between 12.5 mg and 62.5 mg a day) titrating up to a dose at which adequate tremor control can be achieved and tolerated well, which could be up to 750 mg/day.

The long-term use of primidone is supported by studies with 12 month follow-up comparing two different daily doses of primidone (250 and 750mg)[34] or comparing primidone with propranolol.[22] In the latter study, the use of primidone led to a sustained improvement in about 52% of patients, a waning of effect in 13% of the cases, with better chronic tolerability than propranolol.[22] A higher daily dose of primidone (750 mg) is associated with a greater discontinuation rate.[34]

Topiramate: Topiramate is a carbonic anhydrase inhibitor.[35] The CNS action is related to activation of GABA-A-mediated inhibition, modulation of voltage-gated Na + channels and inhibition of excitatory AMPA glutamate mediate transmission.[36] Topiramate was evaluated for ET in four placebo-controlled RCTs with a total of 322 subjects and a mean treatment duration of 10.5 weeks.[37-40] Only two of the studies were parallel in design, and the remaining had a crossover design. Overall, topiramate demonstrated improvement in the tremor amplitude and a significant improvement in functional disability,[37,38,40] but with an increased risk of withdrawal.[41] In fact, at the observed therapeutic daily dose of topiramate (215–333 mg) there was a significant dropout rate (30%–54.2%) in these studies[7] due to side effects. The most common adverse effects included paresthesia, weight loss,

anorexia, and memory difficulties. The latter may be particularly disabling.

Other medications: A variety of other pharmacological interventions have been evaluated for the treatment of ET; however, the results from the studies either do not support a consistent benefit or are limited by tolerability concerns (Table 19.3). Gabapentin and alprazolam have been studied in more detail with some evidence of efficacy, albeit less robust than first-line therapy options. Gabapentin (1200–3600 mg/d) was evaluated in two RCTs with conflicting results.[42,43] Benzodiazepines have been considered for ET. Alprazolam (0.75–1.54 mg/d) is the one most studied with two placebo-controlled RCTs,[44,45] documenting a reduction in tremor severity and improved task performance. Tolerability is an important clinical issue, with as much as 50% of subjects experiencing sedation,[46] along with the known dependence potential with chronic use of the medication.

The acute relief of tremor is a particular therapeutic indication for ET. In clinical practice, patients can start treatment with propranolol with an as needed regimen. The observation that a significant proportion of patients diagnosed with ET report a subjective improvement of the tremor with the ingestion of small amounts of ethanol[47] led to the development of another intervention targeting GABA-A receptor-mediated transmission, which is likely the mechanism of action of ethanol.[47,48] 1-octanol[49,50] and its octanoic acid metabolite[51-53] are long-chain alcohols evaluated in clinical trials for acute symptomatic relief of tremor in ethanol-responsive ET patients. Overall, these compounds seem to be well tolerated and can improve tremors up to 5 hours.[53] The most common adverse events were mild transient dysgeusia in the absence of sedation and intoxication associated with ethanol. Further therapeutic development is required before the role of these compounds can be established in treatment of ET.

The current evidence for ET treatment is mostly for upper limb tremor and less so much for head and voice tremors (Table 19.1, Table 19.2). Pharmacological agents with documented effectiveness for upper limb tremor of ET have not been equally effective for voice and head ET tremor,[54,55] making these symptoms more difficult to treat. Zonisamide may be more effective for isolated head tremor than propranolol.[56]

Parkinsonian tremor

Tremor is one of the cardinal manifestations of Parkinson disease (PD).[57] The classical

TABLE 19.3: DOSES AND COMMON SIDE EFFECTS OF PHARMACOLOGICAL
AGENTS USED FOR THE TREATMENT OF ET*

Medication	Daily dose (mg)	Side effects
Propranolol	40–240	Bradycardia, syncope, fatigue, and erectile dysfunction (most common)
		Caution in patients with asthma, diabetes mellitus or chronic obstructive pulmonary disease
Primidone	62.5–750	Initial acute toxic reaction (~23%), sedation, daytime sleepiness, tiredness, nausea, ataxia, dizziness, and confusion
Topiramate	>200	Weight loss, paresthesias, trouble concentrating, and memory disturbance, increased risk of kidney stones
Alprazolam	0.75–1.5	Sedation, risk of dependence, cognitive dysfunction
Gabapentin	300–3600	Drowsiness, dizziness, loss of coordination, tiredness, fatigue, decreased libido
Zonisamide*	100–225	Headache, nausea, fatigue/sleepiness, diarrhea

* with the exception of zonisamide, the evidence is for upper limb tremor

** Studied in isolated head tremor, at the time classified as a form of ET

parkinsonian tremor is a 4–6 Hz resting tremor that re-emerges with maintained posture.[58] Action tremors are also well recognized in PD and can present isolated or combined with a resting tremor[59] in as much as 92% of cases with PD with tremor.[60] The systematic evaluation of the tremor phenomenology is important, as a resting tremor is likely more bothersome, and an action tremor may lead to significant disability. Most of the studies conducted in PD report the effect of several medications on tremor without a distinction of types of tremor.[61,62]

The approach of treatment of parkinsonian tremor follows the general treatment principles of PD.

Levodopa/carbidopa, the gold standard dopaminergic treatment for PD, is associated with a significant improvement in resting tremor in about 50% of patients.[63,64] Dopamine agonists such as pramipexole and pergolide have demonstrated their efficacy in reducing resting and action parkinsonian tremor,[65–68] even in cases of severe tremor refractory to a stable anti-parkinsonian medications that included levodopa in most of the cases.[68]

Beta-blockers such as propranolol and nadolol have been assessed explicitly for treating tremor in PD,[69–71] with a reported improvement in the action and resting components of PD tremor. A Cochrane review concluded that there was insufficient evidence to determine the efficacy and safety of propranolol or oxprenolol,[69] mainly due to methodological issues. In clinical practice, β-blockers such as propranolol or nadolol can be considered in PD patients with tremor.

Anticholinergic medications were the first symptomatic treatment of PD, namely for tremors. In a Cochrane review, a specific anti-tremor effect was not established in nine double-blind crossover RCTs of various anticholinergic interventions[72] that did not include trihexyphenidyl or benztropine. Nevertheless, the clinical usefulness of anticholinergic medication is limited by tolerability issues, namely those secondary to neuropsychiatric side effects of sedation, confusion, hallucinations, and blurred vision,[72] especially in the aged PD population. Anticholinergic medications may still be considered in young PD patients with a clinically significant tremor.

Other medications like clozapine[73,74] and amantadine[75,76] have shown an improvement of parkinsonian tremor. While amantadine may be less effective than dopaminergic treatments,[75,76] clozapine may play a role in treating refractory severe resting and action PD tremor. The requirement of monitoring white blood cell count weekly at the onset due to the risk of agranulocytosis (0.4 to 1–2%) makes clozapine one of the last choices in the pharmacological armamentarium for parkinsonian tremor.

Orthostatic tremor

Orthostatic tremor (OT) is a rare tremor syndrome characterized by 13–18 Hz low-amplitude tremor, documented by surface EMG in the lower extremities on standing, that can extend to involve trunk and arms.[1,77] The diagnosis of OT can be delayed for many years.[78] Patients complain of leg tremors and unsteadiness on standing with a fear of falling, although falls are rare.[78] Other than a hand tremor, patients can sometimes have additional neurological features like mild to moderate axial and appendicular ataxia and parkinsonism, leading to a subgroup classification of "OT plus."[78]

A very low level of evidence supports the pharmacological treatment of OT. Various medications have been empirically used for the treatment of OT and include clonazepam, gabapentin, primidone, propranolol, valproic acid, phenobarbital, topiramate, pregabalin, carbamazepine, acetazolamide, mirtazapine, and dopaminergic drugs.[78–81] Overall, the clinical benefit is variable, and these options can be used as monotherapy and more commonly combined using a trial-and-error approach. There are a small number of RCTs that evaluated gabapentin,[82,83] and levetiracetam.[84]

The most widely used medication for the treatment of OT is clonazepam, followed by gabapentin.[85] The degree of clinical response is variable[78–81] and can decline with time.[80] In a series of 124 patients with OT, 57.5% had a mild benefit, and 15.3% had marked benefit[80] with clonazepam. Sedation is a main dose-limiting side effect and may lead to discontinuation.[79] The co-existence of parkinsonism in some OT cases leads to the consideration of dopaminergic therapy in OT. As with other interventions, the evidence is low, and the reported clinical benefit is not consistent.[80,81,86–89]

BOTULINUM TOXIN FOR THE TREATMENT OF TREMORS

Botulinum toxin (BoNT) is an exotoxin produced by the anaerobic bacterium *Clostridium perfringens*. BoNT acts pre-synaptically in the neuromuscular junction by inhibiting the release of acetylcholine from motor cholinergic nerve terminals. BoNT binds to high-affinity recognition protein and prevents the release of acetylcholine by inhibiting the fusion of synaptic vesicles.[90] The muscle paralysis can lead to dampening the peripheral oscillations at the muscle level, affecting the reciprocal inhibition at spinal cord level,

and centrally by altering the excitability of cortical motor areas.[91,92] There are eight serotypes (A–H), and serotypes A and B have therapeutic use.[90] Three BoNT-A products are commonly available (onabotulinumtoxinA/ Botox®, abobotulinumtoxinA/ Dysport®, and incobotulinumtoxinA/ Xeomin®), and rimabotulinumtoxinB/ Myobloc® is the only BoNT-B available.

The most common indications of BoNT are the various forms of focal dystonia, including dystonic tremor (DT) syndromes. Other indications explored for BoNT include ET, multiple sclerosis (MS)–related tremor, and parkinsonian tremor.

Dystonic tremor

DT is defined as a postural/kinetic tremor occurring in the body region that has dystonia.[1] The most common form of DT is head tremor in association with cervical dystonia.[93] Other forms of DT include primary writing tremor (PWT), in which tremor consistently occurs during the task of writing, and tremulous spasmodic dysphonia.

BoNT is the mainstay option for DT. There are no controlled trials to support the use of any pharmacological agent for DT, including medications such as trihexyphenidyl, tetrabenazine, or benzodiazepines.[94] BoNT-A was evaluated in a total of 330 patients with PWT, head tremor, tremulous spasmodic dysphonia, or task-specific jaw tremor.[94] Overall, BoNT was more effective than pharmacological therapy.[94]

Essential tremor

BoNT has been explored for the treatment of hand tremor in ET since the 1990s with case series reports.[95,96] The initial placebo-RCTs[97,98] evaluated the efficacy and safety of EMG-guided BoNT-A for hand tremors in ET and reported an improvement in limb tremor. The associated dose-dependent limb weakness in 30–100% of participants and variable functional impact has precluded a wide clinical use.[97,98]

A recent RCT evaluated the use of a customized approach to BoNT-A injections based on clinical observation and EMG data with findings of less frequent forearm weakness (18%) and a significant anti-tremor effect.[99] Sensor-based kinematic analysis has also been used for customization of injections.[100] An open-label trial reported a consistent significant improvement in tremor severity and functional ability after 6 treatment cycles.[101] The discontinuation rate due to limb weakness was 8%.[101] These new techniques are promising but need more evidence to establish utility in the treatment of ET hand tremor. As a general rule, BoNT is not routinely used for the treatment of hand tremor in ET.

Isolated head tremor

There is a lack of evidence from well-designed RCTs to evaluate the effect of BoNT in isolated head tremor. In a small double-blind crossover RCT with ten patients, 100 IU of BoNT-A was associated with a significant clinical improvement compared with placebo without safety concerns.[102]

Parkinsonian tremor

The therapeutic evaluation of BoNT for parkinsonian tremor is minimal and is not used in clinical practice. Similar to ET, customized BoNT-A injection approach based on EMG data[99] or kinematic analysis[103] was evaluated in PD tremor with reports of significant clinical improvement and variable occurrence of hand weakness ranging from 4%[104] to 36%.[103] Older studies have reported less robust efficacy results.[105,106]

Palatal and vocal tremors

Palatal tremor (PT) is a rare disorder and is subdivided into two general categories: "essential" or idiopathic PT and secondary or acquired PT.[107] A common treatment for PT is the administration of BoNT in palate muscles such as the tensor veli palatini or salpingopharyngeus muscles, despite an extremely low level of evidence[108] based on case reports and small case series. The clinical benefit may last for months to almost two years.[108] Associated side effects include transient dysphagia, trans-nasal regurgitation, changes in speech, and aural fullness.

Recently, idiopathic PT has been recognized in the spectrum of functional movement disorder,[109] which widens the therapeutic approaches of PT to include cognitive behavioral therapy, education, management of comorbid psychiatric issues (see Treatment of functional tremors, later in this chapter).

Vocal tremor

Vocal tremor can be found in various neurological disorders with a high prevalence in ET, spasmodic dysphonia, and, to some extent, in PD. Vocal tremor has a significant impact on the life of patients.[110] The management of the tremor depends on the underlying disease. BoNT is the mainstay of treatment for patients with spasmodic dysphonia and medication-refractory vocal tremor in ET. The injections of BoNT are performed under EMG guidance, and the muscles targeted are determined by the characteristics of the tremor. A systematic review of 13 studies evaluating BoNT-A injection in spasmodic adductor dysphonia reported a clinical improvement with a positive impact on quality of life.[111] Non-controlled studies have reported benefit with tremor reduction in vocal tremors for ET[112-114] with lesser clinical benefit than in spasmodic dysphonia.[113]

Multiple sclerosis–related tremor

The prevalence of tremor in MS varies from 25% to 60%.[115-117] MS-related tremor is usually a postural and kinetic tremor and most frequently affects the arms, but may also involve the head, voice, and trunk. There is a lack of controlled studies, and most of the data is from observational series reporting variable results on upper limb tremor reduction with various pharmacological agents.[118] Overall, isoniazid is the most common pharmacologic agent investigated and demonstrated benefit in approximately 60% to 80% of patients.[118] BoNT-A was evaluated in one crossover placebo-RCT that reported significant improvement in tremor severity associated with reversible weakness in around 42% of the cases.[115]

SURGICAL THERAPIES FOR TREMOR

A tremor that is refractory to medical treatment can be generally considered for surgical therapy. As with pharmacological therapies, ET has the most clinical evidence. The surgical treatment of tremor includes lesional surgery and DBS. Radiofrequency thalamotomy, gamma knife (GK®) thalamotomy, and magnetic resonance-guided focused ultrasound (MRgFUS) have been considered to induce therapeutic brain lesioning for tremors. For DBS, the nucleus ventralis intermedius (VIM) thalamic DBS has been classically used. Other targets evaluated and/or used clinically for tremor suppression include the posterior subthalamic area (PSA), zona incerta (ZI), and the ventralis oralis anterior (VoA)/ventralis oralis posterior (VOP) nuclei of the thalamus, as well as the globus pallidus *pars interna* (GPi) and the subthalamic nucleus (STN). The selection of the target depends on the underlying condition. The use of surgical therapies for tremor requires a center of excellence with multidisciplinary teams to ensure an appropriate patient selection, accurate neurosurgical procedures, and appropriate care during follow-up.

Deep brain stimulation

After the first description in the 1980s, DBS has become the preferred surgical treatment for tremors because of less potential of permanent adverse effects, better functional outcome, and the possibility of bilateral treatment.[119,120]

Essential tremor: The most common target for ET is unilateral or bilateral VIM. The VIM nucleus corresponds to the posterior ventrolateral (VL) part of the thalamus and relays contralateral cerebellar inputs to the thalamus and ultimately to the primary motor cortex (Brodmann's area 4) and premotor cortex.[121]

In clinical practice, patients with ET who have tried a maximally tolerated dose of first-line pharmacological interventions (at least two) without satisfactory suppression of tremor and with no significant comorbidities like severe cardiac or respiratory issues can be considered for DBS.

There is a single RCT comparing unilateral VIM-DBS and unilateral thalamotomy in 13 patients. In this study, there was a greater improvement in the functional activity score (Frenchay Activities Index) with VIM-DBS compared with thalamotomy.[122] Additionally, the thalamotomy group experienced more adverse events than the DBS group. Evidence of improvement in clinical rating scales of tremor severity and on task performance was found in the blinded comparison of ON and OFF stimulation conditions in case series.[123–127] A more vertically placed electrode may greatly improve head tremor.[128] Although bilateral VIM-DBS is used in clinical practice, there are few studies comparing unilateral and bilateral procedures. Bilateral VIM-DBS is associated with greater improvement in the severity of arm and leg tremor and midline tremors such as neck or head compared with unilateral VIM-DBS.[129] Nevertheless, unilateral VIM-DBS may be associated with an ipsilateral limb tremor improvement of lesser magnitude than with bilateral VIM-DBS.[130] Long-term studies of VIM-DBS show a consistent tremor suppression[126–128,132–137] for 7–10 years[127,131] with overall patient satisfaction[138] and improved quality of life.[137] The most common side effect of VIM-DBS is transient stimulation-induced paresthesia. More disabling side effects include gait ataxia and dysarthria that are more common with bilateral VIM-DBS.[129,139,140] Current DBS devices allow for utilization of predefined stimulation groups that may provide a better

tremor control or better tolerability according to the patient's lifestyle needs.

A gradual loss of efficacy with time is found in 0%[131]–73%[141] of the cases after VIM-DBS for ET,[142,143] as early as ten weeks[144] and up to ten years.[145] A comprehensive evaluation of different factors is fundamental to address this loss of efficacy with VIM-DBS clinically. The related mechanisms have not been fully established and can be the result of a combination of disease-related factors (tremor etiology and progression); surgery-related factors (sub-optimal electrode location, microlesional effect, and placebo effect); and stimulation-related factors (sub-optimal stimulation, stimulation-induced side effects, habituation, and tremor rebound).[146–148]

Other targets evaluated for neurostimulation include the PSA and its structures located ventrally to the thalamus or other nuclei of the thalamus like the VoA[14] or the centromedian nucleus,[150] a part of the intralaminar nucleus of the thalamus. The STN was also evaluated as a target for DBS in ET with lesser efficacy than other targets like the VIM[151] or ZI.[152]

From an anatomic perspective, the PSA is a region that includes the nucleus of the ZI and the white fiber tracts of the prelemniscal radiations.[153] The ZI serves as a hub for basal ganglia circuitry, thalamocortical, and cerebellar-thalamocortical circuits.[154] The prelemniscal radiations include the pallido-thalamic tract and the dentate-rubro-thalamic tract, which has been evaluated for the treatment of tremor.[155–158]

The PSA and the ZI have received the most attention as alternative targets. The observation that, in patients undergoing VIM-DBS, more ventral contacts could be more effective for tremor suppression[159] hinted at the exploration of PSA as a suitable neurostimulation target in ET and other tremor syndromes. Overall, case series with PSA-DBS have shown consistent improvement in limb[160–162] and voice tremor,[163] up to 6 years of follow-up.[162] A single randomized controlled study comparing PSA and VIM-DBS[164] showed that PSA-DBS is not significantly different from VIM-DBS for tremor suppression up to 12 months of follow-up. Still, a similar clinical benefit in PSA-DBS can be achieved with a lower amplitude of stimulation. The side effect profile of PSA-DBS is similar to VIM-DBS: mainly gait ataxia and speech changes (decreased articulation rate, and voicing).[164,165]

Neurostimulation of ZI consistently suppresses limb tremor[166–168] up to 3–5 years[169] in the absence of tolerance.[166,169] Like PSA, ZI-DBS achieves similar tremor suppression to VIM-DBS with less energy of stimulation,[152] although VIM-DBS may be associated with better outcomes in the long term.[170] ZI-DBS may provide incremental tremor suppression as a rescue procedure for those patients that failed VIM-DBS.[171] In terms of safety, ZI-DBS is associated with a lower complication rate[166] than VIM-DBS, though loss of verbal fluency, either transient or persistent, has been specifically reported for ZI-DBS,[172] as well as stimulation-induced visual phenomena when compared with VIM-DBS.[173,174] There is no RCT comparing ZI-DBS with VIM-DBS for ET.

Other tremor conditions

Neurostimulation has been used for various tremor conditions other than ET using similar targets (see Table 19.4). Examples include parkinsonian tremor, MS-related tremor, OT, DT, PWT, Fragile-X Tremor Ataxia syndrome (FXTAS), neuropathic tremor, and Holmes tremor, among others. More frequently, these tremor syndromes are refractory to pharmacotherapy. Overall, the evidence available is limited to case reports and series. To approach these cases, the accurate identification of movement disorders phenomenology is critical to establish a more appropriate target and identify the co-existence of features such as ataxia that may worsen after thalamic DBS and lead to suboptimal outcomes even with a clinically significant tremor suppression. Also, weighing the expected progression of various clinical features of a tremor syndrome is paramount to establish the overall clinical impact of DBS. For example, the diagnosis of DT would favor the indication for GPi-DBS as an initial target to address the underlying dystonia. In FXTAS, while an initial unilateral VIM-DBS may be considered safer,[175] VIM-DBS is generally associated with either no benefit or worsening of ataxia and balance. Alternate targeting of the VOP and ZI[176] or the PSA[177] have been evaluated in FXTAS with robust tremor suppression and potentially improvement of ataxia.[176]

Dual targeting approaches have been contemplated with lead implantation in different thalamic nuclei for MS-related tremor[178] and post-traumatic Holmes tremor,[179] or with thalamic and pallidal stimulation for secondary tremors of mixed etiologies.[180] In MS-related tremor, an RCT documented that dual-lead thalamic DBS with VIM and VOP location provided greater limb tremor suppression than a single-target approach.[178]

Lesional therapy

Lesional therapy in the form of radiofrequency thermocoagulation of the VIM nucleus of thalamus[181–184] was the main surgical modality for tremor treatment in the mid-twentieth century. With the advent of DBS, lesional therapies became largely secondary due to the lesser clinical utility of unilateral intervention compared with the bilateral treatment option with DBS. Lesional therapies have had a resurgence in the last decades with the emergence of minimally invasive ablation techniques such as radiosurgery (GK*) and, more recently, MRgFUS. These approaches are more appropriate for those with an high surgical risk that precludes DBS, but patient preference and accessibility to treatments are also relevant.

Gamma Knife thalamotomy: GK* uses the convergence of multiple beams of low-dose ionizing radiation onto one defined target point, inducing radio-necrosis. The main limitation of GK* is the possible risk of delayed spread of lesioning which can present with undesirable side effects with high variability in severity, months to years after the procedure.[185] There is no controlled trial, and evidence is supported by case series of reference centers, rarely with blinded assessments. Unilateral GK* VIM thalamotomy has been associated with a significant tremor reduction in as much as 80% of PD patients[185,186] but with latency for clinical benefit of 2–3 months. In ET patients, unilateral GK* VIM thalamotomy has been reported to have a sustained clinical benefit in as much as 88% of patients after four years or more.[187] Another case series with blinded clinical assessments reported a more modest clinical improvement in ET and PD tremor, with delayed neurological side effects in 3 out of 18 patients.[188]

MRI-guided focused ultrasound (MRgFUS) thalamotomy: The MRgFUS procedure delivers a high-intensity ultrasound without craniotomy, producing a controlled lesion in real time through heating in the planned target. MRgFUS has been mostly assessed for tremor reduction in ET with unilateral ablation of the VIM thalamic nucleus. Due to the real-time monitoring of ultrasound delivery, MRgFUS can maximize the benefit of tremor reduction and mitigate the risk of adverse events. For this reason, MRgFUS thalamotomy has generated interest for clinical practice.

Unilateral MRgFUS has shown significant improvement in contralateral limb tremor in ET in both open-label[189,190] and RCTs with sham stimulation,[191] with a positive impact on quality of life

TABLE 19.4: ANATOMICAL TARGETS USED FOR NEUROSTIMULATION IN A SELECTION OF TREMOR SYNDROMES

Tremor syndrome	Target	Type of studies	Comments
Essential tremor	VIM	RCT (most unilateral VIM)	53–63% improvement (unilateral VIM-DBS) vs. 66–78% % improvement (bilateral VIM-DBS) in FTS score[251] Bilateral VIM-DBS: more frequent side effects[129,139,140]
	PSA	RCT	PSA-DBS vs. VIM-DBS PSA: similar tremor improvement, lower stimulation amplitudes for PSA-DBS[164]
	ZI	Retrospective case series	Conflicting results[166–169]
	VIM + VOA	Case series	16.7% improvement compared with either lead in isolation for refractory ET tremor[149]
Dystonic tremor	VIM	Case reports and series	Reports in PWT (85.2%–100% tremor reduction) and other forms of arm DT[94]
	Gpi	Case reports and series	Reduction in arm and head tremor severity[94]
	ZI	Case reports	Improvement of DT in generalized dystonia[9]
	VLp	Case series	Improvement of arm DT[94]
Orthostatic tremor	VIM	Case reports and case series	Tremor amplitude reduction or increased latency to symptom onset after standing in 83.3%[252–254] Most patients experienced a mild/moderate waning of tremor improvement over time
	ZI	Case series	Improvement in symptoms but conflicting results on onset, frequent changes in stimulation settings to maintain benefit[255,256]
	Spinal cord stimulation	Case series	Symptoms of unsteadiness and objective measures on electrophysiology demonstrated improvement[257,258]
Multiple sclerosis–associated tremor	VIM	Case reports and case series	Symptoms improved in 83.6% Transient response in 13.7%[252]
	VIM + (STN, VOP, pre-lemniscal radiations)	Case reports and case series	Improvement of all tremor components most of treated patients[252]
	ZI	Case reports and case series	
	ZI + VOP	Case reports and case series	Improvement in most of treated patients[252]
	VL	Case reports and case series	Improvement reported in all cases but short-term results available (<12 months)[252]
	VL + STN	Case reports	Improvement in all cases[252]

FTS = Fahn-Tolosa-Marin scale; VIM = ventralis intermedius nuclei of the thalamus; RCT = randomized controlled trial; ZI = zona incerta; VL = ventrolateral thalamic nucleus; Gpi = internal globus pallidus; VOP = ventralis oralis posterior; VOA = ventralis oralis anterior; PSA = posterior subthalamic area; PWT = primary writing tremor; STN = subthalamic nucleus; VLp = posterior part of the ventrolateral thalamus.

and disability.[191] In the latter study,[191] MRgFUS was associated with a 47% improvement of the severity of arm tremor at three months, with a between-group difference from the sham arm of 8.3 points in the Clinical Rating Scale for Tremor (CRST), together with improvement in function and quality of life. The improvement in the MRgFUS group was maintained at 12 months. A more recent meta-analysis of nine studies in a total of 160 ET patients, evaluating for the most part the VIM nucleus but also the cerebellothalamic tract as targets,[192] estimated that the pooled percentage improvements in the total CRST, CRST sections A and C, and Quality of Life in Essential **Tremor** Questionnaire QUEST scores were 62.2%, 62.4%, 69.1%, and 46.5%, respectively.[193] In terms of safety, while the procedure is generally well tolerated, MRgFUS unilateral thalamotomy is associated with side effects such as ataxia and paresthesia. Overall, ataxia is the most common complication (29.7%) at three months but tends to improve at 12 months.[194] Still, gait ataxia and limb incoordination may persist in a small but notable percentage of cases. Consequently, patients who have prior balance dysfunction may not be the optimal candidates for MRgFUS.

Long-term prospective studies document a clinical benefit after unilateral MRgFUS VIM thalamotomy up to 4–5 years.[195–197] A multi-center open-label extension prospective study documented a sustained improvement in the hand tremor score up to 2 years, together with improvement in postural tremor, disability, and quality of life. There were no delayed neurological complications.[195]

Alternative targeting such as unilateral MRgFUS of the cerebellothalamic tract was also evaluated in ET with encouraging results.[192] Unilateral MRgFUS VIM thalamotomy has been evaluated for tremor-predominant PD [198] with improvement in medication-refractory tremor[199] in patients with DT,[200] FXTAS,[201] and MS-related tremor.[202]

NON-INVASIVE BRAIN STIMULATION

Non-invasive brain stimulation techniques such as repetitive transcranial magnetic stimulation (rTMS) or transcranial current stimulation (tCS) have been explored for their therapeutic potential.

rTMS applied at varying frequencies and locations might be used to modulate a network and render a symptomatic effect. Low-frequency (1 Hz or less) repetitive stimulation of the motor cortex is thought to be inhibitory, whereas high-frequency stimulation (5 Hz and above) is thought to be excitatory to motor circuits.[203] Non-controlled studies of rTMS applied over the cerebellum area demonstrated variable efficacy in terms of tremor control.[204,205] rTMS to the pre-supplementary motor area has been tested in a sham-controlled pilot study with no significant difference in the improvement in the tremor rating scales between the rTMS and sham interventions.[206] Because rTMS can cause some local discomfort to the posterior head and neck musculature, other electrical stimulation modalities in the form of transcranial direct current (tDCS) have been explored. Experimental paradigms using tDCS have not shown consistent results.[207,208]

OTHER NON-PHARMACOLOGICAL TREATMENT APPROACHES FOR COMMON TREMORS

Different strategies have been evaluated in occupational and physical therapy to reduce the functional impairment of tremor. Neuromuscular physiotherapy, strength training, weighted splints or cuffs,[209–211] forearm cooling,[212] and adaptive equipment and tools are examples.[213]

The use of a weight in the distal extremity has been more extensively evaluated. It may benefit MS-related tremor and other non-progressive cerebellar tremors more than parkinsonian tremor, however, and be less impactful for feeding tasks.[213] Limb cooling is considered too uncomfortable and inconvenient for long-term management. Some authors propose its use for specific tasks. Localized and whole-body vibration have been evaluated in MS-related tremor and parkinsonian tremor.[214–216]

Adaptive equipment and tools can be broadly categorized into exoskeletons (wearable mechatronic systems, in which the physical interface provides a direct transfer of mechanical power and some exchange of information), orthoses (an externally applied device that modifies tremor), and handheld external devices (e.g., spoons or gloves).[217] Adaptive equipment and tools have been used in various tremor etiologies. For example, a handheld orthotic device was evaluated in PWT.[209] A dental splint may be helpful in jaw DT, likely acting as a sensory trick.[218] Exoskeleton systems were evaluated in cerebellar tremor[210] and ET,[211] but development is hampered by cost and the bulkiness of the devices. A non-invasive handheld device in the form of a spoon using Active Cancellation of Tremor was evaluated in patients with ET for three tasks, with an improvement of tremor amplitude.[219] Overall, the level of evidence regarding the efficacy of such devices remains low.

Electrical muscle stimulation therapy administered in a glove has been evaluated for intractable resting tremor in PD. An acute short-lived reduction in tremor amplitude was hypothesized to be associated with the modulation of peripheral reflex mechanisms by electrical muscle stimulation.[220] A wrist-worn peripheral nerve stimulation device (Cala Trio™) was also evaluated in patients with ET, with transient relief of upper limb tremor.[221] Transcutaneous electrical nerve stimulation was used in patients with arm DT[222] and PWT,[223] and is generally discouraged.

TREATMENT OF FUNCTIONAL TREMORS

Functional movement disorders (FMDs) are prevalent, and tremors are the most common functional movement disorders.[224] Overall, FMDs negatively impact patient quality of life even in the absence of psychiatric comorbidities,[225] making adequate treatment paramount.

The therapeutic approach to functional tremor (and FMDs in general) entails a multidisciplinary strategy. The first step is diagnosis based on history and examination findings with particular emphasis on certain phenomenological features.[224] The presence of characteristic phenomenology supports a diagnosis that does not require an exhaustive exclusion of other disorders.[226] Signs of a functional tremor include distractibility, entrainment, variability, tonic coactivation of antagonistic muscles at tremor onset, and the "whack-a-mole" sign.[227] Some of these signs can be further documented by electrophysiological studies available in a few specialized centers.[228] The demonstration of signs of a functional etiology to the patient can play an important role in helping the patient understand the nature of the tremors and, by showing reversibility, provides hope to patients that the tremors can be treated.[229] One important step is explaining the diagnosis to help the patient understand the presenting symptoms and create a patient–physician therapeutic relationship. The patient should be assured that the disorder is real and is experienced by a significant number of people.[230] The potential of recovery should be emphasized during the clinic visit, and follow-up is important to ensure patient's understanding of functional symptoms and preparedness for treatment.[229]

It is important to avoid common errors in the management of FMDs. These include failure to give an explicit diagnosis[229] or not demonstrating physical signs that can be shown to the patient. This form of demonstration helps the patient to understand that the diagnosis is made based on positive signs and not just because the tests are normal. It is common for patients with functional movement disorders to have the "jumping to conclusions" bias, meaning they require less information to make a decision.[231]

A functional tremor diagnosis will be successful if a patient recognizes the clinical presentation, feels that disability was validated, understands the multidisciplinary management, and trusts the treating neurologist with the management plan.[232] It is fundamental for patients to have confidence in the diagnosis, avoiding the unnecessary consumption of medical resources in seeking an alternative diagnosis.[232]

There is limited data on the outcome of functional tremors.[233,234] Negative predictors include long duration of symptoms before diagnosis and personality disorders.[234] Good physical health, positive social life, patients' perception of effective treatment by the physician, elimination of stressors, young age, and early diagnosis have been found to have favorable effects on the long-term outcome.[235] A broader recognition of FMD with an earlier diagnosis and improved access to treatment may contribute to more consistent favorable outcomes.

Isolated interventions evaluated for functional tremors include motor rehabilitation with physiotherapy,[236] motor retraining, cognitive behavioral therapy,[237] and rTMS with standardized suggestion of benefit.[238] Few studies are available in existing literature, and rarely have these interventions been assessed specifically for functional tremors.[237]

The organization of multispecialty approaches has been evaluated using inpatient and outpatient models[239,240] that usually include a neurologist, a psychiatrist, and a physiotherapist. In a comprehensive multidisciplinary clinic, a patient is seen sequentially by the different healthcare professionals, and a management plan is delivered by consensus among team members.[240] An integrated approach has been evaluated in which the neurologist, neuropsychiatrist, and physiotherapist work together in a single medical visit to deliver an individualized treatment plan.[239] These programs have shown good compliance and a positive impact. Overall, the evidence is low and corresponds to case series or small feasibility studies. The effect of these approaches needs to be tested in more robust studies with adequate controls.

CONCLUSIONS AND FUTURE DIRECTIONS

The current treatment modalities for tremors are limited and frequently discouraging. The evidence available for the various therapeutic options covered in this chapter corresponds to a great extent to ET studies and limb tremor. Novel pharmacological interventions being tested in ET include the positive allosteric modulator of GABA-A receptors (SAGE-324, NCT04305275) and SK channels (small conductance, calcium-activated potassium ion channels, CAD-1883, NCT03688685), selective modulator of T-Type calcium channel (CX-8998, NCT03101241), and non-competitive antagonism of AMPA receptors (perampanel). Among these interventions, perampanel was recently evaluated in a small crossover placebo-RCT,[241] with documentation of a significant improvement in performance tasks using blinded video ratings, but without an impact on quality of life. Further, controlled studies with a larger sample size would be required to prove the efficacy of perampanel in the treatment of ET.

New technological advances with innovative lead design and stimulation paradigms have been evaluated to improve efficacy outcome and minimize side effects of DBS.[242,243] Novel energy delivery paradigms have been introduced and are being evaluated. One of them is constant current stimulation. Studies have demonstrated similar tremor reduction with constant current DBS and possibly a wider therapeutic window.[244,245] Square biphasic pulse stimulation, used unilaterally for three hours, showed better or similar tremor control as compared to the conventional stimulation parameters, with no side effects.[246] As mentioned earlier, tolerance to clinical effect is one of the challenges of DBS over time. Beyond the current practice of turning off the stimulator during sleep, a revolutionary change may be delivered using a closed-loop DBS for an on-demand adaptive stimulation.[247] Although there are no studies in patients with ET, the results of studies in PD[248,249] suggest that the technique is feasible and safe and may also help deal with issues of tolerance, as it may decrease the time of stimulation.

One of the greatest gaps in knowledge in the field of ET is a more complete understanding of the pathogenesis of ET. ET is currently considered a clinical syndrome with foreseen heterogeneity.[1] A better understanding of common tremor syndromes and accessibility of diagnostic biomarkers in therapeutic development and clinical practice may open the field to individualized medicine with a higher yield of therapeutic success.

REFERENCES

1. Bhatia KP, Bain P, Bajaj N, et al. Consensus statement on the classification of tremors: from the Task Force on Tremor of the International Parkinson and Movement Disorder Society. *Mov Disord.* 2018;33(1):75–87.
2. Louis ED, Ferreira JJ. How common is the most common adult movement disorder? Update on the worldwide prevalence of essential tremor. *Mov Disord.* 2010;25(5):534–541.
3. Louis ED, Barnes L, Albert SM, et al. Correlates of functional disability in essential tremor. *Mov Disord.* 2001;16(5):914–920.
4. Louis ED, Machado DG. Tremor-related quality of life: a comparison of essential tremor vs. Parkinson's disease patients. *Parkinsonism Relat Disord.* 2015;21(7):729–735.
5. Bain PG, Findley LJ, Thompson PD, et al. A study of hereditary essential tremor. Brain. 1994;117(Pt 4):805–824.
6. Smeltere L, Kuzņecovs V, Erts R. Depression and social phobia in essential tremor and Parkinson's disease. *Brain Behav.* 2017;7(9):e00781.
7. Ferreira JJ, Mestre TA, Lyons KE, et al. MDS evidence-based review of treatments for essential tremor. *Mov Disord.* 2019;34(7):950–958.
8. Diaz NL, Louis ED. Survey of medication usage patterns among essential tremor patients: movement disorder specialists vs. general neurologists. *Parkinsonism Relat Disord.* 2010;16(9):604–607.
9. Owen DA, Marsden CD. Effect of adrenergic beta-blockade on parkinsonian tremor. *Lancet (Lond).* 1965;2(7425):1259–1262.
10. Koller WC. Long-acting propranolol in essential tremor. *Neurology.* 1985;35(1):108–110.
11. Cleeves L, Findley LJ. Propranolol and propranolol-LA in essential tremor: a double blind comparative study. *J Neurol Neurosurg Psychiatry.* 1988;51(3):379–384.
12. Dupont E, Hansen HJ, Dalby MA. Treatment of benign essential tremor with propranolol. A controlled clinical trial. *Acta Neurol Scand.* 1973;49(1):75–84.
13. Tolosa ES, Loewenson RB. Essential tremor: treatment with propranolol. *Neurology.* 1975;25(11):1041–1044.
14. Jefferson D, Jenner P, Marsden CD. Relationship between plasma propranolol levels and the clinical suppression of essential tremor [proceedings]. *Br J Clin Pharmacol.* 1979;7(4):419P–420P.
15. Baruzzi A, Procaccianti G, Martinelli P, et al. Phenobarbital and propranolol in essential tremor: a double-blind controlled clinical trial. *Neurology.* 1983;33(3):296–300.
16. Koller WC, Biary N. Metoprolol compared with propranolol in the treatment of essential tremor. *Arch Neurol.* 1984;41(2):171–172.
17. Gorman WP, Cooper R, Pocock P, Campbell MJ. A comparison of primidone, propranolol, and placebo in essential tremor, using quantitative analysis. *J Neurol Neurosurg Psychiatry.* 1986;49(1):64–68.
18. Yetimalar Y, Irtman G, Kurt T, Başoğlu M. Olanzapine versus propranolol in essential tremor. *Clin Neurol Neurosurg.* 2005;108(1):32–35.

19. Gironell A, Kulisevsky J, Barbanoj M, López-Villegas D, Hernández G, Pascual-Sedano B. A randomized placebo-controlled comparative trial of gabapentin and propranolol in essential tremor. *Arch Neurol.* 1999;56(4):475–480.

20. Mally J, Stone TW. Efficacy of an adenosine antagonist, theophylline, in essential tremor: comparison with placebo and propranolol. *J Neurol Sci.* 1995;132(2):129–132.

21. Koller W, Biary N, Cone S. Disability in essential tremor: effect of treatment. *Neurology.* 1986;36(7):1001–1004.

22. Koller WC, Vetere-Overfield B. Acute and chronic effects of propranolol and primidone in essential tremor. *Neurology.* 1989;39(12):1587–1588.

23. Pozzi R. True and presumed contraindications of beta blockers. Peripheral vascular disease, diabetes mellitus, chronic bronchopneumopathy. *Ital Heart J Suppl.* 2000;1(8):1031–1037.

24. Larsen TA, Teräväinen H, Calne DB. Atenolol vs. propranolol in essential tremor. A controlled, quantitative study. *Acta Neurol Scand.* 1982;66(5):547–554.

25. Koller WC. Nadolol in essential tremor. *Neurology.* 1983;33(8):1076.

26. Hod H, Har-Zahav J, Kaplinsky N. Pindolol-induced tremor. *Postgrad Med J.* 1980;56:346–347.

27. Koller W, Orebaugh C, Lawson L, Potempa K. Pindolol-induced tremor. *Clin Neuropharmacol.* 1987;10(5):449–452.

28. Koller WC, Royse VL. Efficacy of primidone in essential tremor. *Neurology.* 1986;36(1):121–124.

29. Findley LJ, Calzetti S. Double-blind controlled study of primidone in essential tremor: preliminary results. *Br Med J (Clin Res Ed).* 1982;285(6342):608.

30. Findley LJ, Cleeves L, Calzetti S. Primidone in essential tremor of the hands and head: a double blind controlled clinical study. *J Neurol Neurosurg Psychiatry.* 1985;48(9):911–915.

31. Sasso E, Perucca E, Calzetti S. Double-blind comparison of primidone and phenobarbital in essential tremor. *Neurology.* 1988;38(5):808–810.

32. Findley LJ, Calzetti S, Richens A. Benign familial tremor treated with primidone. *Br Med J (Clin Res Ed).* 1981;283(6285):234. doi: 10.1136/bmj.283.6285.234-b

33. O'Suilleabhain P, Dewey RB. Randomized trial comparing primidone initiation schedules for treating essential tremor. *Mov Disord.* 2002;17(2):382–386.

34. Serrano-Dueñas M. Use of primidone in low doses (250 mg/day) versus high doses (750 mg/day) in the management of essential tremor. Double-blind comparative study with one-year follow-up. *Parkinsonism Relat Disord.* 2003;10(1):29–33.

35. Shank RP, Doose DR, Streeter AJ, Bialer M. Plasma and whole blood pharmacokinetics of topiramate: the role of carbonic anhydrase. *Epilepsy Res.* 2005;63(2–3):103–112.

36. Louis ED. A new twist for stopping the shakes? Revisiting GABAergic therapy for essential tremor. *Arch Neurol.* 1999;56(7):807–808.

37. Connor GS. A double-blind placebo-controlled trial of topiramate treatment for essential tremor. *Neurology.* 2002;59(1):132–134.

38. Connor GS, Edwards K, Tarsy D. Topiramate in essential tremor: findings from double-blind, placebo-controlled, crossover trials. *Clin Neuropharmacol.* 2008;31(2):97–103.

39. Frima N, Grünewald RA. A double-blind, placebo-controlled, crossover trial of topiramate in essential tremor. *Clin Neuropharmacol.* 2006;29(2):94–96.

40. Ondo WG, Jankovic J, Connor GS, et al. Topiramate in essential tremor: a double-blind, placebo-controlled trial. *Neurology.* 2006;66(5):672–677.

41. Bruno E, Nicoletti A, Quattrocchi G, et al. Topiramate for essential tremor. *Cochrane Database Syst Rev.* 2017;4:CD009683.

42. Pahwa R, Lyons K, Hubble JP, et al. Double-blind controlled trial of gabapentin in essential tremor. *Mov Disord.* 1998;13(3):465–467.

43. Ondo W, Hunter C, Vuong KD, Schwartz K, Jankovic J. Gabapentin for essential tremor: a multiple-dose, double-blind, placebo-controlled trial. *Mov Disord.* 2000;15(4):678–682.

44. Gunal DI, Afşar N, Bekiroglu N, Aktan S. New alternative agents in essential tremor therapy: double-blind placebo-controlled study of alprazolam and acetazolamide. *Neurol Sci.* 2000;21(5):315–317.

45. Huber SJ, Paulson GW. Efficacy of alprazolam for essential tremor. *Neurology.* 1988;38(2):241–243.

46. Lou JS, Jankovic J. Essential tremor: clinical correlates in 350 patients. *Neurology.* 1991;41(2 (Pt 1)):234–238.

47. Boecker H, Wills AJ, Ceballos-Baumann A, et al. The effect of ethanol on alcohol-responsive essential tremor: a positron emission tomography study. *Ann Neurol.* 1996;39(5):650–658.

48. Glykys J, Peng Z, Chandra D, Homanics GE, Houser CR, Mody I. A new naturally occurring GABA(A) receptor subunit partnership with high sensitivity to ethanol. *Nat Neurosci.* 2007;10(1):40–48.

49. Bushara KO, Goldstein SR, Grimes GJ, Burstein AH, Hallett M. Pilot trial of 1-octanol in essential tremor. *Neurology.* 2004;62(1):122–124.

50. Shill HA, Bushara KO, Mari Z, Reich M, Hallett M. Open-label dose-escalation study of oral 1-octanol in patients with essential tremor. *Neurology.* 2004;62(12):2320–2322.

51. Nahab FB, Wittevrongel L, Ippolito D, et al. An open-label, single-dose, crossover study of the pharmacokinetics and metabolism of two oral

formulations of 1-octanol in patients with essential tremor. *Neurotherapeutics.* 2011;8(4):753–762.

52. Voller B, Lines E, McCrossin G, et al. Dose-escalation study of octanoic acid in patients with essential tremor. *J Clin Invest.* 2016;126(4):1451–1457.

53. Haubenberger D, McCrossin G, Lungu C, et al. Octanoic acid in alcohol-responsive essential tremor: a randomized controlled study. *Neurology.* 2013;80(10):933–940.

54. Koller W, Graner D, Mlcoch A. Essential voice tremor: treatment with propranolol. *Neurology.* 1985;35(1):106–108.

55. Calzetti S, Sasso E, Negrotti A, Baratti M, Fava R. Effect of propranolol in head tremor: quantitative study following single-dose and sustained drug administration. *Clin Neuropharmacol.* 1992;15(6):470–476.

56. Song I-U, Kim J-S, Lee S-B, et al. Effects of zonisamide on isolated head tremor. *Eur J Neurol.* 2008;15(11):1212–1215.

57. Postuma RB, Berg D, Stern M, et al. MDS clinical diagnostic criteria for Parkinson's disease. *Mov Disord.* 2015;30(12):1591–1601.

58. Jankovic J, Schwartz KS, Ondo W. Re-emergent tremor of Parkinson's disease *J Neurol Neurosurg Psychiatry.* 1999;67(5):646–650.

59. Deuschl G, Bain P, Brin M. Consensus statement of the Movement Disorder Society on Tremor ad hoc scientific committee. *Mov Disord.*1998;13(Suppl 3):2–23.

60. Koller WC, Vetere-Overfield B, Barter R. Tremors in early Parkinson's disease. *Clin Neuropharmacol.* 1989;12(4):293–297.

61. Dowzenko A, Buksowicz C, Kuran W. Effect of Coretal Polfa (Oxprenolol) on parkinsonian tremor and benign essential tremor. *Neurol Neurochir Pol.* 1976;10(1):49–53.

62. Marsden CD, Parkes JD, Rees JE. Letter: propranolol in Parkinson's disease. *Lancet (Lond).* 1974;2(7877):410.

63. Martin WE, Loewenson RB, Resch JA, Baker AB. A controlled study comparing trihexyphenidyl hydrochloride plus levodopa with placebo plus levodopa in patients with Parkinson's disease. *Neurology.* 1974;24(10):912–919.

64. Koller WC. Pharmacologic treatment of parkinsonian tremor. *Arch Neurol.* 1986;43(2):126–127.

65. Navan P, Findley LJ, Jeffs JAR, Pearce RKB, Bain PG. Randomized, double-blind, 3-month parallel study of the effects of pramipexole, pergolide, and placebo on Parkinsonian tremor. *Mov Disord.* 2003;18(11):1324–1331.

66. Navan P, Findley LJ, Jeffs JAR, Pearce RKB, Bain PG. Double-blind, single-dose, cross-over study of the effects of pramipexole, pergolide, and placebo on rest tremor and UPDRS part III in Parkinson's disease. *Mov Disord.* 2003;18(2):176–180.

67. Navan P, Findley LJ, Undy MB, Pearce RKB, Bain PG. A randomly assigned double-blind cross-over study examining the relative antiparkinsonian tremor effects of pramipexole and pergolide. *Eur J Neurol.* 2005;12(1):1–8.

68. Pogarell O, Gasser T, van Hilten JJ, et al. Pramipexole in patients with Parkinson's disease and marked drug resistant tremor: a randomised, double blind, placebo controlled multicentre study. *J Neurol Neurosurg Psychiatry.* 2002;72(6):713–720.

69. Crosby NJ, Deane KHO, Clarke CE. Beta-blocker therapy for tremor in Parkinson's disease. *Cochrane Database Syst Rev.* 2003;(1):CD003361.

70. Koller WC, Herbster G. Adjuvant therapy of parkinsonian tremor. *Arch Neurol.* 1987;44(9):921–923.

71. Foster NL, Newman RP, LeWitt PA, Gillespie MM, Larsen TA, Chase TN. Peripheral beta-adrenergic blockade treatment of parkinsonian tremor. *Ann Neurol.* 1984;16(4):505–508.

72. Katzenschlager R, Sampaio C, Costa J, Lees A. Anticholinergics for symptomatic management of Parkinson's disease. *Cochrane Database Syst Rev.* 2003;(2):CD003735.

73. Bonuccelli U, Ceravolo R, Salvetti S, et al. Clozapine in Parkinson's disease tremor. Effects of acute and chronic administration. *Neurology.* 1997;49(6):1587–1590.

74. Friedman JH, Lannon MC. Clozapine-responsive tremor in Parkinson's disease. *Mov Disord.* 1990;5(3):225–259.

75. Fahn S, Isgreen WP. Long-term evaluation of amantadine and levodopa combination in parkinsonism by double-blind crossover analyses. *Neurology.* 1975;25(8):695–700.

76. Butzer JF, Silver DE, Sahs AL. Amantadine in Parkinson's disease. A double-blind, placebo-controlled, crossover study with long-term follow-up. *Neurology.* 1975;25(7):603–606.

77. McManis PG, Sharbrough FW. Orthostatic tremor: clinical and electrophysiologic characteristics. *Muscle Nerve.* 1993;16(11):1254–1260.

78. Gerschlager W, Münchau A, Katzenschlager R, et al. Natural history and syndromic associations of orthostatic tremor: a review of 41 patients. *Mov Disord.* 2004;19(7):788–795.

79. Gates PC. Orthostatic tremor (shaky legs syndrome). *Clin Exp Neurol.* 1993;30:66–71.

80. Hassan A, Ahlskog JE, Matsumoto JY, Milber JM, Bower JH, Wilkinson JR. Orthostatic tremor: Clinical, electrophysiologic, and treatment findings in 184 patients. *Neurology.* 2016;86(5):458–464.

81. Mestre TA, Lang AE, Lang AE, et al. Associated movement disorders in orthostatic tremor *J Neurol Neurosurg Psychiatry.* 2012;83(7):725–729.

82. Onofrj M, Thomas A, Paci C, D'Andreamatteo G. Gabapentin in orthostatic tremor: results of

a double-blind crossover with placebo in four patients. *Neurology.* 1998;51(3):880–882.

83. Rodrigues JP, Edwards DJ, Walters SE, et al. Blinded placebo crossover study of gabapentin in primary orthostatic tremor. *Mov Disord.* 2006;21(7):900–905.

84. Hellriegel H, Raethjen J, Deuschl G, Volkmann J. Levetiracetam in primary orthostatic tremor: a double-blind placebo-controlled crossover study. *Mov Disord.* 2011;26(13):2431–2434.

85. Ganos C, Maugest L, Apartis E, et al. The long-term outcome of orthostatic tremor. *J Neurol Neurosurg Psychiatry.* 2016;87(2):167–172.

86. Wills AJ, Brusa L, Wang HC, Brown P, Marsden CD. Levodopa may improve orthostatic tremor: case report and trial of treatment. *J Neurol Neurosurg Psychiatry.* 1999;66(5):681–684.

87. Katzenschlager R, Costa D, Gerschlager W, et al. [123I]-FP-CIT-SPECT demonstrates dopaminergic deficit in orthostatic tremor. *Ann Neurol.* 2003;53(4):489–496.

88. Gerschlager W, Münchau A, Katzenschlager R, et al. Natural history and syndromic associations of orthostatic tremor: a review of 41 patients. *Mov Disord.* 2004;19(7):788–795.

89. Leu-Semenescu S, Roze E, Vidailhet M, et al. Myoclonus or tremor in orthostatism: an under-recognized cause of unsteadiness in Parkinson's disease. *Mov Disord.* 2007;22(14):2063–2069.

90. Simpson LL. The origin, structure, and pharmacological activity of botulinum toxin. *Pharmacol Rev.* 1981;33(3):155–188.

91. Gilio F, Currà A, Lorenzano C, Modugno N, Manfredi M, Berardelli A. Effects of botulinum toxin type A on intracortical inhibition in patients with dystonia. *Ann Neurol.* 2000;48(1):20–26.

92. Boroojerdi B, Cohen LG, Hallett M. Effects of botulinum toxin on motor system excitability in patients with writer's cramp. *Neurology.* 2003;61(11):1546–1550.

93. Pal PK, Samii A, Schulzer M, Mak E, Tsui JK. Head tremor in cervical dystonia. *Can J Neurol Sci.* 2000;27(2):137–142.

94. Fasano A, Bove F, Lang AE. The treatment of dystonic tremor: a systematic review. *J Neurol Neurosurg Psychiatry.* 2014;85(7):759–769.

95. Pullman SL, Greene P, Fahn S, Pedersen SF. Approach to the treatment of limb disorders with botulinum toxin A. Experience with 187 patients. *Arch Neurol.* 1996;53(7):617–624.

96. Trosch RM, Pullman SL. Botulinum toxin A injections for the treatment of hand tremors. *Mov Disord.* 1994;9(6):601–609.

97. Jankovic J, Schwartz K, Clemence W, Aswad A, Mordaunt J. A randomized, double-blind, placebo-controlled study to evaluate botulinum toxin type A in essential hand tremor. *Mov Disord.* 1996;11(3):250–256.

98. Brin MF, Lyons KE, Doucette J, et al. A randomized, double masked, controlled trial of botulinum toxin type A in essential hand tremor. *Neurology.* 2001;56(11):1523–1528.

99. Mittal SO, Machado D, Richardson D, Dubey D, Jabbari B. Botulinum toxin in essential hand tremor—a randomized double-blind placebo-controlled study with customized injection approach. *Parkinsonism Relat Disord.* 2018;56:65–69.

100. Samotus O, Rahimi F, Lee J, Jog M. Functional ability improved in essential tremor by inco-botulinumtoxina injections using kinematically determined biomechanical patterns—a new future. *PLoS ONE.* 2016;11(4): e0153739.

101. Samotus O, Lee J, Jog M. Long-term tremor therapy for Parkinson and essential tremor with sensor-guided botulinum toxin type A injections. *PLoS ONE.* 2017;12(6):e0178670.

102. Pahwa R, Busenbark K, Swanson-Hyland EF, et al. Botulinum toxin treatment of essential head tremor. *Neurology.* 1995;45(4):822–824.

103. Rahimi F, Samotus O, Lee J, Jog M. Effective management of upper limb Parkinsonian tremor by incobotulinum toxin A injections using sensor-based biomechanical patterns. *Tremor Other Hyperkinet Mov (N Y).* 2015;5:348.

104. Mittal SO, Machado D, Richardson D, Dubey D, Jabbari B. Botulinum toxin in Parkinson disease tremor: a randomized, double-blind, placebo controlled study with a customized injection approach. *Mayo Clin Proc.* 2017;92(9):1359–1367.

105. Pullman SL, Greene P, Fahn S, Pedersen SF. Approach to the treatment of limb disorders with botulinum toxin A. Experience with 187 patients. *Arch Neurol.* 1996;53(7):617–624.

106. Trosch RM, Pullman SL. Botulinum toxin A injections for the treatment of hand tremors. *Mov Disord.* 1994;9(6):601–609.

107. Deuschl G, Mischke G, Schenck E, Schulte-Mönting J, Lücking CH. Symptomatic and essential rhythmic palatal myoclonus. *Brain.* 1990;113 (Pt 6):1645–1672.

108. Slengerik-Hansen J, Ovesen T. Botulinum toxin treatment of objective tinnitus because of essential palatal tremor: a systematic review. *Otol Neurotol.* 2016;37(7):820–828.

109. Stamelou M, Saifee TA, Edwards MJ, Bhatia KP. Psychogenic palatal tremor may be underrecognized: reappraisal of a large series of cases. *Mov Disord.*2012;27(9):1164–1168.

110. Gibbins N, Awad R, Harris S, Aymat A. The diagnosis, clinical findings and treatment options for Parkinson's disease patients attending a tertiary referral voice clinic. *J Laryngol Otol* 2017; 131:357–362.

111. van Esch BF, Wegner I, Stegeman I, Grolman W. Effect of botulinum toxin and surgery among spasmodic dysphonia patients. *Otolaryngol Head Neck Surg.* 2017;156(2):238–254.

112. Estes C, Sadoughi B, Coleman R, Sarva H, Mauer E, Sulica L. A prospective crossover trial of botulinum toxin chemodenervation

versus injection augmentation for essential voice tremor. *Laryngoscope*. 2018;128(2):437–446.

113. Guglielmino G, de Moraes BT, Villanova LC, Padovani M, Biase NGD. Comparison of botulinum toxin and propranolol for essential and dystonic vocal tremors. *Clinics (Sao Paulo, Brazil)*. 2018 16;73:e87.

114. Gurey LE, Sinclair CF, Blitzer A. A new paradigm for the management of essential vocal tremor with botulinum toxin. *Laryngoscope*. 2013;123(10):2497–2501.

115. Van Der Walt A, Sung S, Spelman T, et al. A double-blind, randomized, controlled study of botulinum toxin type A in MS-related tremor. *Neurology*. 2012;79(1):92–99.

116. Alusi SH, Worthington J, Glickman S, Bain PG. A study of tremor in multiple sclerosis. *Brain*. 2001;124(Pt 4):720–730.

117. Pittock SJ, McClelland RL, Mayr WT, Rodriguez M, Matsumoto JY. Prevalence of tremor in multiple sclerosis and associated disability in the Olmsted County population. *Mov Disord*. 2004;19(12):1482–1485.

118. McCreary JK, Rogers JA, Forwell SJ. Upper limb intention tremor in multiple sclerosis. *Int J MS Care*. 2018;20(5):211–223.

119. Benabid AL, Pollak P, Hommel M, Gaio JM, de Rougemont J, Perret J. Treatment of Parkinson tremor by chronic stimulation of the ventral intermediate nucleus of the thalamus. *Rev Neurol* (Paris). 1989;145(4):320–323.

120. Schuurman PR, Bosch DA, Merkus MP, Speelman JD. Long-term follow-up of thalamic stimulation versus thalamotomy for tremor suppression. *Mov Disord*. 2008;23(8):1146–1153.

121. Al-Fatly B, Ewert S, Kübler D, Kroneberg D, Horn A, Kühn AA. Connectivity profile of thalamic deep brain stimulation to effectively treat essential tremor. *Brain*. 2019;142(10):3086–3098.

122. Schuurman PR, Bosch DA, Bossuyt PM, et al. A comparison of continuous thalamic stimulation and thalamotomy for suppression of severe tremor. *N Engl J Med*. 2000;342(7):461–468.

123. Koller WC, Lyons KE, Wilkinson SB, Pahwa R. Efficacy of unilateral deep brain stimulation of the VIM nucleus of the thalamus for essential head tremor. *Mov Disord*. 1999;14(5):847–850.

124. Hubble JP, Busenbark KL, Wilkinson S, et al. Effects of thalamic deep brain stimulation based on tremor type and diagnosis. *Mov Disord*. 1997;12(3):337–341.

125. Koller W, Pahwa R, Busenbark K, et al. High-frequency unilateral thalamic stimulation in the treatment of essential and parkinsonian tremor. *Ann Neurol*. 1997;42(3):292–299.

126. Koller WC, Lyons KE, Wilkinson SB, Troster AI, Pahwa R. Long-term safety and efficacy of unilateral deep brain stimulation of the thalamus in essential tremor. *Mov Disord*. 2001;16(3):464–468.

127. Rehncrona S, Johnels B, Widner H, Törnqvist A-L, Hariz M, Sydow O. Long-term efficacy of thalamic deep brain stimulation for tremor: double-blind assessments. *Mov Disord*. 2003;18(2):163–170.

128. Moscovich M, Morishita T, Foote KD, Favilla CG, Chen ZP, Okun MS. Effect of lead trajectory on the response of essential head tremor to deep brain stimulation. *Parkinsonism Relat Disord*. 2013;19(9):789–794.

129. Ondo W, Almaguer M, Jankovic J, Simpson RK. Thalamic deep brain stimulation: comparison between unilateral and bilateral placement. *Arch Neurol*. 2001;58(2):218–222.

130. Peng-Chen Z, Morishita T, Vaillancourt D, et al. Unilateral thalamic deep brain stimulation in essential tremor demonstrates long-term ipsilateral effects. *Parkinsonism Relat Disord*. 2013;19(12):1113–1117.

131. Cury RG, Fraix V, Castrioto A, et al. Thalamic deep brain stimulation for tremor in Parkinson disease, essential tremor, and dystonia. *Neurology*. 2017;89(13):1416–1423.

132. Zhang K, Bhatia S, Oh MY, Cohen D, Angle C, Whiting D. Long-term results of thalamic deep brain stimulation for essential tremor. *J Neurosurg*. 2010;112(6):1271–1276.

133. Kumar R, Lozano AM, Sime E, Lang AE. Long-term follow-up of thalamic deep brain stimulation for essential and parkinsonian tremor. *Neurology*. 2003;61(11):1601–1604.

134. Pahwa R, Lyons KE, Wilkinson SB, et al. Long-term evaluation of deep brain stimulation of the thalamus. *J Neurosurg*. 2006;104(4):506–512.

135. Blomstedt P, Hariz G-M, Hariz MI, Koskinen L-OD. Thalamic deep brain stimulation in the treatment of essential tremor: a long-term follow-up. *Br J Neurosurg*. 2007;21(5):504–509.

136. Hariz G-M, Blomstedt P, Koskinen L-OD. Long-term effect of deep brain stimulation for essential tremor on activities of daily living and health-related quality of life. *Acta Neurol Scand*. 2008;118(6):387–394.

137. Nazzaro JM, Pahwa R, Lyons KE. Long-term benefits in quality of life after unilateral thalamic deep brain stimulation for essential tremor. *J Neurosurg*. 2012;117(1):156–161.

138. Børretzen MN, Bjerknes S, Sæhle T, et al. Long-term follow-up of thalamic deep brain stimulation for essential tremor—patient satisfaction and mortality. *BMC Neurol*. 2014;14:120.

139. Hwynn N, Hass CJ, Zeilman P, et al. Steady or not following thalamic deep brain stimulation for essential tremor. *J Neurol*. 2011;258(9):1643–1648.

140. Becker J, Barbe MT, Hartinger M, et al. The effect of uni- and bilateral thalamic deep brain stimulation on speech in patients with essential tremor: acoustics and intelligibility. *Neuromodulation*. 2017;20(3):223–232.

141. Shih LC, LaFaver K, Lim C, Papavassiliou E, Tarsy D. Loss of benefit in VIM thalamic deep brain stimulation (DBS) for essential tremor (ET): how prevalent is it? *Parkinsonism Relat Disord.* 2013;19(7):676–679.

142. Favilla CG, Ullman D, Wagle Shukla A, Foote KD, Jacobson CE, Okun MS. Worsening essential tremor following deep brain stimulation: disease progression versus tolerance. *Brain.* 2012;135(Pt 5):1455–1462.

143. Hariz MI, Shamsgovara P, Johansson F, Hariz G, Fodstad H. Tolerance and tremor rebound following long-term chronic thalamic stimulation for Parkinsonian and essential tremor. *Stereotact Funct Neurosurg.* 1999;72(2–4):208–218.

144. Barbe MT, Liebhart L, Runge M, et al. Deep brain stimulation in the nucleus ventralis intermedius in patients with essential tremor: habituation of tremor suppression. *J Neurol.* 2011;258(3):434–439.

145. Paschen S, Forstenpointner J, Becktepe J, et al. Long-term efficacy of deep brain stimulation for essential tremor: an observer-blinded study. *Neurology.* 2019 19;92(12):e1378–e1386.

146. Pilitsis JG, Metman LV, Toleikis JR, Hughes LE, Sani SB, Bakay RAE. Factors involved in long-term efficacy of deep brain stimulation of the thalamus for essential tremor. *J Neurosurg.* 2008;109(4):640–646.

147. Mestre TA, Lang AE, Okun MS. Factors influencing the outcome of deep brain stimulation: placebo, nocebo, lessebo, and lesion effects. *Mov Disord.* 2016;31:290–296.

148. Seier M, Hiller A, Quinn J, Murchison C, Brodsky M, Anderson S. Alternating thalamic deep brain stimulation for essential tremor: a trial to reduce habituation. *Mov Disord Clin Pract.* 2018;5(6):620–626.

149. Isaacs DA, Butler J, Sukul V, et al. Confined thalamic deep brain stimulation in refractory essential tremor. *Stereotact Funct Neurosurg.* 2018;96(5):296–304.

150. Sharma VD, Mewes K, Wichmann T, Buetefisch C, Willie JT, DeLong M. Deep brain stimulation of the centromedian thalamic nucleus for essential tremor: a case report. *Acta Neurochir.* 2017;159(5):789–793.

151. Lind G, Schechtmann G, Lind C, Winter J, Meyerson BA, Linderoth B. Subthalamic stimulation for essential tremor. Short- and long-term results and critical target area. *Stereotact Funct Neurosurg.* 2008;86(4):253–258.

152. Blomstedt P, Sandvik U, Linder J, Fredricks A, Forsgren L, Hariz MI. Deep brain stimulation of the subthalamic nucleus versus the zona incerta in the treatment of essential tremor. *Acta Neurochir.* 2011;153(12):2329–2335.

153. Niemann K, Mennicken VR, Jeanmonod D, Morel A. The Morel stereotactic atlas of the human thalamus: atlas-to-MR registration of internally consistent canonical model. *Neuroimage.* 2000;12(6):601–616.

154. Blomstedt P, Sandvik U, Fytagoridis A, Tisch S. The posterior subthalamic area in the treatment of movement disorders: past, present, and future. *Neurosurgery.* 2009;64(6):1029–1038; discussion 1038–1042.

155. Fenoy AJ, Schiess MC. Deep brain stimulation of the dentato-rubro-thalamic tract: outcomes of direct targeting for tremor. *Neuromodulation.* 2017;20(5):429–436.

156. Yang AI, Buch VP, Heman-Ackah SM, et al. Thalamic deep brain stimulation for essential tremor: relation of the dentatorubrothalamic tract with stimulation parameters. *World Neurosurg.* 2020;137: e89–e97.

157. Coenen VA, Sajonz B, Prokop T, et al. The dentato-rubro-thalamic tract as the potential common deep brain stimulation target for tremor of various origin: an observational case series. *Acta Neurochir.* 2020;162(5):1053–1066.

158. Dembek TA, Petry-Schmelzer JN, Reker P, et al. PSA and VIM DBS efficiency in essential tremor depends on distance to the dentatorubrothalamic tract. *NeuroImage Clin.* 2020;26:102235.

159. Barbe MT, Liebhart L, Runge M, et al. Deep brain stimulation of the ventral intermediate nucleus in patients with essential tremor: stimulation below intercommissural line is more efficient but equally effective as stimulation above. *Exp Neurol.* 2011;230(1):131–137.

160. Blomstedt P, Sandvik U, Tisch S. Deep brain stimulation in the posterior subthalamic area in the treatment of essential tremor. *Mov Disord.* 2010;25(10):1350–1356.

161. Sandvik U, Koskinen L-O, Lundquist A, Blomstedt P. Thalamic and subthalamic deep brain stimulation for essential tremor: where is the optimal target? *Neurosurgery.* 2012;70(4):840–845; discussion 845–846.

162. Degeneffe A, Kuijf ML, Ackermans L, Temel Y, Kubben PL. Comparing deep brain stimulation in the ventral intermediate nucleus versus the posterior subthalamic area in essential tremor patients. *Surg Neurol Int.* 2018;9:244.

163. Sandström L, Blomstedt P, Karlsson F. Voice tremor response to deep brain stimulation in relation to electrode location in the posterior subthalamic area. *World Neurosurg.* 2019;3:100024.

164. Barbe MT, Reker P, Hamacher S, et al. DBS of the PSA and the VIM in essential tremor: a randomized, double-blind, crossover trial. *Neurology.* 2018;91(6):e543–e550.

165. Becker J, Thies T, Petry-Schmelzer JN, et al. The effects of thalamic and posterior subthalamic deep brain stimulation on speech in patients

with essential tremor—a prospective, randomized, double-blind crossover study. *Brain Lang.* 2020;202:104724.

166. Plaha P, Khan S, Gill SS. Bilateral stimulation of the caudal zona incerta nucleus for tremor control. *J Neurol Neurosurg Psychiatry.* 2008;79(5):504–513.

167. Plaha P, Javed S, Agombar D, et al. Bilateral caudal zona incerta nucleus stimulation for essential tremor: outcome and quality of life. *J Neurol Neurosurg Psychiatry.* 2011;82(8):899–904.

168. Murata J, Kitagawa M, Uesugi H, et al. Deep brain stimulation of the posterior subthalamic area (Zi/Raprl) for intractable tremor. *No Shinkei Geka.* 2007;35(4):355–362.

169. Fytagoridis A, Sandvik U, Aström M, Bergenheim T, Blomstedt P. Long term follow-up of deep brain stimulation of the caudal zona incerta for essential tremor *J Neurol Neurosurg Psychiatry.* 2012;83(3):258–262.

170. Eisinger RS, Wong J, Almeida L, et al. Ventral intermediate nucleus versus zona incerta region deep brain stimulation in essential tremor. *Mov Disord Clin Pract.* 2018;5(1):75–82.

171. Blomstedt P, Lindvall P, Linder J, Olivecrona M, Forsgren L, Hariz MI. Reoperation after failed deep brain stimulation for essential tremor. *World Neurosurg.* 2012;78(5):554.e1–554.e5.

172. Fytagoridis A, Sjöberg RL, Åström M, Fredricks A, Nyberg L, Blomstedt P. Effects of deep brain stimulation in the caudal zona incerta on verbal fluency. *Stereotact Funct Neurosurg.* 2013;91(1):24–29.

173. Holslag JAH, Neef N, Beudel M, et al. Deep brain stimulation for essential tremor: a comparison of targets. *World Neurosurg.* 2018;110:e580–e584.

174. Philipson J, Blomstedt P, Hariz M, Jahanshahi M. Deep brain stimulation in the caudal zona incerta in patients with essential tremor: effects on cognition 1 year after surgery. *J Neurosurg.* 2019;1–8.

175. Mehanna R, Itin I. Which approach is better: bilateral versus unilateral thalamic deep brain stimulation in patients with fragile X-associated tremor ataxia syndrome? *Cerebellum (Lond).* 2014;13(2):222–225.

176. dos Santos Ghilardi MG, Cury RG, dos Ângelos JS, et al. Long-term improvement of tremor and ataxia after bilateral DBS of VoP/zona incerta in FXTAS. *Neurology.* 2015;84(18):1904–1906.

177. Oyama G, Umemura A, Shimo Y, et al. Posterior subthalamic area deep brain stimulation for fragile X-associated tremor/ataxia syndrome. *Neuromodulation.* 2014;17(8):721–723.

178. Oliveria SF, Rodriguez RL, Bowers D, et al. Safety and efficacy of dual-lead thalamic deep brain stimulation for patients with treatment-refractory multiple sclerosis tremor: a single-center,

randomised, single-blind, pilot trial. *Lancet Neurol.* 2017;16(9):691–700.

179. Foote KD, Okun MS. Ventralis intermedius plus ventralis oralis anterior and posterior deep brain stimulation for posttraumatic Holmes tremor: two leads may be better than one: technical note. *Neurosurgery.* 2005;56(2 Suppl):E445; discussion E445.

180. Parker T, Raghu ALB, FitzGerald JJ, Green AL, Aziz TZ. Multitarget deep brain stimulation for clinically complex movement disorders. *J Neurosurg.* 2020;1–6.

181. Prajakta G, Horisawa S, Kawamata T, Taira T. Feasibility of staged bilateral radiofrequency ventral intermediate nucleus thalamotomy for bilateral essential tremor. *World Neurosurg.* 2019;125:e992–e997.

182. Jankovic J, Cardoso F, Grossman RG, Hamilton WJ. Outcome after stereotactic thalamotomy for parkinsonian, essential, and other types of tremor. *Neurosurgery.* 1995;37(4):680–686; discussion 686–687.

183. Goldman MS, Ahlskog JE, Kelly PJ. The symptomatic and functional outcome of stereotactic thalamotomy for medically intractable essential tremor. *J Neurosurg.* 1992;76(6):924–928.

184. Martínez-Moreno NE, Sahgal A, De Salles A, et al. Stereotactic radiosurgery for tremor: systematic review. *J Neurosurg.* 2018;1–12.

185. Ohye C, Higuchi Y, Shibazaki T, et al. Gamma knife thalamotomy for Parkinson disease and essential tremor: a prospective multicenter study. *Neurosurgery.* 2012;70(3):526–535; discussion 535–536.

186. Duma CM, Jacques DB, Kopyov OV, Mark RJ, Copcutt B, Farokhi HK. Gamma Kknife radiosurgery for thalamotomy in parkinsonian tremor: a five-year experience. *J Neurosurg.* 1998;88(6):1044–1049.

187. Young RF, Li F, Vermeulen S, Meier R. Gamma Knife thalamotomy for treatment of essential tremor: long-term results. *J Neurosurg.* 2010;112(6):1311–1317.

188. Lim S-Y, Hodaie M, Fallis M, Poon Y-Y, Mazzella F, Moro E. Gamma knife thalamotomy for disabling tremor: a blinded evaluation. *Arch Neurol.* 2010;67(5):584–588.

189. Lipsman N, Schwartz ML, Huang Y, et al. MR-guided focused ultrasound thalamotomy for essential tremor: a proof-of-concept study. *Lancet Neurol.* 2013;12(5):462–468.

190. Chang WS, Jung HH, Kweon EJ, Zadicario E, Rachmilevitch I, Chang JW. Unilateral magnetic resonance guided focused ultrasound thalamotomy for essential tremor: practices and clinicoradiological outcomes. *J Neurol Neurosurg Psychiatry.* 2015;86(3):257–264.

191. Elias WJ, Lipsman N, Ondo WG, et al. A randomized trial of focused ultrasound

thalamotomy for essential tremor. *N Engl J Med.* 2016;375(8):730–739.

192. Schreglmann SR, Bauer R, Hägele-Link S, et al. Unilateral cerebellothalamic tract ablation in essential tremor by MRI-guided focused ultrasound. *Neurology.* 2017;88(14):1329–1333.

193. Mohammed N, Patra D, Nanda A. A meta-analysis of outcomes and complications of magnetic resonance-guided focused ultrasound in the treatment of essential tremor. *Neurosurg Focus.* 2018;44(2):E4.

194. Meng Y, Solomon B, Boutet A, et al. Magnetic resonance-guided focused ultrasound thalamotomy for treatment of essential tremor: a 2-year outcome study. *Mov Disord.* 2018;33(10):1647–1650.

195. Chang JW, Park CK, Lipsman N, et al. A prospective trial of magnetic resonance-guided focused ultrasound thalamotomy for essential tremor: results at the 2-year follow-up. *Ann Neurol.* 2018;83(1):107–114.

196. Park Y-S, Jung NY, Na YC, Chang JW. Four-year follow-up results of magnetic resonance-guided focused ultrasound thalamotomy for essential tremor. *Mov Disord.*2019;34(5):727–734.

197. Sinai A, Nassar M, Eran A, et al. Magnetic resonance-guided focused ultrasound thalamotomy for essential tremor: a 5-year single-center experience. *J Neurosurg.* 2019;1–8.

198. Schlesinger I, Eran A, Sinai A, et al. MRI guided focused ultrasound thalamotomy for moderate-to-severe tremor in Parkinson's disease. *Parkinson's Dis.* 2015;2015:219149.

199. Bond AE, Shah BB, Huss DS, et al. Safety and efficacy of focused ultrasound thalamotomy for patients with medication-refractory, tremor-dominant parkinson disease: a randomized clinical trial. *JAMA Neurol.* 2017;74(12):1412–1418.

200. Fasano A, Llinas M, Munhoz RP, Hlasny E, Kucharczyk W, Lozano AM. MRI-guided focused ultrasound thalamotomy in non-ET tremor syndromes. *Neurology.* 2017;89(8):771–775.

201. Fasano A, Sammartino F, Llinas M, Lozano AM. MRI-guided focused ultrasound thalamotomy in fragile X-associated tremor/ataxia syndrome. *Neurology.* 2016;87(7):736–738.

202. Máñez-Miró JU, Martínez-Fernández R, Del Alamo M, Pineda-Pardo JA, Fernández-Rodríguez B, Alonso-Frech F, et al. Focused ultrasound thalamotomy for multiple sclerosis-associated tremor. *Multiple Scler.* 2020;26(7):855–858.

203. Lefaucheur J-P. Transcranial magnetic stimulation. *Handb Clin Neurol.* 2019;160:559–580.

204. Popa T, Russo M, Vidailhet M, et al. Cerebellar rTMS stimulation may induce prolonged clinical benefits in essential tremor, and subjacent changes in functional connectivity: an open label trial. *Brain Stimul.* 2013;6(2):175–179.

205. Gironell A, Kulisevsky J, Lorenzo J, Barbanoj M, Pascual-Sedano B, Otermin P. Transcranial magnetic stimulation of the cerebellum in essential tremor: a controlled study. *Arch Neurol.* 2002;59(3):413–417.

206. Badran BW, Glusman CE, Austelle CW, et al. A double-blind, sham-controlled pilot trial of pre-supplementary motor area (pre-sma) 1 hz rtms to treat essential tremor. *Brain Stimul.* 2016;9(6):945–947.

207. Gironell A, Martínez-Horta S, Aguilar S, et al. Transcranial direct current stimulation of the cerebellum in essential tremor: a controlled study. *Brain Stimul.* 2014;7(3):491–492.

208. Bologna M, Rocchi L, Leodori G, et al. Cerebellar continuous theta burst stimulation in essential tremor. *Cerebellum (Lond).* 2015;14(2):133–141.

209. Espay AJ, Hung SW, Sanger TD, Moro E, Fox SH, Lang AE. A writing device improves writing in primary writing tremor. *Neurology.* 2005;64(9):1648–1650.

210. Aisen ML, Arnold A, Baiges I, Maxwell S, Rosen M. The effect of mechanical damping loads on disabling action tremor. *Neurology.* 1993;43(7):1346–1350.

211. Rocon E, Manto M, Pons J, Camut S, Belda JM. Mechanical suppression of essential tremor. *Cerebellum (Lond).* 2007;6(1):73–78.

212. Cooper C, Evidente VG, Hentz JG, Adler CH, Caviness JN, Gwinn-Hardy K. The effect of temperature on hand function in patients with tremor. *J Hand Ther.* 2000;13(4):276–288.

213. O'Connor RJ, Kini MU. Non-pharmacological and non-surgical interventions for tremor: a systematic review. *Parkinsonism Relat Disord.* 2011;17(7):509–515.

214. Feys P, Helsen WF, Verschueren S, et al. Online movement control in multiple sclerosis patients with tremor: effects of tendon vibration. *Mov Disord.* 2006;21(8):1148–1153.

215. Haas CT, Turbanski S, Kessler K, Schmidtbleicher D. The effects of random whole-body-vibration on motor symptoms in Parkinson's disease. *Neurorehabilitation.* 2006;21(1):29–36.

216. King LK, Almeida QJ, Ahonen H. Short-term effects of vibration therapy on motor impairments in Parkinson's disease. *Neurorehabilitation.* 2009;25(4):297–306.

217. Castrillo-Fraile V, Peña EC, Gabriel Y, et al. Tremor control devices for essential tremor: a systematic literature review. *Tremor Other Hyperkinet Mov (N Y).* 2019;9. doi: 10.7916/tohm.v0.688

218. Satoh M, Narita M, Tomimoto H. Three cases of focal embouchure dystonia: classifications and successful therapy using a dental splint. *Eur Neurol.* 2011;66(2):85–90.

219. Pathak A, Redmond JA, Allen M, Chou KL. A noninvasive handheld assistive device to accommodate essential tremor: a pilot study. *Mov Disord.* 2014;29(6):838–842.

220. Jitkritsadakul O, Thanawattano C, Anan C, Bhidayasiri R. Tremor's glove-an innovative electrical muscle stimulation therapy for intractable tremor in Parkinson's disease: a randomized sham-controlled trial. *J Neurol Sci.* 2017;381:331–340.

221. Pahwa R, Dhall R, Ostrem J, et al. An acute randomized controlled trial of noninvasive peripheral nerve stimulation in essential tremor. *Neuromodulation.* 2019;22(5):537–545.

222. Bending J, Cleeves L. Effect of electrical nerve stimulation on dystonic tremor. *Lancet (Lond).* 1990;336(8727):1385–1386.

223. Meunier S, Bleton JP, Mazevet D, et al. TENS is harmful in primary writing tremor. *Clin Neurophysiol.* 2011;122(1):171–175.

224. Edwards MJ, Bhatia KP. Functional (psychogenic) movement disorders: merging mind and brain. *Lancet Neurol.* 2012;11(3):250–260.

225. Gendre T, Carle G, Mesrati F, et al. Quality of life in functional movement disorders is as altered as in organic movement disorders. *J Psychosom Res.* 2019;116:10–16.

226. Gasca-Salas C, Lang AE. Neurologic diagnostic criteria for functional neurologic disorders. *Handb Clin Neurol.* 2016;139:193–212.

227. Park JE, Maurer CW, Hallett M. The "whack-a-mole" sign in functional movement disorders. *Mov Disord Clin Pract.* 2015;2(3):286–288.

228. Schwingenschuh P, Saifee TA, Katschnig-Winter P, et al. Validation of "laboratory-supported" criteria for functional (psychogenic) tremor. *Mov Disord.* 2016;31(4):555–562.

229. Stone J, Hoeritzauer I. How do I explain the diagnosis of functional movement disorder to a patient? *Mov Disord Clin Pract.* 2019;6(5):419.

230. Hallett M. Functional (psychogenic) movement disorders—clinical presentations. *Parkinsonism Relat Disord.* 2016;22(0 1):S149–S152.

231. Pareés I, Kassavetis P, Saifee TA, et al. "Jumping to conclusions" bias in functional movement disorders. *J Neurol Neurosurg Psychiatry.* 2012;83(4):460–463.

232. Espay AJ, Aybek S, Carson A, et al. Current concepts in diagnosis and treatment of functional neurological disorders. *JAMA Neurol.* 2018 01;75(9):1132–1141.

233. McKeon A, Ahlskog JE, Bower JH, Josephs KA, Matsumoto JY. Psychogenic tremor: long-term prognosis in patients with electrophysiologically confirmed disease. *Mov Disord.* 2009;24(1):72–76.

234. Gelauff J, Stone J, Edwards M, Carson A. The prognosis of functional (psychogenic) motor symptoms: a systematic review. *J Neurol Neurosurg Psychiatry.*2014;85(2):220–226.

235. Thomas M, Vuong KD, Jankovic J. Long-term prognosis of patients with psychogenic movement disorders. *Parkinsonism Relat Disord.* 2006;12(6):382–387.

236. Nielsen G, Buszewicz M, Stevenson F, et al. Randomised feasibility study of physiotherapy for patients with functional motor symptoms. *J Neurol Neurosurg Psychiatry.* 2017;88(6):484–490.

237. Espay AJ, Ries S, Maloney T, et al. Clinical and neural responses to cognitive behavioural therapy for functional tremor. *Neurology.* 2020;94(10):459.

238. Shah BB, Chen R, Zurowski M, Kalia LV, Gunraj C, Lang AE. Repetitive transcranial magnetic stimulation plus standardized suggestion of benefit for functional movement disorders: an open label case series. *Parkinsonism Relat Disord.* 2015;21(4):407–412.

239. Lidstone SC, MacGillivray L, Lang AE. Integrated therapy for functional movement disorders: time for a change. *Mov Disord Clin Pract.* 2020;7(2):169–174.

240. Jacob AE, Kaelin DL, Roach AR, Ziegler CH, LaFaver K. Motor retraining (more) for functional movement disorders: outcomes from a 1-week multidisciplinary rehabilitation program. *PM R.* 2018;10(11):1164–1172.

241. Handforth A, Tse W, Elble RJ. A pilot double-blind randomized trial of perampanel for essential tremor. *Mov Disord Clin Pract.* 2020;7(4):399–404.

242. Shao MM, Liss A, Park YL, et al. Early experience with new generation deep brain stimulation leads in Parkinson's disease and essential tremor patients. *Neuromodulation.* 2020;23(4):537–542.

243. Moldovan A-S, Hartmann CJ, Trenado C, et al. Less is more—Pulse width dependent therapeutic window in deep brain stimulation for essential tremor. *Brain Stimul.* 2018;11(5):1132–1139.

244. Rezaei Haddad A, Samuel M, Hulse N, Lin H-Y, Ashkan K. Long-term efficacy of constant current deep brain stimulation in essential tremor. *Neuromodulation.* 2017;20(5):437–443.

245. Lettieri C, Rinaldo S, Devigili G, et al. Clinical outcome of deep brain stimulation for dystonia: constant-current or constant-voltage stimulation? A non-randomized study. *Eur J Neurol.* 2015;22(6):919–926.

246. De Jesus S, Almeida L, Shahgholi L, et al. Square biphasic pulse deep brain stimulation for essential tremor: the BiP tremor study. *Parkinsonism Relat Disord.* 2018;46:41–46.

247. Tan H, Debarros J, He S, et al. Decoding voluntary movements and postural tremor based on thalamic LFPs as a basis for closed-loop stimulation for essential tremor. *Brain Stimul.* 2019;12(4):858–867.

248. Arlotti M, Marceglia S, Foffani G, et al. Eight-hours adaptive deep brain stimulation in patients with Parkinson disease. *Neurology.* 2018 13;90(11):e971–e976.

249. Little S, Beudel M, Zrinzo L, et al. Bilateral adaptive deep brain stimulation is effective

in Parkinson's disease. *J Neurol Neurosurg Psychiatry.* 2016;87(7):717–721.

250. Zesiewicz TA, Elble RJ, Louis ED, et al. Evidence-based guideline update: treatment of essential tremor. *Neurology.* 2011;77(19):1752–1755.

251. Dallapiazza RF, Lee DJ, De Vloo P, et al. Outcomes from stereotactic surgery for essential tremor. *J Neurol Neurosurg Psychiatry.* 2019;90(4):474–482.

252. Artusi CA, Farooqi A, Romagnolo A, et al. Deep brain stimulation in uncommon tremor disorders: indications, targets, and programming. *J Neurol.* 2018;265(11):2473–2493.

253. Coleman RR, Starr PA, Katz M, et al. Bilateral ventral intermediate nucleus thalamic deep brain stimulation in orthostatic tremor. *Stereotact Funct Neurosurg.* 2016;94(2):69–74.

254. Espay AJ, Duker AP, Chen R, et al. Deep brain stimulation of the ventral intermediate nucleus of the thalamus in medically refractory orthostatic tremor: preliminary observations. *Mov Disord.* 2008;23(16):2357–2362.

255. Gilmore G, Murgai A, Nazer A, Parrent A, Jog M. Zona incerta deep-brain stimulation in orthostatic tremor: efficacy and mechanism of improvement. *J Neurol.* 2019;266(11):2829–37.

256. Athauda D, Georgiev D, Aviles-Olmos I, et al. Thalamic-caudal zona incerta deep brain stimulation for refractory orthostatic tremor: a report of 3 cases. *Mov Disord Clin Pract.* 2017;4(1):105–110.

257. Krauss JK, Weigel R, Blahak C, et al. Chronic spinal cord stimulation in medically intractable orthostatic tremor. *J Neurol Neurosurg Psychiatry.* 2006;77(9):1013–1016.

258. Blahak C, Sauer T, Baezner H, et al. Long-term follow-up of chronic spinal cord stimulation for medically intractable orthostatic tremor. *J Neurol.* 2016;263(11):2224–2228.

Thinking and Treating Beyond the Tremor

APARNA WAGLE SHUKLA

INTRODUCTION

Tremor, a rhythmic involuntary movement disorder that can affect any body part, is the most prevalent movement disorder that affects millions of people worldwide. Essential tremor and Parkinson disease tremors comprise the more common types, and dystonic tremor and orthostatic tremor as less common types of tremor.[1] When treating tremors, clinicians should not view these disorders as isolated tremor disorders as many additional features such as gait impairment and nonmotor symptoms of cognitive difficulties often co-occur. Furthermore, neuropsychiatric features such as anxiety and depression, physiological factors, and comorbidities may contribute to tremor disabilities and pose additional treatment challenges. The Movement Disorders Society recently provided consensus criteria for diagnosing and classifying essential tremor along the clinical (Axis 1) and etiological axis (Axis 2). According to these criteria, patients presenting with tremor alone are diagnosed with an isolated tremor syndrome. Patients with gait ataxia, dementia, parkinsonism, dystonia, and other systemic or neurological signs co-occurring with tremor are diagnosed with a combined tremor syndrome. For patients with essential tremor, there is an intermediate in-between category of "essential tremor plus" that refers to soft signs of impaired tandem gait, questionable dystonic posturing, memory impairment, or other mild neurologic signs of unknown significance that clinicians may observe in their practice. Notably, the Axis 1 classification is flexible, and as patients develop additional features, they should be recategorized. This chapter will discuss the importance of these co-occurring features, as they have a definite albeit indirect role in determining the treatment outcomes. Many studies discussed in this chapter were conducted before the classification was introduced. Nevertheless, tremor researchers have long thought of considerations beyond the pure motor presentation, and clinicians should provide due attention to these features when formulating a treatment plan. While the focus will be mainly on gait, cognition, and neuropsychiatric features in the context of essential tremor, their implications for Parkinson disease, dystonia, and orthostatic tremor will be discussed under "other tremor disorders."

GAIT

Gait in essential tremor

Essential tremor was viewed as an exclusively motor disorder for many decades given that the primary clinical feature of the disease was postural and action tremor involving the arms.[2] A growing body of evidence has evolved that supports the presence of co-occurring features in essential tremor.[3,4] Abnormalities in gait and balance control are frequently reported.[5,6] While subjective symptoms related to gait and balance have been captured by specific questionnaires; clinicians have also documented objective impairments during bedside physical examination in the clinic. Most studies have used simple bedside 10-step tandem gait test for assessment. Subjects are required to walk ten steps in a straight line, with the heel of the leading foot touching the toe of the following foot.[5,7,8] In these studies, about 30–50% of patients were observed to have two or more missteps during the tandem testing.[5,8,9] In one study, the occurrence of the first misstep was determined to assess the severity of impairment[7] and was found to be more frequently impacted in essential tremor patients compared with controls. Rao et al. pooled data from multiple gait studies (essential tremor n = 784; healthy controls n = 467) to find the odds ratio for tandem walk abnormality was seven times higher in essential tremor compared with a healthy control population.[10]

In a large study (n = 104 patients) that employed instrumented gait analysis, participants with essential tremor compared to age-matched healthy controls revealed several abnormalities on the GAIT rite system.[11] These participants with a mean age of 86.0 ± 4.6 years were found to have a decline in gait speed, increase in double support time (dynamic balance), and increase in step asymmetry during the standard and tandem walk testing. Other studies found that essential tremor patients walked with shorter step lengths and increased step width regardless of whether they were performing routine walks or engaged in walks with increased cognitive demands.[12,13] In one study, an increased stride-to-stride variability was observed; this is an important predictor of falls risk in the elderly.[14] These abnormalities, including slow gait speed, short step length, increased step width, and increased step-to-step variability, are similar to what is seen in cerebellar disorders. In contrast to quantitative gait analysis, posturographic assessment of balance that involves measurement of the center of pressure for patients standing on a force platform has been less frequently studied. In one study, patients with postural abnormality had pronounced head tremor on examination.[15] Other studies have more commonly reported tandem missteps with head tremors compared to arm tremors. Midline tremors are associated with pronounced gait and balance problems and increased susceptibility to experiencing a fall.[8]

Although gait and balance impairment are known consequences of aging, these manifest in patients with essential tremor independent of the age advancement. The prevalence of tandem gait abnormality is estimated to increase three times more in the older healthy population (42%) than in the younger demographic (14%). In one study, while essential tremor patients had a similar prevalence of tandem abnormality to that found in patients below 70 years of age (about 10%), there was a substantial increase (70%) when the older population was examined.[5,16] The pathophysiology of essential tremor has strong ties with the cerebellum which likely explains these abnormalities. Similar observations were made during quantitative analysis of gait and balance. In two large studies (n > 100), there were abnormalities in spatiotemporal gait parameters (speed, cadence, and double support time) that were noted to worsen with age.[11,12] Accelerated worsening with an increase in age may not be related to disease duration, but an additional presence of cognitive abnormalities has detrimental effects on gait. A comprehensive assessment for cognition was performed in a study involving 199 essential tremor cases (mean age 78.6 years), which included Montreal Cognitive Assessment

(MoCA) to measure global cognition, multiple motor-free tests, and Clinical Dementia Rating scores. In a regression model, after due consideration of confounding variables such as age, total tremor score, and medication use, poorer cognition was associated with an increased number of falls and reduced balance confidence on the Activities of the Balance Confidence scale.[17]

To compound further, medications such as primidone, one of the first-line agents for treating essential tremor, has dose-limiting toxicity for gait and balance control. Deep brain stimulation targeted to the ventral intermedius nucleus, an FDA-approved target, is also linked with worsening of gait. Studies have shown that stimulation delivered, especially at higher intensities and bilateral stimulation worsens gait and balance.[18] Some centers advocate for unilateral implantation surgery to treat tremors affecting the dominant arm to mitigate these potential concerns.[19] Despite a growing recognition of gait and balance impairment, there are no clear treatment guidelines. Rehabilitation interventions such as resistance training[20,21] are likely promising, but limited awareness among practicing clinicians has led to only a few studies in the literature. Only a single case report so far found improvement of DBS-therapy-related gait and balance impairment.[22] Interestingly, in one study that used a three-dimensional optoelectronic gait analysis system, oral ingestion of alcohol with a mean blood level of 0.45% led to a significant improvement of the ataxia score and the number of missteps in patients with essential tremor.[23] These treatments need further assessment in larger samples.

Gait in other tremor disorders

Gait impairment is a cardinal manifestation of Parkinson disease. Some patients present with predominant postural instability gait disorder (PIGD) phenotype, whereas some present with disabling tremor (tremor-dominant) phenotype. PIGD patients have slower gait speed, shorter strides, excessive instability, and increased risk for falls, and are usually less responsive to dopaminergic medications.[24,25] Gait symptoms that increase with the progression of disease impact the quality of life. The PIGD phenotype is also more likely to be accompanied by cognitive symptoms.[26] Functional imaging with near-infrared spectroscopy techniques has shown increased frontal lobe activation even during simple, unobstructed walking tasks, indicating that gait automaticity is compromised with the advancement of the disease, and there is an increased dependency on cognitive resources.[27,28] The PIGD subtype is found to progress at a faster pace compared to the tremor-predominant phenotype. Many patients present with a mixed phenotype, thus have both tremor, and gait symptoms. Furthermore, Parkinson disease is accompanied by cognitive decline that contributes to worsening of gait. Advances in the understanding of the interrelationship between gait, cognition, and tremor can potentially lead to the development of effective intervention strategies. There is evidence to support the alleviation of gait symptoms with the treatment of nonmotor symptoms such as anxiety, depression, and cognitive impairment.[29,30]

Orthostatic tremor is a rare progressive disorder characterized by a high frequency of 13–18 Hz leg tremors. Patients commonly report symptoms of unsteadiness during standing that worsen with the progression of tremor. As the disease severity increases, unsteadiness symptoms persist during walking. Physiological studies have recorded tremors during sitting, standing, and walking tasks.[31] Unsteadiness, particularly noted during slow walking, is attributable to the persistence of tremor discharge in the leg muscles during all phases of walking.[31] Many previous studies have proposed that the cerebellum is the primary source of tremor, and this likely explains the symptoms of gait unsteadiness. There is increasing objective evidence to demonstrate postural and gait abnormalities in orthostatic tremor. In a recent study, patients with orthostatic tremor assessed with an instrumented walkway system were observed to have several gait abnormalities that were akin to a cerebellar disorder.[31] Some patients experience falls, which is infrequent or rare, but is increasingly reported by patients with slow frequency tremor (tremor frequency < 13 Hz). Thus, it is prudent to think beyond tremor and provide due attention to gait and balance features that are integral to tremor disorders and are important determinants of quality of life.

COGNITION

Cognition in essential tremor

Many clinical and epidemiological studies have found evidence for cognitive impairment in essential tremor patients compared to age-matched healthy populations.[32-36] While mild cognitive impairment is frequently seen, some patients with essential tremor develop significant worsening, or frank dementia over time.[37] In one study from Spain, 11.4% of older-onset patients had dementia compared to 6.0% of age-matched controls.[38] In another study from New York, the rate of dementia was even higher, with 25.0% in older-onset essential tremor group compared to 9.2% in controls.[39] The brain networks for aging-related tremors have been found to be different from those in essential tremor presenting at a younger age.[40] By contrast, in one study with the mean age of participants as 24.7 ± 6.2 years, the Montreal Cognitive Assessment (MoCA) score was 25.8 ± 2.8 in the essential tremor group compared to 28.2 ± 1.7 in the healthy controls (p < 0.001).[41] Essential tremor has a bimodal distribution for the age of onset. Given the recent definition and classification for essential tremors, we need larger samples to reevaluate the relationship between essential tremor, aging, and cognitive changes.

In one of the earlier studies consisting of 101 patients, Tröster et al. found significant deficits in auditory and visual attention, executive functions, verbal fluency, and immediate recall of a word list even when controlled for the presence of comorbidities, anxiety, or depression in essential tremor.[42] In a large epidemiological study, mild deficits in attention, executive function, information-processing speed, immediate and delayed memory, and verbal fluency were observed in the essential tremor group (n = 232) compared to age-matched controls (n = 696).[43] Collins et al. found impaired recognition memory related to storage and retrieval during a comprehensive neuropsychology assessment.[44] While deficits in attention, concentration, working memory, executive function, language, and global cognitive function are consistently found, impairments in abstract reasoning, planning, processing speed, calculation, and visuospatial abilities are usually spared.

Despite emergence of multiple studies over the past two decades in support of cognitive impairment in essential tremor, there is limited knowledge on rates of worsening (estimated relative risk is about 1.7), and the factors contributing to worsening are not entirely clear.[37,45] In one study, the cognitive change was observed to precede the motor manifestation of essential tremor, thus raising the possibility of a "premotor stage" as seen in Parkinson disease.[4] Impaired cognitive performance is associated with greater functional difficulty and lower activities of daily living scores,[46] which provides evidence for a direct relationship between cognitive impairment and functional disability experienced by these patients. It is also not surprising that cognitive impairment, in conjunction with essential tremor-related motor disability, increases the risk of hospitalization and requirement for nursing home facilities.[36,46]

The neuroanatomical and neuropathological underpinnings for cognitive changes in essential tremor are currently open for discussion. The cerebello-thalamo-cortical pathway, regarded as the central pathway for motor symptoms, is also conceptualized as the source for cognitive impairment in essential tremor. The cognitive deficits could also be a result of cerebellar cognitive affective syndrome observed in patients with acute and chronic cerebellar damage.[47] Multimodal imaging studies have shown changes throughout the brain. In a recent task-based functional MRI study, an increase in visual feedback was observed to increase tremor, which was associated with abnormal signal changes within the cerebello-thalamo-motor cortical pathway, which extended to visual and parietal areas.[48,49] Resting-state functional MRI and diffusion tensor imaging studies have shown a global compromise of functional connectivity and white matter microstructure, respectively, in essential tremor.[50,51] While cerebellar-cortical network dysfunction could potentially lead to executive dysfunction,[52,53] changes in the hippocampus, temporal cortex, and parietal cortex likely explain impairments seen in the language and memory.[54] In an EEG source analysis study, aging-related tremor (onset age > 50 years) was observed to have more pronounced abnormalities in the cortico-thalamic network compared to broader abnormalities in the cortico-brainstem-cerebello-thalamo-cortical network for patients with early onset (onset age < 30 years) essential tremor. Another possibility for cognitive impairment is concomitant pathological change related to aging, vascular comorbidities, and concurrent Parkinson disease or Alzheimer disease. In one study, essential tremor patients had a higher intracellular burden (neuronal tangles) of tau pathology. Still, there were no differences in the extracellular neuritic plaques between patients and controls, suggesting that increased accumulation of tau aggregates may predispose patients to cognitive impairment.[55]

While the underlying causes, risk factors, or progression of symptoms warrants further research, cognitive changes in essential tremor should be routinely included for dialogue between clinicians, patients, and their families. Furthermore, a battery of tests, including mini mental status examination (MMSE) or MoCA for global cognition, verbal fluency tests, the clock-drawing test, and the trail making test, along with a referral to a neuropsychologist, should be incorporated into the routine evaluation to guide the clinicians in managing the tremors more successfully.

Cognition in other tremor disorders

Cognitive dysfunction is one of the most prevalent nonmotor manifestations in Parkinson disease. Unlike essential tremor, cognitive decline affects about 80% of patients with Parkinson disease and is more prevalent older patients with the disease (greater than 70 years old), regardless of the age at onset of motor symptoms.[56] Although subtle and mild cognitive impairment may be noted at the motor onset, the severity of symptoms increases with disease progression.[57,58] The initial deficits involve attention span, problem-solving skills, and mental processing speed; however, as the burden of cognitive pathology increases, there is an emergence of visual-spatial impairment, visual misperceptions, and loss of semantic and episodic memory. Impairments in these cognitive domains are related to pathology in the parietal and temporal lobes.[59] Indeed, cognitive impairment becomes a significant determinant influencing the quality of life for patients with Parkinson disease. An important complicating factor is the use of anticholinergic medications such as benztropine and trihexyphenidyl for control of tremor, and one of their major limitations is cognitive dysfunction. However, patients with the akinetic-rigid or PIGD phenotypes are at a higher risk of cognitive decline compared to those with the tremor-predominant phenotype.[60] Thus, the relationship between tremor and cognitive dysfunction in Parkinson disease is intricate and warrants a careful approach when planning the treatment.

There is also early data to support cognitive dysfunction in other tremor disorders. In one study involving extensive neuropsychological testing for patients with orthostatic tremor poor performance was observed on tests of executive function, visuospatial ability, verbal memory, visual memory, and language tests when compared with healthy controls and adjusted for age in years, sex, years of education, comorbidity index, current smoker, and depressive symptoms, diagnosis. Older-onset (> 60 years) patients had poorer scores on cognitive and personality testing compared with their younger-onset counterparts.[61] Although there is increasing evidence for nonmotor impairments in dystonia, no study to date has focused on the prevalence and the specific challenges influencing treatment in dystonic tremor. Minimal data published for dystonia points toward deficits in executive, attentional, or visuospatial function; however, for most of the studies the sample size has been small, the patient population recruited was heterogeneous, and the confounding effects of age, form of dystonia, the severity of dystonia, education level, and medications used for treatment have not been included.[62]

ROLE OF NEUROPSYCHIATRIC FACTORS

Anxiety and depression in healthy populations can lead to tremor that either manifests as a fine, low amplitude, high-frequency physiological tremor involving the hands when the patient is engaged in day-to-day activities, or is sometimes evident in the voice. At the time of physical examination, tremor is mostly observed during the postural elevation of the arm and when the arms are observed during writing, drawing, and pouring tasks. An intentional component during the finger-nose-finger maneuver is not observed, and tremor does not seem to involve the head, trunk, or legs. Physiological tremor is also enhanced in the presence of stimulant intake, medications, or hormonal disturbances such as hyperthyroidism and hypoglycemia.[63] While these tremors often respond to beta-blocker medications, it is essential for clinicians to recognize the presence of underlying physiological factors that could potentially confound the assessment and treatment of pathological tremors.

Neuropsychiatric disturbances such as anxiety, depression, and personality changes have been reported frequently by studies in essential tremor. About 30% or more of patients may report mild depression, with concentration difficulties and lassitude as primary symptoms.[64,65] The pathophysiological basis for anxiety and depression symptoms in essential tremor is not clear and warrants further investigation. Then, anxiety and depression are some of the most frequently reported nonmotor manifestations of Parkinson disease. Anxiety, encompassing symptoms of apprehension, worry, fear, panic attacks, and social phobias, is seen in about 60% of patients, especially in females, patients with young-onset disease, and patients with advanced disease.[66] Anxiety commonly co-occurs with depression.[67,68] Depression alone affects about

35% of the patient population and can predate the onset of motor symptoms.[69] Symptoms of depression correlate with disease duration and disease severity, and, in some patients, is related to the dosage of dopaminergic medications. Anxiety and depression are biological, clinical manifestations related to Parkinson disease pathology.[66] Anxiety and depression are also linked to symptoms of cognitive decline and dementia, and together these can impact assessment and management of tremor in the clinic. While recent studies have identified nonmotor subtypes based on predominant cholinergic dysfunction (cognitive decline and falls), serotonergic dysfunction (somnolence and fatigue), or noradrenergic dysfunction (autonomic dysfunction),[70] it remains to be seen whether anxiety and depression are more prevalent in the tremor-predominant motor subtype. There is also evidence for the manifestation of depression before the motor symptoms of essential tremor.[71,72] Premorbid personality traits including "depressive," "introverted," "rigid," and "lonely" are observed in both essential tremor and Parkinson disease populations.[73] The prevalence of anxiety and depression in focal or generalized dystonia is similar to that of essential tremor and throughout a lifetime falls in the range of about 25–50%; however, to date, there is no data for dystonic tremor. In a comparative study, the frequency and intensity of depression were of similar magnitude in patients with essential tremor, Parkinson disease, and dystonia.[74] Patients reporting comorbid anxiety and depression likely underappreciate the benefits of tremor-controlling medications.

Tremor is an outwardly visible symptom. Studies have found a high prevalence of social embarrassment, as patients with essential tremor are negatively judged on a repeated basis by observers (e.g., as nervous, incompetent, defective, or intoxicated).[75–77] These patients have low self-esteem and lack confidence in navigating social situations.[78] Social embarrassment is often accompanied by emotional and autonomic consequences such as sweating, stuttering, increased heart rate and blood pressure, and blushing.[78] While tremor leads to social embarrassment, an increased level of emotional and autonomic activation associated with social embarrassment leads to a tremor's worsening. Thus, there is a self-perpetuating vicious cycle of tremor–social embarrassment–anxiety–tremor, a cycle that may be challenging to break.

CONCLUSIONS

In summary, with increasing evidence for non-motor manifestations, tremor disorders should no longer be regarded as monosymptomatic disorders. These nonmotor manifestations are critical determinants during evaluation and for managing tremor symptoms. Gait disturbances, balance impairment, cognitive dysfunction, and neuropsychiatric symptoms are common co-occurring features in patients with essential tremor and Parkinson disease. Cognition and gait disturbances are also relevant in the context of orthostatic tremor. While there is increasing support for nonmotor manifestations in dystonia, there is minimal data in dystonic tremor. Most studies have focused on dystonia and have not necessarily included patients with tremor. Physiological factors and medications exacerbate tremor and are additional important considerations. Clinicians should give due attention to co-occurring features in tremor disorders when formulating a treatment plan. While the importance of addressing these issues continues to increase, the underlying mechanistic and biological basis warrants further research to develop effective disease-specific treatments.

REFERENCES

1. Bhatia KP, Bain P, Bajaj N, et al. Consensus Statement on the classification of tremors from the task force on tremor of the International Parkinson and Movement Disorder Society. *Mov Disord.* 2018;33:75–87.
2. Marshall J. Observations on essential tremor. *J Neurol Neurosurg Psychiatry.* 1962;25:s.
3. Benito-León J. Essential tremor: from a monosymptomatic disorder to a more complex entity. *Neuroepidemiology.* 2008;31:191–192.
4. Louis ED, Benito-León J, Vega-Quiroga S, Bermejo-Pareja F. Cognitive and motor functional activity in non-demented community-dwelling essential tremor cases. *J Neurol Neurosurg Psychiatry.* 2010;81:997–1001.
5. Singer C, Sanchez-Ramos J, Weiner WJ. Gait abnormality in essential tremor. *Mov Disord.* 1994;9:193–196.
6. Kronenbuerger M, Konczak J, Ziegler W, et al. Balance and motor speech impairment in essential tremor. *Cerebellum (Lond).* 2009;8:389–398.
7. Cinar N, Sahin S, Okluoglu Onay T, Karsidag S. Balance in essential tremor during tandem gait: is the first mis-step an important finding? *J Clin Neurosci.* 2013;20:1433–1437.
8. Louis ED, Rios E, Rao AK. Tandem gait performance in essential tremor: clinical correlates and association with midline tremors. *Mov Disord.* 2010;25:1633–1638.
9. Hubble JP, Busenbark KL, Pahwa R, Lyons K, Koller WC. Clinical expression of essential tremor: effects of gender and age. *Mov Disord.* 1997;12:969–972.
10. Rao AK, Louis ED. Ataxic gait in essential tremor: a disease-associated feature? *Tremor Other Hyperkinet Mov (N Y).* 2019;9. doi: 10.7916/d8-28jq-8t52
11. Rao AK, Gillman A, Louis ED. Quantitative gait analysis in essential tremor reveals impairments that are maintained into advanced age. *Gait Posture.* 2011;34:65–70.
12. Rao AK, Uddin J, Gillman A, Louis ED. Cognitive motor interference during dual-task gait in essential tremor. *Gait Posture.* 2013;38:403–409.
13. Roemmich RT, Zeilman PR, Vaillancourt DE, Okun MS, Hass CJ. Gait variability magnitude but not structure is altered in essential tremor. *J Biomech.* 2013;46:2682–2687.
14. Hausdorff JM, Rios DA, Edelberg HK. Gait variability and fall risk in community-living older adults: a 1-year prospective study. *Arch Phys Med Rehab.* 2001;82:1050–1056.
15. Bove M, Marinelli L, Avanzino L, Marchese R, Abbruzzese G. Posturographic analysis of balance control in patients with essential tremor. *Mov Disord.* 2006;21:192–198.
16. Lim ES, Seo MW, Woo SR, Jeong SY, Jeong SK. Relationship between essential tremor and cerebellar dysfunction according to age. *J Clin Neurol.* 2005;1:76–80.
17. Louis ED, Kellner S, Morgan S, et al. Cognitive dysfunction is associated with greater imbalance and falls in essential tremor. *Front Neurol.* 2017;8:154.
18. Fasano A, Herzog J, Raethjen J, et al. Gait ataxia in essential tremor is differentially modulated by thalamic stimulation. *Brain.* 2010;133:3635–3648.
19. Wagle Shukla A, Okun MS. State of the art for deep brain stimulation therapy in movement disorders: a clinical and technological perspective. *IEEE Rev Biomed Eng.* 2016;9:219–233.
20. Kavanagh JJ, Wedderburn-Bisshop J, Keogh JW. Resistance training reduces force tremor and improves manual dexterity in older individuals with essential tremor. *J Mot Behav.* 2016;48:20–30.
21. Sequeira G, Keogh JW, Kavanagh JJ. Resistance training can improve fine manual dexterity in essential tremor patients: a preliminary study. *Arch Phys Med Rehab.* 2012;93:1466–1468.
22. Ulanowski EA, Danzl MM, Sims KM. Physical therapy for a patient with essential tremor and prolonged deep brain stimulation: a case report. *Tremor Other Hyperkinet Mov (N Y).* 2017;7:448.
23. Klebe S, Stolze H, Grensing K, Volkmann J, Wenzelburger R, Deuschl G. Influence of alcohol on gait in patients with essential tremor. *Neurology.* 2005;65:96–101.

24. van der Heeden JF, Marinus J, Martinez-Martin P, Rodriguez-Blazquez C, Geraedts VJ, van Hilten JJ. Postural instability and gait are associated with severity and prognosis of Parkinson disease. *Neurology.* 2016;86:2243–2250.

25. Herman T, Weiss A, Brozgol M, Giladi N, Hausdorff JM. Gait and balance in Parkinson's disease subtypes: objective measures and classification considerations. *J Neurol.* 2014;261:2401–2410.

26. Nieuwboer A, Giladi N. Characterizing freezing of gait in Parkinson's disease: models of an episodic phenomenon. *Mov Disord.* 2013;28:1509–1519.

27. Maidan I, Bernad-Elazari H, Gazit E, Giladi N, Hausdorff JM, Mirelman A. Changes in oxygenated hemoglobin link freezing of gait to frontal activation in patients with Parkinson disease: an fNIRS study of transient motor-cognitive failures. *J Neurol.* 2015;262:899–908.

28. Maidan I, Nieuwhof F, Bernad-Elazari H, et al. The role of the frontal lobe in complex walking among patients with Parkinson's disease and healthy older adults: an FNIRS study. *Neurorehabil Neural Repair.* 2016;30:963–971.

29. Arie L, Herman T, Shema-Shiratzky S, Giladi N, Hausdorff JM. Do cognition and other non-motor symptoms decline similarly among patients with Parkinson's disease motor subtypes? Findings from a 5-year prospective study. *J Neurol.* 2017;264:2149–2157.

30. Gilat M, Ehgoetz Martens KA, Miranda-Domínguez O, et al. Dysfunctional limbic circuitry underlying freezing of gait in Parkinson's disease. *Neuroscience.* 2018;374:119–132.

31. Opri E, Hu W, Jabarkheel Z, et al. Gait characterization for patients with orthostatic tremor. *Parkinsonism Relat Disord.* 2020;71:23–27.

32. Lombardi WJ, Woolston DJ, Roberts JW, Gross RE. Cognitive deficits in patients with essential tremor. *Neurology.* 2001;57:785–790.

33. Lacritz LH, Dewey Jr. R, Giller C, Cullum CM. Cognitive functioning in individuals with "benign" essential tremor. *J Int Neuropsychol Soc.* 2002;8:125–129.

34. Kim JS, Song IU, Shim YS, et al. Impact of tremor severity on cognition in elderly patients with essential tremor. *Neurocase.* 2010;16:50–58.

35. Benito-León J, Louis ED, Posada IJ, et al. Population-based case-control study of cognitive function in early Parkinson's disease (NEDICES). *J Neurol Sci.* 2011;310:176–182.

36. Bermejo-Pareja F. Essential tremor--a neurodegenerative disorder associated with cognitive defects? *Nat Rev Neurol.* 2011;7:273–282.

37. Bermejo-Pareja F, Louis ED, Benito-León J. Risk of incident dementia in essential tremor: a population-based study. *Mov Disord.* 2007;22:1573–1580.

38. Benito-León J, Louis ED, Bermejo-Pareja F. Elderly-onset essential tremor is associated with dementia. *Neurology.* 2006;66:1500–1505.

39. Thawani SP, Schupf N, Louis ED. Essential tremor is associated with dementia: prospective population-based study in New York. *Neurology.* 2009;73:621–625.

40. Muthuraman M, Deuschl G, Anwar AR, Mideksa KG, von Helmolt F, Schneider SA. Essential and aging-related tremor: differences of central control. *Mov Disord.* 2015;30:1673–1680.

41. Sengul Y, Sengul HS, Yucekaya SK, et al. Cognitive functions, fatigue, depression, anxiety, and sleep disturbances: assessment of nonmotor features in young patients with essential tremor. *Acta Neurologica Belgica.* 2015;115:281–287.

42. Troster AI, Woods SP, Fields JA, et al. Neuropsychological deficits in essential tremor: an expression of cerebello-thalamo-cortical pathophysiology? *European Journal of Neurology.* 2002;9:143–151.

43. Benito-León J, Louis ED, Bermejo-Pareja F. Population-based case-control study of cognitive function in essential tremor. *Neurology.* 2006;66:69–74.

44. Collins K, Rohl B, Morgan S, Huey ED, Louis ED, Cosentino S. Mild Cognitive Impairment Subtypes in a Cohort of Elderly Essential Tremor Cases. *Journal of the International Neuropsychological Society: JINS.* 2017;23:390–399.

45. Louis ED, Joyce JL, Cosentino S. Mind the gaps: what we don't know about cognitive impairment in essential tremor. *Parkinsonism Relat Disord.* 2019;63:10–19.

46. Frisina PG, Tse W, Hälbig TD, Libow LS. The pattern of cognitive-functional decline in elderly essential tremor patients: an exploratory-comparative study with Parkinson's and Alzheimer's disease patients. *J Am Med Dir Assoc.* 2009;10:238–242.

47. Schmahmann JD, Sherman JC. The cerebellar cognitive affective syndrome. *Brain.* 1998;121(Pt 4):561–579.

48. Archer DB, Coombes SA, Chu WT, et al. A widespread visually-sensitive functional network relates to symptoms in essential tremor. *Brain.* 2018;141:472–485.

49. DeSimone JC, Archer DB, Vaillancourt DE, Wagle Shukla A. Network-level connectivity is a critical feature distinguishing dystonic tremor and essential tremor. *Brain.* 2019;142(6):1644–1659. doi: 10.1093/brain/awz085. PMID: 30957839; PMCID: PMC6536846.

50. Fang W, Lv F, Luo T, et al. Abnormal regional homogeneity in patients with essential tremor revealed by resting-state functional MRI. *PLoS ONE.* 2013;8:e69199.

51. Feinberg DA, Moeller S, Smith SM, et al. Multiplexed echo planar imaging for sub-second whole brain FMRI and fast diffusion imaging. *PLoS ONE*. 2010;5:e15710.

52. Wallesch CW, Horn A. Long-term effects of cerebellar pathology on cognitive functions. *Brain Cogn*. 1990;14:19–25.

53. Louis ED. Essential tremor: evolving clinicopathological concepts in an era of intensive post-mortem enquiry. *Lancet Neurol*. 2010;9:613–622.

54. Rajput AH, Rajput A. Significance of cerebellar Purkinje cell loss to pathogenesis of essential tremor. *Parkinsonism Relat Disord*. 2011;17:410–412.

55. Pan JJ, Lee M, Honig LS, Vonsattel JP, Faust PL, Louis ED. Alzheimer's-related changes in nondemented essential tremor patients vs. controls: links between tau and tremor? *Parkinsonism Relat Disord*. 2014;20:655–658.

56. Hely MA, Reid WG, Adena MA, Halliday GM, Morris JG. The Sydney multicenter study of Parkinson's disease: the inevitability of dementia at 20 years. *Mov Disord*. 2008;23:837–844.

57. Kempster PA, O'Sullivan SS, Holton JL, Revesz T, Lees AJ. Relationships between age and late progression of Parkinson's disease: a clinicopathological study. *Brain*. 2010;133:1755–1762.

58. Schapira AHV, Chaudhuri KR, Jenner P. Nonmotor features of Parkinson disease. *Nat Rev Neurosci*. 2017;18:509.

59. Churchyard A, Lees AJ. The relationship between dementia and direct involvement of the hippocampus and amygdala in Parkinson's disease. *Neurology*. 1997;49:1570–1576.

60. Marras C, Chaudhuri KR. Nonmotor features of Parkinson's disease subtypes. *Mov Disord*. 2016;31:1095–1102.

61. Benito-León J, Louis ED, Puertas-Martín V, et al. Cognitive and neuropsychiatric features of orthostatic tremor: a case-control comparison. *J Neurol Sci*. 2016;361:137–143.

62. Kuyper DJ, Parra V, Aerts S, Okun MS, Kluger BM. Nonmotor manifestations of dystonia: a systematic review. *Mov Disord*. 2011;26:1206–1217.

63. Louis ED. Tremor. *Continuum (Minneapolis, Minn.)*. 2019;25:959–975.

64. Li ZW, Xie MJ, Tian DS, et al. Characteristics of depressive symptoms in essential tremor. *J Clin Neurosci* 2011;18:52–56.

65. Bermejo-Pareja F, Puertas-Martin V. Cognitive features of essential tremor: a review of the clinical aspects and possible mechanistic underpinnings.

66. *Tremor Other Hyperkinet Mov (N Y)*. 2012;2:02-74-541-1. doi: 10.7916/D89W0D7W.

67. Schapira AHV, Chaudhuri KR, Jenner P. Nonmotor features of Parkinson disease. *Nat Rev Neurosci*. 2017;18:435–450.

68. Lin CH, Lin JW, Liu YC, Chang CH, Wu RM. Risk of Parkinson's disease following anxiety disorders: a nationwide population-based cohort study. *Eur J Neurol*. 2015;22:1280–1287.

69. Brown RG, Landau S, Hindle JV, et al. Depression and anxiety related subtypes in Parkinson's disease. *J Neurol Neurosurg Psychiatry*. 2011;82:803–809.

70. Shiba M, Bower JH, Maraganore DM, et al. Anxiety disorders and depressive disorders preceding Parkinson's disease: a case-control study. *Mov Disord*. 2000;15:669–677.

71. Marras C, Chaudhuri KR, Titova N, Mestre TA. Therapy of Parkinson's Disease Subtypes. *Neurotherapeutics*. 2020;17:1366–1377.

72. Louis ED, Benito-León J, Bermejo-Pareja F. Self-reported depression and anti-depressant medication use in essential tremor: cross-sectional and prospective analyses in a population-based study. *Eur J Neurol*. 2007;14:1138–1146.

73. Dogu O, Sevim S, Camdeviren H, et al. Prevalence of essential tremor: door-to-door neurologic exams in Mersin Province, Turkey. *Neurology*. 2003;61:1804–1806.

74. Poewe W, Karamat E, Kemmler GW, Gerstenbrand F. The premorbid personality of patients with Parkinson's disease: a comparative study with healthy controls and patients with essential tremor. *Adv Neurol*. 1990;53:339–342.

75. Miller KM, Okun MS, Fernandez HF, Jacobson CE, Rodriguez RL, Bowers D. Depression symptoms in movement disorders: comparing Parkinson's disease, dystonia, and essential tremor. *Mov Disord*. 2007;22:666–672.

76. Louis ED, Rios E. Embarrassment in essential tremor: prevalence, clinical correlates and therapeutic implications. *Parkinsonism Relat Disord*. 2009;15:535–538.

77. Holding SJ, Lew AR. Relations between psychological avoidance, symptom severity and embarrassment in essential tremor. *Chronic Illn*. 2015;11:69–71.

78. Louis ED, Rohl B, Rice C. Defining the treatment gap: what essential tremor patients want that they are not getting. *Tremor Other Hyperkinet Mov (N Y)*. 2015;5:331.

79. Keltner D, Buswell BN. Embarrassment: its distinct form and appeasement functions. *Psychol Bull*. 1997;122:250–270.

Tremor: Emerging and Investigational Treatments

WILLIAM ONDO

INTRODUCTION

Tremor is defined by rhythmic oscillations around a point. Human tremor is segregated into rest tremor, most commonly seen in Parkinson disease (PD), and action tremor. Action tremor is subsequently segregated by phenomenology (postural tremor, kinetic tremor, intention tremor) and by specific diagnostic labels (cerebellar outflow tremor, task specific tremor, dystonic tremor, orthostatic tremor, and most commonly essential tremor (ET). There is almost no active therapeutic research specifically evaluating rest tremor, except as part of overall PD treatment, or cerebellar outflow tremor, apart from overall ataxia treatment. Likewise, specific action tremor disorders such as dystonic tremor, task specific tremor, and orthostatic tremor have no clear therapeutic pipelines. Therefore, the chapter will focus on future treatments for ET.

ET, also known as benign essential tremor, familial tremor, or senile tremor is a common neurologic syndrome manifested by involuntary rhythmic oscillatory movement with volitional muscle action. Exact diagnostic criteria have varied modestly over time, and the clinical syndrome is likely pathophysiologically heterogeneous. The most recent tremor consensus tremor classification system emphasizes a 2-axis classification based on clinical characteristics (anatomy, frequency, quality, etc.) and etiology (acquired, genetic, or idiopathic).[1] The condition is common, impacting up to 4% of all people, can occur at any age with bimodal peaks in the second and sixth decades, and gradually worsens over time.

The pathophysiology of ET is only partially illuminated. There is some understanding of culpable macro-circuitry, mostly based on functional PET/SPECT studies, functional MRI, tractography, transcranial stimulation, and other electrophysiological techniques.[2] However, there is very little understanding at the cellular level. Postmortem pathology of ET is inconsistent; variably being normal, demonstrating Lewy body pathology, cerebellar Purkinje cell degeneration,[3,4] and altered inferior olivary climbing fiber anatomy in the Purkinje cell layer.[5]

No currently available medication used for ET was specifically developed for this purpose. The most commonly used oral treatments are non-cardiac selective beta-adrenergic antagonists (B-blockers), primidone, and topiramate. [Table 21.1] If these are not adequate, deep brain stimulation, most commonly of the ventral intermediate (VIM) thalamus, can markedly improve symptoms. Recently, however, improved physiologic understanding, improved technology, and improved assessment techniques are facilitating rationally designed ET drug development and more sophisticated surgical and peripheral electromechanical treatments. This chapter will review recently developed and investigational medications, devices, and surgical treatments of ET.

ALCOHOLS

Ethanol reduces ET severity in approximately two-thirds of patients.[6] Improvement can be rapid and robust. Onset to tremor suppression typically takes 10–15 minutes and lasts 3–4 hours. A rebound tremor exacerbation is reported by many patients. Improvement is mostly derived from the central nervous system (CNS), based on weight loading studies and reduced cerebellar activity on PET following ingestion.[7] The exact cellular mechanism by which alcohol improves ET is unclear, but GABAergic agonism and cellular decoupling are possible explanations.[8]

Octanol, an 8-carbon alcohol used as a food flavoring agent is metabolized to octanoic acid, which is now thought to be its active metabolite. Several open label and controlled studies have shown a short duration benefit (90–120 minutes) in tremor without problematic side effects.[9–11] The medicine has minimal adverse effects and has a long-established use at smaller doses in humans.

TABLE 21.1 LEVEL OF EFFICACY, MECHANISM OF ACTION, DAILY DOSAGE, AND COMMON SIDE EFFECTS OF CURRENTLY USED AND INVESTIGATIONAL MEDICATIONS IN ESSENTIAL TREMOR

Medication	Efficacy	Mechanism of action	Daily dose Doses per day	Common side effects
Ethanol	+++	GABAo	1 drink	Intoxication
Topiramate	+++	GABAo, CAI, Na, AMPA GABAs	50–400 2/day	Paresthesia, altered taste, weight loss, worse cognition
Primidone	+++	GABAo, Na	50–300 2–3/day	Sedation, dizzy, ataxia
Propranolol	+++	*Beta*	20–240 1–3/day	Fatigue, hypotension, bradycardia
Phenobarbital	++	GABAo, AMPA	30–180 1/day	Sedation, balance
Benzodiazepines	++	GABAo	variable	Sedation, ataxia
Dihydropyridines Nicardipine nifedipine nimodipine	+	Ca^{2+}	variable	Low BP, flushing
Gabapentin	+	Ca^{2+} α2γ	300–3600 2–3/day	Sedation, dizziness, edema
Pregabalin	+	Ca^{2+} α2γ	100–400 2–3/day	Sedation, dizziness, edema, weight gain
Zonisamide	+	Ca^{2+} LVA, Na	100–300 2/day	Malaise, weight loss
Levetiracetam	+	AMPA, GABAo, Na	500–3000 2/day	Agitation
Acetazolamide	+	CAI		Diuresis
CX-8998	?	Ca^{2+} T	Not available	Dizziness
PRAX-944	?	Ca^{2+} T	Not available	?
CAD-1883	?	PAM SK	Not available	?
Sage-324	?	GABAo	Not available	?

AMPA = *blocks glutamate release and/or inhibits* AMPA alpha-amino-3-hydroxy-5-methylisoxazole-4-propionic acid, Beta = blocks *B*1 and *B*2 adrenergic receptors, CAI = carbonic anhydrase inhibitor, Ca^{2+} = non-selective Calcium channel inhibition, usually more affinity for Ca^{2+} L, Ca^{2+} α2γ = inhibits alpha-2 delta subunit of calcium channel blocker, Ca^{2+} L = L-type (Ca_v1) antagonist, Ca^{2+} T = T-type (Ca_v3) antagonist, GABAo = opens or potentiates GABA receptors, GABAs = increases GABA synthesis, GABAr = inhibits GABA re-uptake or metabolism, NA = inhibits sodium channels, PAM SK = positive allosteric modulator of small conductance Ca^{2+} activated K^+ channels (SK channels), SV2A = inhibits synaptic vesicle glycoprotein receptor

Future development for tremor is unclear. Methylpentynol, a six-carbon chain alcohol, proved clinically ineffective when compared to placebo.[12] Therefore, it is not clear whether alcohols improve tremor as a class or whether it is specific to individual compounds.

Sodium oxybate (Xyrem®) is the sodium salt of δ-hydroxybutyric acid (GHB) a powerful sedating hypnotic currently approved for cataplexy. GHB can be a precursor to GABA and glutamate, but the mechanism of action (MOA) is unclear. It has similar but exaggerated clinical properties as ethanol. Sodium oxybate has been reported to improve tremor but is unlikely to have much utility secondary to extreme sedation and abuse potential.[13] Recently, a new salt solution (ZZP-258, Xywav™), using much less sodium, was approved for narcolepsy/cataplexy, but has not been tested in tremor.

A longer-acting deuterated version (JZP-386) is being developed, but there are no current plans for its development as a tremor treatment.

AMPA RECEPTOR ANTAGONISTS

Glutamate is the most common excitatory neurotransmitter and has wide brain distribution. The main receptors for glutamate are kainate, N-methyl-D-aspartate (NMDA), and alpha-aminon-3-hydroxy-5-methylisoxazole-4-proprionic acid (AMPA). AMPA receptors are prominent in the cerebellum cortex and seem to increase Purkinje cell spike synchrony.[14] Furthermore, AMPA antagonists have demonstrated reduced tremor in harmaline models.[15] Topiramate, levetiracetam, and phenobarbital all modestly effect AMPA receptors.

The AMPA receptor antagonist perampanel, a relatively new anti-epileptic drug (AED), markedly and specifically inhibits AMPA receptors. In an open label study, Gironell et al. reported that perampanel titrated up to 4mg/day markedly improved tremor in 8/12 subjects using several tremor assessments.[16] The other 4 subjects dropped out secondary to adverse events. Handforth et al. published a placebo-controlled crossover trial of 26 randomized subjects titrating up to 8mg/day.[17] The primary efficacy point was a videotaped TETRAS scale[18] rated by an independent examiner. This study also suffered from frequent dropouts secondary to adverse events (AEs), 11 subjects on drug, most commonly imbalance, sedation, fatigue, irritability, and worsening cognition. AEs were dose dependent resulting in a mean finishing dose of 6 mg/day. Nevertheless, intention to treat analysis showed significant improvement in the videotaped TETRAS performance (motor exam) and TETRAS Activities of Daily Living (ADL) scales, but not the quality of life in essential tremor (QUEST) scale.

Overall, preliminary data reports intriguing benefit of perampanel for ET, although the drug is poorly tolerated. Future plans for development are unknown.

OLDER CALCIUM CHANNEL BLOCKERS

There are many overlapping calcium channel subtypes, some of which have been implicated in tremor genesis. Although calcium channel antagonists are historically used for cardiovascular purposes, there is literature supporting use for tremor.

Flunarizine, a piperazine derivative diphenylalkylamine slow channel calcium channel blocker widely available outside the United States, demonstrated clinical and electrophysiologic efficacy, at 10 mg/d, in one 15-subject placebo-controlled crossover trial[19] but not in another trial for refractory patients.[20] Flunarizine commonly causes parkinsonism, so it should be used with caution. Nicardipine demonstrated short-term accelerometry amplitude reduction over placebo but failed to sustain statistical improvement over a one-month period.[21] A separate placebo-controlled trial comparing propranolol 160 mg/day to nicardipine 1mg/kg/day reported that both medications were superior to placebo but that propranolol tended to show greater efficacy than nicardipine on a clinical scale.[22] Nimodipine at 30mg Q.I.D, another dihydropyridine-sensitive calcium channel blocker, was superior to placebo in one small, controlled crossover trial using accelerometry and subjective reporting.[23] Ethosuximide, a

moderate affinity T-type Ca blocker, did not show benefit in a small trial.[24] Despite these data, available Ca blockers have not been widely used for tremor. However, several novel T-type Ca blockers are currently under investigation.

INVESTIGATIONAL CALCIUM CHANNEL BLOCKERS

T-type calcium channel blocking medications are being investigated for ET. T-type (a.k.a. low voltage) and Cav3 calcium channels are predominately neuronal and have minimal cardiovascular impact. They are especially abundant in the thalamus, cerebellum, and cortex; are thought to play a role in rhythmic neuronal firing; and can mitigate spontaneous action potentials in vitro by altering the resting membrane potential.[25] In the murine harmaline tremor model, Cav3.1 knockout mice demonstrate essentially no tremor. One Cav3.1 subunit gene (*CACNA1G*) segregates with tremor in whole genome sequencing studies,[26] but is also implicated in other phenotypes including ataxia.

CX-8998/JZP-385 (Cavion, now owned by Jazz Pharmaceuticals) is a highly selective Cav3 antagonist with good CNS penetration and a 10- to 13-hour $T_{1/2}$, previously tested for schizophrenia. In preclinical trials, CX-8998 improved harmaline and GABA-A knockout tremor models.[27]

A 95-subject, Phase-2 trial randomized CX-8998 (10 mg BID) 1:1 against placebo for 28 days showed benefit in some tremor measures.[28] Subjects (18–75 years) could concurrently take one other stable ET drug, except primidone. Efficacy points included a videotaped centrally rated blinded TETRAS[29] performance scale, locally done TETRAS performance scale, subjective TETRAS-ADL scale, clinical global impressions (CGI), and accelerometry. Safety data in this study, and previous studies, was generally good; however, dropout secondary to AE was 17% in CX-8998 vs. 6% in placebo in this trial. Dizziness was the adverse evet that most separated from placebo (42% vs. 21%). The locally rated TETRAS performance ($p<0.05$), TETRAS-ADL section ($p<0.05$), and CGI ($p<0.05$) favored drug, whereas centrally rated TETRAS performance and accelerometry did not. The compound was purchased by Jazz Pharmaceuticals and future studies are starting.

PRAX-944 (Praxis Precision Medicines) is also a T-type calcium channel antagonist that shows similar affinity to Cav 3.1, 3.2, and 3.3 receptors. It has been shown to interrupt burst and rhythmic firing in several animal models including the harmaline model and a T channel gain of function model.[30] In humans, the drug reduces rhythmic sigma firing seen in non-REM sleep, which is analogous to spindle activity seen on polysomnogram.[31]

Preliminary Phase 1 human safety data from approximately 100 subjects is unremarkable. A small, multi-center, Phase 2A study using a once-daily, sustained-release dose of 20 and 40 mg is ongoing in Australia. [ACTRN12619001052123] and another is planned for North America. PRAX-944 is also being evaluated for epilepsy.

SK CHANNEL POSITIVE ALLOSTERIC MODULATOR: CAD-1883

CAD-1883 recently renamed Rimtuzalcap, (Cadent Pharmaceuticals, now owned by Novartis) is a positive allosteric modulation (PAM) of small-conductance Ca^{2+} activated K^+ channels (SK channels). SK channels are activated by increasing intracellular Ca^{2+} concentrations and play a central role in neuronal repolarization following a spike and in the fast component of the after-hyperpolarization.[32,33] They seem to regulate somatic excitability and have been most studied in the context of synaptic plasticity.

ET may be caused by, or at least associated with, hypersynchronized firing of Purkinje cells in the cerebellar cortex.[34] Since SK channels mediate after-hyperpolarization and burst termination in cerebellar Purkinje cells, modulation of the SK channel could restore a normalized firing pattern and reduce tremor by desynchronizing Purkinje cell output.

The starting chemical points for CAD-1883 contained a 1,3-pyrimidyl chemical core similar to CyPPA, a modestly potent SK PAM.[33] The drug modulates cerebellar Purkinje cell firing in mouse brain slices and reduces forepaw and axial tremor in the harmaline murine model of tremor. [Kuo, S. personal communication 2020]

In Phase 1 controlled trials with healthy volunteers, CAD-1883 was well tolerated at doses up to 1200 mg/day, demonstrated no food nor gender effect, and achieved steady-state plasma concentrations several-fold higher than the level projected to be required for efficacy based on animal models. A small Phase 2a trial is in progress. [ClinicalTrials.gov Identifier: NCT03688685]

POSITIVE ALLOSTERIC MODULATORS OF GABA RECEPTORS

Gamma-aminobutyric acid (GABA-A) receptors are ligand gated ion channels resulting in

chloride (Cl-) influx that hyperpolarizes cells, and therefore inhibit their downstream signaling. The GABA-A receptor is a pentamer, variably employing 5 of 19 different proteins (*alpha* 1–6, *beta* 1–3, *gamma* 1–3, *delta, epsilon, theta, pi, rho* 1–3).[35,36] The most common arrangement is two *alpha*, two *beta*, and one *gamma*. Alpha-1 is the overall most common subunit, and is especially present in synaptic receptors, which rapidly open and close. Extra-synaptic GABA-A receptors actually have higher affinity for endogenous GABA, and contain more *delta* subunits.[37] Stimulation of these extra-synaptic receptors causes more tonic receptor opening and subsequent inhibition.

Sage Therapeutics developed a series of positive allosteric steroid modulators of GABA-A receptors, several of which have been evaluated for ET. These drugs potentiate both synaptic and extra-synaptic receptors, in contrast to benzodiazepines and barbiturates (primidone), which largely stimulate only synaptic receptors. The active site transverses alpha and beta subunits at a point within the cellular membrane, and is distinct from that of benzodiazepines, barbiturates, or endogenous GABA.

Physiologically, this class reduces occipital *beta* activity, a possible biomarker for tremor. Despite the steroid structure backbone, these drugs do not have immunologic properties, hormonal properties, or mineralocorticoid properties. Brexanolone (Sage 547), an intravenous preparation, and Zuranolone (Sage 217), an oral preparation, both underwent small exploratory ET trials. [ClinicalTrials.gov Identifier: NCT02277106]. However, future tremor studies are not planned for either drug. Brexanolone was recently approved for postpartum depression in the US. Zuranolone is being studied in several depression trials. Sage 324, an oral allosteric modulator with a very long $T_{1/2}$, is currently being investigated in a large placebo-controlled Phase 2 ET trial. [ClinicalTrials.gov Identifier: NCT04305275]. Previously, a small 6-subject open label trial showed improved accelerometry scores, which correlated with reduction in *beta* frequency occipital EEG activity. [Takahashi, K. Personal Communication 2020]

BOTULINUM TOXIN INJECTIONS

Botulinum toxin A and B (BoNT) successfully treat a variety of involuntary movements. Currently there are 4 widely available BoNT: 3 type A toxins (ona-, inco-, and abobotulinum toxinA), and 1 type B (rimabotulinum toxinB).

A fourth type A toxin, daxi-botulinum toxinA, is pending approval. The goal is to weaken the muscle generating tremor without inducing functional weakness.

Numerous open label studies and a few controlled trials have reported benefits of BoNT for hand tremor associated with ET, but also for PD, dystonic tremor, and to a lesser extent cerebellar outflow tremor.[38] In ET, open label studies that allow for flexible dosing demonstrate greater subjective benefits and improved quality of life scales. Treatment requires individualized muscle selection, necessitating a good understanding of anatomy. The role of electromyographic and ultrasound guidance to improve injection accuracy is not clearly established but may improve the efficacy to side effect ratio in some cases. Computerized kinematic tremor analysis guidance localization has also been recently advocated.[39] There are no prospective comparative trials evaluating either different injection techniques or different toxins in ET.

Head tremor in ET may respond particularly well to BoNT, although there is limited controlled data.[40] In general, posterior muscles such as capitus splenius are most targeted. Vocal cord injections (thyroarytenoid, cricothyroid, or thyrohyoid muscles) can variably improve voice tremor to a similar degree overall as propranolol.[41] Vocal cord injections are done via EMG or direct visualization and muscle selection, especially whether to inject a smaller dose bilaterally or larger dose unilaterally, is individualized.

In the author's experience, BoNT often effectively treats head tremor, jaw tremor, and hand tremor that oscillates mostly around the wrist. Larger amplitude proximal arm tremors and tremor oscillating around finger joints (metacarpophalangeal, and proximal and distal interphalangeal joints) are more difficult to inject secondary to functional weakness side effects. A large, multi-center, controlled trial of incobotulinumtoxin-A for ET is being planned.

DEEP BRAIN STIMULATION AND LESIONING THERAPIES

VIM DBS is a long-established treatment for ET and will be discussed in detail elsewhere. Numerous series have reported marked contralateral tremor reduction in 68%–100% of patients.[42] Head and voice tremor also improve but this may not be as robust. DBS into the subthalamic nucleus (STN) and zona incerta (ZI) are less established for ET.[43] DBS is also used for other tremor types but results for dystonic

tremor and cerebellar outflow tremor show less functional improvement compared to ET.[44,45] Recent advances in DBS include different lead configurations allowing greater adjustment fidelity, improved and smaller batteries, and a device that reads local field potentials attempting to identify beta frequency which may eventually auto-adjust stimulation patterns in real time based on those local field potentials. Improved battery function and lead density could improve ET, although the beta band identification is specific to PD.

Stereotaxic radiofrequency thalamotomy is also a safe and effective treatment of ET, used for almost 70 years. One large prospective study comparing VIM DBS to thalamotomy found that they were equally effective, but that DBS had a better safety profile.[46] So, despite the fact that stereotactic thalamotomy is faster, cheaper, and requires only minimal subsequent care, traditional radiofrequency thalamotomy, which requires insertion of a probe to electrically burn a lesion, has been little used over the past two decades.

More recently, focused ultrasound (FUS) lesioning has been developed to create highly targeted brain lesioning. The device (Exablate, InSightec) uses up to 1,080 transcranial, synchronized ultrasound waves that coalesce to create a targeted thermal lesion. [Figure 21.1] The procedure is done in an MRI scanner and lesion location can be adjusted in almost real time by slightly heating the area, then identifying it on a specially sequenced MRI. The lesion can then be adjusted in any dimension prior to increasing power enough to raise temperature to 55 C for approximately 40 seconds, making a permanent lesion. The partial warming often also reduces tremor, thus adding a physiologic clinical assessment, similar to DBS intraoperative stimulation, prior to permanent lesioning. Target fidelity based on postoperative MRI is excellent, usually within 1 mm of the planned target.

A large, sham-controlled, well blinded, clinical trial demonstrate marked tremor reduction in the targeted arm.[47] Adverse events were modest, usually transient sensory disturbance, transient balance problems, with rare cases of dysarthria. Potential loss of effect over time has been a concern but one recent 4-year open label report showed continued benefit in most subjects.[48] Repeat procedures are also possible.[49] No prospective FUS vs. DBS trial exists but retrospective data and published study comparisons show equal efficacy and an overall equal adverse event burden.[50] FUS appears cost effective, especially compared to

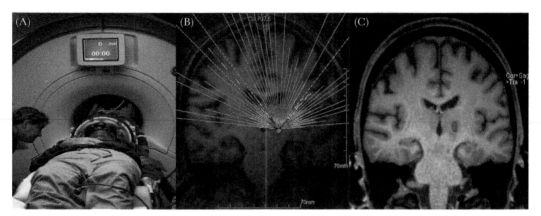

FIGURE 21.1: (A) Exablate™ device with procedure done in MRI; (B) Computer-Simulated targeting into the VIM Nucleus; (C) Post-procedure lesion.

DBS, and the device is currently approved by U.S. regulatory agencies for ET.[51] Bilateral FUS VIM lesioning trials are ongoing but this is not yet recommended. Alternative lesion targets specifically the posterior part of the subthalamus also show benefit in ET.[52] VIM lesioning is also reported to improve tremor in PD.[53] Cases of improved dystonic tremor are also reported.[54] The same technique is also used for lesions in the GPI and STN for dystonia and Parkinson disease.

Although "incisionless," FUS creates a permanent lesion so is not "non-invasive." It requires patients to completely shave their head and importantly, about 8% of the population is not eligible secondary to skull thickness and lack of skull windows, which in eligible patients might also mitigate efficacy.[55] Potential high initial costs to purchase the device, and relatively modest reimbursement compared to DBS, have limited use to date.

One group reported marked benefit of ET after unilateral laser thalamotomy.[56] Localization is MRI guided using the Clearpoint stereotactic system. The procedure requires electrode penetration into the VIM thalamus, similar to traditional radiofrequency thalamotomy, but uses a laser instead of electrically generated thermal ablation, potentially resulting in more consistent and accurate localization. A 13-subject open label trial for tremor (8 with ET) showed a mean 62% reduction in target limb tremor scores maintained at 3–17 months.

Gamma knife thalamotomy uses extracranial cobalt radiation from a circular collimator to create a lesion, thus obviating the need for surgical craniotomy. It has been used in ET for many years, and some open label data report good long-term results,[57] although the only blinded trial did not show any statistical benefit.[58] The functional lesion can take months to develop, and targeting can't be refined, so fidelity is not consistent, sometimes resulting in permanent neurological deficits. A potentially more accurate and localizing linear accelerator radiosurgery technique is called virtual cone, which uses a multileaf collimator.[59] The VIM is targeted with 130 Gy delivered through a high-definition multi-lead collimator. The radiation is delivered in 20 half-arches with the goal of creating a 4 mm sphere.

NOVEL PERIPHERAL ELECTRIC AND MECHANICAL HAND TREMOR TREATMENTS

Peripheral nerve stimulation can create field potentials in the brain and has been used for many years to treat pain. Alternating peripheral nerve stimulation is thought to impact CNS neural circuits involved in ET, potentially interfering with CNS tremor circuit pathways.[60] Therefore, Transcutaneous Afferent Patterned Stimulation (TAPS) neuromodulation of peripheral nerves could improve CNS-generated tremor. The Cala Trio™ is a small wrist-worn device that delivers current alternating over the medial and radial nerve at a frequency synced to the patient's tremor. The device voltage is titrated up as tolerated and typically worn for 40 minutes/day.

A short, 77-subject, single-treatment, sham-controlled trial showed improved TETRAS and simulated ADL scores, but not improved spiral ratings, immediately after stimulation in the target limb.[61,62] A large, 263 subject, 3-month open label study employed 2 stimulation periods/day.

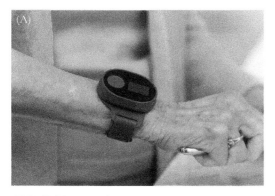 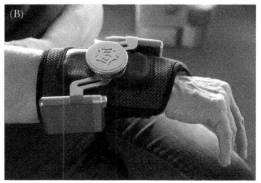

FIGURES 21.2A AND B: (A) CALA Trio™ device; (B) 5 Micron Tremelo™ device.

In the 205 completers, examination (TETRAS) and ADL scales improved.[63] Accelerometry scores, measured by the device, also improved. Results were similar in patients taking and not taking ET medications. Irritation at the electrode site, the only common AE, was reported by 18% of subjects. The Cala Trio™ device is available via prescription (Figure 21.2A).

Low-frequency transcranial magnetic stimulation to the cerebellum[64,65] and supplementary motor area[66] have shown modest or no benefit in short-term trials. The treatments consist of daily sessions of 1-Hz stimulation for weeks. Adverse events appear negligible.

Spring-operated counterbalance dampening devices, using the same principle employed in building construction to minimize wind-induced sway, have been tested in tremor patients with mixed results [Nguyen L. Personal Communication 2020]. In 2020, Five Microns began marketing their Tremelo™ device, which uses 2 mechanical spring dampeners, tuned with tremor frequency, to physically suppress hand tremor (Figure 21.2B). There is no published data, and the device is available for purchase without prescription.

Simple limb weighting (strapping a weight to the hand/wrist) may dampen tremor, but is not generally considered to improve function secondary to loss of coordination and dexterity. Many of these weights are available without prescription.

Accelerometer-engineered eating utensils, which shift the utensil tip opposite to the immediate hand tremor vector in order to lessen the total displacement of the utensil tip, have been developed and are generally preferred to simple weighted devices.[67] Several of these, including Majic Spoon™, Liftware™, and Gyenno™, are currently marketed without prescription. Controlled trials are lacking.

A gyroscope glove that dampens movement in all directions is being developed for hand tremor (Gyrogear™). The single gyroscope revolves at very high speed and reduces movement in all directions. Preliminary data with several prototypes are encouraging, but no published data exists. Phase 2/3 trials are being planned [Ong F. Personal Communication 2020].

Specific devices to physically dampen tremor specifically while writing have also been developed but are not commercially available.

CONCLUSION

ET treatments include oral medications, botulinum injections, CNS surgical interventions, and peripheral devices. Although existing treatments are effective in many cases, additional treatment options are clearly needed.[68] Multiple oral agents including JZP-385/CX-8998, ZPRAX-944, CAD-1883, and Sage 324 are undergoing Phase 2/3 trials for ET. Advances in lesioning strategies with focused ultrasound, laser lesioning, and possibly improved Gamma knife methods, as well as continued improvement in DBS technologies, will continue to help patients with severe tremor. Peripheral devices, including counterweighting strategies, accelerometry compensatory tools, gyroscope gloves, and peripheral stimulation with the Cala Trio, will likely lessen disability from tremor in many cases. Although there is little in development for non-ET tremor, some of these treatments will likely be tried for other tremor types.

REFERENCES

1. Bhatia KP, Bain P, Bajaj N, et al. Consensus statement on the classification of tremors. from the task force on tremor of the International Parkinson and Movement Disorder Society. *Mov Disord.* 2018;33(1):75–87.

2. Buijink AW, van der Stouwe AM, Broersma M, et al. Motor network disruption in essential tremor: a functional and effective connectivity study. *Brain.* 2015;138(Pt 10):2934–2947.

3. Erickson-Davis CR, Faust PL, Vonsattel JP, Gupta S, Honig LS, Louis ED. "Hairy baskets" associated with degenerative Purkinje cell changes in essential tremor. *J Neuropathol Exp Neurol.* 2010;69(3):262–271.

4. Rajput AH, Adler CH, Shill HA, Rajput A. Essential tremor is not a neurodegenerative disease. *Neurodegener Dis Manag.* 2012;2(3):259–268.

5. Louis RJ, Lin CY, Faust PL, Koeppen AH, Kuo SH. Climbing fiber synaptic changes correlate with clinical features in essential tremor. *Neurology.* 2015;84(22):2284–2286.

6. Koller WC, Biary N. Effect of alcohol on tremors: comparison with propranolol. *Neurology.* 1984;34(2):221–222.

7. Boecker H, Wills AJ, Ceballos-Baumann A, et al. The effect of ethanol on alcohol-responsive essential tremor: a positron emission tomography study. *Ann Neurol.* 1996;39(5):650–658.

8. Zeuner KE, Molloy FM, Shoge RO, Goldstein SR, Wesley R, Hallett M. Effect of ethanol on the central oscillator in essential tremor. *Mov Disord.* 2003;18(11):1280–1285.

9. Bushara KO, Goldstein SR, Grimes GJ, Jr., Burstein AH, Hallett M. Pilot trial of 1-octanol in essential tremor. *Neurology.* 2004;62(1):122–124.

10. Voller B, Lines E, McCrossin G, et al. Dose-escalation study of octanoic acid in patients with essential tremor. *J Clin Invest.* 2016;126(4):1451–1457.

11. Shill HA, Bushara KO, Mari Z, Reich M, Hallett M. Open-label dose-escalation study of oral 1-octanol in patients with essential tremor. *Neurology.* 2004;62(12):2320–2322.

12. Teravainen H, Huttunen J, Lewitt P. Ineffective treatment of essential tremor with an alcohol, methylpentynol. *J Neurol Neurosurg Psychiatry.* 1986;49(2):198–199.

13. Frucht SJ, Bordelon Y, Houghton WH, Reardan D. A pilot tolerability and efficacy trial of sodium oxybate in ethanol-responsive movement disorders. *Mov Disord.* 2005;20(10):1330–1337.

14. Lang EJ. GABAergic and glutamatergic modulation of spontaneous and motor-cortex-evoked complex spike activity. *J Neurophysiol.* 2002;87(4):1993–2008.

15. Mignani S, Bohme GA, Birraux G, et al. 9-Carboxymethyl-5H,10H-imidazo[1,2-a]indeno[1,2-e]pyrazin-4-one-2-carbocylic acid (RPR117824): selective anticonvulsive and neuroprotective AMPA antagonist. *Bioorg Med Chem.* 2002;10(5):1627–1637.

16. Gironell A, Pascual-Sedano B, Marin-Lahoz J. Perampanel, a new hope for essential tremor: an open label trial. *Parkinsonism Relat Disord.* 2019;60:171–172.

17. Handforth A, Tse W, Elble RJ. A pilot double-blind randomized trial of perampanel for essential tremor. *Mov Disord Clin Pract.* 2020;7(4):399–404.

18. Elble R. The essential tremor rating scale. *J Neuro Neuromed.* 2016;1(4):34–38.

19. Biary N, al Deeb SM, Langenberg P. The effect of flunarizine on essential tremor. *Neurology.* 1991;41(2 (Pt 1)):311–312.

20. Curran T, Lang AE. Flunarizine in essential tremor. *Clin Neuropharmacol.* 1993;16(5):460–463.

21. Garcia Ruiz PJ, Garcia de Yebenes Prous J, Jimenez Proust J. Effect of nicardipine on essential tremor: brief report. *Clin Neuropharmacol.* 1993;16(5):456–459.

22. Mitsuda M, Nomoto M, Iwata S. Effects of beta-blockers and nicardipine on oxotremorine-induced tremor in common marmosets. *Jpn J Pharmacol.* 1999;81(2):244–246.

23. Biary N, Bahou Y, Sofi MA, Thomas W, al Deeb SM. The effect of nimodipine on essential tremor. *Neurology.* 1995;45(8):1523–1525.

24. Gironell A, Marin-Lahoz J. Ethosuximide for essential tremor: an open-label trial. *Tremor Other Hyperkinet Mov (N Y).* 2016;6:378.

25. Dreyfus FM, Tscherter A, Errington AC, et al. Selective T-type calcium channel block in thalamic neurons reveals channel redundancy and physiological impact of I(T)window. *J Neurosci.* 2010;30(1):99–109.

26. Odgerel Z, Sonti S, Hernandez N, et al. Whole genome sequencing and rare variant analysis in essential tremor families. *PLoS ONE.* 2019;14(8):e0220512.

27. Handforth A, Homanics GE, Covey DF, et al. T-type calcium channel antagonists suppress tremor in two mouse models of essential tremor. *Neuropharmacology.* 2010;59(6):380–387.

28. Papapetropoulos S, Lee M, Versavel S, et al. A phase 2, proof-of-concept, randomized, placebo-controlled trial of CX-8998 in essential tremor. *Mov Disord.* 2021. doi: 10.1002/mds.285842

29. Elble R, Comella C, Fahn S, et al. Reliability of a new scale for essential tremor. *Mov Disord.* 2012;27(12):1567–1569.

30. Cain SM, Tyson JR, Jones KL, Snutch TP. Thalamocortical neurons display suppressed burst-firing due to an enhanced Ih current in a genetic model of absence epilepsy. *Pflugers Arch.* 2015;467(6):1367–1382.

31. Scott L, Puryear CB, Belfort GM, Raines S, Hughes ZA, Matthews LG, Ravina B, Wittmann M. Translational pharmacology of PRAX-944, a novel T-type calcium channel blocker in development for the treatment of essential tremor. *Mov Disord.* 2022 Mar 7. doi: 10.1002/mds.28969. Epub ahead of print. PMID: 35257414.

32. Adelman JP, Maylie J, Sah P. Small-conductance Ca2+-activated K+ channels: form and function. *Annu Rev Physiol*. 2012;74:245–269.

33. Brown BM, Shim H, Christophersen P, Wulff H. Pharmacology of small- and intermediate-conductance calcium-activated potassium channels. *Annu Rev Pharmacol Toxicol*. 2019 Jul 23. doi:10.1146/annurev-pharmtox-010919-023420

34. Lin CY, Louis ED, Faust PL, Koeppen AH, Vonsattel JP, Kuo SH. Abnormal climbing fibre-Purkinje cell synaptic connections in the essential tremor cerebellum. *Brain*. 2014;137(Pt 12):3149–3159.

35. Kumar S, Porcu P, Werner DF, et al. The role of GABA(A) receptors in the acute and chronic effects of ethanol: a decade of progress. *Psychopharmacology*. 2009;205(4):529–564.

36. Olsen RW, Sieghart W. GABA A receptors: subtypes provide diversity of function and pharmacology. *Neuropharmacology*. 2009;56(1):141–148.

37. Zheleznova NN, Sedelnikova A, Weiss DS. Function and modulation of delta-containing GABA(A) receptors. *Psychoneuroendocrinology*. 2009;34 (Suppl 1):S67–S73.

38. Mittal SO, Lenka A, Jankovic J. Botulinum toxin for the treatment of tremor. *Parkinsonism Relat Disord*. 2019. pii: S1353–8020(19)30023-9. doi: 10.1016/j.parkreldis.2019.01.023

39. Samotus O, Lee J, Jog M. Personalized bilateral upper limb essential tremor therapy with botulinum toxin using kinematics. *Toxins (Basel)*. 2019;11(2). doi: 10.3390/toxins11020125

40. Pahwa R, Busenbark K, Swanson-Hyland EF, et al. Botulinum toxin treatment of essential head tremor. *Neurology*. 1995;45(4):822–824.

41. Justicz N, Hapner ER, Josephs JS, Boone BC, Jinnah HA, Johns MM, 3rd. Comparative effectiveness of propranolol and botulinum for the treatment of essential voice tremor. *Laryngoscope*. 2016;126(1):113–117.

42. Flora ED, Perera CL, Cameron AL, Maddern GJ. Deep brain stimulation for essential tremor: a systematic review. *Mov Disord*. 2010;25(11):1550–1559.

43. Wong JK, Hess CW, Almeida L, et al. Deep brain stimulation in essential tremor: targets, technology, and a comprehensive review of clinical outcomes. *Expert Rev Neurother*. 2020;20(4):319–331. doi: 10.1080/14737175.2020.1737017

44. Tsuboi T, Jabarkheel Z, Zeilman PR, et al. Longitudinal follow-up with VIM thalamic deep brain stimulation for dystonic or essential tremor. *Neurology*. 2020;94(10):e1073–e1084. doi: 10.1212/WNL.0000000000008875

45. Raina GB, Cersosimo MG, Folgar SS, et al. Holmes tremor: clinical description, lesion localization, and treatment in a series of 29 cases. *Neurology*. 2016;86(10):931–938.

46. Schuurman PR, Bosch DA, Bossuyt PM, et al. A comparison of continuous thalamic stimulation and thalamotomy for suppression of severe tremor [see comments]. *N Engl J Med*. 2000;342(7):461–468.

47. Elias WJ, Lipsman N, Ondo WG, et al. A randomized trial of focused ultrasound thalamotomy for essential tremor. *N Engl J Med*. 2016;375(8):730–739.

48. Park YS, Jung NY, Na YC, Chang JW. Four-year follow-up results of magnetic resonance-guided focused ultrasound thalamotomy for essential tremor. *Mov Disord*. 2019;34(5):727–734.

49. Weidman EK, Kaplitt MG, Strybing K, Chazen JL. Repeat magnetic resonance imaging-guided focused ultrasound thalamotomy for recurrent essential tremor: case report and review of MRI findings. *J Neurosurg*. 2019;1–6. doi: 10.3171/2018.10.JNS181721

50. Harary M, Segar DJ, Hayes MT, Cosgrove GR. Unilateral thalamic deep brain stimulation versus focused ultrasound thalamotomy for essential tremor. *World Neurosurg*. 2019;pii: S1878–8750(19)30400-0. doi: 10.1016/j.wneu.2019.01.281

51. Li C, Gajic-Veljanoski O, Schaink AK, et al. Cost-effectiveness of magnetic resonance-guided focused ultrasound for essential tremor. *Mov Disord*. 2019;34(5):735–743.

52. Gallay MN, Moser D, Jeanmonod D. MR-guided focused ultrasound cerebellothalamic tractotomy for chronic therapy-resistant essential tremor: anatomical target reappraisal and clinical results. *J Neurosurg*. 2020;1–10. doi: 10.3171/2019.12.JNS192219

53. Zur G, Lesman-Segev OH, Schlesinger I, et al. Tremor relief and structural integrity after MRI-guided focused US thalamotomy in tremor disorders. *Radiology*. 2020;294(3):676–685.

54. Fasano A, Llinas M, Munhoz RP, Hlasny E, Kucharczyk W, Lozano AM. MRI-guided focused ultrasound thalamotomy in non-ET tremor syndromes. *Neurology*. 2017;89(8):771–775.

55. D'Souza M, Chen KS, Rosenberg J, et al. Impact of skull density ratio on efficacy and safety of magnetic resonance-guided focused ultrasound treatment of essential tremor. *J Neurosurg*. 2019;1–6. doi: 10.3171/2019.2.JNS183517

56. Harris M, Steele J, Williams R, Pinkston J, Zweig R, Wilden JA. MRI-guided laser interstitial thermal thalamotomy for medically intractable tremor disorders. *Mov Disord*. 2019;34(1):124–129.

57. Young RF, Li F, Vermeulen S, Meier R. Gamma Knife thalamotomy for treatment of essential tremor: long-term results. *J Neurosurg*. 2010;112(6):1311–1317.

58. Lim SY, Hodaie M, Fallis M, Poon YY, Mazzella F, Moro E. Gamma knife thalamotomy for disabling tremor: a blinded evaluation. *Arch Neurol*. 2010;67(5):584–588.

59. Popple RA, Wu X, Brezovich IA, et al. The virtual cone: A novel technique to generate spherical

dose distributions using a multileaf collimator and standardized control-point sequence for small target radiation surgery. *Adv Radiat Oncol.* 2018;3(3):421–430.

60. Brittain JS, Cagnan H, Mehta AR, Saifee TA, Edwards MJ, Brown P. Distinguishing the central drive to tremor in Parkinson's disease and essential tremor. *J Neurosci.* 2015;35(2):795–806.

61. Pahwa R, Dhall R, Ostrem J, et al. An acute randomized controlled trial of noninvasive peripheral nerve stimulation in essential tremor. *Neuromodulation.* 2019;22(5):537–545.

62. Lin PT, Ross EK, Chidester P, et al. Noninvasive neuromodulation in essential tremor demonstrates relief in a sham-controlled pilot trial. *Mov Disord.* 2018;33(7):1182–1183.

63. Isaacson SH, Peckham E, Tse W, et al. Prospective home-use study on non-invasive neuromodulation therapy for essential tremor. *Tremor Other Hyperkinet Mov (N Y).* 2020;10:29.

64. Shin HW, Hallett M, Sohn YH. Cerebellar repetitive transcranial magnetic stimulation for patients with essential tremor. *Parkinsonism Relat Disord.* 2019;pii: S1353–8020(19)30179-8. doi: 10.1016/j.parkreldis.2019.03.019

65. Gironell A, Kulisevsky J, Lorenzo J, Barbanoj M, Pascual-Sedano B, Otermin P. Transcranial magnetic stimulation of the cerebellum in essential tremor: a controlled study. *Arch Neurol.* 2002;59(3):413–417.

66. Badran BW, Glusman CE, Austelle CW, et al. A double-blind, sham-controlled pilot trial of pre-supplementary motor area (Pre-SMA) 1 Hz rTMS to treat essential tremor. *Brain Stimul.* 2016;9(6):945–947.

67. Sabari J, Stefanov DG, Chan J, Goed L, Starr J. Adapted feeding utensils for people with Parkinson's-related or essential tremor. *Am J Occup Ther.* 2019;73(2):7302205120p7302205121-7302205120p7302205129.

68. Ferreira JJ, Mestre TA, Lyons KE, et al. MDS evidence-based review of treatments for essential tremor. *Movement Disorders.* 2019 May 2. doi: 10.1002/mds.27700.

INDEX

For the benefit of digital users, indexed terms that span two pages (e.g., 52–53) may, on occasion, appear on only one of those pages.

Tables, figures, and boxes are indicated by *t*, *f*, and *b* following the page number.